ACUTE PHASE PROTEINS – REGULATION AND FUNCTIONS OF ACUTE PHASE PROTEINS

Edited by **Francisco Veas**

Acute Phase Proteins – Regulation and Functions of Acute Phase Proteins
Edited by Francisco Veas

Published by InTech

Janeza Trdine 9, 51000 Rijeka, Croatia

Publishing Process Manager Davor Vidic

Technical Editor Teodora Smiljanic

Cover Designer InTech Design Team

Additional hard copies can be obtained from orders@intechopen.com

Acute Phase Proteins – Regulation and Functions of Acute Phase Proteins,
Edited by Francisco Veas
p. cm.
ISBN 978-953-307-252-4

For EU product safety concerns:
IN TECH d.o.o., Prolaz Marije Krucifikse Kozulić 3, 51000 Rijeka, Croatia,
info@intechopen.com or visit our website at intechopen.com.

Meet the editor

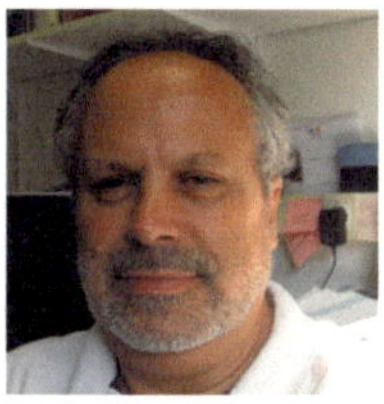

Dr. Francisco Veas, Ph.D. is a Viral Immuno-Physiopathologist and is currently a Research Professor at the Health Department of the French Institute for Development (IRD). He is also in charge of Comparative Molecular Immuno-Physiopathology Lab and Deputy Director of the research unit UMR-MD3-Université Montpellier 1 in Montpellier, France. Professor Veas received his PhD in Comparative Pathology in 1986 at the University Montpellier II. Between January 1987 and June 1988 he held a post-doctoral position on molecular biology of the protozoan Leishmania sp and Trypanosoma cruzi at the Research Centre on Macromolecular Biology of the centre National de la Recherche Scientifique (CNRS), Montpellier. In 1988, he was a laureate of the Fondation pour la Recherche Médicale and from July 1988 up to 1990 he served as Assistant Professor in the Parasites' population genetics lab at the IRD in Montpellier. From 1991-1995 he was in charge of viral experimental research of the AIDS program at IRD. From 1996 to 2000, he was director of the Retroviral Immunology Lab at the IRD CNRS Unit 5087 in Montpellier. In 2000, he cofounded the ApoH-Technologies biotech spin-off of IRD. From 2001 to 2009 he was in charge of studies on viral physiopathology of HIV and Dengue virus at the IRD research Unit "Viral Emerging Diseases Unit". In 2009, Professor Veas has been appointed CSO of ApoH-Technologies and in 2010 has been appointed head of Comparative Molecular Immuno-Physiopathology Lab at the Unit MD3 which he co-directs. From 1998, different French institutions, including Foundation pour la Recherche Médicale, SIDACTION, ANRS, CNRS, IRD, Region Languedoc Roussillon, have been supporting and funding his research. Recently, he was promoter, member of the executive board and reporter of the USDEP European Project (Ultrasensitive detection of emerging pathogens, 2006-2010). Professor Veas has also created several technological platforms including sequencing, high biosafety labs (BSL2 and BSL3), proteomics, etc. His scientific activities and publication and patents have been mainly dedicated to conserved aspects of host and pathogens including innate immunity, viral physiopathology, vaccines and diagnostics.

Contents

Preface

A dynamic physiological equilibrium known under the name of homeostasis is determined by endogenous factors and by interactions of organisms with their exogenous environment. To preserve this equilibrium state, which reflects a healthy state of the individual, the organism is constantly sensing and adjusting levels of factors involved in these mechanisms participating to the equilibrium. Most of these homeostatic factors are well preserved because of their highly relevant functional importance for life.

Depending on species, some of them could vary in their expression, and will be adapted to the encountered situations. These conserved innate strategies will not only have effects on individuals, but also on populations and moreover in their relations with the environmental stimuli (temperature, humidity, chemical, infections, diet).

A broad and conserved response to internal or external stimuli will very quickly be induced, in a matter of minutes, to generate a cascade of inflammatory processes in order to reestablish the homeostatic state in the organism as soon as possible. Stimuli inducing homeostatic changes can be of different nature: trauma, toxin, infection, genetic dysfunction, childbirth, etc.

The process of acute inflammation is initiated by cells already present in all tissues, including macrophages, dendritic cells, Kupffer cells. These cells harbor surfaces pattern recognition receptors (PRRs), which recognize at the beginning of the infectious process, exogenous molecules broadly shared by pathogens (pathogen-associated molecular patterns, PAMPs), but not by the host. Important addition to PAMPs, but to a lesser extent, are non-pathogenic microorganisms which also harbor the highly conserved molecules recognized as non-self that will induce a very low level of local inflammation. This response is amplified by endogenously released mediators and by co-factors or concomitant stressful events (burn, trauma, apoptosis, etc.) as well as molecular mechanisms involved in the vicious circle of destruction-reconstruction of vessels and tissues, acting through injury-associated signals known as Damage-Associated Molecular Patterns (DAMPs or Alarmins) and acute phase proteins. Moreover, some of the APP are also antimicrobials exhibiting a wide range of defensive functions, that alongside their repair functions help to reduce pathologic damage, and consequently help to restore the homeostasis.

The maintaining of homeostasis requires rapid and short acute inflammatory responsiveness. Inflammatory mediators, including APP, exhibit short half-lives, which ensures that the inflammatory phenomenon ceases as soon as the stimulus disappears. In contrast, the presence of APP at increased levels can be considered as sensitive sensor of homeostasis disruption. Persisting levels of APP are observed in chronic diseases.

The inflammation process is strongly associated with vascular changes as vasodilation and its resulting increased blood flow causes the redness (rubor) and increased heat (calor) as well as an augmented permeability resulting in a plasma protein leakage into the tissue causing edema, observed as swelling (tumor) and pain (dolor). Activated cells will then migrate the injury site. Depending on the intensity of inflammation and the organ in question, it is possible to observe the fifth component of inflammation as described by Aulus Cornelius Celsus in his treatise On Medicine (1st century BC) - loss of function (functio laesa) that results from cross talk between inflammation process and the central nervous system.

The two volumes of Acute Phase Proteins book consist of chapters that give a large panel of fundamental and applied knowledge on one of the major elements of the inflammatory process during the acute phase response, i.e., the acute phase proteins expression and functions that regulate homeostasis. We have organized this book in two volumes - the first volume, mainly containing chapters on structure, biology and functions of APP, the second volume discussing different uses of APP as diagnostic tools in human and veterinary medicine.

By using an open access publishing model, we wanted to facilitate a large access to readers from different places all over the world, notably developing countries, with the aim of contributing to a better world of knowledge. We also wanted to dedicate this book to our colleagues from both academia and industry in order to create values of knowledge in the field of control of inflammatory processes occurring in diverse diseases to improve the management efficacy of a more personalized medicine.

At present, CRP and SAA are the most responsive APP during inflammatory processes in humans. In most cases they are associated with the erythrocyte sedimentation rate (ESR) marker, which strongly depends on high fibrinogen concentration allowing the sticking between erythrocytes. In mice, some changes are also reported for SAA. Despite the fact that the field of inflammation and its associated factors, including APP, cytokines antimicrobial peptides, etc., have been observed and studied from very ancient times, a detailed and updated knowledge is urgently needed as well as pivotal in future research for an integrative personalized medicine that takes into account several parameters including nutritional and systemic factors. Particularly, with the help of large-scale identification methods, such as proteomics, transcriptomics, metabolomics and interactomics, it should be important to get more precise data on kinetic and on the individual role of each APP within the network of the acute phase responsive elements. Thus, it should be important, in this research, to consider organs involved in this complex network - the central nervous system that reflects its involvement by fever, somnolence, anorexia, over-secretion of some hormones, liver being the main provider of APP, epithelial cells that produce cationic antimicrobials, bone being the site of erythropoiesis suppression and thrombosis induction, and the adrenal gland that produces cortisol to regulate inflammatory inducers, adipose tissue that induces changes in lipids metabolism.

As a final note, I would like to thank InTech's editorial staff, particularly Mr. Vidic who managed, with patience, difficult tasks in helping the organization of chapter reviewing and finalization process.

Francisco Veas, PhD
Comparative Molecular Immuno-Physiopathology Lab
UMR-MD3 Faculty of Pharmacy, University Montpellier 1
Montpellier, France

1

Transcriptional Regulation of Acute Phase Protein Genes

Claude Asselin and Mylène Blais
Département d'anatomie et biologie cellulaire,
Faculté de médecine et des sciences de la santé,
Université de Sherbrooke, Sherbrooke, Québec,
Canada

1. Introduction

Inflammation is an adaptive mechanism to insure restoration of tissue and cell homeostasis after injury, infection or stress. The inflammatory response leads to differential recruitment of immune cells in organs, as well as cell-specific modifications by inflammation-induced signaling pathways. All these inflammatory-specific changes establish cell- and lineage-context dependent gene expression programs characterized by gene-specific temporal regulation, resulting in waves of induced or repressed gene expression. These regulatory programs are established by the coordination of cell- and signal-specific transcription factors, co-activator or co-repressor recruitment and chromatin modifications that act through proximal promoter elements and enhancers. Here, we will review recent data uncovering the role of transcription factors in the regulation of the inflammatory response, in macrophages. With these general notions, we will discuss about the acute-phase response, as part of a repertoire of the inflammatory response, and we will review knowledge obtained in the last ten years about the regulatory transcriptional mechanisms of selected acute phase protein genes.

2. LPS/TLR4-dependent macrophage inflammatory responses are coordinated by combinations of transcription factors

Macrophages are important regulators of the inflammatory response, and sense bacterial products through Toll-like receptors (TLR). For example, TLR4 senses the presence of Gram negative bacterial lipopolysaccharide (LPS). LPS, in a complex with LPS-binding protein (LBP), is transferred by CD14 to a TLR4/MD-2 cell surface receptor. Ligand binding leads to MyD88 signaling through IRAK1/IRAK2/IRAK4 and TAK1 kinase activation, and subsequent activation of downstream signaling kinases, such as IKKs, MAPkinases ERK1/2, p38 and JNK, which affect NF-κB and AP-1 transcription factor activities. In addition, a TRIF-dependent pathway activates kinases such as TAK1 and TBK1 and IKKε non-canonical IKKs, leading respectively to NF-κB and IRF3 activation (Kumar et al., 2011). As a result, TLR4 activation induces acute inflammation in macrophages, characterized by the expression of a series of genes, such as cytokines, chemokines and antibacterial peptides, among others. These genes are temporally regulated, with early expressed or primary response genes, and late expressed or secondary response genes. In contrast to primary response genes, secondary response genes need new protein synthesis to establish full expression patterns.

This complex regulation depends on an array of transcription factors that may be divided in four classes (Medzhitov and Horng, 2009) (Table 1). The first two classes of transcription factors are ubiquitous stress sensors that respond to external stress signals. Class I includes constitutively expressed transcription factors, such as NF-κB and IRF3, activated by signal-dependent post-translational modifications that affect their activation properties and nuclear localization. For example, cytoplasmic NF-κB is rapidly translocated to the nucleus after LPS stimulation, and is involved in the induction of primary genes. Other transcription factors of this class include latent nuclear AP-1 transcription factors, such as c-Jun phosphorylated rapidly after LPS stimulation. Class II transcription factors, including C/EBP and AP-1 transcription factor family members, need new protein synthesis for LPS-dependent stimulation. In addition to inducing secondary late gene expression, these transcription factors play a role in determining waves of time-dependent levels of gene expression. In macrophages, CCAAT/enhancer-binding protein δ (C/EBPδ) expression is increased late after LPS induction (see below).

The two last classes comprise tissue-restricted and cell-lineage transcription factors. The third category includes the macrophage-differentiation transcription factors PU.1 and C/EBPβ. Transcription factors of this class establish inducible cell-specific responses to stress and inflammation, by generating macrophage-specific chromatin domain modifications. The fourth category includes metabolic sensors of the nuclear receptor family, such as peroxisome proliferator-activated receptors (PPARs) and liver X receptors (LXR), activated respectively by fatty acids and cholesterol metabolites (Glass and Saijo, 2010). These ligand-dependent transcription factors are anti-inflammatory and link metabolism and tissue inflammation.

Recent findings have uncovered a general view of the various regulatory mechanisms establishing differential gene-specific patterns of primary and secondary gene expression after LPS stimulation in macrophages. These studies have determined the role of transcription factors, chromatin modifications and structure in gene regulation from transcription start sites and proximal promoter elements, or from enhancers, with microarray data generating genome-wide expression patterns, global chromatin immunoprecipitation experiments (ChIP-on-ChIP), real-time PCR analysis and massively parallel sequencing.

	Macrophage IR	**Acute Phase Response**
signal	LPS	IL-1, IL-6, TNF
class I	NF-κB, IRF3, AP1	STAT3, NF-κB, AP1
class II	C/EBPδ, ATF3, AP1	C/EBPβ, C/EBPδ, AP1
class III	PU.1, C/EBPβ, RUNX1, BCL-6	HNF1, HNF4α, GATA4
class IV	PPARγ, LXR	PPARα, PPARδ, PPARγ, LXR, LRH1

Table 1. Transcription factors involved in macrophage inflammatory response (IR) or acute phase response according to their classes.

3. Stress sensor transcriptional regulatory networks control LPS/TLR4-dependent macrophage inflammatory responses

LPS-dependent macrophage-specific primary and secondary gene expression depends on regulatory networks implicating the transcription factors NF-κB, C/EBPδ and ATF3, a member of the CREB/ATF family of transcription factors (Gilchrist et al., 2006; Litvak et al., 2009) (Figure 1). Indeed, transcriptomic analysis has defined clusters of early, intermediate and late patterns of gene expression in response to LPS. Included in the early phase cluster is ATF3. Promoter analysis has uncovered the juxtaposition of NF-κB and ATF3 DNA-binding sites, in a subset of promoters, including Il6 and Nos2. Chromatin immunoprecipitation experiments have shown that LPS-induced chromatin acetylation allows NF-κB recruitment at the Il6 promoter, and subsequent activation. ATF3 then binds to the promoter, and by recruiting histone deacetylase activities, inhibits transcription. Thus, ATF3 acts as a transcriptional repressor in a NF-κB-dependent negative feedback loop. The same group observed that LPS induced C/EBPδ promoter NF-κB binding after 1 hour, and ATF3 binding after four hours. Chromatin immunoprecipitation experiments showed that C/EBPδ and ATF3 bound the Il6 promoter later than NF-κB. Mathematical modeling of this regulatory network indicated that, while NF-κB initiates and ATF3 attenuates C/EBPδ and Il6 expression, C/EBPδ synergizes only with NF-κB to insure maximal Il6 transcription. This transcriptional network may be maintained by C/EBPδ's ability to induce its own expression by autoregulation. It has been proposed that C/EBPδ acts as an amplifier of the LPS response, distinguishing transient from persistent TLR4 signals and enabling the innate immune system to detect the duration of the inflammatory response. Thus, regulatory networks implicating combinatorial gene controls with subsets of transcription factors, such as C/EBPδ and ATF3, specify the proper NF-κB regulatory yield to unique gene subsets.

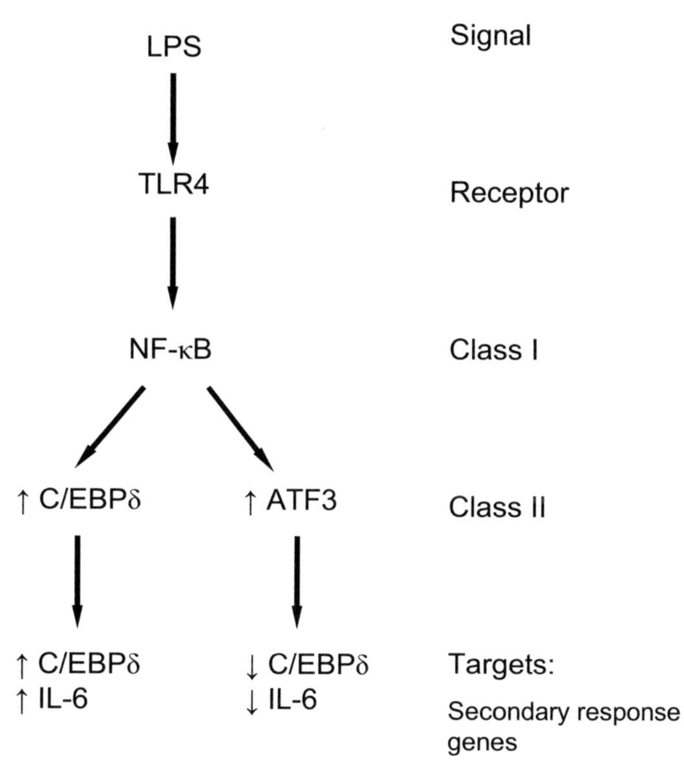

Fig. 1. Transcriptional network regulating LPS/TLR4-dependent secondary gene expression.

4. Distinct proximal promoter elements and chromatin modifications regulate LPS/TLR4-dependent macrophage inflammatory responses

Promoter, as well as chromatin structure, differentiates LPS-dependent macrophage-specific primary and secondary gene expression. Inflammatory gene expression has been divided in three classes, namely early primary, late primary and secondary response genes, depending on expression kinetics, the secondary gene expression being dependent on new protein synthesis. Ramirez-Carrozzi et al. (2006) have shown different chromatin remodeling requirements between these three classes. Both ATP-dependent remodeling complexes SWI/SNF and Mi-2/NURD were involved. SWI/SNF contains ATPase subunits BRG1 or BRM, and the Mi-2/NURD complex contains the Mi-2α or Mi-2β ATPase subunit associated with histone deacetylases, among others (Hargreaves and Crabtree, 2011). While constitutively associated BRG1 and Mi-2β complexes correlate with primary response gene accessible chromatin structure, both BRG1 and Mi-2β-containing complexes are recruited in an LPS-dependent manner to late primary and secondary gene promoters. As opposed to primary gene activation, secondary gene expression requires BRG1/BRM-containing SWI/SNF complexes for activation. In addition, Mi-2β recruitment depends on prior chromatin remodeling by SWI/SNF. While SWI/SNF-dependent remodeling positively regulates secondary gene expression, Mi-2β-mediated chromatin alterations inhibit late primary as well as secondary gene LPS-dependent induction.

These data suggest that basic promoter element signatures may be differently decoded in order to establish contrasting chromatin remodeling requirements. Indeed, genome-wide analysis has uncovered two promoter classes based on normalized CpG dinucleotide content between observed and expected ratios (Saxonov et al., 2006). While CpG is underrepresented in the genome, CpG islands, originally discovered in housekeeping gene promoters, occur at or near transcription start sites. Indeed, 72% of human gene promoters are characterized with high CpG concentrations, and 28% with low CpG content. In unstimulated cells, one class of primary response genes is characterized by CpG-island promoters and SWI/SNF independence, with constitutively active chromatin demonstrating reduced histone H3 levels, but high basal levels of acetylated H3K9/K14 (H3K9ac, H3K14ac) and trimethylated H3K4 (H3K4me3) positive regulatory marks and increased presence of RNA polymerase II and TATA-binding protein (Ramirez-Carrozzi et al., 2009). It is proposed that nucleosome destabilization on CpG-island promoters could result from the binding of transcription factors, such as the GC-rich DNA-binding Sp1 transcription factor (Wierstra, 2008). Thus, high CpG-containing promoters display reduced nucleosome stability that favor increased basal chromatin availability and facilitate further induction. Indeed, these genes are favored targets of TNFα-mediated induction. A subset of non-CpG primary response genes and secondary response genes are characterized by low CpG content in their promoter. Non-CpG primary response gene promoters form stable nucleosomes and require for their induction, recruitment of SWI-SNF activity and IRF3 activation through TLR4 signaling. These promoters, as well as secondary response gene promoters, are not associated with active chromatin or RNA polymerase II before induction. Thus, the correlation between CpG content of primary and secondary response gene promoters with basal levels of RNA polymerase II, as well as H3K4me3 and H3ac modifications, suggests that chromatin's transcriptional potential may depend in part on variations of CpG proportions. In addition, promoter structure may preferentially target gene expression to specific signaling pathways. Of note, two acute-phase protein genes, namely Lcn2 and Saa3, display properties of non-CpG island promoters, with SWI/SNF-dependent LPS activation (Ramirez-Carrozzi et al., 2009).

While the transcriptional initiation phase depends on Ser5 TFIIH-dependent phosphorylation of the C-terminal domain (CTD) of the recruited polymerase, the elongation phase occurs after Ser2 phosphorylation by the P-TEFb cyclin T1/cdk9 complex (Sims et al., 2004). Short RNAs are produced by the initiating RNA polymerase II because of transcriptional pausing before elongation (Fuda et al., 2009). Hargreaves et al. (2009) have determined the transcriptional state of RNA polymerase II complexes recruited to primary response gene promoters. Indeed, at the basal state, there is enrichment for the Ser5-phosphorylated form of RNA polymerase II associated with transcriptional initiation (Sims et al., 2004). The Ser2-phosphorylated form, associated with transcriptional elongation, is only induced after LPS stimulation and recruitment of the Ser2 P-TEFb phosphorylation complex (Hargreaves et al., 2009). Basal RNA polymerase II recruitment is insured by the Sp1 transcription factor which binds GC-rich DNA elements more frequently found in GC-rich promoter sequences (Li and Davie, 2010). Interestingly, only full-length unspliced precursor transcripts are detected at the basal state, suggesting that the RNA polymerase II Ser5-phosphorylated form is competent for full transcription, but not for RNA processing. Thus, continuous basal primary response gene expression insures a permissive chromatin environment. LPS stimulation leads to recruitment of the Brd4 bromodomain-containing protein and its interacting P-TEFb partner (Yang et al., 2005), through binding to co-activator PCAF- or GCN5-generated H4K5/K8/K12 acetylated marks. This results in Ser2 RNA polymerase II phosphorylation and productive transcriptional processing. In addition to Brd4/P-TEFb, NF-κB, while not implicated in transcriptional events related to initiation, is required for effective elongation of primary response gene transcripts. Basal expression of primary response genes is further regulated by HDAC-containing co-repressor complexes NCoR and CoREST (Cunliffe, 2008). Indeed, NCoR, CoREST, HDAC1 and HDAC3 are present at the basal state, and keep H4K5/K8/K12 in an unacetylated state, therefore inhibiting P-TEFb recruitment and subsequent productive elongation. Upon LPS stimulation, co-repressors are removed. NF-κB p50/p50 dimers, which do not transactivate, are present on primary response gene promoters, in the absence of the NF-κB p65 transactivating partner, and may assure a H4K5/K8/K12 unacetylated state by recruiting co-repressor complexes at non-induced promoters (Hargreaves et al., 2009). Thus, primed CpG-rich primary response genes, with basal active chromatin, Sp1 and co-repressor recruitment, among others, are ubiquitously regulated by multiple signals. In contrast, GC-poor primary and secondary response genes require further chromatin modifications, including SWI/SNF-dependent remodeling, to insure inflammatory gene expression. A summary of the different modifications associated with inflammatory primary response genes is presented in Table 2.

5. Distal enhancer elements and chromatin modifications differentially regulate LPS/TLR4-dependent macrophage inflammatory responses

In addition to proximal sequences, distal elements, such as enhancers, are important to establish proper inflammatory gene-specific and cell-specific regulation. Enhancer-specific signature elements, namely high levels of the H3K4 monomethylated mark as opposed to the trimethylated mark (Heintzman et al., 2007), and bound acetyltransferase coregulator p300, have allowed genome-wide enhancer identification (Heintzman et al., 2009; Visel et

		primary response gene protein synthesis not required SWI/SNF independent GC rich promoters	
		- LPS	+ LPS
Chromatin modification	H3K9Ac	+	+
	H3K4me3	+	+
	H4K5/K8/K12Ac		+
Transcription factors	Sp1	+	+
	NF-κB		+
	C/EBPβ	+	+
Coactivator	p300/CBP	+	+
	PCAF/Gcn5		+
Corepressor	HDAC1	+	
	HDAC3	+	
	NCoR	+	
	CoREST	+	
Pol II phosphorylated	ser 5	+	+
	ser 2		+
Elongation regulator	P-TEFb		+
	Brd 4		+
Pol II status	Initiation/paused	+	
	elongating		+
Transcripts	full lenght unspliced	+	
	mature processed		+
SWI/SNF remodeling complexes	Mi2-beta (CHD4)	+	+
	BRG	+	+

+ indicates high levels detected on promoters, based on Hargreaves et al. (2009) and Ramirez-Carrozzi et al. (2006).

Table 2. Basal and LPS-induced chromatin modifications of primary response gene promoters.

al., 2009). Ghisletti et al. (2010) have used LPS-stimulated p300 chromatin binding in order to isolate and characterize enhancer regions, in macrophages, by chromatin immunoprecipitation experiments followed by high-throughput sequencing (ChIP-seq). Enhancers are associated with known LPS-induced primary and secondary response genes, among others. While binding site motifs for inflammatory transcription factors such as NF-κB, AP-1 and IRFs are enriched in these inflammatory enhancers, the most enriched transcription factor is PU.1, a cell-lineage-restricted transcription factor required for macrophage differentiation (Friedman, 2007). Enhancer elements are characterized by constitutive PU.1 binding, nucleosome depletion, high H3K4me1, low H3K4me3 and LPS-inducible p300 and NF-κB recruitment (Ghisletti et al., 2010). Nucleosome alterations as well as positioning of the H3K4me1 modification require PU.1 recruitment to the enhancers (Heinz et al., 2010). Thus, PU.1 binding in collaboration with other cell-lineage transcription factors such as C/EBPβ, primes and marks cell-specific regulatory enhancer elements. The PU.1 macrophage-specific transcription factor targets not only cell-specific enhancers, but also inducible enhancers, in order to insure cell- and signal-specific regulation of the inflammatory response by ubiquitous stress sensors, such as NF-κB and IRFs, or by metabolic sensors, such as liver X receptors (LXR). Indeed, enhancer-specific binding of these oxysterol-inducible nuclear receptors (Rigamonti et al., 2008) requires PU.1-mediated enhancer recognition and modification as well (Heinz et al., 2010). Similar ChIP-seq experiments have uncovered B-cell lymphoma 6 (Bcl-6) as a negative regulator of TLR4/NF-κB activation of the inflammatory response in macrophages. Indeed, in addition to PU.1, both NF-κB and Bcl-6 DNA-binding sites co-localize in a large subset of LPS-inducible enhancers. Bcl-6, through HDAC3 recruitment and histone deacetylation, attenuates NF-κB- and p300 acetyltransferase-mediated transcriptional activation in response to LPS, in Bcl-6/NF-κB containing enhancers (Barish et al., 2010). Thus, lineage-specific transcription factors, through the establishment of enhancer-specific chromatin domains, allow the proper cell-specific reading of environmental and metabolic stimuli by ubiquitous transcription factors, including stress and metabolic sensors.

6. Metabolic sensors repress LPS/TLR4-dependent macrophage inflammatory responses

Co-repressor complexes negatively regulate the inflammatory response. The NCoR and SMRT co-repressors form complexes including the histone deacetylase HDAC3, transducin β-like 1 (TBL1) and TBL-related 1 (TBLR1) and G protein-pathway suppressor 2 (GPS2). The importance of NCoR in the regulation of the inflammatory response has been uncovered in NCoR-deficient macrophages displaying derepression of AP-1 and NF-κB regulated genes in response to inflammatory stimuli (Ogawa et al., 2004). NCoR and SMRT complexes are recruited to chromatin, where they establish repressive chromatin domains by mediating deacetylation of nucleosomal histones. NCoR and SMRT co-repressors do not interact directly with DNA. Recruitment of NCoR and SMRT complexes is insured by various transcription factors, including NF-κB and AP-1 subunits, ETS factors and nuclear receptors. Indeed, in addition to NF-κB p50, as discussed above, unphosphorylated c-Jun recruits NCoR while the Ets repressor TEL recruits SMRT (Ghisletti et al., 2009), thus guaranteeing specific recruitment to subsets of inflammatory gene promoters. NCoR and/or SMRT may be recruited not only to SWI/SNF-independent primary response gene promoters, such as Il1b, Tnf and Cxcl2, but also to SWI/SNF-dependent primary and secondary response gene promoters, such as Nos2, Ccl2 and Mmp13 (Hargreaves et al., 2009; Ghisletti et al., 2009). In order to achieve TLR4-dependent gene activation, NCoR and SMRT complexes must be removed and replaced by co-activators. A common nuclear receptor and signal-dependent transcription factor derepression pathway involves the activation of NCoR/SMRT subunits TBL1 and TBLR1, which act as recruiters of ubiquitin-conjugating enzymes, such as the UbcH5 E2 ligase. This leads to NCoR/SMRT ubiquitylation and ensuing disposal by the 19S proteasome complex (Ogawa et al., 2004; Perissi et al., 2004). Recent analysis of Nos2 activation by LPS in macrophages suggests that c-Jun phosphorylation is central to insure

NCoR promoter discharge (Huang et al., 2009). Indeed, LPS treatment leads to recruitment of NF-κB p65 to a NF-κB DNA-binding site near the AP-1 element. NF-κB p65 recruits the inhibitor of κB kinase IKKε (Nomura et al., 2000) which phosphorylates c-Jun and triggers NCoR removal (Huang et al., 2009). In addition to Nos2, other composite NF-κB- and AP-1-containing promoters are regulated by NF-κB p65/IKKε-dependent c-Jun phosphorylation, such as Cxcl2, Cxcl9, Cxcl10 and Ccl4 (Huang et al., 2009).

Peroxysome proliferator-activated receptors (PPARs) and liver X receptors ((LXRs) are nuclear receptors forming dimers with retinoid X receptors (RXRs). These metabolic sensors bind specific hormone responsive elements, and ligand binding leads to transcriptional activation (Glass and Saijo, 2010). In addition, PPARs and LXRs repress inflammatory gene expression by a mechanism of transrepression. Indeed, PPARγ and LXR ligands inhibit TLR4/LPS-mediated inflammatory gene expression by counteracting NCoR disposal. PPARγ agonists stimulate PPARγ sumoylation by the SUMO E3 ligase PIAS1, which adds SUMO1. Sumoylated PPARγ binds NCoR and inhibits NCoR removal normally induced in response to TLR4/LPS signaling (Pascual et al., 2005). Likewise, LXR agonists stimulate LXR sumoylation by HDAC4, which acts as a SUMO E3 ligase adding SUMO2/3. As for PPARγ, sumoylated LXRs bind NCoR and inhibit NCoR removal induced by TLR4/LPS signaling (Ghisletti et al., 2007). Thus, NCoR and SMRT complexes integrate both cell-extrinsic and –intrinsic signals, resulting in stress and metabolic activation or repression of specific inflammatory response gene expression programs.

7. The acute phase-response and acute phase proteins

Tissue injury, trauma or infection lead to complex and systemic reactions referred to as the acute-phase reaction (APR) (Epstein, 1999). The APR is part of a repertoire of cell responses to inflammation, characterized by increased or decreased plasma concentrations of acute phase proteins (APPs). These plasma proteins, mostly synthesized by the liver, participate in blood coagulation, maintenance of homeostasis, defense against infection, transport of nutrients, metabolite and hormone transport, among others. Marked changes in APP gene expression vary from 0.5-fold to 1000-fold, with either rapid or slow expression kinetics, and depend on signals generated at the site of injury or distributed via the bloodstream to remote sites. Indeed, cytokines produced locally or by circulating activated mononuclear cells in response to inflammatory stimuli elicit the diverse effects characteristic of the APR: regulating and amplifying the immune response, restoring homeostasis or inducing chronic tissue injury. Mediators of APP gene expression include pro-inflammatory cytokines such as IL-6, IL-1β and TNFα, glucocorticoids and growth factors. APPs are divided as positive and negative APPs, respectively increasing or decreasing during the APR. Positive APPs include CRP, HP, AGT, ORM, SAA, LBP, FBG, VTN, among others. ALB and TRR are examples of negative APPs (Epstein, 1999; Gruys et al., 2005; Khan and Khan, 2010).

Hepatocytes are considered as the primary cell type expressing APPs. However, APP production is induced after lipopolysaccharide- or cytokine-mediated systemic inflammation in other cell types, including intestinal epithelial cells, adipocytes, endothelial cells, fibroblasts and monocytes. Thus, local APP production may be important. Of note, APP expression is increased in various chronic inflammatory diseases, such as atherosclerosis (Packard and Libby, 2008). Obesity, through the formation of stressed fat tissue, contributes to both local and systemic inflammation by releasing pro-inflammatory cytokines, such as TNFα and IL-1, and APPs, such as HP and CRP. These APPs are useful as inflammatory biomarkers for these conditions (Rocha and Libby, 2009).

Depending on their cytokine responsiveness, class I APPs are induced by IL-1β and IL-6, while class II APPs are expressed in response to IL-6. Pro-inflammatory signaling converges on APP gene regulatory regions, by activating various classes of transcription factors acting as stress sensors. The IL-1 pathway shares many signal transduction components with TLR pathways. IL-1 binding to the IL-1 receptor leads to the association of the IL-1 receptor accessory protein. This complex leads to MyD88 signaling through IRAK1/IRAK2/IRAK4 and TAK1 kinase activation, and subsequent activation of downstream signaling kinases, such as IKKs, MAPkinases ERK1/2, p38 and JNK, which affect NF-κB, AP-1 and C/EBP transcription factor activities (Weber et al., 2010). The IL-6 pathway is activated by IL-6 binding to the IL-6 receptor, followed by induced recruitment of gp130. This complex activates Janus kinase 1 (JAK1)/STAT3 and ERK1/2 kinase signaling pathways. JAK1-dependent STAT3 tyrosine phosphorylation leads to STAT3 dimerization, nuclear translocation and regulation of genes with STAT3-responsive promoter elements (Murray, 2007). ERK1/2 signaling activates AP-1, C/EBPβ and ELK1 that again, target specific promoter elements (Kamimura et al., 2003).

From a selected list of 28 human APPs (Epstein, 1999), we have found that 27 APP gene promoters displayed low CpG content, under normalized CpG values of 0.35, as assessed by Saxonov et al. (2006): CRP, HP, FGG, A2M, SAA1, ORM, TTR, FGG, CP, SERPINE1, SERPING1, SERPINA1, SERPINC1, SERPINA3, APCS, KNG1, LCN2, ALB, CFP, C3, TF, C9, IL1RN, CSF3, MBL2, IGF1, VTN. This observation suggests that most APP genes may be considered as late primary or secondary response genes, that RNA polymerase II pre-loading, as found for primary response genes, may not be the norm, and that chromatin modifications including remodeling, may be important for APP gene induction during the APR.

In the next section, we will review some examples of APP gene regulation mostly in hepatocytes. We will discuss the role of Class I constitutively expressed (NF-κB, STAT3) and Class II regulated (C/EBP, AP-1) stress-induced transcription factors, as well as tissue-restricted and cell lineage-specific Class III transcription factors (GATA4, HNF-1α, HNF4α) and Class IV metabolic sensors (PPARs, LXR) (Table 1).

8. Stress sensors and APP gene regulation

8.1 CRP promoter structure and APP gene regulation

Plasma C-reactive protein levels (CRP) are induced more than 1000-fold in response to APR (Mortensen, 2001). Human CRP synergistic induction in response to IL-1β and IL-6 depends on a combination of transcription factors, including STAT3, C/EBP family members and NF-κB. The proximal 300 bp promoter element binds C/EBPβ and C/EBPδ at two sites. The more proximal site is a composite C/EBP site with a non-consensus NF-κB site. While C/EBPβ binding in vitro is not efficient, NF-κB p50 binds to the non-consensus NF-κB site, increases C/EBPβ binding and transcriptional activation by cytokines (Cha-Molstad et al., 2000; Agrawal et al., 2001; Agrawal et al., 2003a; Agrawal et al., 2003b; Cha-Molstad et al., 2007). This site is essential for CRP expression. In the absence of C/EBPβ, this element is bound by a negative regulator of C/EBP activities, namely C/EBPζ (Oyadomari and Mori, 2004), and by RBP-Jκ, a transcriptional repressor of Notch signaling (Sanalkumar et al., 2010), which insures C/EBPζ binding to the C/EBP site (Singh et al., 2007). Cytokine stimulation leads to a replacement of the repressor complex by the p50/C/EBP positive regulatory complex. An upstream element consisting of an overlapping NF-κB/OCT-1 DNA-binding site has also been uncovered (Voleti and Agrawal, 2005). OCT-1 binding is increased in response to transient NF-κB p50-p50 dimer levels, resulting in CRP repression. Cytokine stimulation leads to a switch to NF-κB p50-p65 dimers which replace OCT-1, and in conjunction with C/EBPs, mediate CRP transcriptional activation. Chromatin immunoprecipitation (ChIP) assays show that cytokine treatment increases binding of C/EBPβ, STAT3, NF-κB p50, c-Rel and TBP to the CRP promoter, while low levels of these transcription factors are present on the unstimulated CRP promoter (Young et al., 2008). C/EBPβ recruitment appeared after 2 hours, in contrast to later induced recruitment for STAT3 and NF-κB p50. Of note, no expression of CRP was observed in basal conditions, suggesting that pre-bound transcription factors are not sufficient to insure basal transcription. Thus, APP regulation depends on the promoter structure, which acts as a platform characterized by specific transcription factor DNA-binding site arrangements, allowing the exact response to inflammatory stimuli.

8.2 STAT3 and APP gene regulation

STAT3 is the major class I stress sensor induced in response to IL-6. STAT3 mouse knockout results in decreased inducible expression of APP genes, including serum amyloid A (SAA) and γ-fibrinogen (γ-FBG) (Alonzi et al., 2001). STAT3 transcriptional activity is regulated by posttranscriptional modifications altering STAT3 localization and interactions with co-activators or co-repressors. Recent data have uncovered the role of STAT3 in the regulation of APP expression. IL-6 is a major regulator of the acute-phase protein γ-FBG (Duan and Simpson-Haidaris, 2003, 2006). Hou et al. (2007) have found that IL-6-inducible γ-FBG expression mediated by STAT3 involves the formation of a stable enhanceosome including STAT3, p300, and phosphorylation of RNA polymerase II on Ser2 of the C-terminal domain. The γ-FBG promoter contains three IL-6 response elements. IL-6-induced Tyr-phosphorylated and acetylated nuclear STAT3 interacts with the TEFb complex composed of CDK9 and cyclin T1, as determined by co-immunoprecipitation. Although the STAT3 N-terminal region is sufficient for TEFb complex formation, both N- and C-terminal domains participate in complex formation. CDK9 silencing decreases IL-6-induced γ-FBG expression. In addition, ChIP experiments show that STAT3, CDK9, RNA polymerase II and its phosphorylated form are recruited rapidly to the γ-FBG promoter. Inhibition of CDK9 activity reduces both basal and IL-6-inducible phosphoSer2 CTD RNA polymerase II formation. Thus, activated STAT3 interacts with TEFb, and recruits TEFb to the γ-FBG promoter. TEFb phosphorylates recruited RNA polymerase II, and renders RNA polymerase II competent for transcriptional elongation. In addition, the p300 bromodomain mediates p300 interaction with the acetylated STAT3 N-terminal domain. This strengthened interaction between p300 and acetylSTAT3, stimulated by IL-6, further stabilizes the recruitment of other transcription factors, including RNA polymerase II, to insure correct initiation and elongation (Hou et al., 2008). Thus, STAT3 induces APP gene regulation, in part by recruiting competent RNA polymerase II forms for transcriptional initiation and elongation,

IL-6-mediated angiotensinogen (AGT) gene expression in hepatocytes is regulated by IL-6 at the transcriptional level (Brasier et al., 1999). The proximal AGT promoter contains distinct elements binding STAT3 (Sherman and Brasier, 2001). Using an acetyl-lysine antibody, it was found that IL-6 treatment of hepatocytes leads to STAT3 acetylation, and that the p300 acetyltransferase mediates this acetylation (Ray et al., 2005). Proteomic analysis uncovered STAT3 N-terminal lysines 49 and 87 as being acetylated. While mutation of STAT3 K49 and K87 does not alter IL-6-mediated STAT3 translocation, the double mutant acts as a dominant-negative inhibitor of endogenous STAT3 transactivation and AGT expression in response to IL-6. Mutation of the acetylated lysines, while not affecting DNA-binding ability, decreases STAT3 interaction with the p300 co-activator, thereby leading to decreased transcriptional activation. ChIP assays show that, at the basal state, the AGT promoter is occupied by unacetylated STAT3 and p300, and displays acetylated H3 modifications. Recruitment of STAT3 and its acetylated forms to the AGT promoter is increased after IL-6 treatment, correlating with a slight increase in p300 engagement. Induction of an APR in mice by LPS injection induces STAT3 acetylation in liver nuclear extracts. Treatment with the HDAC inhibitor Trichostatin A increases STAT3-dependent AGT expression in the absence of IL-6 (Ray et al., 2002). It was found by co-immunoprecipitation that histone deacetylase HDAC1, HDAC2, HDAC4 and HDAC5 interact with STAT3, and that HDAC overexpression inhibits IL-6 mediated AGT transcriptional activity. Thus, HDACs associate with STAT3 and inhibit IL-6 signaling and hepatic APR. While the HDAC1 C-terminal domain is necessary to repress IL-6-induced STAT3 signaling, the STAT3 N-acetylated domain is required for HDAC1 interaction. HDAC1 overexpression in hepatocytes reduces nuclear STAT3 amounts after IL-6 treatment while HDAC1 silencing increases STAT3 nuclear accumulation. HDAC1 knockdown augments IL-6 stimulated AGT expression. This suggests that HDAC1 may be required to insure proper STAT3 cytoplasmic-nuclear distribution and to restore non-induced expression levels after inflammation (Ray et al., 2008).

It has been recently shown that STAT3 activates apurinic/apyrimidinic endonuclease 1 (APE/Ref-1), involved in base-excision repair (Izumi et al., 2003). This activation may protect against Fas-induced liver injury (Haga et al., 2003). It was found that IL-6 induces a nuclear STAT3-APE1 complex (Ray et al., 2010). Indeed, co-immunoprecipitation studies show that APE1 interacts with the acetylated STAT3 N-terminus, leading to increased transactivation of the STAT3-containing AGT promoter, in response to IL-6. RNAi knockdown experiments show that APE1 enables IL-6-mediated STAT3 DNA-binding. APE1 knockdown in hepatocytes decreases CRP and SAA APP gene expression in response to IL-6. This is confirmed in APE1 heterozygous knockout mice in which liver LPS-induced expression of α-acid glycoprotein (ORM) is decreased. Finally, ChIP assays show that APE1 is important for γ-FBG promoter enhanceosome formation, as shown by a decrease in STAT3, p300 and phosphorylated RNA polymerase II when APE1 levels are decreased by shRNAs. Thus, APE1 may represent a novel co-activator of APP gene expression and APR, as p300 and TEF-b, through STAT3-mediated activation.

In addition to STAT3-mediated activation of APP genes, STAT3 synergizes with NF-κB to attain full APP gene expression. Indeed, although there is no consensus STAT3 DNA-binding in the SAA1 and SAA2 promoters, IL-1 and IL-6 stimulation of HepG2 cells leads to the formation of a complex between NF-κB p65 and STAT3, as assessed by co-immunoprecipitation. STAT3 interacts with a non-consensus STAT3 site in a NF-κB-STAT3 composite element (Hagihara et al., 2005). This synergistic element requires the co-activator p300. IL-1 and IL-6 treatment leads to NF-κB p65, STAT3 and p300 recruitment to the SAA1 promoter. Thus, protein interactions with members of different stress sensor categories are involved in mediating transcriptional synergy.

A2M is regulated by IL-6 through STAT3. STAT3 cooperates with the glucocorticoid receptor (GR) induced by dexamethasone (Dex) for full A2M induction in rat hepatocytes. While there is no GR DNA-binding site, the A2M proximal promoter contains DNA-binding sites for STAT3, AP-1 and OCT-1 (Zhang and Darnell, 2001). GR binds both STAT3 and c-Jun (Lerner et al., 2003). IL-6 and Dex synergize for full transcriptional activation. Double immunoprecipitation ChIP assays have been used to assess the sequential recruitment of transcription factors to the A2M promoter and their role in enhanceosome formation. At the basal state, both OCT-1 and c-Jun are constitutively bound. Dex-activated GR is first recruited by c-Jun interaction. Then, IL-6 dependent STAT3 is recruited, leading to histone acetylation and RNA polymerase II recruitment, rendering the gene transcriptionnally active. While IL-6 signaling alone, through STAT3 recruitment is sufficient to insure RNA polymerase II recruitment and low levels of A2M expression, both IL-6 and Dex are more effective to recruit RNA polymerase II and achieve maximal transcription.

8.3 C/EBPs and APP gene regulation in intestinal epithelial cells

C/EBP isoforms regulate APP gene expression in intestinal epithelial cells (IEC). Indeed, APP transcriptional response to glucocorticoids, cAMP, TGFβ and IL-1β is mediated in part by C/EBP isoforms (Boudreau et al., 1998; Pelletier et al., 1998; Yu et al., 1999; Désilets et al., 2000). C/EBP isoform overexpression increases IL-1β-mediated induction of the APP gene haptoglobin (HP), and C/EBPs are the major regulator of HP expression in IEC (Gheorghiu er al., 2001). We have found that a functional interaction between C/EBPδ and the p300 co-activator is necessary for HP IL-1β-mediated transactivation (Svotelis et al., 2005). In addition, we have shown that C/EBPδ interacts with HDAC1 and HDAC3. HDAC1 interaction necessitates both N-terminal transactivation and C-terminal DNA-binding domain. HDAC1 represses C/EBPδ-dependent HP transactivation. ChIP assays show that, at the basal state, the HP promoter is characterized by the presence of HDAC1, with low levels of C/EBPβ and C/EBPδ. HDAC1 recruitment is inhibited by IL-1β, and this correlates with increased occupation by C/EBPβ and C/EBPδ, and increased H3 and H4 acetylation (Turgeon et al., 2008). To determine whether C/EBP isoforms are sufficient to establish a proper chromatin environment for transcription, we have studied HP and T-kininogen (KNG1) expression in IECs. IL-1β treatment leads to late HP and KNG1 expression, as assessed by semi-quantitative RT-PCR after 24 h (Fig. 2A). Kinetics of expression suggests that both HP and KNG1 are secondary response genes (Désilets et al., 2000; Turgeon et al., 2008; Rousseau et al., 2008). C/EBP isoform overexpression increases both basal and IL-1β-mediated HP and KNG1 expression (Figure 2A). ChIP experiments show that HP and KNG1 promoter sequences in non-stimulated control cells are not associated with RNA polymerase II binding or H3/H4 acetylation, but with low levels of C/EBP isoforms. In contrast, IL-1β treatment leads to increased RNA polymerase II and C/EBP isoform recruitment after 4 hours, correlating with increased H3/H4 acetylation (Figure 2B). In the absence of IL-1β, C/EBP isoform overexpression is sufficient to induce RNA polymerase II recruitment to both promoters (Figure 2C). This suggests that C/EBP isoform overexpression leads to chromatin changes compatible with RNA polymerase II recruitment and transcriptional activity. Whether recruitment of co-activators, such as p300 and CBP (Kovacs et al., 2003; Svotelis et al., 2005), and/or of remodeling SWI/SNF complexes (Kowenz-Leutz et al., 2010) are required, needs to be addressed. Thus, C/EBPs are a major regulator of APP inflammatory secondary responses in IECs.

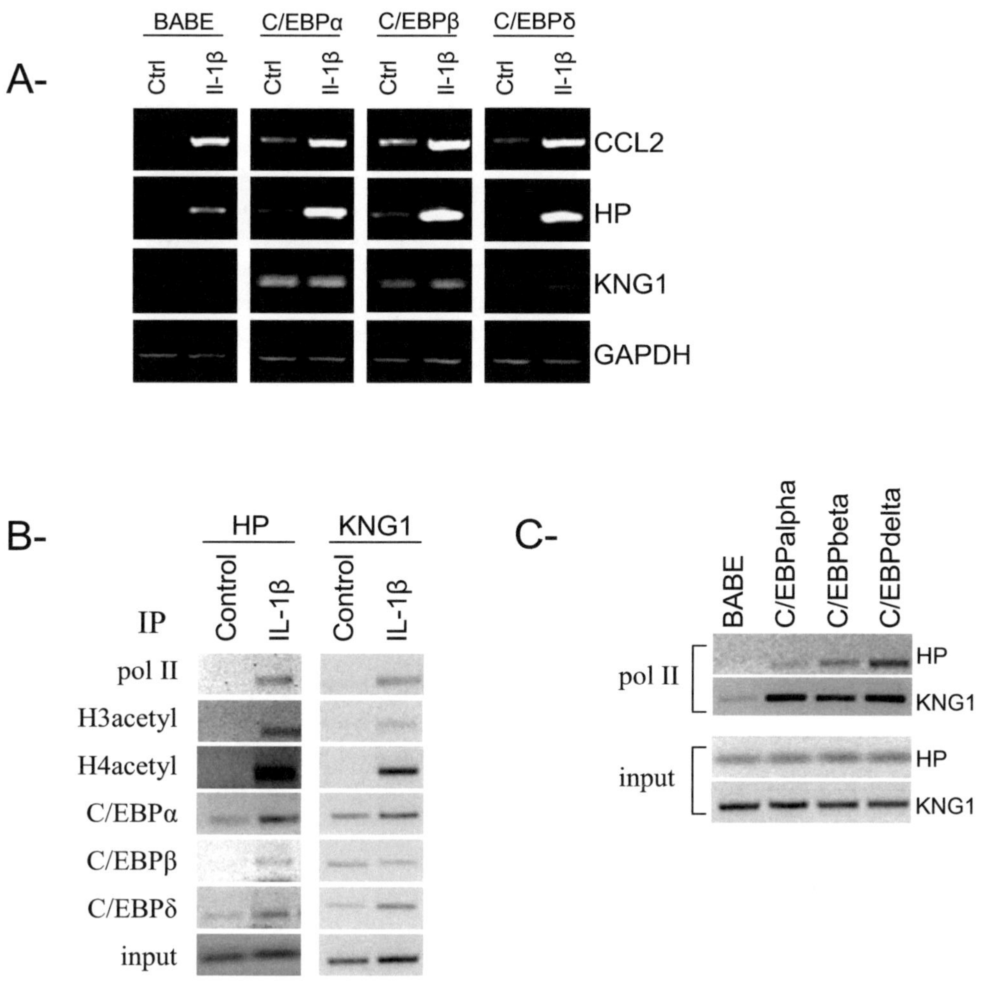

A) Rat intestinal epithelial IEC-6 cells stably transfected with C/EBP isoforms α, β and δ were treated for 24 h with IL-1β. Expression levels of APP genes Chemokine ligand 2 (CCL2), Haptoglobin (HP) and T-Kininogen 1 (KNG1) were evaluated by semi-quantitative RT-PCR. HP and KNG1 proximal promoter modifications were assessed by chromatin immunoprecipitation with IEC-6 cells treated for 4 h with IL-1β (B) or with IEC-6 cells stably transfected with C/EBP isoforms α, β and δ (C).

Fig. 2. Regulation of APP gene expression by C/EBP isoforms involves chromatin remodeling.

9. Cell lineage-specific transcription factors and APP gene regulation

9.1 HNF-1α and APP gene regulation

Liver-specific gene expression is regulated by tissue-restricted transcription factors, including hepatocyte nuclear factor 1 (HNF-1α and HNF-1β) and hepatocyte nuclear factor 4α (HNF4α) (Nagaki and Moriwaki, 2008). The POU homeodomain-containing transcription factor HNF-1α regulates bile acid, cholesterol and lipoprotein metabolism as well as glucose and fatty acid metabolism (Shih et al., 2001; Armendariz and Krauss, 2009). In addition, HNF-1α activates numerous APP genes, including SERPINA1, ALB, TRR, CRP, FBG, LBP and VTN. Indeed, expression of these APP genes is reduced in HNF-1α knockout mice (Armendariz and Krauss, 2009).

CRP proximal promoter binds the HNF-1α transcription factor. While HNF-1α is required but not sufficient for CRP expression (Toniatti et al., 1990), HNF-1α, along with a complex composed of STAT3 and c-Fos, regulates cytokine-dependent CRP expression synergistically (Nishikawa et al., 2008). Indeed, c-Fos is recruited to the CRP promoter in the late induction phase of IL-1β and IL-6 stimulation. Since there is no AP-1 site found on the CRP promoter, it is proposed that c-Fos may bridge STAT3 and HNF-1α transcription factors bound to their respective site. A similar interaction between HNF-1α, IL-6-induced STAT3 and AP-1 regulates the expression of the HNF-1α-regulated APP gene α-FBG (Hu et al., 1995; Leu et al., 2001). Interestingly, unlike the CRP promoter which contains a STAT3 DNA-binding element, STAT3 does not bind the α-FBG proximal promoter (Liu and Fuller, 1995), suggesting that HNF-1α may act as a STAT3 recruiter. HNF-1α plays also an important role in IL-6-induced AGT expression (Jain et al., 2007). Of the three putative STAT3 DNA-binding sites identified (Sherman and Brasier, 2001), the most proximal site indeed binds STAT3, and when mutated, decreases IL-6-mediated AGT transactivation, while a secondary STAT3 DNA-binding site binds HNF-1α instead. ChIP assays indicate that, indeed, HNF-1α occupies the AGT promoter and that IL-6 treatment increases HNF-1α recruitment. While HNF-1α positively regulates AGT expression in the absence of IL-6, mutation of the HNF-1α DNA-binding site reduces IL-6 induced promoter activity. STAT3 or HNF-1α reduction by siRNAs inhibits AGT promoter activity as well as AGT endogenous protein levels. These results suggest that, in addition to the STAT3 DNA-binding site, the HNF-1α DNA-binding site acts as an IL-6 inducible element, playing an important role in both basal as well as IL-6 induced AGT expression.

9.2 HNF4α and APP gene regulation

The nuclear hormone receptor HNF4α is one of the major modulator of hepatocyte differentiation and regulates the expression of a number of liver-specific transcription factors, including C/EBPs and HNF-1α (Nagaki and Moriwaki, 2008). HNF4α regulates APP gene targets. Indeed, basal human AGT expression is regulated by HNF4α through two responsive sites (Yanai et al., 1999; Oishi et al., 2010). In addition, the HNF4α-regulated TTR and SERPINA1 genes are respectively downregulated and upregulated in response to cytokines (Wang and Burke, 2007). HNF4α DNA-binding activity decreases following cytokine IL-1β, IL-6 and TNFα treatment, leading to decreased HNF4α-dependent transcriptional activation (Li et al., 2002). In addition, ChIP assays demonstrate diminished HNF4α recruitment to the TTR promoter in response to cytokines, and a lesser decrease at the SERPINA1 promoter. HNF4α knockdown with shRNAs reduces SERPINA1 and TTR basal mRNA levels, and cancels the cytokine-dependent increase or decrease of SERPINA1 and TTR expression respectively. This is specific for HNF4α-regulated APP genes since cytokine-dependent expression of SAA, which is devoid of an HNF4α DNA-binding site, is not altered. It is proposed that cytokine-induced phosphorylation of HNF4α modulates HNF4α DNA-binding ability.

Recruitment of the peroxysome-proliferator-activated receptor-γ co-activator 1α (PGC-1α) may be important to modulate the action of HNF4α. In contrast to the p300 co-activator,

PGC-1α increases the HNF4α-dependent transactivation of TTR and SERPINA1, while HNF4α silencing impairs PGC-1α co-activation (Wang and Burke, 2008). Interestingly, PGC-1α overexpression cancels cytokine-mediated HNF4α DNA-binding capacity. ChIP assays indicate that, as for HNF4α, cytokine treatment reduces PGC-1α recruitment. Thus, HNF4α may control a subset of APP genes in response to inflammatory stimuli.
The TTR proximal promoter contains, in addition to HNF4α, DNA-binding sites for tissue-restricted transcription factors HNF-1α and HNF-3/HNF-6 (Wang and Burke, 2010). Mutation of the HNF4α DNA-binding site decreases the TTR transcriptional response induced not only by HNF4α, but also by HNF-1α and HNF-6. Mutation of the respective HNF DNA-binding sites reduces their specific binding, without affecting other HNF binding in vitro. However, cytokine treatment decreases HNF4α, but also HNF-1α and HNF-6 recruitment to the TTR proximal promoter, as assessed by ChIP assays. This indicates that HNF4α may serve as an interacting element organizing interactions between HNFs, to insure basal expression levels.
HNF4α may also regulate the inflammatory response in liver by regulating tissue-restricted transcription factors involved in inflammation. One of these transcription factors is CREB3L3 (CREBH). CREB3L3 is a membrane-bound transcription factor related to ATF6, an endoplasmic reticulum (ER) transmembrane transcription factor normally retained in the ER through interaction with the BIP/GRP78 chaperone, but released and cleaved after accumulation of misfolded proteins. Activated ATF6 then induces the expression of unfolded protein response (UPR) genes, to insure homeostasis (Inagi, 2010). CREB3L3 is a liver-specific bZIP-containing transcription factor of the cyclic-AMP response element binding protein (CREB/ATF) family. ER stress induces a cleaved form of CREB3L3 that translocates to the nucleus and mediates UPR gene expression in response to ER stress. Interestingly, CREB3L3 knockdown in mice reduces the expression of APP genes, such as CRP, serum amyloid P (SAP) and SAA3. In addition, serum SAP and CRP levels are reduced in IL-6/IL-1β or LPS stimulated CREB3L3 knockout mice, as compared to wild-type mice. Pro-inflammatory cytokines and LPS induce CREB3L3 cleavage during APR activation. CREB3L3 and ATF6 form heterodimers and synergistically activate the expression of target genes, including a subset of APR genes, in response to ER stress. Indeed, CREB3L3 responsive elements have been found in the CRP and SAP promoter regions (Zhang et al., 2006). One major regulator of CREB3L3 expression is HNF4α. Indeed, CREB3L3 is a direct target of HNF4α transcriptional activity, and HNF4α binds the CREB3L3 promoter, as determined by ChIP assays. While mice with liver CREB3L3 targeted deletion do not show hepatocyte differentiation defects, loss of CREB3L3 results in reduced expression of APP genes induced by tunicamycin, an UPR inducer. Thus, CREB3L3 controls APP gene expression induced by ER stress. In addition, a cell-lineage specific transcription factor, namely HNF4α, may link both APR and ER stress response, by insuring liver-specific CREB3L3 expression (Luebke-Wheeler et al., 2008).

9.3 GATA4 and APP gene regulation

GATA4 is a zinc-finger-containing transcription factor whose expression is restricted to certain tissues, such as heart and intestine (Viger et al., 2008). IEC-expressed GATA4 is required to maintain proximal-to-distal identities along the gastrointestinal tract (Bosse et al., 2006). We have found that IEC-restricted GATA4 modulates C/EBP-dependent transcriptional activation of APP genes (Rousseau et al., 2008). Indeed, GATA4 represses

C/EBP isoform activation of the KNG1 and HP promoters. GATA4 interacts with the C/EBPδ C-terminal DNA-binding domain. GATA4 overexpression leads to decreases in C/EBPβ and C/EBPδ basal as well as IL-1β-induced protein levels. This results in decreased IL-1β-dependent induction of KNG1. This correlates with decreased IL-1β-dependent C/EBPδ recruitment and H4 acetylation, as assessed by ChIP assays. Thus, the lineage-specific transcription factor GATA4 may insure specific regulation of APP genes in IECs.

10. Metabolic sensors and APP gene regulation

Nuclear receptors have been shown to play a regulatory role in APP gene expression. For example, the nuclear receptor liver receptor homolog 1 (LRH-1) regulates bile acid biosynthesis and cholesterol homeostasis (Fayard et al., 2004). LRH-1 inhibits IL-1β- and IL-6-mediated induction of the APP genes HP, SAA, FBG and CRP. LRH-1 negatively regulates specifically C/EBP activation by IL-1β and IL-6, without affecting STAT3 and NF-κB transactivation. Indeed, mutation of the HP C/EBP DNA-binding site decreases basal expression levels, as well as IL-1β and IL-6 induction levels, and abolishes LRH-1 negative repression. LRH-1 reduces C/EBPβ DNA-binding capacity. Increased LPS-stimulated APP plasma gene concentrations are reduced in heterozygous LRH-1 mice, as compared to wild-type mice. These results indicate that LRH-1 regulates the hepatic APR at least in part by down-regulating C/EBP-mediated transcriptional activation (Venteclef et al., 2006).

The oxysterol receptors LXRα and LXRβ play similar roles in CRP regulation in hepatocytes (Blaschke et al., 2006). Indeed, LXR agonists inhibit IL-1β and IL-6-mediated CRP induction. A portion of the promoter including a C/EBP DNA-binding site is necessary. The N-CoR co-repressor complex, with the histone deacetylase HDAC3, is necessary to mediate LXR negative regulation. Indeed, ligand-activated LXR prevents cytokine-induced removal of N-CoR on the CRP promoter, as assessed by ChIP assays. In vivo, LXR agonists inhibit the LPS-induced hepatocyte APR, as assessed by reduction of CRP and SAP mRNA levels specifically in wild-type mice, as opposed to LXRα/LXRβ knockout mice. Thus, both LRH-1 and LXR nuclear hormone receptors regulate negatively APP gene expression in hepatocytes.

Recent data suggest that LXRβ is the main LXR subtype regulating APP gene expression (Venteclef et al., 2010). Ligand-activated LRH-1 and LXR inhibit HP, SAA and SERPINE1 expression by preventing NcoR complex removal. ChIP experiments indicate that components of the NcoR complex, but not of the SMRT co-repressor complex, are present on the non-stimulated HP promoter, namely HDAC3, GPS2 and TBLR1. HP transrepression is dependent on sumoylation of both LRH-1 and LXRβ receptors. Indeed, an increased hepatic APR is observed in SUMO-1 knockout mice. ChIP experiments have been done with liver extracts of control as well as LXR knockout mice treated with agonists before LPS induction. Results show that while N-CoR and GPS2 recruitment is decreased by LPS treatment, LXR agonists prevent N-CoR and GPS2 removal, and increase HDAC4, LXR and SUMO-2/3 recruitment to the HP promoter. In contrast, LRH-1 transrepression depends on SUMO-1. Thus, LRH-1 and LXR repress APP gene expression by ligand- and SUMO-dependent nuclear receptor interactions with N-CoR/GPS2-containing co-repressor complexes, resulting in inhibition of complex removal after cytokine induction. Ligand activation leads to increased SUMOylated nuclear receptors, either through stabilization of LRH-1 SUMOylated levels, or through induction of specific LXRβ SUMOylation. These modified

nuclear receptors interact with GPS2, associate with the N-CoR complex and prevent its disposal following the inflammatory response.
Another nuclear receptor, namely PPARδ, is involved in negative regulation of IL-6 mediated APR in hepatocytes (Kino et al., 2007). Indeed, treatment of liver cells with PPARδ agonists inhibits IL-6 induction of A2M, ORM, CRP, FBG and SERPINA3. PPARδ depletion by siRNAs, but not that of PPARα or PPARγ, attenuates agonist-dependent suppression. ChIP experiments suggest that PPARδ agonist treatment inhibits IL-6-dependent STAT3 recruitment to the SERPINA3 promoter. Thus, both C/EBP and STAT3 recruitment is altered by nuclear agonist treatment, respectively by LRH-1 (Venteclef et al., 2006) and PPARδ (Kino et al., 2007), explaining in part the nuclear receptor-dependent regulation of hepatocyte APP expression during the inflammatory response.

11. Conclusion

APP genes form a subset of inflammatory genes, with promoters associated with low CpG content, and rather late response expression patterns. Most APPs are considered late primary or secondary response genes. In response to stimulus from IL-1β and IL-6, among others, proximal promoters, with specific transcription factors, such as STAT3, AP-1 and C/EBPs, form an enhanceosome, through DNA-protein and protein-protein interactions. Tissue-restricted transcription factors, such as HNF-1α, HNF4α or GATA4 are involved in establishing proper tissue-specific inflammatory responses. Transcriptional activation depends on co-activator complexes with chromatin and transcription factor modifying activities, such as p300, and on chromatin remodeling complexes, such as SWI/SNF. Transcriptional repression depends on co-repressor complexes, like NCoR and SMRT complexes, with chromatin modifying activities as well. In addition, metabolic sensors, such as PPARs, LXRs and LRH-1, through the induction of post-translational modifications, such as sumoylation, may cancel APP induction by inflammatory signaling pathways. In contrast to primary response genes, much remains to be done to understand the mechanisms behind specific late primary and secondary APP gene regulation. Basal as well as signal-specific chromatin modifications (methylation and acetylation of various lysines on histones), RNA polymerase II status and presence of remodeling complexes remain to be determined. What is the temporal activation of these modifications during APR induction? How are these modifications established? How do tissue-specific transcription factors affect chromatin structure before and after the APR? What is the basis of the APR tissue-specific response? What is the promoter specificity of co-repressor complexes with HDAC3 activity (NCoR, SMRT) versus HDAC1/HDAC2 activity (NURD, CoREST)? What is the exact role of the various stress sensors in establishing proper chromatin structure? In addition to binding to proximal promoter sequences, do tissue-specific transcription factors, such as HNF-1α and HNF4α, mediate part of the inflammatory response through the establishment of enhancer-specific chromatin domains, like PU.1 in macrophages?

12. Acknowledgement

This work is supported by the Crohn's and Colitis Foundation of Canada. Claude Asselin is a member of the FRSQ-funded Centre de recherche clinique Étienne-Lebel.

13. References

Agrawal, A., Cha-Molstad, H., Samols, D., & Kushner, I. (2001). Transactivation of C-reactive protein by IL-6 requires synergistic interaction of CCAAT/enhancer binding protein beta (C/EBP beta) and Rel p50. *J. Immunol.*, 166(4): 2378-2384.

Agrawal, A., Cha-Molstad, H., Samols, D., & Kushner, I. (2003a). Overexpressed nuclear factor-kappaB can participate in endogenous C-reactive protein induction, and enhances the effects of C/EBPbeta and signal transducer and activator of transcription 3. *Immunology*, 108(4); 539-547.

Agrawal, A., Samols, D., & Kushner, I. (2003b). Transcription factor c-Rel enhances C-reactive protein expression by facilitating the binding of C/EBPbeta to the promoter. *Mol. Immunol.*, 40(6): 373-380.

Alonzi, T., Maritano, D., Gorgoni, B., Rizzuto, G., Libert, C., & Poli, V. (2001). Essential role of STAT3 in the control of the acute-phase response as revealed by inducible gene activation in the liver. *Mol. Cell. Biol.*, 21(5): 1621-1632.

Armandariz, A. D., & Krauss, R. M. (2009). Hepatic nuclear factor 1-alpha : inflammation, genetics, and atherosclerosis. *Curr. Opin. Lipidol.*, 20(2): 106-111.

Barish, G. D., Yu, R. T., Karunasiri, M., Ocampo, C. B., Dixon, J., Benner, C., Dent, A. L., Tangirala, R. K., & Evans, R. M. (2010). Bcl-6 and NF-kappaB cistromes mediate opposing regulation of the innate immune response. *Genes Dev.*, 24(24): 2760-2765.

Blaschke, F., Takata, Y., Caglayan, E., Collins, A., Tontonoz, P., Hsueh, W. A., & Tangirala, R. K. (2006). A nuclear receptor corepressor-dependent pathway mediates suppression of cytokine-induced C-reactive protein gene expression by liver X receptor. *Circ. Res.*, 99(12): e88-e99.

Bosse, T., Piaseckyj, C. M., Burghard, E., Fialkovich, J. J., Rajagopal, S., Pu, W. T., & Krasinski, S. D. (2006). Gata4 is essential for the maintenance of jejunal-ileal identities in the adult mouse small intestine. *Mol. Cell. Biol.*, 26(23): 9060-9070.

Boudreau, F., Yu, S. J., & Asselin, C. (1998). CCAAT/enhancer binding proteins beta and delta regulate alpha1-acid glycoprotein gene expression in rat intestinal epithelial cells. *DNA Cell Biol.*, 17(8): 669-677.

Brasier, A. R., Han, Y., & Sherman, C. T. (1999). Transcriptional regulation of angiotensinogen gene expression. *Vitam. Horm.* 57: 217-247.

Cha-Molstad, H., Agrawal, A., Zhang, D., Samols, D., & Kushner, I. (2000). The Rel family member P50 mediates cytokine-induced C-reactive protein expression by a novel mechanism. *J. Immunol.*, 165(8): 4592-4597.

Cha-Molstad, H., Young, D. P., Kushner, I, & Samols, D. (2007). The interaction of C-Rel with C/EBPbeta enhances C/EBPbeta binding to the C-reactive protein gene promoter. *Mol. Immunol.*, 44(11): 2933-2942.

Cunliffe, V. T. (2008). Eloquent silence: developmental functions of Class I histone deacetylases. *Curr. Opin. Genet. Dev.*, 18(5): 404-410.

Désilets, A., Gheorghiu, I., Yu, S. J., Seidman, E. G., & Asselin, C. (2000). Inhibition by deacetylase inhibitors of IL-1-dependent induction of haptoglobin involves CCAAT/enhancer-binding protein isoforms in intestinal epithelial cells. *Biochem. Biophys. Res. Commun.*, 276(2): 673-679.

Duan, H. O., & Simpson-Haidaris, P. J. (2003). Functional analysis of interleukin 6 response elements (IL-6REs) on the human gamma-fibrinogen promoter : binding of hepatic

Stat3 correlates negatively with transactivation potential of type II IL-6REs. *J. Biol. Chem.* 278(42): 41270-41281.

Duan, H. O., & Simpson-Haidaris, P. J. (2006). Cell type-specific differential induction of the human gamma-fibrinogen promoter by interleukin-6. *J. Biol. Chem.*, 281(18): 12451-12457.

Epstein, F. H. (1999). Acute-phase proteins and other systemic responses to inflammation. *New Engl. J. Med.*, 340(6); 448-454.

Fayard, E., Auwerx, J., & Schoonjans, K. (2004). LRH-1: an orphan nuclear receptor involved in development, metabolism and steroidogenesis. *Trends Cell Biol.*, 14(5): 250-260.

Friedman, A. D. (2007). Transcriptional control of granulocyte and monocyte development. *Oncogene*, 26(47): 6816-6828.

Fuda, N. J., Ardehali, M. B., & Lis, J. T. (2009). Defining mechanisms that regulate RNA polymerase II transcription in vivo. *Nature*, 461(7621): 186-192.

Gheorghiu, I., Deschênes, C., Blais, M., Boudreau, F., Rivard, N., & Asselin, C. (2001). Role of specific CCAAT/enhancer-binding protein isoforms in intestinal epithelial cells. *J. Biol. Chem.*, 276(47): 44331-44337.

Ghisletti, S., Huang, W., Ogawa, S., Pascual, G., Lin, M. E., Wilson, T. M., Rosenfeld, M. G., & Glass, C. K. (2007). Parallel SUMOylation-dependent pathways mediate gene- and signal-specific transrepression by LXRs and PPARgamma. *Mol. Cell*, 25(1): 57-70.

Ghisletti, S., Huang, W., Jepsen, K., Benner, C., Hardiman, G., Rosenfeld, M. G., & Glass, C. K. (2009). Cooperative NCoR/SMRT interactions establish a corepressor-based strategy for integration of inflammatory and anti-inflammatory signaling pathways. *Genes Dev.*, 23(6): 681-693.

Ghisletti, S., Barozzi, I., Mietton, F., Polletti, S., De Santa, F., Venturini, E., Gregory, L., Lonie, L., Chew, A., Wei, C. L., Ragoussis, J., & Natoli, G. (2010). Identification and characterization of enhancers controlling the inflammatory gene expression program in macrophages. *Immunity*, 32(3): 317-328.

Gilchrist, M., Thorsson, V., Li, B., Rust, A. G., Korb, M., Kenedy, K., Hai, T., Bolouri, H., & Aderem, A. (2006). Systems biology approaches identify ATF3 as a negative regulator of Toll-like receptor 4. *Nature*, 441(7090): 173-178.

Glass, C. K., & Saijo, K. (2010). Nuclear receptor transrepression pathways that regulate inflammation in macrophages and T cells. *Nat. Rev. Immunol.*, 10(5): 365-376.

Gruys, E., Toussaint, M. J. M., Niewold, T. A., & Koopmans, S. J. (2005). Acute phase reaction and acute phase proteins. *J. Zhejiang Univ.*, 6B(11): 1045-1056.

Haga, S., Terui, K., Zhang, H. Q., Enosawa, S., Ogawa, W., Inoue, H., Okuyama, T., Takeda, K., Akira, S., Ogino, T., Irani, K., & Ozaki, M. (2003). Stat3 protects against Fas-induced liver injury by redox-dependent and –independent mechanisms. *J. Clin. Invest.*, 112(7): 989-998.

Hagihara, K., Nishikawa, T., Sugamata, Y., Song, J., Isobe, T., Taga, T., & Yoshizaki, K. (2005). Essential role of STAT3 in cytokine-driven NF-kappaB-mediated serum amyloid A gene expression. *Genes Cells*, 10(11): 1051-1063.

Hargreaves, D. C., & Crabtree, G. R. (2011). ATP-dependent chromatin remodeling: genetics, genomics and mechanisms. *Cell Res.*, 21(3): 396-420.

Hargreaves, D. C., Horng, T., & Medzhitov, R. (2009). Control of inducible gene expression by signal-dependent transcriptional elongation. *Cell*, 138(1): 129-145.

Heintzman, N. D., Stuart, R. K., Hon, G., Fu, Y., Ching, C. W., Hawkins, R. D., Barrera, L. O., Van Calcar, S., Qu, C., Ching, K. A., Wang, W., Weng, Z., Green, R. D., Crawford, G.E., & Ren, B. (2007). Distinct and predictive signatures of transcriptional promoters and enhancers in the human genome. *Nat. Genet.*, 39(3); 311-318.

Heintzman, N. D., Hon, G. C., Hawkins, R. D., Kheradpour, P., Stark, A., Harp, L. F., Ye, Z., Start, R. K., Ching, C. W., Ching, K. A., Antosiewicz-Bourget, J. E., Liu, H., Zhang, X., Gree, R. D., Lobanenkov, V. V., Stewart, R., Thomson, J. A., Crawford, G. E., Kellis, M., & Ren, B. (2009). Histone modifications at human enhancers reflect global cell-type-specific gene expression. *Nature*, 459(7243): 108-112.

Heinz, S., Benner, C., Spann, N., Bertolino, E., Lin, Y. C., Laslo, P., Cheng, J. X., Murre, C., Singh, H., & Glass, C. K. (2010). Simple combinations of lineage-determining transcription factors prime cis-regulatory elements required for macrophage and B cell identities. *Mol. Cell*, 38(4): 576-589.

Hou, T., Ray, S., & Brasier, A. R. (2007). The functional role of an interleukin 6-inducible CDK9·STAT3 complex in human gamma-fibrinogen gene expression. *J. Biol. Chem.*, 282(51): 37091-37102.

Hou, T., Ray, S., Lee, c., & Brasier, A. R. (2008). The STAT3 NH_2-terminal domain stabilizes enhanceosome assembly by interacting with the p300 bromodomain. *J. Biol. Chem.*, 283(45): 30725-30734.

Hu, C. H., Harris, J. E., Davie, E. W., & Chung, D. W. (1995). Characterization of the 5'-flanking region of the gene for the alpha chain of human fibrinogen. *J. Biol. Chem.*, 270(47): 28342-28349.

Huang, W., Ghisletti, S., Perissi, V., Rosenfeld, M. G., & Glass, C. K. (2009). Transcriptional integration of TLR2 and TLR4 signaling at the NCoR derepression checkpoint. *Mol. Cell*, 35(1): 48-57.

Inagi, R. (2010). Endoplasmic reticulum stress as a progression factor for kidney injury. *Curr. Opin. Pharmacol.*, 10(2): 156-165.

Izumi, T., Wiederhold, L. R., Roy, G., Roy, R., Jaiswal, A., Bhakat, K. K., Mitra, S., & Hazra, T. K. (2003). Mammalian DNA base excision repair proteins: their interactions and role in repair of oxidative DNA damage. *Toxicology*, 193(1-2): 43-65.

Jain, S., Patil, S., & Kumar, A. (2007). HNF-1alpha plays an important role in IL-6-induced expression of the human angiotensinogen gene. *Am. J. Physiol.*, 293(1): C401-C410.

Kamimura, D., Ishihara, K., & Hirano, T. (2003). IL-6 signal transduction and its physiological roles: the signal orchestration model. *Rev. Physiol. Biochem. Pharmacol.*, 149: 1-38.

Khan, F.A., & Khan, M. F. (2010). Inflammation and acute phase response. *Int. J. Appl. Biol. Pharmaceut. Technol.*, 1(2): 312-321.

Kino, T., Rice, K. C., & Chrousos, G. P. (2007). The PPARdelta agonist GW501516 suppresses interleukin-6-mediated hepatocyte acute phase reaction via STAT3 inhibition. *Eur. J. Clin, Invest.*, 37(5): 425-433.

Kovacs, K. A., Steinmann, M., Magistretti, P. J., Halfon, O., & Cardinaux, J. R. (2003). CCAAT/enhancer-binding protein family members recruit the coactivator CREB-binding protein and trigger its phosphorylation. *J. Biol. Chem.*, 278(38): 36959-36965.

Kowenz-Leutz E., Pless, O., Dittmar, G., Knoblich, M., & Leutz, A. (2010). Crosstalk between C/EBPbeta phosphorylation, arginine methylation, and SWI/SNF/Mediator implies an indexing transcription factor code. *EMBO J.*, 29(6): 1105-1115.

Kumar, H., Kawai, T., & Akira S. (2011). Pathogen recognition by the innate immune system. *Int. Rev. Immunol.*, 30: 16-34.

Lerner, L., Henriksen, M. A., Zhang, X., & Darnell, J. E. (2003). STAT3-dependent enhanceosome assembly and disassembly: synergy with GR for full transcriptional increase of the alpha2-macroglobulin gene. *Genes Dev.*, 17(20): 2564-2577.

Leu, J. I., Crissey, M. A. S., Leu, J. P., Ciliberto, G., & Taub, R. (2001). Interleukin-6-induced STAT3 and AP-1 amplify hepatocyte nuclear factor 1-mediated transactivation of hepatic genes, an adaptive response to liver injury. *Mol. Cell. Biol.*, 21(2): 414-424.

Li, L., & Davie, J. R. (2010). The role of Sp1 and Sp3 in normal and cancer cell biology. *Ann. Anat.*, 192(5); 275-283.

Li, X., Salisbury-Rowswell, J., Murdock, A. D., Forse, R. A., & Burke, P. A. (2002). Hepatocyte nuclear factor 4 response to injury involves a rapid decrease in DNA binding and transactivation via a JAK2 signal transduction pathway. *Biochem. J.*, 368(1): 203-211.

Litvak, V., Ramsey, S. A., Rust, A. G., Zak, D. E., Kennedy, K. A., Lampano, A. E., Nykter, M., Shmulevich, I., & Aderem, A. (2009). *Nature Immunol.*, 10(4): 437-443.

Liu, Z., & Fuller, G. M. (1995). Detection of a novel transcription factor for the A alpha-fibrinogen gene in response to interleukin-6. *J. Biol. Chem.*, 270(13): 7580-7586.

Luebke-Wheeler, J., Zhang, K., Battle, M., Si-Tayeb, K., Garrison, W., Chhinder, S., Li, J., Kaufman, R. J., & Duncan, S. A. (2008). Hepatocyte nuclear factor 4 alpha is implicated in endoplasmic reticulum stress-induced acute phase response by regulating expression of cyclic adenosine monophosphate responsive element binding protein H. *Hepatology*, 48(4): 1242-1250.

Medzhitov, R., & Horng, T. (2009). Transcriptional control of the inflammatory response. *Nat. Rev. Immunol.*, 9(10): 692-703.

Mortensen, R. F. (2001). C-reactive protein, inflammation, and innate immunity. *Immunol. Res.*, 24(2): 163-176.

Murray, P. J. (2007). The JAK-STAT signaling pathway: input and output integration. *J. Immunol.*, 178(5): 2623-2629.

Nagaki, M., & Moriwaki, H. (2008). Transcription factor HNF and hepatocyte differentiation. *Hepatol. Res.*, 38(10): 961-969.

Nishikawa, T., Hagihara, K., Serada, S., Isobe, T., Matsumura, A., Song, J., Tanaka, T., Kawase, I., Naka, T., & Yoshizaki, K. (2008). Transcriptional complex formation of c-Fos, STAT3, and Hepatocyte NF-1alpha is essential for cytokine-driven C-reactive protein gene expression. *J. Immunol.*, 180(5): 3492-3501.

Nomura, F., Kawai, T., Nakanishi, K., & Akira, S. (2000). NF-kappaB activation through IKK-i-dependent I-TRAF/TANK phosphorylation. *Genes Cells*, 5(3): 191-202.

Ogawa, S., Lozach, J., Jepsen, K., Sawka-Verhelle, D., Perissi, V., Rose, D. W., Johnson, R. S., Rosenfeld, M. G., & Glass, C. K. (2004). A nuclear receptor corepressor transcriptional checkpoint controlling activator protein 1-dependent gene networks required for macrophage activation. *Proc. Natl. Acad. Sci. USA*, 101(40): 14461-14466.

Oishi, T., Date, S., Shimamoto, Y., Saito, T., Hirota, K., Sugaya, T., Kon, Y., Fukamizu, A., & Tanimoto, K. (2010). A nuclear receptor, hepatocyte nuclear factor 4, differently contributes to the human and mouse angiotensinogen promoter activities. *J. Recept. Signal Transduct.*, 30(6): 484-492.

Oyadomari, S., & Mori M. (2004). Roles of CHOP/GADD154 in endoplasmic reticulum stress. *Cell Death Differ.*, 11(4): 381-389.

Pascual, G., Fong, A. L., Ogawa, S., Gamliel, A., Li, A. C., Perissi, V., Rose, D. W., Wilson, T. M., Rosenfeld, M. G., & Glass, C. K. (2005). A SUMOylation-dependent pathway mediates transrepression of inflammatory response genes by PPAR-gamma. *Nature*, 437(7059): 759-763.

Pelletier, N., Boudreau, F., Yu, S. J., Zannoni, S., Boulanger, V., & asselin, C. (1998). Activation of haptoglobin gene expression by cAMP involves CCAAT/enhancer-binding protein isoforms in intestinal epithelial cells. *FEBS Lett.*, 439(3): 275-280.

Perissi, V., Aggarwal, A., Glass, C. K., Rose, D. W., & Rosenfeld, M. G. (2004). A corepressor/coactivator exchange complex required for transcriptional activation by nuclear receptors and other regulated transcription factors. *Cell*, 116(4): 511-526.

Ramirez-Carrozzi, V. R., Nazarian, A. A., Li, C. C., Gore, S. L., Sridharan, R., Imbalzano, A. N., & Smale, S. T. (2006). Selective and antagonistic functions of SWI/SNF and Mi-2beta nucleosome remodeling complexes during an inflammatory response. *Genes Dev.*, 20(3): 282-296.

Ramirez-Carrozzi, V. R., Braas, D., Bhatt, D. M., Cheng, C. S., Hong, C., Doty, K. R., Black, J. C., Hoffman, A., Carey, M., & Smale, S. T. (2009). A unifying model for the selective regulation of inducible transcription by CpG islands and nucleosome remodeling. *Cell*, 138(1): 114-128.

Ray, S., Sherman, C. T., Lu, M., & Brasier, A. R. (2002). Angiotensinogen gene expression is dependent on signal transducer and activator of transcription 3-mediated p300/cAMP response element binding protein-binding protein coactivator recruitment and histone acetyltransferase activity. *Mol. Endocrinol.*, 16(4): 824-836.

Ray, S., Boldogh, I., & Brasier, A. R. (2005). STAT3 NH2-terminal acetylation is activated by the hepatic acute-phase response and required for IL-6 induction of angiotensinogen. *Gastroenterology*, 129(5): 1616-1632.

Ray, S., Lee, C., Hou, T., Boldogh, I., & Brasier, A. R. (2008). Requirement of histone deacetylase1 (HDAC1) in signal transducer and activator of transcription 3 (STAT3) nucleocytoplasmic distribution. *Nucleic Acids Res.*, 36(13): 4510-4520.

Ray, S., Lee, C., Hou, T., Bhakat, K. K., & Brasier, A. R. (2010). Regulation of signal transducer and activator of transcription 3 enhanceosome formation by apurinic/apyrimidinic endonuclease 1 in hepatic acute phase response. *Mol. Endocrinol.*, 24(2): 391-401.

Rigamonti, E., Chinetti-Gbaguidi, G., & Staels, B. (2008). Regulation of macrophage functions by PPAR-alpha, PPAR-gamma, and LXRs in mice and men. *Arterioscler. Thromb. Vasc. Biol.*, 28(6): 1050-1059.

Rocha, V. Z., & Libby, P. (2009). Obesity, inflammation, and atherosclerosis. *Nat. Rev. Cardiol.*, 6(4): 399-409.

Rousseau, D., Turgeon, N., D., Roy, E., & Asselin, C. (2008). GATA-4 modulates C/EBP-dependent transcriptional activation of acute phase protein genes. *Biochem. Biophys. Res. Commun.*, 370(2): 371-375.

Sanalkumar, R., Dhanesh, S. B., & James, J. (2010). Non-canonical activation of Notch signaling/target genes in vertebrates. *Cell. Mol. Life Sci.*, 67(17): 2957-2968.

Saxonov, S., Berg, P., & Brutlag, D. L. (2006). A genome-wide analysis of CpG dinucleotides in the human genome distinguishes two distinct classes of promoters. *Proc. Natl. Acad. Sci. USA*, 103(5): 1412-1427.

Sherman, C. T., & Brasier, A. R. (2001). Role of signal transducers and activators of transcription 1 and -3 in inducible regulation of the human angiotensinogen gene by interleukin-6. *Mol. Endocrinol.*, 15(3): 441-457.

Shih, D. Q., Bussen, M., Sehayek, E., Ananthanarayanan, M., Shneider, B. L., Suchy, F. J., Shefer, S., Bollileni, J. S., Gonzalez, F. J., Breslow, J. L., & Stoffel, M. (2001). Hepatocyte nuclear factor-1alpha is an essential regulator of bile acid and plasma cholesterol metabolism. *Nat. Genet.*, 27(4): 375-382.

Sims, R. J., Belotserkovskaya, R., & Reinberg, D. (2004). Elongation by RNA polymerase II: the short and long of it. *Genes Dev.*, 18(20): 2437-2468.

Singh, P. P., Voleti, B., & Agrawal, A. (2007). A novel RBP-Jkappa-dependent switch from C/EBPbeta to C/EBPzeta at the C/EBP binding site on the C-reactive protein promoter. *J. Immunol.*, 178(11): 7302-7309.

Svotelis, A., Doyon, G., Bernatchez, G., Désilets, A., Rivard, N., & Asselin, C. (2005). IL-1 beta-dependent regulation of C/EBP delta transcriptional activity. *Biochem. Biophys. Res. Commun.*, 328(2): 461-470.

Toniatti, C., Demartis, A., Monaci, P., Nicosia, A., & Ciliberto, G. (1990). Synergistic trans-activation of the human C-reactive protein promoter by transcription factor HNF-1 binding at two distinct sites. *EMBO J.*, 9(13): 4467-4475.

Turgeon, N., Valiquette, C., Blais, M., Routhier, S., Seidman, E. G., & Asselin, C. (2008). Regulation of C/EBPdelta-dependent transactivation by histone deacetylases in intestinal epithelial cells. *J. Cell. Biochem.*, 103(5): 1573-1583.

Viger, R. S., Guittot, S. M., Anttonen, M., Wilson, D. B., & Heikinheimo, M. (2008). Role of GATA family of transcription factors in endocrine development, function, and disease. *Mol. Endocrinol.*, 22: 781-798.

Venteclef, N., Smith, J. C., Goodwin, B., & Delerive, P. (2006). Liver receptor homolog 1 is a negative regulator of the hepatic acute-phase response. *Mol. Cell. Biol.*, 26(18): 6799-6807.

Venteclef, N., Jakobsson, T., Ehrlund, A., Damdimopoulos, A., Mikkonen, L., Ellis, E., Nilsson, L. M., Parini, P., Janne, O. A., Gustafsson, J. A., Steffensen, K. R., & Treuter, E. (2010). GPS2-dependent corepressor/SUMO pathways govern anti-inflammatory actions of LRH-1 and LXRbeta in the hepatic acute phase response. *Genes Dev.*, 24(4): 381-395.

Visel, A., Rubin, E. M., & Pennacchio, L. A. (2009). Genomic views of distant-acting enhancers. *Nature*, 461(7261): 199-205.

Voleti, B., & Agrawal, A. (2005). Regulation of basal and induced expression of C-reactive protein through an overlapping element for OCT-1 and NF-kappaB on the proximal promoter. *J. Immunol.*, 175(5): 3386-3390.

Wang, Z., & Burke, P. A. (2007). Effects of hepatocye nuclear factor-4alpha on the regulation of the hepatic acute phase response. *J. Mol. Biol.*, 371(2): 323-335.

Wang, Z., & Burke, P. A. (2008). Modulation of hepatocyte nuclear factor-4alpha function by the peroxisome-proliferator-activated receptor-gamma co-activator-1alpha in the acute-phase response. *Biochem. J.*, 415(2): 289-296.

Wang, Z., & Burke, P. A. (2010). Hepatocyte nuclear factor-4alpha interacts with other hepatocyte nuclear factors in regulating transthyretin gene expression. *FEBS J.*, ,277(19): 4066-4075.

Weber, A., Wasiliew, P., & Kracht, M. (2010). Interleukin (IL-1) pathway. *SCIENCESIGNALING*, 3(105 cm1): 1-6.

Wierstra, I. (2008). Sp1: emerging roles- beyond constitutive activation of TATA-less housekeeping genes. *Biochem. Biophys. Res. Commun.*, 372(1): 1-13.

Yanai, K., Hirota, K., Taniguchi-Yanai, K., Shigematsu, Y., Shimamoto, Y., Saito, T., Chowdhury, S., Takiguchi, M., Arakawa, M., Nibu, Y., Sugiyama, F., Yagami, K., & Fukamizu, A. (1999). Regulated expression of human angiotensinogen gene by hepatocyte nuclear factor 4 and chicken ovalbumin upstream promoter-transcription factor. *J. Biol. Chem.*, 274(49): 34605-34612.

Yang, Z., Yik, J. H., Chen, R., He, N., Jang, M. K., Ozato, K., & Zhou, Q. (2005). Recruitment of P-TEFb for stimulation of transcriptional elongation by the bromodomain protein Brd4. *Mol. Cell*, 19(4): 535-545.

Young, D. P., Kushner, I., & Samols, D. (2008). Binding of C/EBPbeta to the C-reactive protein (CRP) promoter in Hep3B cells is associated with transcription of CRP mRNA. *J. Immunol.*, 181(4): 2420-2427.

Yu, S. J., Boudreau, F., Désilets, A., Houde, M., Rivard, N., & Asselin, C. (1999). Attenuation of haptoglobin gene expression by TGFbeta requires the MAP kinase pathway. *Biochem. Biophys. Res. Commun.*, 259(3): 544-549.

Zhang, X., & Darnell, J. E. (2001). Functional importance of Stat3 tetramerization in activation of the alpha2-macroglobulin gene. *J. Biol. Chem.*, 276(36): 33576-33581.

Zhang, K., Shen, X., Wu, J., Sakaki, K., saunders, T., Rutkowski, D. T., Back, S. H., & Kaufman, R. J. (2006). Endoplasmic reticulum stress activates cleavage of CREBH to induce a systemic inflammatory response. *Cell*, 124(3): 587-599.

2

Acute Phase Proteins: Structure and Function Relationship

Sabina Janciauskiene[1], Tobias Welte[1] and Ravi Mahadeva[2]
[1]Department of Respiratory Medicine, Hannover Medical School, Hannover,
[2]Department of Respiratory Medicine, University of Cambridge, Cambridge,
[1]Germany
[2]England

1. Introduction

The acute-phase response is critical to the body's ability to successfully respond to injury. It normally lasts only few days; however, if continued unchecked, the acute phase response may contribute to the development of chronic inflammatory states, tissue damage and disease. The acute phase response is typically characterized by fever and changes in vascular permeability, along with profound changes in the biosynthetic profile of various acute phase proteins (APPs) (Hack et al., 1997, Gabay & Kushner, 1999). APPs are an evolutionarily conserved family of proteins produced mainly in the liver in response to infection and inflammation. In all mammalian species, the synthesis of the APPs is mainly regulated by inflammatory cytokines, such as interleukin-6 (IL-6), interleukin-1 (IL-1) and tumor necrosis factor (TNF). For instance, haptoglobin (Hp), C-reactive protein (CRP), serum amyloid A (SAA), alpha-1 acid glycoprotein (AGP) and hemopexin are regulated mainly by IL-1 or combinations of IL-1 and IL-6, whereas fibrinogen, alpha-1 antichymotrypsin (ACT) and alpha-1 antitrypsin (AAT) are regulated by IL-6 (Koj, 1985; Kushner & Mackiewicz, 1993). Exogenous glucocorticoids can also influence APPs by their effect on cytokines. The decreased synthesis of albumin during the inflammatory reaction has also been shown to be the result of monocyte/macrophage-derived products, such as IL-1 (Moshage et al., 1987). The concentration of specific blood APPs varies during inflammatory states; increasing or decreasing by at least 25 percent (Kushner et al., 1982). Indeed, ceruloplasmin concentrations can increase by 50 percent and CRP and serum amyloid A by a 1000-fold (Kushner et al., 1981; Dinarello, 1983; Blackburn, 1994; Gruys et al., 1994; Ingenbleek & Bernstein, 1999).

The rise in the plasma concentration of APPs can assist host defense by aiding recognition of invading microbes, mobilization of leukocytes into the circulation, and increasing blood flow to injured or infected sites. These actions favor the accumulation of effector molecules and leukocytes at locally inflamed sites; in essence, they enhance local inflammation and antimicrobial defense. Concurrently, the APPs also prevent inflammation in uninvolved tissues by neutralizing inflammation-induced molecules (such as cytokines, proteases, and oxidants) that enter the bloodstream, by diminishing the proinflammatory responses of circulating leukocytes, and by forestalling endothelial activation.

A particularly important role for APPs in the establishment of host defense is also suggested by the magnitude and rapidity of changes in concentrations of APPs, together with their short half-life. This is also supported by the known functional capabilities of the APPs, and hence theories as to how they might serve useful purposes in inflammation, healing, or adaptation to a noxious stimulus. The functional activities of APPs as well as the relationship between protein structure and function are discussed in this chapter.

2. Diverse functional activities of acute phase proteins (APPs)

APPs are regarded as both mediators and inhibitors of inflammation operating at multiple possible sites. The classic complement components, many of which are APPs, have central proinflammatory roles in immunity. Complement activation leads to chemotaxis, plasma protein exudation at inflammatory sites, and opsonization of infectious agents and damaged cells. Other APPs such as fibrinogen, plasminogen, tissue plasminogen activator (tPA), urokinase and plasminogen activator inhibitor-I (PAI-1) play an active role in tissue repair and tissue remodelling (Gabay & Kushner, 1999). APPs also have antiinflammatory actions. For example, the antioxidants haptoglobin and hemopexin protect against reactive oxygen species, and AAT and ACT both antagonize the activity of proteolytic enzymes (Janciauskiene, 2001). Some metal chelating proteins, such as ceruloplasmin, that binds copper, and hemopexin, that binds heme, act more directly against pathogens. Other proteins are directly involved in the innate immunity against pathogens. LPS-binding protein (LPS-BP), for example, interacts with bacterial lipopolysaccharide (LPS) transferring it to CD14, a receptor on the surface of macrophages and B-cells. Following the presentation of LPS by LBP, a lipopolysaccharide recognition complex is formed on the membrane via the recruitment of a second receptor, Toll Like Receptor 4. These events drive the TLR signaling pathway that induces the activation of several inflammatory and immune-response genes, including pro-inflammatory cytokines (Gutsmann et al., 2001). Some APPs might act as protectors against cell death by apoptosis. For example, alpha 1-acid glycoprotein (AGP) and AAT have been shown to inhibit the major mediators of apoptosis, namely caspase-3 and caspase-7 (Van Molle et al., 1999). There are many diseases where induction of specific APPs parallels the degree and evolution of the inflammatory processes, hence, elevated APPs can be of diagnostic and prognostic value. The pathogenic role of fibrin in thrombosis is well known. CRP has been demonstrated to enhance ischemia/reperfusion injury by activating the complement system (Lu et al., 2009). Elevated serum values of CRP are known to be associated with an increased risk of human atherosclerosis. Ferritin, another APP, is a primary iron-storage protein and often measured to assess a patient's iron status. Procalcitonin (PCT), was discovered recently as a marker of bacterial infection (Assicot et al., 1993). On the other hand, APPs can be considered as putative drugs for the treatment of various inflammatory diseases. Different experimental studies have demonstrated how the administration of a specific APP prior to or after the initiation of an acute-phase response can switch the pro-inflammatory to the anti-inflammatory pathway necessary for the resolution of inflammation. In this regard, purified plasma AAT is used for the treatment of emphysema and other diseases in patients with inherited AAT deficiency and shows anti-inflammatory and immune modulatory effects.

3. Multifunctional activities of single APP

Despite vast pro- and anti-inflammatory properties ascribed to individual APPs, their role during infections remains incompletely defined as to the functional advantages acquiring from changes in plasma concentrations of the APPs. So far, existing data provide evidence that APPs act on a variety of cells involved in the early and late stages of inflammation and that their effects are time, concentration and molecular conformation-dependent (Figure 1). Many APPs have a duel function; amplifying inflammatory responses when the inciting pathogen is present within the host and down-regulating the response when the pathogen has been eradicated.

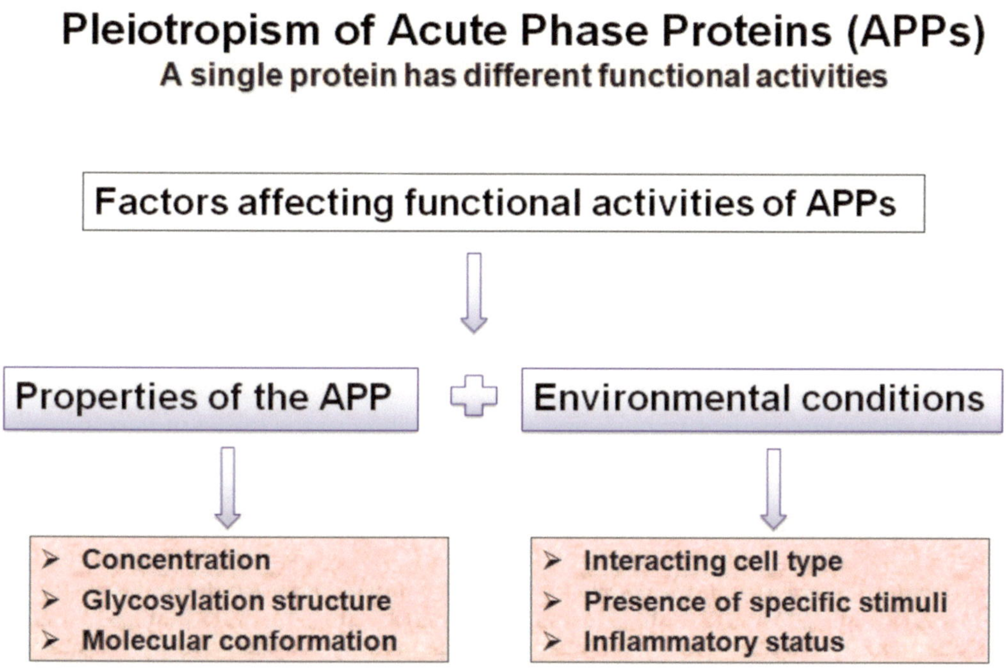

Fig. 1. Schematic presentation of factors that may affect activities of APPs.

3.1 C-reactive protein (CRP)

C-reactive protein (CRP) is a member of the pentraxin family of proteins, which are serum opsonins, which bind to damaged membranes and nuclear autoantigens. CRP has an ability to recognize pathogens and to mediate their elimination by recruiting the complement system and phagocytic cells, thus making it an important member of the first line of innate host defense. The normal concentration in healthy human serum is usually lower than 10 mg/L, increasing slightly with age. Current research suggests that subjects with elevated basal levels of CRP are at an increased risk of diabetes (Pradhan et al., 2001, Dehghan et al., 2007), hypertension and cardiovascular disease (Koenig et al., 2006). CRP is an ancient protein whose biological role appears quite complex. Although, originally CRP was suggested to be purely a biomarker, recent studies have pointed that it may in fact be a direct mediator of patho-physiological processes. It is likely that the activity of CRP in humans, either pro- or anti-inflammatory is dependent on the context in which it is acting, and thus CRP may be more versatile than previously thought.

3.1.1 Pro-inflammatory effects of CRP

CRP displays pro-inflammatory effects by activating the complement system and inducing inflammatory cytokines and tissue factor production in monocytes. The binding of phosphocholine and the complement pathway component (C1q) by CRP is part of innate immunity that activates the classical complement pathway (Gabay & Kushner, 1999; Du Clos, 2000). Data on the consumption of complement components and cell lysis have indicated that CRP-initiated complement activation is restricted to the formation of the C3 convertase (Berman et al., 1986). Formation of the alternative pathway amplification convertase and of C5 convertases is inhibited by factor H (Mold et al., 1984), which binds directly to CRP (Mold et al., 1999). The interactions between CRP and its diverse ligands, such as phosphocholine or Fcγ receptors, has the potential to influence a variety of cells and pathways with the potential to affect: apoptotic cells (Gershov et al., 2000), damaged cell membranes (Volanakis & Wirtz, 1979), phagocytic cells (Ballou & Lozanski, 1992), smooth muscle cells (Hattori et al., 2003), and endothelial cells (Pasceri et al., 2000). Experimental evidence for the binding of CRP to apoptotic cells was provided recently (Gershov et al., 2000). The distribution of CRP on the surface of such cells is similar to that of the complement membrane attack complex. In addition to the membrane of intact injured cells, CRP also binds to membranes and nuclear constituents of necrotic cells. Several nuclear constituents, including histones (Du Clos et al., 1988), small nuclear ribonucleoproteins (Du Clos, 1989) and ribonucleoprotein particles (Pepys et al., 1994) have been shown to bind CRP in a calcium-dependent fashion, and CRP deposition to the nuclei of necrotic cells at sites of inflammation has been observed (Gitlin et al., 1977).

To date, experiments with monocytes have shown that CRP induces the production of inflammatory cytokines (IL-1, IL-6, TNFα, IL-8) (Ballou & Lozanski, 1992; Xie et al., 2005), the generation of reactive oxygen species (Zeller & Sullivan, 1992), leads to increased expression of tissue factor (Cermak et al., 1993), and affects cell chemotaxis (Whisler et al., 1986; Kew et al., 1990). Recently, Hanriot et al. (2008), investigating human monocytes exposed to CRP have confirmed the results of earlier studies on CRP-mediated induction of expression of numerous proinflammatory cytokine genes (with the exception of TNFα) and further evidenced increased expression of PAI-2, MCP-1, GRO-α, GRO-β, and the chemokine receptors CCR8 and CXCR4. It has also been demonstrated that isolated from serum and recombinant CRP can stimulate expression of the monocytic surface integrin CD11b and downregulate that of CD31 antigen (Woollard et al., 2002). Numerous reports in the literature document the role of CRP in atherogenesis. Epidemiological evidence reveals an association between elevated plasma CRP and atherosclerosis (Haverkate et al., 1997; Ridker et al., 1997; Koenig et al., 1999). Infusion of recombinant CRP in healthy men results in the activation of inflammation and coagulation (Bisoendial *et al.*, 2005). *In vitro*, CRP has been shown to exert a direct proinflammatory and proatherosclerotic effect on vascular cells, as exemplified by: (1) induction of an increased expression of adhesion molecules, such as vascular cell adhesion molecule-1 (VCAM-1), intercellular adhesion molecule- 1 (ICAM-1), and E-selectin (Pasceri et al., 2000); (2) stimulation of secretion of monocyte chemoattractant protein-1 (MCP-1) (Pasceri et al., 2001); and (3) facilitation of macrophage low-density lipoprotein (LDL) uptake (Verma et al., 2002a). Transcription of genes encoding the cell adhesion molecules (VCAM-1, ICAM-1, E-selectin) and chemokines is tightly regulated by the transcription factor NF-κB, which has been implicated as a key mediator of atherosclerosis (Brand et al., 1996; Marumo et al., 1997; Thurberg & Collins, 1998; De Martin et al., 2000). However, with regard to the effects of CRP on endothelial cells, published studies are somewhat controversial. CRP has been shown to promote production of pro-angiogenic molecules such as endothelin-1 and IL-6 in human saphenous vein endothelial cells (Verma et al., 2002), and activate NF-κB signalling through the CD32 receptor (Liang et al., 2006). However, other studies suggested that endothelial cell activation by CRP is due to contamination of the commercially obtained protein with LPS and/or sodium azide (Liu et al., 2005, Taylor et al., 2005).

3.1.2 Anti-inflammatory effects of CRP

3.1.2.1 *In vitro*

CRP appears to express anti-inflammatory properties. For example, in monocytic cells CRP has been shown to increase the synthesis of interleukin-1-receptor antagonist (IL-1ra), to up-regulate vascular endothelial growth factor A (VEGF-A) expression (Tilg et al, 1993), to increase the release of the anti-inflammatory cytokine IL-10 (Mold et al, 2002; Szalai et al, 2002) and to repress the synthesis of IFN-γ (Szalai et al, 2002). Furthermore, CRP has been reported to display anti-inflammatory effects in monocytes through down-regulation of alpha2-macroglobulin expression and up-regulation of liver X receptor α expression (Hanriot et al., 2008). CRP was found to bind to a ligand on Leishmania donovani and phosphorylcholine-expressing Neisseria meningitides, and hence increase their uptake by human phagocytes (Culley et al., 1996, Casey et al., 2008). Thomas-Rudolph et al (2007) have also reported that innate recognition by CRP enhances effective uptake and presentation of bacterial antigens through Fc-gamma receptors on dendritic cells and stimulates protective adaptive immunity. CRP has been shown to express multiple anti-inflammatory effects on neutrophils. CRP down-regulates the generation of superoxide by activated neutrophils which leads to a significant reduction of intracellular protein phosphorylation. IL-8-, formyl-methionyl-leucyl-phenylalanine (fMLP)-, and the complement component C5a-induced chemotactic responses of neutrophils are also found to be inhibited by CRP (Zhong et al., 1998). Inhibition of neutrophil chemotactic responses by CRP correlates with a reduction of chemotactic peptide-induced p38 kinase activity (Heuertz et al., 1999). In addition, CRP has been reported to induce cleavage and shedding of L-selectin from the surface of neutrophils, and markedly attenuate the attachment of human neutrophils to endothelial cells (Zouki et al., 1997). Finally, CRP has been shown to mediate shedding of the membrane-bound IL-6 receptor from neutrophils (Jones et al., 1999). The combined data on the effects of CRP on neutrophils indicate that this protein can limit the inflammatory response.

3.1.2.2 *In vivo*

A variety of studies utilizing exogenous or transgenic CRP have probed the effects of CRP *in vivo*. The ability of CRP to protect mice against bacterial infection by various species has been well established. These species include *S. pneumoniae* (Mold et al., 1981; Szalai et al., 1995) and *Haemophilus influenza* (Weiser et al., 1998; Lysenko et al., 2000), which have phosphocholine-rich surfaces, and *Salmonella enterica* serovar Typhimurium, which has no known surface phosphocholine, although its cell membrane is known to be rich in another

CRP ligand, phosphoethanolamine (Szalai et al., 2000). Protection is presumably mediated through CRP binding to phosphocholine or phosphoethanolamine, followed by activation of the classical complement pathway. CRP protection of mice infected with *S. pneumoniae* has been shown to require an intact complement system, but does not require interaction with FcγRs (Mold et al., 2002; Szalai et al., 2002). CRP`s protective effects are not limited to bacteria. It has been shown to play a protective role in a variety of inflammatory conditions, including endotoxin-mediated shock (Mold et al., 2002; Xia et al., 1997). Transgenic mice expressing human CRP are resistant to experimental allergic encephalomyelitis (Szalai et al, 2002). The study by Heuertz and collaborators has demonstrated that pretreatment of rabbits with purified human CRP intravenously significantly reduces neutrophil infiltration and C5a-induced alveolitis (Heuertz at al., 1993). One of the most commonly studied animal models of human systemic lupus erythematosus (SLE) is the female NZB x NZW F mouse model (B/W). These mice, as with human SLE patients, develop high levels of autoantibodies to nuclear antigens, leading to circulating immune complexes, the renal deposition of immune complexes and renal pathology. In this experimental model a single injection of human CRP not only markedly delayed the development of proteinuria, but also reversed ongoing active nephritis. The half-life of CRP in mice is only 4 hours (Kushner et al, 1978), however, despite the rapid clearance of injected CRP, the downregulation of the inflammatory process in the kidney persisted for more than 2 months. This suggests that CRP is most likely to be a direct regulator of the inflammation induced by immune complex deposition. In support of this B/W mice transgenic for human CRP also show a delayed onset of proteinuria and enhanced survival compared with non-transgenic B/W mice (Rodriguez et al., 2005). A single injection of CRP both prevents and reverses accelerated nephrotoxic nephritis (NTN) in C57BL/6 mice (Rodriguez et al., 2005) indicating that CRP-induced suppression of immune complex-mediated inflammation is not limited to autoimmune nephritis. Protection from NTN by CRP was associated with a decrease in inflammatory and pathologic changes in glomeruli and a marked reduction in renal expression of IL-1β and other macrophage chemoattractants (Rodriguez et al, 2007).

3.2 Alpha1-acid glycoprotein (AGP)

AGP is another example of an APP with multiple biological effects. AGP belongs to the lipocalin family, a group of proteins sharing a similar three-dimensional structure capable of binding and carrying hydrophobic molecules. The normal range of AGP concentration in the serum is 0.5-1.0 g/L, which can be increased several-fold in response to inflammation, infection, and systemic tissue injury (Engstrom et al., 2004; Lind et al., 2004). AGP function is still unknown; however, this protein is suggested to have a complex role by differentially regulating inflammatory responses (Logdberg & Wester, 2000; Fournier et al., 2000). So far, the most important function of AGP is linked to its ability to inhibit platelet aggregation (Snyder & Coodley, 1976; Costello et al., 1979).

3.2.1 Pro-inflammatory effects of AGP

Earlier studies have shown that AGP can activate monocytes, induce T cell proliferation (Singh & Fudenberg, 1986) and enhance TNFα, IL-1, and IL-6 secretion (Boutten et al., 1992; Drenth et al., 1996; Su & Yeh, 1996). More recently it has been demonstrated that AGP activates human monocytes to secrete TNFα through a tyrosine kinase dependent pathway and this can be enhanced in the presence of serum AGP-binding proteins. Since TNFα can also trigger the synthesis and secretion of AGP, the increase in TNFα secretion by AGP-stimulated monocytes may represent a positive feedback of APPs to amplify the inflammatory signal (Su et al., 1999). A current study evaluated the effects of bovine AGP on neutrophil pro-inflammatory responses, including respiratory burst activity and cytokine production, and found that bovine AGP enhanced neutrophil production of IL-8 in a dose-dependent manner (Rinaldi et al., 2008)

3.2.2 Anti-inflammatory effects of AGP

3.2.2.1 *In vitro*

AGP has been shown to induce macrophage expression of IL-1ra and soluble TNF receptor, which antagonize the activity of IL-1β and TNFα, respectively (Tilg et al., 1993, Hochepied et al., 2003). Sorensson and colleagues (1999) reported that endothelial barrier functions are dependent on the presence of AGP. A number of studies have investigated the effects of AGP on neutrophil function. At physiological concentrations, human AGP has inhibitory effects on neutrophil chemotactic responses after stimulation with fMLP and the complement component C5a (Laine et al., 1990, Vasson et al., 1994). Moreover, it has been shown that low doses of AGP promote neutrophil aggregation, while higher doses inhibit this response (Laine et al., 1990). Neutrophil respiratory burst activity is also reported to be modulated by AGP, and several studies have demonstrated that human AGP can inhibit the extracellular release of superoxide anion after activation with opsonized zymosan or phorbol 12-myristate,13-acetate (PMA) (Costello et al., 1984; Vasson et al., 1994). Bovine AGP inhibited zymosan-induced neutrophil extracellular release of superoxide anion and hydrogen peroxide without affecting the capacity of neutrophils to engulf and kill *Staphylococcus aureus*. Interestingly, AGP exerted its effect on free radical production regardless of whether neutrophils were exposed to AGP prior to or after activation (Rinaldi et al., 2008).

3.2.2.2 *In vivo*

Several studies have shown that AGP may function as an immune modulator displaying a protective effect in different models of shock. In a model of bacterial septic shock, using the gram-negative *Klebsiella pneumoniae*, AGP showed clear protection when given prior to the lethal challenge (Fournier et al., 2000). Furthermore, AGP was found to inhibit apoptosis and inflammation in murine models, and to induce cAMP-dependent signaling in the endothelial cells (Libert et al., 1994; Costello et al., 1979). Using *Escherichia coli* LPS, an initiator of the acute inflammatory response associated with septic shock, Morre DF and coworkers (1997) demonstrated that AGP-LPS complexes can activate mouse macrophages *in vitro* and that AGP protects against sepsis. It has also reported that AGP protects mice from lethal shock induced by TNFα or endotoxin. The protection was observed in both normal and in galactosamine-sensitized mice; with optimal desensitization requiring at least 3 mg of AGP administered 2 hours before the lethal challenge. Under these conditions, complete inhibition of all TNF-induced metabolic changes was observed (Libert et al., 1994). In another model, AGP has been found to significantly increase survival rate (48 hours) in rats with septic peritonitis. This effect was seen when AGP (200 mg/kg i.v.) was given 15 min prior to and 24 hours after cecal puncture. In a hemorrhagic/hypovolemic shock model (including a defined trauma) in rats treated with 200 mg/kg AGP resulted in significantly higher values of mean arterial blood pressure, cardiac output and stroke volume when compared to corresponding values obtained after resuscitation with Ringer's solution or-intravenous albumin (Muchitsch et al., 1998). In addition, AGP has been found to be protective against ischemia reperfusion in kidneys (Daemen et al., 2000). According to the results of this study AGP and AAT administered at reperfusion prevented apoptosis at 2 hours and 24 hours and exerted anti-inflammatory effects, as indicated by reduced renal TNF-α expression and neutrophil influx after 24 hours leading to improved renal function. Administration of AGP and AAT 2 hours after reperfusion resulted in a similar trend but without functional improvement. Moreover ischemia reperfusion elicited an acute phase response, as reflected by elevated serum AGP and serum amyloid P (SAP) levels after 24 hours, and increased hepatic acute phase protein mRNA levels after 18 hours of renal reperfusion. Other useful physiological effects of AGP include protection against brain edema formation after experimental stroke (Pichler et al., 1999), and injuries after intestinal ischemia (Williams et al., 1997).

3.3 Alpha1-antitrypsin (AAT)

Alpha1-Antitrypsin (AAT), also referred to as alpha$_1$-proteinase inhibitor or SERPINA1, is the prototypical member of the SERPIN (an acronym for serine proteinase inhibitor) family of protease inhibitors (Carrell, 1986). The normal plasma concentration of AAT ranges from 0.9 to 1.75 g/L. AAT is present in all tissues and biological fluids including cerebrospinal fluid, saliva, tears, breast milk, semen, urine and bile. Over 100 alleles of AAT have been identified to date, of which at least 20 affect either the amount or the function of the AAT molecule *in vivo* (Gooptu & Lomas, 2009). The genes are inherited as co-dominant alleles (products of both genes can be found in the circulation). Individuals with plasma AAT values below 0.7 g/L are considered to be AAT deficient. In very rare circumstances individuals may inherit AAT null alleles which are characterized by very low levels of serum AAT. AAT deficiency typically results from point mutations causing a perturbation in protein structure and resulting in increased intracellular polymerization and retention in the cell of synthesis. Retained AAT polymers in the endoplasmic reticulum of hepatocytes can promote liver damage with a variable clinical presentation, from neonatal hepatitis to liver cirrhosis and hepatocellular carcinoma in adults. The lack of circulating protein predisposes to the development of early-onset COPD (Carrell & Lomas, 1997). AAT deficiency has also been associated with a number of other inflammatory diseases, although the association is only moderate or weak. These include bronchial asthma, bronchiectasis, systemic vasculitis, rheumatoid arthritis, inflammatory bowel diseases, intracranial and abdominal aneurysms, arterial dissections, psoriasis, chronic urticaria, mesangiocapillary glomerulonephritis, pancreatitis and pancreatic tumors, multiple sclerosis, and other occasionally reported conditions (Janciauskiene et al., 2011).

3.3.1 Anti-inflammatory effects of AAT

3.3.1.1 *In vitro*

It was previously thought that the primary function of AAT was to inhibit neutrophil elastase and proteinase 3 (Gettings, 2002). However, current studies demonstrate that AAT is an irreversible inhibitor for kallikreins 7 and 14 (Schapira et al., 1982; Luo et al., 2006), and that AAT also inhibits intracellular and cell-surface proteases. Matriptase, a cell surface serine protease involved in the activation of epithelial sodium channels, is one such protease (Tseng et al., 2008; Janciauskiene et al., 2008). AAT also inhibits the activity of caspase-3, an intracellular cysteine protease which plays an essential role in cell apoptosis (Petrache et al., 2006). A recent study provides new evidence that AAT inhibits ADAM-17 activity, also called TACE (tumor necrosis factor-α-converting enzyme) (Bergin et al, 2010). We recently found that AAT inhibits calpain I which is implicated in numerous pathological conditions including Alzheimer's disease, demyelination events of multiple sclerosis, neuronal damage after spinal cord injury and hypoxic/ischaemic injury to brain, kidney and heart organs, and tumour development and invasion (Al-Omari et al., 2011). The ability of AAT to inhibit neutrophil calpain I was related to intracellular entry of AAT via lipid rafts (Subramaniyam et al., 2010), a transient rise in intracellular calcium, increase in intracellular cholesterol esters, activation of the Rho GTPases, Rac1 and Cdc42, and extracellular signal-regulated kinase (ERK1/2). Furthermore, AAT caused a significant inhibition of non-stimulated as well as formyl-met-leu-phe (fMLP)-stimulated neutrophil adhesion to fibronectin, inhibited lipopolysaccharide (LPS)-induced IL-8 release and slightly delayed neutrophil apoptosis (Al-Omari M et al 2011). Recently, AAT was found to bind to IL-8 and to inhibit IL-8 interaction with its receptor CXCR1 (Bergin et al., 2010). AAT plays an immunoregulatory role, to inhibit neutrophil superoxide production, to enhance insulin-induced mitogenesis in various cell lines, and to induce IL-1ra expression (Bucurenci et al., 1992; She et al., 2000; Tilg et al., 1993). Findings that AAT enhances the synthesis of both transferrin receptor and ferritin revealed a role of AAT in iron metabolism (Graziadei et al, 1997). Interestingly, AAT has been shown to regulatete heme oxygenase-1 activity in Alzheimer´s disease patients (Maes et al., 2006). AAT has also been found to bind to the secreted enteropathogenic *Escherichia coli* proteins (EspB, EspD), thereby reducing their hemolysis of red blood cells (Knappstein et al., 2004). An interaction between AAT and *Cryptosporidium parvum* (Forney et al., 1996), a protozoan parasite, has been shown to inhibit Cryptosporidium parvum infection, suggesting a potential role for AAT in cryptosporidiosis. AAT inhibits endotoxin-stimulated TNFα, IL-6, IL-1β and enhances IL-10 expression in human monocytes, neutrophils, endothelial cells (Janciauskiene et al., 2007) AAT also expresses a broad anti-inflammatory profile in gene expression studies on primary human lung microvascular endothelial cells, including the suppression of self-induced TNFα expression (Subramaniyam et al., 2008). Current studies provide further evidence that AAT therapy prolongs islet graft survival in transplanted allogeneic diabetic mice (Lewis et al., 2008) and show that AAT stimulates insulin secretion and protects β-cells against cytokine-induced apoptosis, and these effects of AAT also seem to be mediated through the cAMP pathway (Kalis et al., 2010). In view of these novel findings, it is suggested that AAT may act as an anti-inflammatory compound to protect β-cells under immunological attack in type 1diabetes, and also raise the possibility of a new therapeutic strategy to potentiate insulin secretion in type 2 diabetes (Koulmanda et al., 2008).

AAT has also been found to express dual, time-dependent effects. Both *in vitro* and *in vivo* studies have shown that within a short time (2 to 4 hours) AAT amplifies endotoxin (LPS)-induced pro-inflammatory responses whereas after 18-48 hours AAT significantly inhibits LPS-induced TNFα, IL-1β and IL-8 expression and release, and enhances IL-10 synthesis (Subramaniyam et al., 2010).This finding point to hypothesis that AAT can regulate the progression and resolution of the acute-phase reaction in a time-dependent manner. The overall view that arises from the current data is that short-term enhancement of LPS-induced cell activation may be the key mechanism by which the function of AAT is accomplished. In keeping with this, several *in vitro* and *in vivo* studies have been published in which prior initiation of an acute-phase response or administration of a specific APP has been shown to switch the pro-inflammatory to the anti-inflammatory pathways necessary for the resolution of inflammation.

3.3.1.2 *In vivo*

AAT has been found to significantly protect against the lethality induced by TNFα or endotoxin in mice (Libert et at., 1996). The protection is optimal with a single dose of at least 300 μg i.p. or 100 μg i.v. given 2 hours before a lethal challenge, either with a low dose of TNFα in the presence of galactosamine or a higher dose of murine TNF alone. Under optimal conditions, the drop in body temperature, the release of liver transaminases, and the increase in clotting time are also inhibited. Similarly, Jie and co-workers (2003) have shown that pretreatment with AAT (120 mg/kg) can attenuate acute lung injury in rabbits induced with endotoxin. The pretreatment of AAT attenuated the deterioration of oxygenation, the reduction of compliance and the deterioration of other physiological and biochemical parameters mentioned above. In agreement, we currently found that pre-treatment with AAT protects mice against LPS-induced lung injury, inhibits LPS-induced pro-inflammatory genes and enhances the expression of genes associated with tissue repair and regeneration (unpublished data). In another model, Churg et al, (2001) have demonstrated that at 2 hours after dust administration, AAT completely suppressed silica-induced neutrophil influx into the lung and macrophage inflammatory protein-2 (MIP-2)/monocyte chemotactic protein-1 (MCP-1) (neutrophil/macrophage chemoattractant) gene expression, partially suppressed nuclear transcription factor -kB (NF-kB) translocation, and increased inhibitor of NF-kB (IkB) levels. By 24 hours, PMN influx and connective tissue breakdown measured as lavage desmosine or hydroxyproline were still at, or close to, control levels after AAT treatment. In the recent study by Lewis e al., (2005), diabetic mice were grafted with allogeneic islets and treated with AAT monotherapy. After 14 days of treatment, mice remained normoglycemic and islet allografts were functional for up to 120 treatment-free days. After graft removal and retransplantation, mice accepted same-strain islets but rejected third-strain islets, thus confirming that specific immune tolerance had been induced. Explanted grafts exhibited a population of T regulatory cells in transplant sites. Grafts also contained high levels of mRNA for foxp3, cytotoxic T lymphocyte antigen-4, TGF-β, IL-10, and IL-1 receptor antagonist, but expression of pro-inflammatory mediators was low or absent. After implantation of skin allografts, AAT-treated mice had greater numbers of foxp3-positive cells in draining lymph nodes compared with control treatment mice. Moreover, dendritic cells exhibited an immature phenotype with a decrease in the activation marker CD86. Although the number of CD3 transcripts decreased in the DLNs, AAT did not affect IL-2 activity *in vitro*. AAT monotherapy provides allografts with anti-inflammatory conditions that favor development of antigen-specific T regulatory cells. AAT treatment in humans is known to be safe, hence its use during human transplantation may be considered.

3.3.1.3 Augmentation therapy with AAT in patients

Based on the protease-antiprotease hypothesis, augmentation therapy was introduced for COPD patients with severe (ZZ) AAT deficiency during the 1980s. The major concept behind augmentation therapy was that raising the levels of blood and tissue AAT would protect the lungs from continuous destruction by proteases, particularly neutrophil elastase. Whether this biochemical normalization of AAT levels influences the pathogenic processes of COPD is still under debate. However, recent results do suggest that augmentation therapy may have beneficial effects including reducing the frequency of lung infections and reducing the rate of decline of lung function. Several non-randomized observational studies and one meta analysis on the clinical effectiveness of AAT augmentation treatment showed a favorable result regarding lung function (FEV_1) in AAT-deficient COPD patients with moderate disease undergoing augmentation therapy (Chapman et al, 2009; Stockley et al, 2009).

Clinical studies provide evidence that augmentation therapy with AAT reduces the incidence of lung infections in patients with AAT deficiency-related emphysema and reduces levels of the chemoattractant leukotriene B4. A study by Lieberman and co-workers (2000) showed that augmentation therapy with AAT is associated with a marked reduction in the frequency of lung infections in the majority of patients. Most patients reported a frequency of three to five infections per year before starting AAT therapy, which dropped to zero to one infection per year while receiving AAT. In two patients with a prior history of continuous lung infections, AAT therapy was associated with the complete absence of infection in one patient and with one to two infections per year in the second. It was also reported that aerosolized AAT suppresses bacterial proliferation in a rat model of chronic *Pseudomonas aeruginosa* lung infection (Kueppers et al., 2011)

Several case reports support the beneficial effects of AAT augmentation therapy in other clinical conditions. Two ZZ AAT Spanish sisters with fibromyalgia experienced a rapid, progressive, and constant control of their fibromyalgia symptoms during AAT augmentation therapy (Blanco et al, 2006). Another report described a 21yr old a ZZ AAT female with septal panniculitis which was poorly responsive to dapsone and doxycycline treatment, who was successfully treated with intravenous infusion of AAT (Gross et al., 2008). Recently Chowdhury and collaborators have described a 33-year-old ZZ AAT woman with rapidly progressing panniculitis and extensive skin necrosis. Augmentation therapy with AAT proved to be life saving (Chrowdhury et al., 2002). Cutaneous vasculitis in a 49-year-old man with AAT deficiency persisted despite treatment with colchicine, prednisone, and antibiotics, but has been effectively controlled with the administration of AAT (Dowd et al., 1995). In addition, Griese et al, 2007 examined the effect of 4 weeks of AAT inhalation on lung function, protease-antiprotease balance and airway inflammation in Cystic Fibrosis (CF) patients. In a prospective, randomised study, 52 CF patients received a daily inhalation of 25 mg AAT for 4 weeks targeting their peripheral or bronchial compartment. Inhalation of AAT increased AAT levels and decreased the levels of elastase activity, neutrophils, pro-inflammatory cytokines and the numbers of *P. aeruginosa*. However, it had no effect on lung function. No difference was found between the peripheral and bronchial mode of administration. In conclusion, although no effect on lung function was observed, the clear reduction of airway inflammation after AAT treatment may precede pulmonary structural changes.

3.4 Other examples of multifunctional APPs

3.4.1 Haptoglobin (Hp)

Haptoglobin (Hp) is homologous to the serine proteases of the chymotrypsinogen family but has no serine protease activity (Kurosky et al, 1980). Hp exists in two allelic forms in the human population, so-called Hp1 and Hp2, the latter one having arisen due to the partial duplication of the Hp1 gene. Plasma haptoglobin levels change during life, with Hp levels in healthy infants being lower than in healthy adults. In healthy adults, the haptoglobin concentration in plasma is 0.38-2.08 g/L (Javid, 1978). Hp, by binding hemoglobin and removing it from the circulation, prevents iron-stimulated formation of oxygen radicals and has an important role as an antioxidant (Sadrzadek & Bozorgmehr, 2004). Both *in vitro* and *in vivo* studies have established that subjects with the Hp1-1 phenotype are more likely to resist cellular oxidative stress than those with the Hp2-2 phenotype, with Hp2-1 being intermediate (Tseng et al., 2004). Hp has been shown to play an antioxidant/anti-inflammatory role, to contribute to neutrophil activation, to maintain reverse cholesterol transport, to modulate the inhibition of cyclooxygenase and lipooxygenase, and to inhibit monocyte and macrophage functions amongst other activities. For instance, Hp inhibited respiratory burst activity in neutrophils stimulated with fMLP, arachidonic acid, and opsonized zymosan (Oh et al, 1990), inhibited phagocytosis and reduced intracellular bactericidal activities of granulocytes (Rossbacher et al, 1999). Moreover, Hp has been found to stimulate the formation of prostaglandin E2 in osteoblast-like cells, and to potentiate the stimulatory effect of bradykinin and thrombin on PGE2 formation (Frohlander et al, 1991, Lerner & Frohlander, 1992). Hp has also been shown to support angiogenesis (Cid et al, 1993). It has been suggested that the increased levels of Hp found in chronic inflammatory conditions may play an important role in tissue repair. In systemic vasculitis, Hp might also compensate for ischemia by promoting the development of collateral vessels. By enhancing the Th1 cellular response, Hp establishes Th1-Th2 balance *in vitro* (Arredouani et al., 2003). Hp also inhibits epidermal Langerhans cells in the skin and might have a role in preventing T cell–dependent skin disorders (Pagano et al., 1982). In addition, Hp inhibits cathepsin B and L and decreases neutrophil metabolism and antibody production in response to inflammation (Oh et al., 1990, Pagano et al., 1982). Iron is one of the essential elements for bacterial growth. However, once bound to Hp, hemoglobin and iron are no longer available to bacteria that require iron, such as *Escherichia coli*. Indeed, Eaton and collaborators showed that a fatal consequence of intra-peritoneally injected *Escherichia coli* and hemoglobin in rats can be prevented by the administration of Hp (Eaton et al, 1982). In the lungs, Hp is synthesized locally and is a major source of antimicrobial activity in the mucous layer and alveolar fluid and also has an important role in protecting against infection (Yang et al., 1995). Hp-hemoglobin complexes in human plasma inhibit endothelium dependent relaxation (Edwards et al, 1986).

3.4.2 Serum amyloid A (SAA)

SAA structurally resembles an apolipoprotein, and is mainly transported in association with lipoprotein particles, particularly high-density lipoprotein (HDL) (Eriksen & Benditt, 1980). The SAA concentration of serum/plasma samples ranges from 1-5 µg/ml. During an acute phase response, SAA becomes the main apolipoprotein on HDL, and the displaced Apo-AI then becomes available to extract cellular free cholesterol upon interacting with cell-surface (Tam et al., 2008). For this reason, and because SAA itself may also extract cholesterol from cells (Stonik et al., 2004), it is thought that SAA plays a role in cholesterol metabolism and atherosclerosis (Jahangiri et al., 2009). Whether SAA is pro- or anti-atherogenic is not yet clear, since putative beneficial effects on cholesterol metabolism may be mitigated by effects on inflammation- a known risk factor for atherosclerosis (Libby et al., 2002). Some of the effects described for SAA seem to be minimized or abolished by its association with HDL (Barter et al, 2004). The very high expression of SAA gives rise to a completely different pathological problem: the continuous high expression of SAA is the prerequisite for the development of secondary amyloidosis, caused by the conformational change of SAA in an insoluble proteolytic peptide, AA, that deposits as insoluble plaque in major organs (Malle & De Beer, 2003). In attempt to understand the biological role of SAA and of its association with HDL, it was demonstrated that SAA is able, for instance, to induce leukocyte migration (Connolly et al, 2010) and collagenase (Brinckerhoff et al., 1989), and to inhibit the TNFα and IL-1β- induced hypothalamic PGE2 synthesis (Tilg et al., 1993). Several other SAA activities have been described including increasing cleavage of triacylglycerols into glycerol and fatty acids on HDL_3 by enhancing the activity of secretory phospholipase (Sullivan et al., 2009). SAA also directly acts on the cholesterol molecule by decreasing its esterification, and increases its uptake by hepatocytes (Steinmetz et al., 1989). Recent studies reveal that serum SAA also has a dual role in modulating neutrophil function. SAA induces the differentiation of interleukin 10 (IL-10)-secreting neutrophils via signaling dependent on the G protein-coupled protein FPR2 (formyl peptide receptor 2), but also promotes the interaction of neutrophils with invariant natural killer T cells (iNKT cells), restoring T cell proliferation by abolishing IL-10 secretion. The final process is dependent on the antigen-presenting molecule CD1d and co-stimulatory molecule CD40 and results in less production of IL-10 and enhanced production of IL-12, thus limiting the suppressive activity of neutrophils (De Santo et al., 2010). SAA may affect inflammatory responses by activating its putative receptor on neutrophils (FPRL1), leading to increased production of IL-8 (He et al., 2003). SAA is also thought to be able to activate TLR2- and TLR4- dependent signaling (Cheng et al., 2008). Recent reports suggest that SAA may also play a role in host defense, notably in the clearance of Gram-negative bacteria. Shah et al. demonstrated that SAA binds to the outer membrane protein A of *Escherichia coli*, which facilitates bacterial clearance by phagocytes (Shah et al., 2006). Such a bactericidal effect of SAA is intriguing in light of the reported expression of SAA in intestinal epithelia of rodents and humans, since these cells are exposed to many gram-negative bacteria (Berg, 1996). Intestinal epithelial expression of SAA protects from colitis by reducing bacterial load (Eckhardt et al., 2010).

3.5 Importance of the co-ordinated expression and biological activity of APPs

APP expression represents one of the most important and highly effective mechanisms of innate immunity. The wide range of defensive and repair functions fulfilled by APPs not only reduces pathologic damage, but also acts as a homeostatic mechanism. On the other hand APPs may also play pro-inflammatory roles and produce detrimental effects. Importantly, changes in different APPs occur at different rates and to different degrees. Ceruloplasmin and the complement components C3 and C4 exhibit relatively modest acute-phase behaviour (typically about a 50% increases). Concentrations of Hp, AGP, AAT, ACT, and fibrinogen ordinarily increase about 2–5-fold. CRP and SAA are normally present in only trace amounts, but may exhibit a dramatic increase (1000-fold or more) in individuals with severe infections. In contrast, plasma concentrations of negative APPs such as albumin, transferrin, transthyretin, alpha-fetoprotein, typically decrease during the acute-phase response. These orchestrated alterations in specific APP production during inflammatory states are not completely understood. However, the known functional capabilities of many of the APPs leads to the logical speculation that specific changes in APP expression serve useful purposes in inflammation, healing or adaptation to infection or injury. Moreover, current knowledge clearly indicates that during the acute phase reaction a single APP can play multiply roles, and that diverse APPs can possess very similar biological activities (Figure 3). The combined action of two or more APPs may produce effects that no single protein would be able to achieve.

For example, diverse APPs like AAT, AGP, Hp, and CRP can have similar anti-inflammatory and immuno- modulatory roles in experimental models *in vitro* and *in vivo*. AAT which is an archetypal member of the SERPIN superfamily, a main inhibitor of neutrophil elastase, and AGP a member of the lipocalin family, a group of proteins sharing a similar three-dimensional structure capable of binding and carrying hydrophobic molecules, both inhibit cell apoptosis, inhibit neutrophil chemotaxis and adhesion, inhibit neutrophil activation and induce macrophage-derived interleukin-1 receptor antagonist release, and protects mice from endotoxin-induced septic shock. Similarly, CRP (opsonin) and Hp (hemoglobin binder) inhibit neutrophil activation, including chemotaxis and superoxide production and degranulation. Thus, it seems that all these APPs, specifically in neutrophil models, show very similar effects. It cannot be excluded that these proteins may have more common characteristics and biological effects however the lack of high quality purified endotoxin or contaminant-free proteins limits expanding our current understanding.
A more detailed knowledge of the separate and combined APP functional pathways is essential in order to prevent or control development of various pathological conditions as well as to develop safe and effective anti-inflammatory therapies.

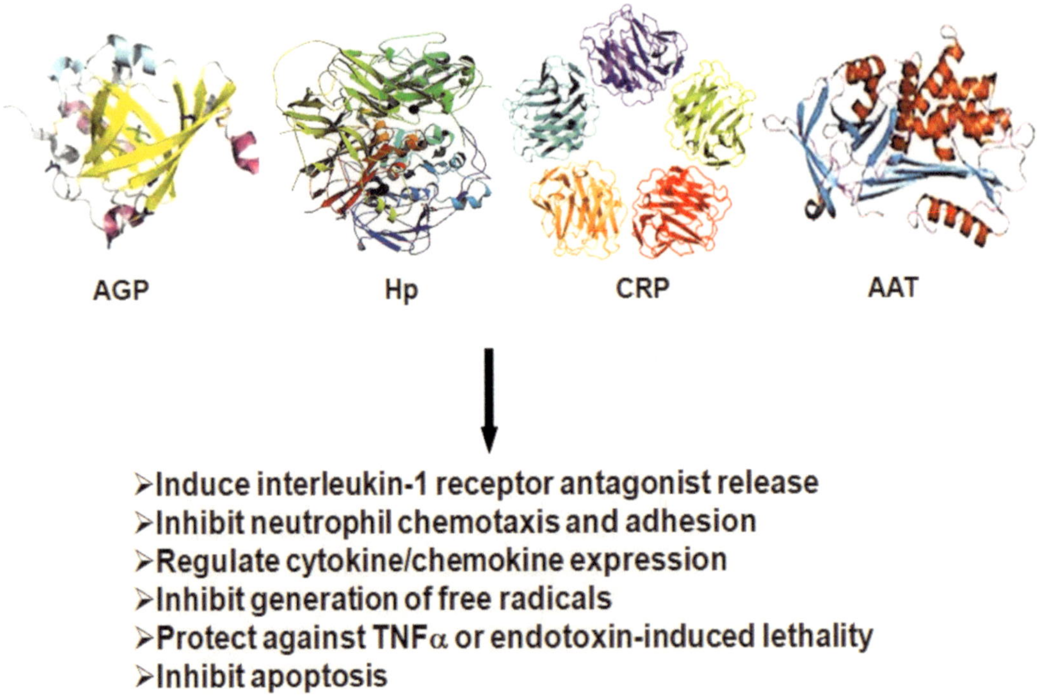

Fig. 3. Diverse APPs express similar anti-inflammatory activities.

4. APPs structure-function relationship

Post-translational modifications of proteins can regulate their function by causing changes in protein activity, their cellular location and dynamic interaction with other proteins. Virtually all proteins function by interacting with other molecules and these interactions can have numerous effects on the physical, structural, biochemical and functional properties of proteins. There are also different types of interactions on a protein-protein and protein-environment level which lead to complex formation, protein degradation, self-assembly or other modifications in protein structures, such as oxidation. The ability to undergo post-translational conformational changes is crucial for the physiological function of many proteins, including APPs. Similarly, such changes could alter both physicochemical and functional properties of the proteins with potential unforeseen physiological or pathological consequences. Conformational modification may lead to an acquired deficiency of specific APP, but also to the generation of new molecular forms with potent biological activities. The altered forms of APPs are detected in tissues and fluids recovered from inflammatory sites, but the important questions of how they are generated, what their biological activities are, and which of them are directly linked to pathological processes and/or may be useful markers to characterise disease states, remain to be answered. Glycosylation is one of the most important post-translational modifications of APPs, and has been widely acknowledged as one of the most important ways to modulate both protein function and lifespan. Glycosylation of APPs which is partially regulated by cytokines may be distinct in disease and provide useful disease markers.

4.1 Glycosylation of APPs

The N-glycan chains of APP glycoproteins differ in their branching, showing bi-, tri-, and tetra-antennary structures. Inflammatory states are usually associated with changes in the glycosylation profile of APPs. It has been demonstrated that there is an increased concentration of the conA-reactive microheterogeneous forms of APPs in patients with acute inflammation, *e.g.* acute bacterial infections and burns. Conversely, a shift in the population of APPs towards those with a higher content of conA-nonreactive tri- and tetra-antennary carbohydrates has been shown in the sera of patients with chronic inflammatory diseases (*e.g.* chronic bacterial infections, rheumatoid arthritis, ankylosing spondylitis) (Hrycaj et al., 1996; Stibler et al., 1998). An intriguing question is whether the changes in the glycosylation profile of APPs might affect their biological activity and/or function.

4.1.1 AGP

AGP purified from human plasma consists of a mixture of AGP with different degrees of sialylation and glycosylation. It has been demonstrated that microheterogeneity variants of AGP differ with regard to their immunomodulatory properties: the conA-nonreactive variant of AGP is more effective in modulating of lymphocyte proliferation than conA-reactive AGP variants. It has also been shown that AGP has an affinity for E-selectin and that this affinity can be changed by *in vitro* fucosylation of AGP (Mackiewicz et al. 1987). The highly branched and sialylated form of AGP which is the ligand for cell adhesion molecules such as E-selectin and P-selectin, inhibits migration of neutrophils, monocytes and T-cells, and modifies complement activity (Hrycaj et al., 1993).
Marked changes in AGP glycoforms are observed during acute-phase reactions. The changes comprise alterations in branching pattern as revealed by reactivity with concanavalin A and the fucose-binding lectin (Elliott *et al.*, 1997). Thus analysis of sialo- and asialo-oligosaccharides of AGP as well as its glycoforms is important for understanding the biological roles of AGP (Kakehi et al., 2002; Sei et al., 2002). For example, the asialylated carbohydrate-deficient variant of AGP appears mainly in sera of patients after acute inflammation, infection, burns or other severe tissue damage (Fournier et al., 2000).

The expression of a sialyl Lewis x{sLe^x, NeuAcα2-3Galβ1-4(Fucα1-3)GlcNAc-} portion in the carbohydrate chains of human AGP molecules has been shown to be of importance in inflammation. De Graaf et al. (1993) found a direct relationship between the reactivity of human AGP to the fucose-specific binding lectin (*Aleuria auranita*) and staining of human AGP by anti-sLe^x monoclonal antibody under healthy and disease conditions.

In a recent study a recombinant form of sialyl Lewis^x(sLe^x)-bearing (sAGP) was administered intravenously to rats after 50 min of intestinal ischemia just before 4 h of reperfusion. A non-sLe^x-bearing form of AGP (nsAGP) was used as control. sAGP-treated animals had a 62% reduction in remote lung injury, assessed by ^{125}I-albumin permeability, compared with those treated with nsAGP. There was a reduction in pulmonary myeloperoxidase levels in sAGP-treated rats compared with nsAGP-treated rats. Complement-dependent intestinal injury, assessed by ^{125}I-albumin permeability was reduced by 28% in animals treated with sAGP compared with those treated with nsAGP leading the authors to conclude that sAGP ameliorates both complement- and neutrophil-mediated injury (Williams et al., 1997).

The changes in the glycosylation pattern of AGP has been found in patients with ulcerative colitis (Ryden et al., 1997), and in patients with various liver diseases (alcoholic liver disease, hepatitis B, hepatitis C cirrhosis). For example, hyperfucosylation occurred in all cases of liver disease, although the hepatitis B and C samples showed a more significant increase in comparison with the others. Additionally N-acetylgalactosamine (GalNAc) was detected in the majority of the hepatitis C samples, which was unexpected since this monosaccharide is not a usual component of the N-linked oligosaccharide chains (Anderson et al., 2002).

In the group of Type I diabetic patients with increased urinary albumin excretion, a significant increase in alpha3-fucosylation of AGP could be detected. Therefore, the increased alpha3-fucosylation of AGP can be used as a putative marker for the development of vascular complications in Type I diabetic patients (Poland et al., 2001).

AGP and its derivatives, prepared by sequential enzymatic cleavage of the carbohydrate units, were tested for their nerve-growth-promoting activities with explants of whole dorsal root ganglia from chick embryos. The results showed that the AGP derivatives with terminal galactose, N-acetylglucosamine, or mannose have marked neurite-promoting activities (Liu et al., 1988).

4.1.2 Other APPs

AAT has a molecular weight of M_r 52 000, and is ~12% carbohydrate by weight. The AAT molecule carries a high negative charge because of sialic acid residues on the three complex glycans attached to asparagine residues 46, 83, and 247. Isoelectric focusing of plasma AAT leads to the detection of eight bands, which are numbered M1 to M8 (anodal-low pH to cathodal-high pH). The bands M4 and M6 are the most abundant of the isoforms, making up 40% and 34% of the total plasma AAT, respectively, whereas M3 and M5 are present in only trace amounts (Mills et al., 2001). Fucosylated AAT was analyzed individually and in combination with the currently used marker, alpha-fetoprotein, for the ability to distinguish between a diagnosis of cirrhosis and hepatocellular carcinoma (HCC). The levels of fucosylated AAT were significantly higher in patients with HCC compared to those with cirrhosis (Wang et al., 2009). Remarkably, non-glycosylated AAT showed shorter half life and no ability to interact with IL-8 than compared to glycosylated form of AAT (Bergin et al., 2010). This suggests an importance of AAT glycosylation for its biological activities.

ACT (alpha 1-antichymotrypsin), a serine anti-protease with specificity against neutrophil cathepsin G, is homologous with AAT, plasminogen activator inhibitor and angiotensinogen. ACT is an APP with carbohydrate content 24% of molecular weight. As for other glycoproteins, micro-heterogeneity of ACT may be ascribed to differences in carbohydrate structure, and indeed different patterns of ACT micro-heterogeneity has been shown in different diseases including cancer, heart failure and rheumatoid arthritis (Saldova et al., 2008; Kazmierczak et al.,1995; Havenaar et al., 1998). A low content of terminal GlcNac glycans and sialic acid in peripheral ACT has been suggested as a marker of progression in Alzheimer's disease (Ianni et al., 2010). The changes in patterns of glycosylation of transferrin (Tf) towards highly branched glycans have been observed in iron deficiency anaemia, rheumatoid arthritis, liver cirrhosis or in physiological state such as pregnancy. Differences in glycosylation of Tf seems to alter the metabolism of iron (Yang et al., 2005; van Pelt J et al., 1996; Dupre et al., 2001). Changes in the glycosylation pattern of major serum APPs such as Hp, AGP, AAT, Tf and alpha-fetoprotein have been recently shown in patients with pancreatic cancer and chronic pancreatitis (Sarrats et al., 2010)

4.2 Cleaved forms of AAPs

The cleaved modifications of APPs may lead to a functional deficiency of the protein, but the cleaved forms of APPs may themselves express new biological activities. For example, antithrombin which functions as an inhibitor of thrombin and other enzymes, has potent antiangiogenic and antitumour activity in its cleaved conformation.

4.2.1 CRP

CRP comprises five identical, non-covalently bound subunits of 206 amino acids (23,017 daltons) arranged in cyclic symmetry (Oliveira et al., 1979). One side of the pentamer participates in binding ligands such as phosphorylcholine, and the other side binds effector molecules such as C1q. When CRP is exposed to denaturing conditions in the presence of a chelating agent, the CRP pentamer is altered to form both individual subunits and aggregates (Gotschlich & Edelman, 1967) designated as modified-CRP (mCRP) (Potempa et al., 1983). The half-life of mCRP in the circulation is <5 min in mice (Motie et al., 1998). These findings indicate that the transport of mCRP from circulation to various sites in the body most likely to be faster than pentameric CRP. mCRP displays antigenic, electrophoretic, and ligand binding reactivities distinct from pentameric CRP (Potempa et al., 1987). Currently has been reported that mCRP is much more potent than pentameric CRP in binding to modified LDL (Singh & Fudenberg, 2009).

Since extravasation and activation of neutrophil granulocytes are essential in the inflammatory response, the effects of CRP on these cells are of particular importance. Stimulation of neutrophils activates a membrane-associated serine protease which leads to the cleavage of biologically active peptides from CRP. CRP peptides 77–82 and 201–206 have been found to inhibit neutrophil chemotaxis to fMLP *in vitro* and to diminish neutrophil influx and protein leakage into alveoli after fMLP induced inflammation in mice (Zouki et al., 1997).

Neutrophil extravasation into inflamed or injured areas involves a complex interaction of leukocytes with endothelial cells *via* regulated expression of surface adhesion molecules. The initial attachment of neutrophils to endothelium is mediated by L-selectin (CD62L) (Díaz-González et al., 1995; Walcheck et al., 1996). L-Selectin is constitutively expressed by neutrophils and is released from neutrophils by proteolytic cleavage within minutes after activation with a concomitant upregulation of Mac-1 (CD11b/CD18). The monomeric CRP (but not nCRP) has been found to up-regulate CD11b/CD18 expression and extracellular signal regulated kinase (ERK) activity, suggesting that mCRP may participate in the promotion of neutrophil adhesion to endothelial cells (Zouki et al., 2001). In contrast to CRP, mCRP induces IL-8 secretion in neutrophils (Khreiss et al, 2005) and human coronary artery endothelial cells (Devaraj S et al., 2004), promotes neutrophil-endothelial cell adhesion (Zouki et al., 2001), and delays apoptosis of human neutrophils (Schwedler et al., 2006).

mCRP binds to a number of different ligands to CRP and also exhibits a different set of biologic activities. More recently, it has been shown that mCRP has profound inhibitory effects on tumor growth and metastatic ability of an adenocarcinoma in mice (Kresl et al., 1999). Cross-reactive epitopes of mCRP have also been detected in the fibrous elements of blood vessels and lymphatic organs suggesting that mCRP may be present in extracellular spaces (Samberg et al., 1988). Since mCRP can self-associate into a matrix-like structure (Motie et al., 1996), the naturally occurring antigen may be self-associated aggregates of mCRP, and thus represent a tissue-based as opposed to a blood based form of CRP. mCRP, but not CRP, binds immune complexes (Khreiss et al., 2004), potentiates the activities of activated leukocytes and platelets (Zouki et al., 2001) and stimulates megakaryocyte differentiation in mice (Potempa et al, 1996).

Additionally, both CRP conformations interact differently with components of the complement cascade. M Mihlan et al., 2009, identified for the first time that mCRP, but not pCRP, has a complement-modulating effect. mCRP recruits the complement inhibitor Factor H to the surface of damaged cells or particles, and enhances local complement inhibition both in the fluid phase and on the cellular surface. Thus, by recruiting C1q to the surface of damaged cells, mCRP triggers complement activation resulting in the formation of C3 convertases and C3b surface deposition. However, by binding inhibitor Factor H and enhancing the inhibitory activity, further complement activation, amplification, cytokine release, C9 deposition and terminal membrane attack assembly are inhibited. Furthermore, the phagocytosis of apoptotic particles is increased. This shows how CRP can contribute to an anti-inflammatory scenario and explains how mCRP contributes to the safe removal of damaged apoptotic particles and necrotic cells which may be relevant for diseases such as atherosclerosis (Zipfel& Skerka, 2009).

Using immunofluorescence microscopy (Eisenhardt et al., 2009) have shown the generation of mCRP from CRP on adherent activated platelets, together with the immunohistological colocalization of mCRP with the CD41 antigen in atherosclerotic plaques. These findings suggest that in atherosclerosis mCRP is generated from circulating CRP, and mCRP is then deposited at the atherosclerotic plaque, exerting strong proinflammatory effects (Agrawal et al., 2010).

Despite the growing interest in mCRP, it remains unclear how mCRP is generated and whether it contributes to inflammatory processes such as atherosclerosis. Thus, it appears that both CRP and altered forms of CRP, including mCRP, may each serve important distinct functions in the acute phase and the host defense response to trauma and infectious agents. Therefore, it is important to ascertain the extent of conversion and reversion of CRP to mCRP and possible intermediate forms to help define and understand the biological function(s) of the CRP molecule.

4.2.2 AAT

AAT is another example of AAP which can be found *in vivo* in cleaved forms. Cleaved forms of AAT are know to occur when AAT forms an inhibitor complex with serine protease which subsequently dissociates or is degraded, or when it is cleaved by non-target proteases, usually at sites in its reactive loop, without the formation of stable inhibitor complexes. Such cleavage generates a 4 kDa carboxyl-terminal fragment of 36 residues, which remains non-covalently bound to the cleaved AAT. Human cathepsin L, collagenase and stromelysin, and bacterial proteinases from *Staphylococcus aureus*, *Serratia marcescens* metalloproteinase and *Pseudomonas aeruginosa* elastase (Rapala-Kozik et al., 1999) all fall into the latter class and exhibit efficient AAT degrading activity. Recent studies established AAT as a key substrate for gelatinase B (MMP-9) *in vivo* (Liu et al., 2000). It has long been hypothesized that neutrophil elastase-mediated tissue destruction in certain inflammatory diseases such as emphysema, is caused by an imbalance in the ratio of elastase to AAT (Weiss, 1989). The studies of Liu and collaborators provide *in vivo* evidence that this mechanism, mediated by the proteolytic inactivation of AAT by gelatinase B, underlies the pathology of the inflammatory skin disorder called bullous pemphigoid which is initiated by deposit formation at the basement membrane (Jordon et al., 1985). Generated cleaved forms of AAT may contribute to the later phase of polymorphonuclear leukocyte infiltration. Indeed, cleaved AAT was shown to form fibrillar structures and to be a potent chemoattractant for monocytes (Janciauskiene et al., 1995; Banda et al., 1988).

Fragments of AAT have been found in human bile, atherosclerotic plaque, urine and plasma, and have been shown to regulate lipid metabolism, inflammatory cell activation and even to inhibit human HIV-1 expression. It has recently been demonstrated that a specific 20-residue fragment of AAT (C-terminal peptide, residues 377–396, referred to as VIRIP) binds to the gp41 fusion peptide of HIV-1 and prevents the virus from entering target cells, thereby inhibiting HIV-1 infection (Münch et al, 2007). These findings suggest that AAT may play a protective role in HIV-1-infected individuals (Forssmann et al., 2010). We found that the C-terminal fragment of AAT, C-36 peptide, corresponding to residues 359-394 suppresses bile acid synthesis *in vitro* and *in vivo*. The DNA element involved in the C-36-mediated regulation of 7alpha- and 12alpha-hydroxylase promoters mapped to the alpha1-fetoprotein transcription factor site in both promoters. The C-36 peptide prevented binding of FTF to its target DNA recognition site by direct interaction with FTF (Gerbod-Giannone et al., 2002). Hence, the effects of AAT peptides as potential drugs for systemic lupus erythematosus are being studied (Shapira et al., 2011).

4.3 Oxidized and nitrosylated forms of APPs

Under conditions of compromised oxygen supply, such as occurs in injury, infection or malignancy, oxygen species with free unpaired electrons are generated during mitochondrial electron transport. Referred to as highly reactive oxygen species (ROS), their production causes damage to cell membranes and macromolecules (lipids, proteins and DNA) (Valko et al., 2007). Oxidative changes of protein structure can have a wide range of downstream functional consequences, such as inhibition of enzymatic and binding activities, increased susceptibility to aggregation and proteolysis, increased or decreased uptake by cells, and altered immunogenicity. It is now recognized that oxidation of proteins plays an essential role in the pathogenesis of an important number of degenerative diseases. Compared to controls more oxidized proteins are found in tissues from animals and patients

suffering from Alzheimer's disease, rheumatoid arthritis, atherosclerosis or amyotrophic lateral sclerosis (Banfi et al., 2008). For example, in plasma from patients with Alzheimer`s disease the most obviously oxidized proteins were identified as isoforms of AAT and fibrinogen γ-chain precursor proteins. Both these proteins have been suggested to be involved in inflammation processes in Alzheimer's disease (Choi et al., 2002).
S-nitrosylation is another important post-transcriptional modification of the APPs and their peptides, which may be involved in NO-dependent signal transductions. For example, a recent study indicates that *S*-nitrosylation can be effectively catalyzed by the copper ion of ceruloplasmin, a major multicopper-containing plasma protein, under physiological conditions (Mani et al., 2004). It is now also conceivable that nitrosylation of thiols is involved in modulation of various biological events, such as functional regulation of receptors, ion channels and synaptic vesicle fusion (Miyamoto et al., 2000).

4.3.1 AAT

Oxidized AAT has been found in inflammatory exudates at levels of ~5–10% that of total AAT (Wong &Travis, 1988), and AAT recovered from BAL fluid in smokers is 40% less active compared with non-smokers due to oxidation of the P1 methionine (methionine 358 at the active site) to methionine sulfoxide (Carp et al., 1982). The oxidation of AAT by cigarette smoke or free radicals in vivo has been proposed as a mechanism by which elastin and thus alveolar destruction occurs in COPD (Gadek et al., 1979; Beatty et al., 1984). Oxidation of the P1 methionine (methionine 358) or methionine 351 to methionine sulfoxide significantly reduces the ability of AAT to inhibit neutrophil elastase (Taggart et al., 2000). Hydrogen peroxide in cigarette smoke and N-chloroamines and hypochlorous acid in neutrophils can oxidize and inactivate AAT (Ossanna et al., 1986; Scott et al., 1999). Thus the oxidation of AAT by cigarette smoke or free radicals in vivo could lead to a relative deficiency of elastase inhibitors and has been suggested as a mechanism contributing to the development of emphysema and other diseases such as cystic fibrosis, adult respiratory distress syndrome, and bronchiectasis (McGuire et al., 1982; Roum et al., 1993; Izumi-Yoneda et al., 2009). In addition, oxidative inactivation can enhance the susceptibility of AAT to proteolytic attack, particularly by neutrophil elastase and certain bacterial proteases, including thermolysin, aureolysin, serralysin, pseudolysin, *Staphylococcus aureus* serine proteinase, streptopain and periodontain. Thus, oxidation and proteolytic processes in some cases may work synergistically. Moreover, oxidized AAT by itself amplifies and perpetuates the inflammatory processes by directly affecting the functional activities of structural and inflammatory cells or by interacting with other molecules such as IgA and low-density lipoproteins. It has been shown that oxidized AAT significantly induces the production of IL-8 and MCP-1 from a lung epithelial cell line (A549 cells) and in a time- and dose-dependent manner and attracts macrophages (Li et al., 2009). Release of oxidants by these inflammatory cells could oxidize newly synthesized AT, which has diffused into the airways and would perpetuate the cycle. This process may be amplified by oxidized AAT induction of MCP-1 synthesis from monocytes (Moraga & Janciauskiene, 2000). These pathways may be one explanation as to why inflammation persists after smoking cessation in chronic obstructive pulmonary disease (Retamales et al., 2001). A complex of oxidized AAT and LDL was isolated from human plasma and was detected in human atherosclerotic lesions of the coronary artery (Donners et al., 2005). The product of AAT nitrosylation, S-NO-AAT, has been shown to have multiple biological functions, including potent anti-microbial activity and inhibition of cysteine protease. In a study by Ikebe and co-workers (Ikebe et al., 2000) it was suggested that S-NO-AAT exerted a potent cytoprotective effect in liver ischemia-reperfusion injury by maintaining the tissue blood flow, inducing hemeoxygenase 1, and suppressing neutrophil-induced liver damage and apoptosis. Interestingly, it was verified that S-NO-AAT expressed similar serine protease inhibitory activity towards pancreatic trypsin and pancreatic and neutrophil elastase as native AAT. Thus, S-NO-AAT may function not only as a simple NO (nitroso) donor but also as a protease inhibitor with a broad inhibitory spectrum.

4.4 Complexed and polymerized forms of APPs

Function of some APPs is dependent on their complex formation with other molecules and/or on their polymerization. For example, CRP binds to phosphocholine, as well as phosphoethanolamine, microbial surface proteins, chromatin and other ligands (Thompson et al., 1999; Agrawal et al., 2002, Okemefuna et al, 2010). CRP activates the classical pathway of complement by binding to C1q, but its binding to CFH in the alternative pathway has turned out to be more controversial. CRP–ligand interactions lead to the recognition of damaged or apoptotic cells and bacterial pathogens. Ca^{2+} and phosphocholine bind to the B (binding) face of the pentameric ring, whereas the other A (α-helix) face binds to macromolecular ligands such as C1q. The complex between Hp and Hemoglobin has been studied for decades and represents one of the strongest non-covalent interactions reported in plasma (Nielsen & Moestrup, 2009). Hp also binds apolipoprotein A-I (ApoA-I), and impairs its stimulation of lecithin: cholesterol acyltransferase (LCAT) which plays a major role in reverse cholesterol transport (Cigliano et al., 2009). Hp binds and protects ApoE from oxidative damage (Salvatore et al., 2009). Some APPs are regulated by co-factors which are needed to expose or maintain the functional conformation of the APP. The best example of this phenomenon is antithrombin, which is activated by heparin through induced and transmitted conformational changes that stabilise the proteinase-sensitive active site (Jodan et al., 1987). Another APP, PAI-1, which normally exists in a latent form, can be maintained in its functional form in the presence of plasma vitronectin (Wiman et al., 1988). As well as stabilising PAI-1 in the active conformation, vitronectin also alters the specificity of PAI-1, making it an efficient inhibitor of thrombin. The finding that active PAI-1 specifically inhibits integrin attachment to vitronectin (Stefansson & Lawrence, 1996) further illustrates the unique functional interdependence that exists between PAI-1 and vitronectin. Complexes between APPs and other proteins are also found to be associated with specific diseases. For example, in sera from patients with myeloma and Bence-Jones proteinuria, complexes between AAT and the kappa light chain of immunoglobulins were detected (Laurell et al., 1974). In plasma from diabetic subjects, complexes between AAT and factor Xia, and AAT and heat shock protein-70 (HSP70), as well as glycosylated forms of AAT were detected (Austin et al., 1987; Scott et al., 1998; Finotti et al., 2004). Moreover, complexes between immunoglobulin A and AAT have been detected in the sera and synovial fluid of patients with rheumatoid arthritis, systemic lupus erythematosus and ankylosing spondylitis (Scott et al., 1998). Human tissue kallikrein 3, a serine proteinase commonly known as a prostate-specific antigen (PSA) which correlates with prostate hypertrophy and malignancy, is also known to bind to AAT in sera of subjects with high PSA concentrations (Zhang et al., 2000). Localization of AAT-low-density-lipoprotein (LDL) complexes in atherosclerotic lesions and enhanced degradation of AAT-LDL by macrophages suggested the involvement of the complex in atherogenesis (Donners et al., 2005). Alpha1-antichymotrypsin/Alzheimer's peptide Abeta (1-42) complexes and ACT polymers have been associated with Alzheimer's disease (Licastro et al., 1997; Sun et al., 2002).Studies of the functional and conformational polymorphism of inhibitory APPs clearly show that some proteins can undergo polymerization due to an inherited mutation, or chemical modification, and obtain new biological activities or reflect undergoing pathological process. A well-characterised example of a mutant APP associated with a disease state is AAT. The most widely studied deficiency variants of AAT are Z and S, which have E342K and E264V mutations respectively (Carrell et al., 1996; Carrell et al., 1892). Polymerisation of these mutants of AAT is known to be involved in AAT deficiency-related diseases such as emphysema, liver cirrhosis, neonatal hepatitis, hepatocellular carcinoma and lung emphysema (Eriksson, 1990) The liver pathology is characterised by the formation of intracellular inclusions of polymerised AAT. Recent studies now indicate that extra-hepatic AAT polymerization may also occur. For example, AAT polymers have been identified in the lungs and circulation of Z AAT deficiency subjects. Importantly, like other modified forms, AAT polymers lack protease inhibitor activity which will exaggerate the severe deficiency, but also exhibit additional biological functions that may be relevant in pathological processes (Mahadeva et al., 2005; Mulgrew et al., 2004) (Figure 5). The susceptibility of Z AAT individuals who smoke to develop chronic obstructive pulmonary disease is in part related to the combination of the severe anti-elastase deficiency arising from an absolute and functional reduction in neutrophil elastase inhibitory capacity (Stoller & Aboussouan, 2005), and the independent multiple effects of cigarette smoke on inflammatory cells and molecules (Barnes et al., 2003). Our current data clearly demonstrate that cigarette smoke promotes polymerization of Z mutant AAT, but not of the normal, M variant of AAT. Thus cigarette smoke directly accelerates polymerization of Z AAT *via* oxidation of the protein leading to further depletion of the neutrophil protease protection in the lung and enhanced neutrophil influx (Alam et al., 2010). The data uniquely suggests that rather than the major risk factors for chronic obstructive pulmonary disease namely cigarette smoke and Z AAT deficiency having independent additive effects, they directly interact to create an effect greater than the sum of the individual risks.

5. General conclusions

Inflammation is a complex, highly orchestrated process involving many cell types and molecules, some of which initiate, amplify, or sustain the process, some of which attenuate it, and some of which aid resolution. A number of the participating AAPs are multifunctional and contribute to both the enhancement and the inhibition of inflammation at different points in its evolution. The outcome of the acute inflammatory response is most likely to be determined by the orchestrated generation of a specific profile of APPs, their concentrations and molecular forms in the microenvironment. Diseases associated with chronic inflammation may be due to an inadequate acute-phase response driven by APPs, their concentration and molecular form and/or an inability to eliminate invading pathogens and to rapidly to resolve the inflammatory processes. Often, a single APP is regarded as a marker for inflammation to aid in diagnosis and assesses response to treatement, however we believe one needs to see the profile of several APPs in action to understand function in relation to disease which may help in turn to determine prognosis.

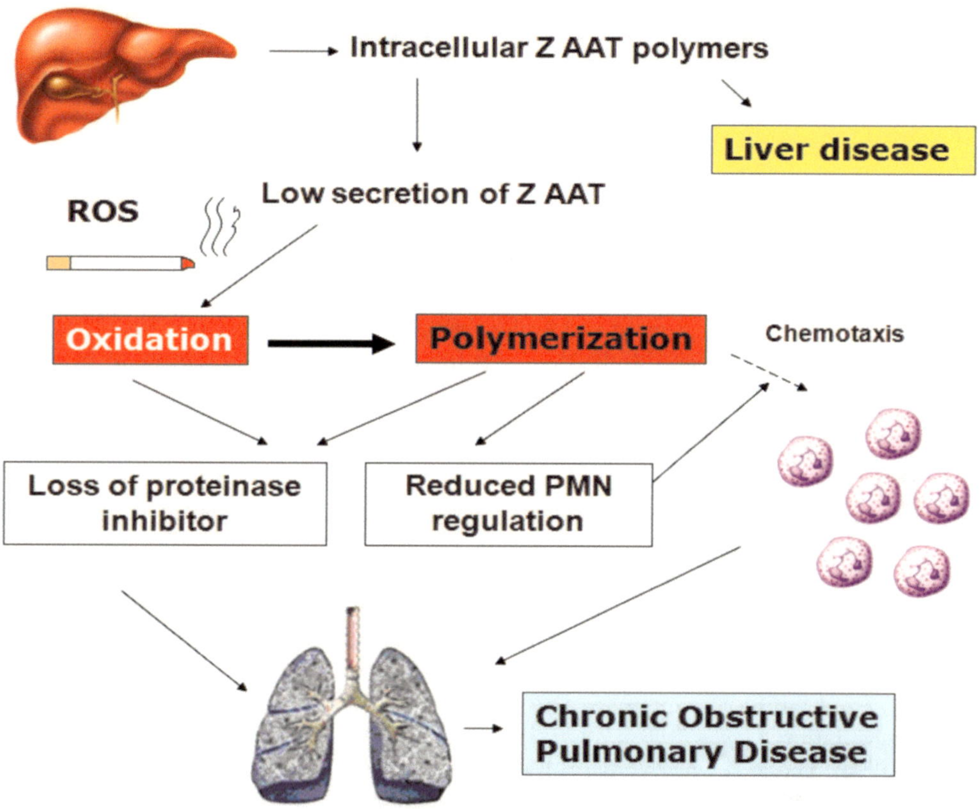

Fig. 4. Schematic diagram showing proposed model for the pathogenesis of emphysema in patients with inherited Z AAT deficiency. Cigarette smoke induces significant oxidation of Z AAT, which accelerates AAT protein polymerization. The plasma deficiency and reduced inhibitory activity of Z AAT would be exacerbated by the oxidation and polymerization of AAT within the lungs, thereby further reducing the antiproteinase screen. This together with the loss of the normal inhibitory effect of AAT on neutrophil chemotaxis and the chemoattractant ability of AAT polymers thereby increase tissue damage and accelerate emphysema progression.

6. Acknowledgment

RM is supported by the Cambridge NIHR Biomedical Research centre. SJ is supported by Hannover Medical School, Germany.

7. References

Agrawal, A, Elhanan, G & Halper, M. (2010). Dissimilarities in the Logical Modeling of Apparently Similar Concepts in SNOMED CT. *AMIA Annu Symp Proc* 2010, 212-216.

Alam, S, Li Z, Janciauskiene, S, & Mahadeva, R. (2010). Oxidation of Z {alpha}1-antitrypsin by Cigarette Smoke Induces Polymerization: A Novel Mechanism of Early-onset Emphysema. *Am J Respir Cell Mol Biol Epub ahead of print.*

Al-Omari, M, et al. (2011). The acute phase protein, alpha1-antitrypsin, inhibits neutrophil calpain I and induces random migration. *Mol Med* Apr 11 [Epub ahead of print].

Anderson, N, et al. (2002). A preliminary evaluation of the differences in the glycosylation of alpha-1-acid glycoprotein between individual liver diseases. *Biomed Chromatogr* 16, 365-372.

Arredouani, M, et al. (2003). Haptoglobin directly affects T cells and suppresses T helper cell type 2 cytokine release. *Immunology* 108, 144-151.

Assicot, M, et al. (1993). High serum procalcitonin concentrations in patients with sepsis and infection. *Lancet* 341, 515-518.

Austin, GE, Mullins, RH & Morin, LG. (1987). Non-enzymic glycation of individual plasma proteins in normoglycemic and hyperglycemic patients. *Clin Chem* 33, 2220-2224.

Ballou, SP& Lozanski G. (1992). Induction of inflammatory cytokine release from cultured human monocytes by C-reactive protein. *Cytokine* 4, 361-368

Banda, MJ, Rice, AG, Griffin, GL, & Senior, RM. (1988). Alpha 1-proteinase inhibitor is a neutrophil chemoattractant after proteolytic inactivation by macrophage elastase. *J Biol Chem* 263, 4481-4484.

Banfi, C, et al. (2008). Oxidized proteins in plasma of patients with heart failure: role in endothelial damage. *Eur J Heart Fail* 10, 244-251.

Barnes, PJ. (2003). New treatments for chronic obstructive pulmonary disease. *Ann Ist Super Sanita* 39, 573-582.

Barter ,PJ, et al. (2004). Antiinflammatory properties of HDL. *Circ Res* 95, 764-772.

Beatty, K, Matheson, N, & Travis, J. (1984). Kinetic and chemical evidence for the inability of oxidized alpha 1-proteinase inhibitor to protect lung elastin from elastolytic degradation. *Hoppe Seylers Z Physiol Chem* 365, 731-736.

Berg, RD. (1996). The indigenous gastrointestinal microflora.*Trends Microbiol* 4, 430-435.

Bergin, DA, et al. (2010). α-1 Antitrypsin regulates human neutrophil chemotaxis induced by soluble immune complexes and IL-8. *J Clin Invest* 120, 4236-4250.

Berman, S, Gewurz, H, & Mold, C. (1986). Binding of C-reactive protein to nucleated cells leads to complement activation without cytolysis. *J Immunol* 136, 1354-1359.

Bisoendial, R, et al. (2005). In vivo effects of C-reactive protein (CRP)-infusion into humans. *Circ Res* 97, e115-116.

Blackburn, WD. (1994). Validity of acute phase proteins as markers of disease activity. *J Rheumatol* 42, 9–13.

Blanco, I, et al. (2006). Estimated numbers and prevalence of PI*S and PI*Z alleles of alpha1-antitrypsin deficiency in European countries. *Eur Respir J* 27, 77-84.

Boutten, A, et al. (1992). Alpha 1-acid glycoprotein potentiates lipopolysaccharide-induced secretion of interleukin-1 beta, interleukin-6 and tumor necrosis factor-alpha by human monocytes and alveolar and peritoneal macrophages. *Eur J Immunol* 22, 2687-2695.

Brand, K, et al. (1996). Activated transcription factor nuclear factor-kappa B is present in the atherosclerotic lesion. *J Clin Invest* 97, 1715-1722.

Brinckerhoff, CE, et al. (1989). Autocrine induction of collagenase by serum amyloid A-like and beta 2-microglobulin-like proteins. *Science* 243, 655-7.

Bucurenci, N, et al. (1992). Inhibition of neutrophil superoxide production by human plasma alpha 1-antitrypsin. *FEBS Lett* 300, 21-24.

Carp, H, et al. (1982). Potential mechanism of emphysema: alpha 1-proteinase inhibitor recovered from lungs of cigarette smokers contains oxidized methionine and has decreased elastase inhibitory capacity. *Proc Natl Acad Sci U S A* 79, 2041-2045.

Carrell , R. (1986). alpha 1-Antitrypsin: molecular pathology, leukocytes, and tissue damage. *J Clin Invest* 78, 1427-1431.

Carrell, RW, & Lomas, DA. (1997). Conformational disease. *Lancet 350*, 134-138.

Carrell, RW, et al. (1996). Alpha 1-antitrypsin deficiency. A conformational disease. *Chest* 110, 243S-247S.

Casey, R, et al. (2008). The acute-phase reactant C-reactive protein binds to phosphorylcholine-expressing Neisseria meningitidis and increases uptake by human phagocytes. *Infect Immun* 76, 1298-1304.

Cermak, J, et al. (1993). Cell heme uptake induces ferritin synthesis resulting in altered oxidant sensitivity: possible role in chemotherapy efficacy. *Tumor Cancer Res* 53, 5308-5313.

Chapman, KR, Stockley, RA, Dawkins, C, Wilkes, MM, & Navickis, RJ. (2009). Augmentation therapy for alpha1 antitrypsin deficiency: a meta-analysis. *COPD* 6, 177-184.

Cheng, N, et al. (2008). Cutting edge: TLR2 is a functional receptor for acute-phase serum amyloid A. *J Immunol.* 181, 22-26.

Choi, J, et al. (2002). Identification of oxidized plasma proteins in Alzheimer's disease. *Biochem Biophys Res Commun* 293, 1566-1570.

Chowdhury, MM, et al. (2002). Severe panniculitis caused by homozygous ZZ alpha1-antitrypsin deficiency treated successfully with human purified enzyme (Prolastin). *Br J Dermatol* 147, 1258-1261.

Churg, A, et al. (2001). Alpha-1-antitrypsin and a broad spectrum metalloprotease inhibitor, RS113456, have similar acute anti-inflammatory effects. *Lab Inves* 81, 1119-1131.

Cid, MC, et al. (1993). Identification of haptoglobin as an angiogenic factor in sera from patients with systemic vasculitis. *J Clin Invest* 91, 977-985.

Cigliano, L, et al. (2009). Haptoglobin binds the antiatherogenic protein apolipoprotein E-impairment of apolipoprotein E stimulation of both lecithin:cholesterol acyltransferase activity and cholesterol uptake by hepatocytes. *FEBS J* 276, 6158-6171.

Connolly, M, et al. (2010). Acute serum amyloid A induces migration, angiogenesis, and inflammation in synovial cells in vitro and in a human rheumatoid arthritis/SCID mouse chimera model. *J Immunol* 184, 6427-6437.

Costello M, Fiedel BA & Gewurz H. (1979). Inhibition of platelet aggregation by native and desialised alpha-1 acid glycoprotein. *Nature* 281, 677-678.

Costello, MJ, Gewurz, H & Siegel, JN. (1984). Inhibition of neutrophil activation by alpha1-acid glycoprotein. *Clin Exp Immunol* 55, 465-472.

Culley, FJ, et al. (1996). C-reactive protein binds to a novel ligand on Leishmania donovani and increases uptake into human macrophages. *J Immunol* 156, 4691-4696.

Daemen, MA, et al. (2000). Functional protection by acute phase proteins alpha(1)-acid glycoprotein and alpha(1)-antitrypsin against ischemia/reperfusion injury by preventing apoptosis and inflammation. *Circulation* 102, 1420-1426.

De Graaf, TW, et al. (1993). Inflammation-induced expression of sialyl Lewis X-containing glycan structures on alpha 1-acid glycoprotein (orosomucoid) in human sera. *J Exp Med* 177, 657-666.

Dehghan, A, et al. (2007). Risk of type 2 diabetes attributable to C-reactive protein and other risk factors. *Diabetes Care* 30, 2695-2699.

De Martin, R, et al. (2000). The transcription factor NF-kappa B and the regulation of vascular cell function. *Arterioscler Thromb Vasc Biol* 20, E83-88.

Devaraj, S, Kumaresan, PR & Jialal, I. (2004). Effect of C-reactive protein on chemokine expression in human aortic endothelial cells. *J Mol Cell Cardiol* 36, 405-410.

De Santo, C, et al. (2010). Invariant NKT cells modulate the suppressive activity of IL-10-secreting neutrophils differentiated with serum amyloid A. *Nat Immunol* 11, 1039-1046.

Díaz-González, F, et al. (1995). Prevention of in vitro neutrophil-endothelial attachment through shedding of L-selectin by nonsteroidal antiinflammatory drugs. *J Clin Invest* 95, 1756-1765.

Dinarello, CA. (1983). Pathogenesis of fever during hemodialysis. *Contrib Nephrol* 36, 90–99.

Donners, MM, et al. (2005). Proteomic analysis of differential protein expression in human atherosclerotic plaque progression. *J Pathol 206*, 39-45.

Dowd, SK, Rodgers, GC, & Callen, JP. (1995). Effective treatment with alpha 1-protease inhibitor of chronic cutaneous vasculitis associated with alpha 1-antitrypsin deficiency. *J Am Acad Dermatol* 33, 913-916.

Drenth JP, van der Meer JW & Kushner I. (1996). Unstimulated peripheral blood mononuclear cells from patients with the hyper-IgD syndrome produce cytokines capable of potent induction of C-reactive protein and serum amyloid A in Hep3B cells. *J Immunol* 157, 400-404.

Du Clos, TW. (1989). C-reactive protein reacts with the U1 small nuclear ribonucleoprotein. *J Immunol* 143, 2553-2559.

Du Clos, TW. (2000). Function of C-reactive protein. *Ann Med* 32, 274-278.

Du Clos, TW, Zlock, LT, & Rubin, RL. (1988). Analysis of the binding of C-reactive protein to histones and chromatin. *J Immunol* 141, 4266-4270.

Dupre, T, et al. (2001). Congenital disorder of glycosylation Ia with deficient phosphomannomutase activity but normal plasma glycoprotein pattern. *Clin Chem* 47, 132-134.

Eaton, JW, et al. (1982). Haptoglobin: a natural bacteriostat. *Science* 215, 691-693.

Eckhardt ER, et al. (2010). Intestinal epithelial serum amyloid A modulates bacterial growth in vitro and pro inflammatory responses in mouse experimental colitis. *BMC Gastroenterol* 10, 133.

Edwards, DH, et al. (1986). Haptoglobin-haemoglobin complex in human plasma inhibits endothelium dependent relaxation: evidence that endothelium derived relaxing factor acts as a local autocoid. *Cardiovasc Res* 20, 549-556.

Eisenhardt, SU, Habersberger, J & Peter, K. (2009). Monomeric C-reactive protein generation on activated platelets: the missing link between inflammation and atherothrombotic risk. *Trends Cardiovasc Med* 19, 232-237.

Elliott, MA, et al. (1997). Investigation into the concanavalin A reactivity, fucosylation and oligosaccharide microheterogeneity of alpha 1-acid glycoprotein expressed in the sera of patients with rheumatoidarthritis. *J Chromatogr B Biomed Sci Appl* 688, 229-237.

Engström, G, et al. (2004). Incidence of fatal or repaired abdominal aortic aneurysm in relation to inflammation-sensitive plasma proteins. *Arterioscler Thromb Vasc Biol* 24, 337-341

Eriksen, N, & Benditt, EP. (1980). Isolation and characterization of the amyloid-related apoprotein (SAA) from human high density lipoprotein. *Proc Natl Acad Sci U S A* 77, 6860-6864.

Finotti, P, & Pagetta, A. (2004). A heat shock protein70 fusion protein with alpha1-antitrypsin in plasma of type 1 diabetic subjects. *Biochem Biophys Res Commun* 315, 297-305.

Fournier, T, Medjoubi-N, N & Porquet, D. (2000). Alpha-1-acid glycoprotein. *Biochim Biophys Acta* 1482, 157-171.

Forney, JR, Yang, S, & Healey, MC. (1996). Interaction of the human serine protease inhibitor alpha-1-antitrypsin with Cryptosporidium parvum. *J Parasitol* 82, 496-502.

Fröhlander, N, Ljunggren, O, & Lerner, UH. (1991). Haptoglobin synergistically potentiates bradykinin and thrombin induced prostaglandin biosynthesis in isolated osteoblasts. *Biochem Biophys Res Commun* 178, 343-351.

Gabay, C, & Kushner, I. (1999). Acute-phase proteins and other systemic responses to inflammation. *N Engl J Med* 340: 448-454.

Gadek, JE, Fells, GA, & Crystal, RG. (1979). Cigarette smoking induces functional antiprotease deficiency in the lower respiratory tract of humans. *Science* 206, 1315-1316.

Gerbod-Giannone, MC, et al. (2002). Suppression of cholesterol 7alpha-hydroxylase transcription and bile acid synthesis by an alpha1-antitrypsin peptide via interaction with alpha1-fetoprotein transcription factor. *J Biol Chem* 277, 42973-42980.

Gershov, D, et al. (2000). C-Reactive protein binds to apoptotic cells, protects the cells from assembly of the terminal complement components, and sustains an antiinflammatory innate immune response: implications for systemic autoimmunity. *J Exp Med* 192, 1353-1364.

Gettins, PG. (2002). Serpin structure, mechanism, and function. *Chem Rev* 102, 4751-4804.

Graziadei, I, et al. (1997). Unidirectional upregulation of the synthesis of the major iron proteins, transferrin-receptor and ferritin, in HepG2 cells by the acute-phase protein alpha1-antitrypsin. *J Hepatol* 27, 716-725.

Gitlin, JD, Gitlin, JI, & Gitlin, D. (1977). Localizing of C-reactive protein in synovium of patients with rheumatoid arthritis. *Arthritis Rheum* 20, 1491-1499.

Griese, M, et al. (2007). alpha1-Antitrypsin inhalation reduces airway inflammation in cystic fibrosis patients. *J Eur Respir* 29, 240-250.

Gooptu, B, & Lomas, DA. (2009). Conformational pathology of the serpins: themes, variations, and therapeutic strategies. *Annu Rev Biochem* 78, 147-176.

Gross, B, et al. (2009). New Findings in PiZZ alpha1-antitrypsin deficiency-related panniculitis.Demonstration of skin polymers and high dosing requirements of intravenous augmentation therapy. *Dermatology* 218, 370-375.

Gruys, E, Obwolo, MJ, & Toussaint, MJ. (1994) Diagnostic significance of the major acute phase proteins in veterinary clinical chemistry: a review. *Vet Bull* 64, 1009–1018.

Gotschlich, EC & Edelman, GM. (1967). Binding properties and specificity of C-reactive protein. *Proc Natl Acad Sci U S A* 57, 706-712.

Gutsmann, T, et al. (2001). Dual role of lipopolysaccharide (LPS)-binding protein in neutralization of LPS and enhancement of LPS-induced activation of mononuclear cells. *Infect Immun* 69, 6942-6950.

Hack, CE, et al. (1997). Role for secretory phospholipase A2 and C-reactive protein in the removal of injured cells. *Immunol Today* 18, 111-115.

Hanriot, D, et al. (2008). C-reactive protein induces pro- and anti-inflammatory effects, including activation of the liver X receptor alpha, on human monocytes. *Thromb Haemost.* 99, 558-569.

Hattori, Y, Matsumura, M, Kasai, K. (2003). Vascular smooth muscle cell activation by C-reactive protein. *Cardiovasc Res* 58, 186-195.

Havenaar, EC, et al. (1998). Severe rheumatoid arthritis prohibits the pregnancy-induced decrease in alpha3-fucosylation of alpha1-acid glycoprotein. *Glycoconj J* 15, 723-729.

Haverkate, F, et al. (1997). Production of C-reactive protein and risk of coronary events in stable and unstable angina. European Concerted Action on Thrombosis and Disabilities Angina Pectoris Study Group. *Lancet* 349, 462-466.

He, R, Sang, H & Ye, RD. (2003). Serum amyloid A induces IL-8 secretion through a G protein-coupled receptor, FPRL1/LXA4R. *Blood* 101, 1572-1581.

Heuertz, RM, et al. (1999). C-reactive protein inhibits chemotactic peptide-induced p38 mitogen-activated protein kinase activity and human neutrophil movement. *J Biol Chem* 274, 17968-17974.

Hochepied, T, et al. (2003). Alpha(1)-acid glycoprotein: an acute phase protein with inflammatory and immunomodulating properties. *Cytokine Growth Factor Rev* 14, 25-34.

Hrycaj, P, et al. (1996). Microheterogeneity of acute-phase glycoproteins in patients with pulmonary sarcoidosis. *Eur Respir J* 9, 313-318

Ianni, M, et al. (2010). Altered glycosylation profile of purified plasma ACT from Alzheimer's disease. *Immun Ageing 7* Suppl, S6.

Ikebe, N, et al. (2000). Protective effect of S-nitrosylated alpha(1)-protease inhibitor on hepatic ischemia-reperfusion injury. *J Pharmacol Exp Ther* 295, 904-911.

Ingenbleek, Y, & Bernstein L. (1999). The stressful condition as a nutritionally dependent adaptive dichotomy. *Nutrition* 15, 305–320.

Izumi-Yoneda, N, et al. (2009). Alpha-1 antitrypsin activity is decreased in human amnion in premature rupture of the fetal membranes. *Mol Hum Reprod* 15, 49-57.

Jahangiri, A, et al. (2009). HDL remodeling during the acute phase response. *Arterioscler Thromb Vasc Biol* 29, 261-267.

Janciauskiene, S. (2001). Conformational properties of serine proteinase inhibitors (serpins) confer multiple pathophysiological roles. *Biochim Biophys Acta* 1535, 221-235.

Janciauskiene, S, Carlemalm, E, & Eriksson, S. (1995). In vitro fibril formation from alpha1-antitrypsin-derived C-terminal peptides. *Biol Chem Hoppe Seyler* 376, 415-423.

Janciauskiene, SM, Nita, IM, & Stevens, T. (2007). Alpha1-antitrypsin, old dog, new tricks. Alpha1-antitrypsin exerts in vitro anti-inflammatory activity in human monocytes by elevating cAMP. *J Biol Chem* 282, 8573-8582.

Janciauskiene, S, et al. (2008). Alpha1-antitrypsin inhibits the activity of the matriptase catalytic domain in vitro. *Am J Respir Cell Mol Biol* 39, 631-637.

Janciauskiene, SM, et al. (2011). The discovery of α1-antitrypsin and its role in health and disease. *Respir Med. [Epub ahead of print].*

Javid, J. (1978). Human haptoglobins. *Curr Top Hematol* 1, 151-192.

Jie, Z, et al. (2003). Protective effects of alpha 1-antitrypsin on acute lung injury in rabbits induced by endotoxin. *Chin Med J (Engl)* 116, 1678-1682.

Jones, SA, et al. (1999). C-reactive protein: a physiological activator of interleukin 6 receptor shedding. *J Exp Med* 189, 599-604.

Jordon, RE, Kawana, S, & Fritz, KA. (1985). Immunopathologic mechanisms in pemphigus and bullous pemphigoid. *J Invest Dermatol* 85, 72s-78s.

Kalis, M, et al. (2010). α 1-antitrypsin enhances insulin secretion and prevents cytokine-mediated apoptosis in pancreatic β-cells. *Islets* 2, 185-189.

Kakehi, K, Kinoshita, M & Nakano, M. (2002). Analysis of glycoproteins and the oligosaccharides thereof by high-performance capillary electrophoresis-significance in regulatory studies on biopharmaceutical products. *Biomed Chromatogr* 16, 103-115.

Kaźmierczak, M, et al. (1995). Changes of acute phase proteins glycosylation profile as a possible prognostic marker in myocardial infarction. *Int J Cardiol* 49, 201-207.

Kew, RR, Hyers, TM, & Webster, RO. (1990). Human C-reactive protein inhibits neutrophil chemotaxis in vitro: possible implications for the adult respiratory distress syndrome. *J Lab Clin Med* 115, 339-345.

Khreiss, T, et al. (2004). Opposing effects of C-reactive protein isoforms on shear-induced neutrophil-platelet adhesion and neutrophil aggregation in whole blood. *Circulation* 110, 2713-2720.

Khreiss, T, et al. (2005). Loss of pentameric symmetry inC-reactive protein induces interleukin-8 secretion through peroxynitrite signaling in human neutrophils. *Circ Res* 97, 690-697.

Knappstein, S, et al. (2004). Alpha 1-antitrypsin binds to and interferes with functionality of EspB from atypical and typical enteropathogenic Escherichia coli strains. *Infect Immun* 72, 4344-4350.

Koenig, W, et al. (1999). C-Reactive protein, a sensitive marker of inflammation, predicts future risk of coronary heart disease in initially healthy middle-aged men: results from the MONICA (Monitoring Trends and Determinants in Cardiovascular Disease) Augsburg Cohort Study, 1984 to 1992. *Circulation* 99, 237-242.

Koenig, W, et al. (2006). Increased concentrations of C-reactive protein and IL-6 but not IL-18 are independently associated with incident coronary events in middle-aged men and women: results from the MONICA/KORA Augsburg case-cohort study, 1984-2002. *Arterioscler Thromb Vasc Biol* 26, 2745-2751.

Koulmanda, M, et al. (2008). Curative and beta cell regenerative effects of alpha1-antitrypsin treatment in autoimmune diabetic NOD mice. *Proc Natl Acad Sci U S A* 105, 16242-16247.

Koj , A. (1985) Cytokines regulating acute inflammation and synthesis of acute phase proteins. *Blut* 51, 267-274.

Kresl, JJ, Potempa, LA, Anderson, B & Radosevich, JA.(1999). Inhibition of mouse mammary adenocarcinoma (EMT6) growth and metastases in mice by a modified form of C-reactive protein. *Tumour Biol* 20, 72-87.

Kueppers, F. (2011). The role of augmentation therapy in alpha-1 antitrypsin deficiency. *Curr Med Res Opin* 27, 579-588.

Kurosky, A, et al. (1980). Covalent structure of human haptoglobin: a serine protease homolog. *Proc Natl Acad Sci U S A* 77, 3388-3392.

Kushner, I. (1982). The phenomenon of the acute phase response. *Ann N Y Acad Sci* 389, 39-48.

Kushner, I & Feldmann, G. (1978). Control of the acute phase response. Demonstration of C-reactive protein synthesis and secretion by hepatocytes during acute inflammation in the rabbit. *J Exp Med* 148, 466-77.

Kushner, I, Gewurz, H, & Benson, MD. (1981). C-reactive protein and the acute-phase response. *J Lab Clin Med* 97, 739-749.

Kushner, I, & Mackiewicz, A. (1993). The acute-phase response: an overview. In: *Acute Phase Proteins Molecular Biology, Biochemistry and Clinical Applications* pp: 3-19. CRC Press, Boca Raton, FL.

Laine, A, et al. (1990). Comparison of the effects of purified human alpha 1-antichymotrypsin and alpha 1-proteinase inhibitor on NK cytotoxicity: only alpha 1-proteinase inhibitor inhibits natural killing. *Clin Chim Acta* 190, 163-173.

Laurell, CB, & Thulin, E. (1974). Complexes in plasma between light chain kappa immunoglobulins and alpha 1-antitrypsin respectively prealbumin. *Immunochemistry* 11, 703-709.

Lerner, UH, & Fröhlander, N. (1992). Haptoglobin-stimulated bone resorption in neonatal mouse calvarial bones in vitro. *Arthritis Rheum* 35, 587-591.

Lewis, EC, et al. (2008). Alpha1-Antitrypsin monotherapy induces immune tolerance during islet allograft transplantation in mice. *Proc Natl Acad Sci U S A* 105, 16236-16241.

Liang, YJ, et al. (2006). C-reactive protein activates the nuclear factor-kappaB pathway and induces vascular cell adhesion molecule-1 expression through CD32 in human umbilical vein endothelial cells and aortic endothelial cells. *J Mol Cell Cardiol* 40, 412-420.

Libby ,P. (2002). Inflammation in atherosclerosis. *Nature* 420, 868-874.

Libert, C, Brouckaert, P & Fiers, W. (1994). Protection by alpha 1-acid glycoprotein against tumor necrosis factor-induced lethality. *J Exp Med* 180, 1571-1575.

Libert, C, et al. (1996). alpha1-Antitrypsin inhibits the lethal response to TNF in mice. *J Immunol* 157, 5126-5129.

Li, Z, et al. (2009). Oxidized{alpha}1-antitrypsin stimulates the release of monocyte chemotactic protein-1 from lung epithelial cells: potential role in emphysema. *Am J Physiol Lung Cell Mol Physiol* 297, L388-400.

Licastro, F, et al. (1997). Monomeric and polymeric forms of alpha-1 antichymotrypsin in sera from patients with probable late onset Alzheimer's disease. *Dement Geriatr Cogn Disord* 8, 337-342.

Lieberman J. (2000). Augmentation therapy reduces frequency of lung infections in antitrypsin deficiency: a new hypothesis with supporting data. *Chest* 118, 1480-1485.

Lind, P, et al. (2004). Risk of myocardial infarction and stroke in smokers is related to plasma levels of inflammation-sensitive proteins. *Arterioscler Thromb Vasc Biol* 24, 577-582.

Liu, HM, Takagaki, K & Schmid, K. (1988). In vitro nerve-growth-promoting activity of human plasma alpha 1-acid glycoprotein. *J Neurosci Res* 20, 64-72.

Liu, Z, et al. (2000). The serpin alpha1-proteinase inhibitor is a critical substrate for gelatinase B/MMP-9 in vivo. *Cell* 102, 647-655.

Liu, C, et al. (2005). Proapoptotic, antimigratory, antiproliferative, and antiangiogenic effects of commercial C-reactive protein on various human endothelial cell types in vitro: implications of contaminating presence of sodium azide in commercial preparation. *Circ Res* 97, 135-143.

Lu X, LY, et al. (2009). Decay-Accelerating Factor Attenuates C-Reactive Protein-Potentiated Tissue Injury After Mesenteric Ischemia/Reperfusion. *J Surg Res* [Epub ahead of print].

Luo, LY, et al. (2006). Characterization of human kallikreins 6 and 10 in ascites fluid from ovarian cancer patients. *Tumour Biol* 27, 227-234.

Lysenko, E, et al. (2000). The position of phosphorylcholine on the lipopolysaccharide of Haemophilus influenzae affects binding and sensitivity to C-reactive protein-mediated killing. *Mol Microbiol* 35, 234-245.

Lögdberg, L & Wester, L. (2000). Immunocalins: a lipocalin subfamily that modulates immune and inflammatory responses. *Biochim Biophys Acta* 1482, 284-297.

Mackiewicz, A, et al. (1987). Monokines regulate glycosylation of acute-phase proteins. *J Exp Med* 166, 253-258.

Maes, OC, et al. (2006). Characterization of alpha1-antitrypsin as a heme oxygenase-1 suppressor in Alzheimer plasma. *Neurobiol Dis* 24, 89-100.

Mahadeva, R, et al., (2005) Polymers of Z alpha1-antitrypsin co-localize with neutrophils in emphysematous alveoli and are chemotactic in vivo. *Am J Pathol* 166, 377-386

Malle, E, & De Beer, FC. (1996). Human serum amyloid A (SAA) protein: a prominent acute-phase reactant for clinical practice. *Eur J Clin Invest* 26, 427-435.

Mani, K, et al. (2004). Involvement of glycosylphosphatidylinositol-linked ceruloplasmin in the copper/zinc-nitric oxide-dependent degradation of glypican-1 heparan sulfate in rat C6 glioma cells. *J Biol Chem* 279, 12918-12923

Marumo, T, et al. (1997). Platelet-derived growthfactor-stimulated superoxide anion production modulates activation of transcription factor NF-kappaB and expression of monocyte chemoattractant protein1 in human aortic smooth muscle cells. *Circulation* 96, 2361-2367.

McGuire, WW, et al. (1982). Studies on the pathogenesis of the adult respiratory distress syndrome. *J Clin Invest* 69, 543-553.

Mills, K, et al. (2001). Identification of alpha(1)-antitrypsin variants in plasma with the use of proteomic technology. *Clin Chem* 47, 2012-22.

Miyamoto, Y, Akaike, T, & Maeda, H. (2000). S-nitrosylated human alpha(1)-protease inhibitor. *Biochim Biophys Acta* 1477, 90-97.

Mold, C, Gewurz, H, & Du Clos, TW. (1999). Regulation of complement activation by C-reactive protein. *Immunopharmacology* 42, 23-30.

Mold, C, Kingzette, M, & Gewurz, H. (1984). C-reactive protein inhibits pneumococcal activation of the alternative pathway by increasing the interaction between factor H and C3b. *J Immunol* 133, 882-885.

Mold, C, et al. (1981). C-reactive protein is protective against Streptococcus pneumoniae infection in mice. *J Exp Med* 54, 1703-8.

Mold, C, et al. (2002). C-reactive protein mediates protection from lipopolysaccharide through interactions with Fc gamma R. *J Immunol Today* 169, 7019-7025.

Moore, DF, et al. (1997). Alpha-1-acid (AAG,orosomucoid) glycoprotein: interaction with bacterial lipopolysaccharide and protection from sepsis. *Inflammation* 21, 69-82.

Moraga, F, & Janciauskiene S. (2000). Activation of primary human monocytes by the oxidized form of alpha1-antitrypsin. *J Biol Chem* 275, 7693-7700.

Moshage, HJ, et al. (1987). Study of the molecular mechanism of decreased liver synthesis of albumin in inflammation. *J Clin Invest* 79, 1635-1641.

Motie, M, Schaul, KW & Potempa, LA. (1998). Biodistribution and clearance of 125I-labeled C-reactive protein and 125I-labeled modified C-reactive protein in CD-1 mice. *Drug Metab Dispos* 26, 977-981.

Muchitsch, EM, Auer, W & Pichler, L. (1998). Effects of alpha 1-acid glycoprotein in different rodent models of shock. *Fundam Clin Pharmacol.* 12, 173-181.

Mulgrew, AT, et al., (2004) Z alpha1-antitrypsin polymers in the lung and acts as a neutrophil chemoattractant. *Chest*, 125, 1952-1957.

Nielsen, MJ, & Moestrup, SK. (2009). Receptor targeting of hemoglobin mediated by the haptoglobins: roles beyond heme scavenging. *Blood* 114, 764-771.

Oh, SK, Pavlotsky, N, & Tauber, AI. (1990). Specific binding of haptoglobin to human neutrophils and its functional consequences. *J Leukoc Biol* 47, 142-148.

Oliveira, EB, Gotschlich, C & Liu, TY. (1979). Primary structure of human C-reactive protein. *J Biol Chem* 254, 489-502.

Okemefuna, AI, et al. (2010). C-reactive protein exists in an NaCl concentration-dependent pentamer-decamer equilibrium in physiological buffer. *J Biol Chem* 285, 1041-1052.

Ossanna, PJ, et al. (1986). Oxidative regulation of neutrophil elastase-alpha-1-proteinase inhibitor interactions. *J Clin Invest* 77, 1939-1951.

Pagano, M, Nicola, MA, & Engler, R. (1982). Inhibition of cathepsin L and B by haptoglobin, the haptoglobin-hemoglobin complex, and asialohaptoglobin. "In vitro" studies in the rat. *Can J Biochem* 60, 631-637.

Pasceri, V, et al. (2001). Modulation of C-reactive protein-mediated monocyte chemoattractant protein-1 induction in human endothelial cells by anti-atherosclerosis drugs. *Circulation* 103, 2531-2534.

Pradhan, AD, et al. (2001). C-reactive protein, interleukin 6, and risk of developing type 2 diabetes mellitus. *JAMA* 286, 327-334.

Pasceri, V, Willerson, JT, & Yeh, ET. (2000). Direct proinflammatory effect of C-reactive protein on human endothelial cells. *Circulation* 102, 2165-2168.

Pepys, MB, et al. (1994). Binding of pentraxins to different nuclear structures: C-reactive protein binds to small nuclear ribonucleoprotein particles, serum amyloid P component binds to chromatin and nucleoli. *Clin Exp Immunol* 97, 152-157.

Petrache, I, et al. (2006). alpha-1 antitrypsin inhibits caspase-3 activity, preventing lung endothelial cell apoptosis. *Am J Pathol* 169, 1155-1166.

Pichler, L, Muchitsch,EM & Schwarz, HP. (1999). [Preclinical investigation of alpha 1-acid glycoprotein (orosomucoid)]. *Wien Klin Wochenschr* 111, 192-198.

Poland, DC, et al. (2001). Increased alpha3-fucosylation of alpha1-acid glycoprotein in Type I diabetic patients is related to vascular function. *Glycoconj J* 18, 261-268.

Potempa, LA, et al. (1983). Antigenic,electrophoretic and binding alterations of human C-reactive protein modified selectively in the absence of calcium. *Mol Immunol* 20, 1165-1175.

Potempa, LA, et al. (1996). Stimulation of megakaryocytopoiesis in mice by human modified C-reactive protein (mCRP). *Exp Hematol* 24, 258-264.

Potempa, LA, et al. (1987). Expression, detection and assay of a neoantigen (Neo-CRP) associated with a free, human C-reactive protein subunit. *Mol Immunol* 24, 531-541.

Potthoff, AV, et al. (2007). HIV infection in a patient with alpha-1 antitrypsin deficiency: a detrimental combination? *AIDS* 21, 2115-2116.

Rapala-Kozik, M, et al. (1999). Comparative cleavage sites within the reactive-site loop of native and oxidized alpha1-proteinase inhibitor by selected bacterial proteinases. *Biol Chem* 380, 1211-1216.

Retamales, I, et al. (2001). Amplification of inflammation in emphysema and its association with latent adenoviral infection. *Am J Respir Crit Care Med* 164, 469-473.

Ridker, PM, et al. (1997). Alu-repeat polymorphism in the gene coding for tissue-type plasminogen activator (t-PA) and risks of myocardial infarction among middle-aged men. *Arterioscler Thromb Vasc Biol* 17, 1687-1690.

Rinaldi, M, et al. (2008). Differential effects of alpha1-acid glycoprotein on bovine neutrophil respiratory burst activity and IL-8 production. *Vet Immunol Immunopathol* 126, 199-210.

Rodriguez, W, et al. (2005). Reversal of ongoing proteinuria in autoimmune mice by treatment with C-reactive protein. *Arthritis Rheum* 52, 642-650.

Rodriguez, W, et al. (2007). C-reactive protein-mediated suppression of nephrotoxic nephritis: role of macrophages, complement, and Fcgamma receptors. *J Immunol* 178, 530-538.

Rossbacher, J, Wagner, L, & Pasternack, MS. (1999). Inhibitory effect of haptoglobin on granulocyte chemotaxis, phagocytosis and bactericidal activity. *Scand J Immunol* 50, 399-404.

Roum, JH, et al. (1993). Systemic deficiency of glutathione in cystic fibrosis. *J Appl Physiol* 75, 2419-2424.

Rydén, I, et al. (1997). Glycosylation of alpha1-acid glycoprotein in inflammatory disease: analysis by high-pH anion-exchange chromatography and concanavalin A crossed affinity immunoelectrophoresis. *Glycoconj J* 14, 481-488.

Sadrzadeh, SM, & Bozorgmeh, J. (2004). Haptoglobin phenotypes in health and disorders. *Am J Clin Pathol* 121 *Suppl.*

Salvatore A, et al. (2009). Haptoglobin binds apolipoprotein E and influences cholesterol esterification in the cerebrospinal fluid.*J Neurochem.* 110, 255-263.

Saldova, R, et al. (2008). Glycosylation changes on serum glycoproteins in ovarian cancer may contribute to disease pathogenesis. *Dis Markers* 25, 219-232.

Samberg, NL, et al. (1988). Preferential expression of neo-CRP epitopes on the surface of human peripheral blood lymphocytes. *Cell Immunol* 116, 86-98.

Sarrats, A, et al. (2010). Glycosylation of liver acute-phase proteins in pancreatic cancer and chronic pancreatitis. *Proteomics Clin Appl* 4, 432-448.

Scott, LJ, et al. (1998). Comparison of IgA-alpha1-antitrypsin levels in rheumatoid arthritis and seronegative oligoarthritis: complex formation is not associated with inflammation per se. *Br J Rheumatol* 37, 398-404.

Sei, K, et al. (2002). Collection of alpha1-acid glycoprotein molecular species by capillary electrophoresis and the analysis of their molecular masses and carbohydrate chains. Basic studies on the analysis of glycoprotein glycoforms. *J Chromatogr A* 958, 273-281.

Shah, C, Hari-Dass, R & Raynes, JG. (2006). Serum amyloid A is an innate immune opsonin for Gram-negative bacteria. *Blood* 108, 1751-1757.

Shapira, I, et al. (2011). Novel peptides as potential treatment of systemic lupus erythematosus. *Lupus [Epub ahead of print].*

Schapira, M, et al. (1982). Purified human plasma kallikrein aggregates human blood neutrophils. *J Clin Invest* 69, 1199-1202.

She QB, et al. (2000). alpha(1)-antitrypsin can increase insulin-induced mitogenesis in various fibroblast and epithelial cell lines. *FEBS Lett* 473, 33-36.

Schwedler, SB, et al. (2006). C-reactive protein: a family of proteins to regulate cardiovascular function. *Am J Kidney Dis* 47, 212-222.

Singh, VK & Fudenberg, HH. (1986). Lymphocyte stimulation in vitro by orosomucoid glycoprotein. *Immunol Lett* 14, 9-13.

Snyder, S & Coodley, EL. (1976). Inhibition of platelet aggregation by alpha1-acid glycoprotein. *Arch Intern Med* 136, 778-781.

Stefansson, S, & Lawrence, DA. (1996). The serpin PAI-1 inhibits cell migration by blocking integrin alpha V beta 3 binding to vitronectin. *Nature* 383, 441-443.

Steinmetz, A, et al. (1989). Influence of serum amyloid A on cholesterol esterification in human plasma. *Biochim Biophys Acta* 1006, 173-178.

Stibler, H, Holzbach, U & Kristiansson, B. (1998). Isoforms and levels of transferrin, antithrombin, alpha(1)-antitrypsin and thyroxine-binding globulin in 48 patients with carbohydrate-deficient glycoprotein syndrome type I. *Scand J Clin Lab Invest* 58, 55-61.

Stoller, JK, et al. (2007). Primary care diagnosis of alpha-1 antitrypsin deficiency: issues and opportunities. *Cleve Clin J Med* 74, 869-874.

Stonik, JA, et al. (2004). Serum amyloid A promotes ABCA1-dependent and ABCA1-independent lipid efflux from cells. *Biochem Biophys Res Commun* 32, 936-941.

Su, SJ, et al. (1999). Alpha 1-acid glycoprotein-induced tumor necrosis factor-alpha secretion of human monocytes is enhanced by serum binding proteins and depends on protein tyrosine kinase activation. *Immunopharmacology*. 41, 21-29.

Su, SJ & Yeh, TM. (1996). Effects of alpha 1-acid glycoprotein on tissue factor expression and tumor necrosis factor secretion in human monocytes. *Immunopharmacology* 34, 139-145.

Sun, YX, Wright, HT, & Janciauskiene, S. (2002). Alpha1-antichymotrypsin/Alzheimer's peptide Abeta(1-42) complex perturbs lipid metabolism and activates transcription factors PPARgamma and NFkappaB in human neuroblastoma (Kelly) cells. *J Neurosci Respir Med* 67, 511-522.

Subramaniyam, D., et al. (2010). Cholesterol rich lipid raft microdomains are gateway for acute phase protein, SERPINA1. *Int J Biochem Cell Biol* 42, 1562-1570.

Subramaniyam, D, et al. (2008). TNF-alpha-induced self expression in human lung endothelial cells is inhibited by native and oxidized alpha1-antitrypsin. *Int J Biochem Cell Biol* 40, 258-271.

Subramaniyam, D., et al. (2010). Effects of alpha 1-antitrypsin on endotoxin-induced lung inflammation in vivo. *Inflamm Res* 59, 571-578.

Sullivan, CP, et al. (2010). Secretory phospholipase A2, group IIA is a novel serum amyloid A target gene: activation of smooth muscle cell expression by an interleukin-1 receptor-independent mechanism. *J Biol Chem* 285, 565-575.

Szalai, AJ, Briles, DE & Volanakis, JE. (1995). Human C-reactive protein is protective against fatal Streptococcus pneumoniae infection in transgenic mice. *J Immunol* 155, 2557-2563.

Szalai, AJ, et al. (2002). Experimental allergic encephalomyelitis is inhibited in transgenic mice expressing human C-reactive protein. *J Immunol* 168, 5792-5797.

Szalai, AJ, et al. (2000). Human C-reactive protein is protective against fatal Salmonella enterica serovar typhimurium infection in transgenic mice. *Infect Immun* 68, 5652-5656.

Sörensson, J, et al. (1999). Human endothelial cells produce orosomucoid, an important component of the capillary barrier. *Am J Physiol* 276, H530-534.

Tam, SP, Kisilevsky, R, & Ancsin, JB. (2008). Acute-phase-HDL remodeling by heparan sulfate generates a novel lipoprotein with exceptional cholesterol efflux activity from macrophages. *PLoS One* 3, e3867.

Taggart, C, et al. (2000). Oxidation of either methionine 351 or methionine 358 in alpha 1-antitrypsin causes loss of anti-neutrophil elastase activity. *J Biol Chem* 275, 27258-27265.

Taylor, KE, Giddings, JC, & van den Berg, CW. (2005). C-reactive protein-induced in vitro endothelial cell activation is an artefact caused by azide and lipopolysaccharide. *Arterioscler Thromb Vasc Biol* 25, 1225-1230.

Thompson, D, Pepys, MB, & Wood, SP. (1999). The physiological structure of human C-reactive protein and its complex with phosphocholine. *Structure* 7, 169-177.

Thomas-Rudolph, D, et al. (2007). C-reactive protein enhances immunity to Streptococcus pneumoniae by targeting uptake to Fc gamma R on dendritic cells. *J Immunol* 178, 7283-7291.

Thurberg, BL, & Collins, T. (1998). The nuclear factor-kappa B/inhibitor of kappa B autoregulatory system and atherosclerosis. *Curr Opin Lipidol* 9, 387-396.

Tilg H, et al. (1993) Antiinflammatory properties of hepatic acute phase proteins: preferential induction of interleukin 1 (IL-1) receptor antagonist over IL-1 beta synthesis by human peripheral blood mononuclear cells. *J Exp Med* 178, 1629-1636.

Tseng, CF, et al. (2004). Antioxidant role of human haptoglobin. *Proteomics* 4, 2221-2228.

Tseng, IC, et al. (2008). Purification from human milk of matriptase complexes with secreted serpins: mechanism for inhibition of matriptase other than HAI-1. *Am J Physiol Cell Physiol* 295, C423-C431.

Valko, M, et al. (2007). Free radicals and antioxidants in normal physiological functions and human disease. *Int J Biochem Cell Biol.* 39, 44-84.

Van Molle, W, et al. (1999). Activation of caspases in lethal experimental hepatitis and prevention by acute phase proteins. *J Immunol* 163, 5235-5241.

van Pelt, J, et al. (1996). Carbohydrate-deficient transferrin values in neonatal and umbilical cord blood. *J Inherit Metab Dis* 19, 253-266.

Verma, S, et al. (2002). Endothelin antagonism and interleukin-6 inhibition attenuate the proatherogenic effects of C-reactive protein. *Circulation* 105, 1890-1896.

Volanakis, JE, & Wirtz, KW. (1979). Interaction of C-reactive protein with artificial phosphatidylcholine bilayers. *Nature* 281, 155-157.

Walcheck, B, et al. (1996). Neutrophil-neutrophil interactions under hydrodynamic shear stress involve L-selectin and PSGL-1. A mechanism that amplifies initial leukocyte accumulation of P-selectin in vitro. *J Clin Invest* 98, 1081-1087.

Wang, M, et al. (2009). Novel fucosylated biomarkers for the early detection of hepatocellular carcinoma. *Cancer Epidemiol Biomarkers Prev* 18, 1914-1921.

Weiser ,JN, et al. (1998). Phosphorylcholine on the lipopolysaccharide of Haemophilus influenzae contributes to persistence in the respiratory tract and sensitivity to serum killing mediated by C-reactive protein. *J Exp Med* 187, 631-640.

Weiss, SJ. (1989). Tissue destruction by neutrophils *N Engl J Med* 320, 365-376.

Whisler, RL, Newhouse, YG, & Mortensen, RF. (1986). C-reactive protein reduces the promotion of human B-cell colony formation by autoreactive T4 cells and T-cell proliferation during the autologous mixed-lymphocyte reaction. *Cell Immunol* 102, 287-298.

Wiman, B, et al. (1988). Plasminogen activator inhibitor 1 (PAI) is bound to vitronectin in plasma. *FEBS Lett* 242, 125-128.

Williams JP, et al. (1997). Alpha1-Acid glycoprotein reduces local and remote injuries after intestinal ischemia in the rat. *Am J Physiol* 273, G1031-10335.

Woollard, KJ, Phillips, DC, & Griffiths, HR. (2002). Direct modulatory effect of C-reactive protein on primary human monocyte adhesion to human endothelial cells. *Clin Exp Immunol Today* 130, 256-262.

Wong, PS, & Travis, J. (1980). Isolation and properties of oxidized alpha-1-proteinase inhibitor from human rheumatoid synovial fluid. *Biochem Biophys Res Commun* 96, 1449-1454.

Xia, D & Samols, D. (1997). Transgenic mice expressing rabbit C-reactive protein are resistant to endotoxemia. *Proc Natl Acad Sci U S A* 94, 2575-2580.

Xie, L, et al. (2005). C-reactive protein augments interleukin-8 secretion in human peripheral blood monocytes. *J Cardiovasc Pharmacol* 46, 690-696.

Yang, F, et al. (1995). Cell type-specific and inflammatory-induced expression of haptoglobin gene in lung. *Lab Invest. 73*, 433-440.

Yang, Z & Hancock, WS. (2005). Monitoring glycosylation pattern changes of glycoproteins using multi-lectin affinity chromatography. *J Chromatogr A* 1070, 57-64.

Zeller, JM, & Sullivan, BL. (1992). C-reactive protein selectively enhances the intracellular generation of reactive oxygen products by IgG-stimulated monocytes and neutrophils. *J Leukoc Biol* 52, 449-455.

Zhang, WM, et al. (2000). Characterization and determination of the complex between prostate-specific antigen and alpha 1-protease inhibitor in benign and malignant prostatic diseases. *Scand J Clin Lab Invest Suppl* 233, 51-58.

Zhong, W, et al. (1998) Effect of human C-reactive protein on chemokine and chemotactic factor-induced neutrophil chemotaxis and signaling. *J Immunol* 161, 2533-2540.

Zipfel, PF & Skerka, C. (2009). Complement regulators and inhibitory proteins. *Nat Rev Immunol* 9, 729-740.

Zouki, C, et al. (1997). Prevention of In vitro neutrophil adhesion to endothelial cells through shedding of L-selectin by C-reactive protein and peptides derived from C-reactive protein. *J Clin Invest* 100, 522-529.

Zouki, C, et al. (2001). Loss of pentameric symmetry of C-reactive protein is associated with promotion of neutrophil-endothelial cell adhesion. *J Immunol* 167, 5355-5361.

3

Regulatory Mechanisms Controlling Inflammation and Synthesis of Acute Phase Proteins

Jolanta Jura and Aleksander Koj
Faculty of Biochemistry, Biophysics and Biotechnology
Jagiellonian University, Krakow,
Poland

1. Introduction

Inflammation is usually defined as a complex response of the animal organism to tissue injury or to invasion of foreign pathogens. Although inflammation often starts as a local reaction it can easily develop into a generalized systemic response involving the whole organism. Participation of inflammatory reactions in the pathogenesis of many diseases is today a generally accepted medical paradigm. These ideas have been thoroughly discussed in numerous excellent monographs and specialized recent publications (Nathan, 2002; Dinarello, 2008, 2010; Medzhitov, 2010) whereas our presentation is just a brief account focused on regulatory mechanisms involved in the initiation, development and termination of the "generalized inflammatory response" (**GIR**) and its relations to the induced synthesis of certain plasma and tissue proteins.

The results obtained by techniques of modern genomics indicate that these three phases of response to injury are tightly controlled and are characterized by distinct profiles of hundreds of activated genes. The fine tuning of gene expression during initiation, development and resolution of inflammation occurs at many levels starting from transcription and followed by changes in mRNA decay, receptors cross-talk, intracellular signaling cascades and posttranslational protein modifications. Disturbances in the regulatory network lead to either acute pathological states such as septic shock, or to various chronic autoimmune and auto-inflammatory diseases.

Discovery of C-reactive protein (**CRP**) in the blood of patients with febrile diseases some 80 years ago (Tillett & Francis, 1930) was seminal for the development of the idea of "acute phase reaction" (**APR**) and the concept of "acute phase proteins" (**APPs**) reflected as profound rearrangement of plasma protein profile accompanying systemic inflammatory reaction (Kushner, 1982). The so called "positive AP-proteins" increase their plasma concentration in a broad range – from barely 25 per cent above the control up to several hundred fold - at the expense of "negative APPs" which go down in comparison to control. Other metabolic changes during this response include fever, leukocytosis, negative nitrogen balance, altered levels of some ions and hormones, activation of clotting and complement pathways, as well as certain less defined phenomena (for references see (Gordon and Koj, 1985)). The principal features of APR resemble the unspecific innate immunological reaction and some authors assume that in fact we are dealing with synonyms corresponding to the two sides of the same biological phenomenon (Koj, 2008). From historic perspective however, the APR corresponds to the metabolic response of liver, manifested predominantly as induced synthesis of acute phase proteins. For several years it was silently assumed that the term APP is limited to plasma proteins synthesized by and secreted from liver parenchymal cells. However, many resident proteins are also affected by inflammatory response and they are called "acute phase regulated intracellular proteins" i.e. APRIPs (Ruminy et al., 2001), or even more broadly - cytokine-responsive cellular proteins (Koj, 2008).

2. Initiation of generalized inflammatory response

Inflammation can be induced by two types of noxious stimuli: invasion of foreign pathogens of biological origin, or sterile tissue damage. In reality, however, the most common is mixed type of GIR. The pathogens include bacteria, fungi, yeasts, viruses or parasites as well as their products which after penetrating of the organism are present either in the extracellular space, or already in the cell compartments. In the first case they can be recognized by a special class of cell membrane receptors abounding on the surface of sentinel cells exposed to the environment. Receptors of this type were first discovered in *Drosophila* fruit fly and named Toll receptors, being important for embryonic development and protection against invading fungi. Their mammalian counterparts named Toll-like receptors **(TLRs)** have been extensively studied during last 15 years (Medzhitov et al., 1997). TLRs are able to discriminate between self and non-self by recognizing pathogen-associated molecular patterns **(PAMPs)** (Medzhitov, 2010). Typical examples of this class of PAMPs are lipopolysaccharides of the bacterial wall, or mannans from the yeasts cells (Takeuchi & Akira, 2010). Today more than ten mammalian TLRs are known and depending on their cellular localization and type of the ligand they are divided into two subgroups. TLRs from the first group are localized at the cell membrane (TLRs 1, 2, 4, 5, 6, 10), whereas others (TLRs 3, 7, 8, 9) are expressed intracellularly anchoring vesicles of the endoplasmic reticulum, endosomes and lysosomes (Kawai & Akira, 2010; Ospelt & Gay, 2010). Toll-like receptors are important in the initiation of molecular alarm during pathogen invasion of the host and also in response to other danger signals expressed in a variety of immune as well as non-immune cells. Effector or "sentinel" cells, such as neutrophils, dendritic cells and macrophages express almost all types of TLRs, in distinction to other specialized cells. The first group of TLRs recognizes mainly microbial membrane components (lipids, lipoproteins and proteins) whereas the other group responds to microbial nucleic acids. For example TLR1 acts mainly as a heterodimer together with TLR2 and recognizes lipopeptides originating from *Mycobacteria*. TLR2 responds also to material derived from bacteria, fungi, parasites and viruses (lipopeptides, peptidoglycan, lipoarabinomannan, zymosan or hemagglutinins), whereas the heterodimer TLR2/TLR6 binds lipopeptides. TLR4 was the first TLR identified in human cells and we know that it responds to bacterial lipopolysaccharides (LPS) from the membrane of Gram-negative bacteria (Akira et al., 2006). Another receptor from this group, TLR5, recognizes bacterial protein, flagellin, essential for movement of bacteria (Akira et al., 2006). The recently discovered human TLR10 was found to heterodimerize with TLR1 (Hasan et al., 2005) but so far its ligand was not determined. As already mentioned, TLRs from intracellular compartments may recognize nucleic acids: TLR3 binds double stranded RNA of viral origin, but also similar endogenous ligands from necrotic cells (Brentano et al., 2005). On the other hand, TLR7 and TLR8 respond to single-stranded

RNA from viruses and endogenous sources. Finally, TLR9 recognizes DNA-containing unmethylated CpG motifs. All the discussed TLRs differ not only in structure and ligand affinity but also in the intracellular signaling cascades. Their ability to form dimers certainly expands the array of recognized PAMPs. Signals generated by the formation of a PAMP-TLR complex activate at least one out of five specific adaptor cytoplasmic proteins (MyD88, MAL, TRIF, TRAF or SARM) (O'Neill & Bowie, 2007). These adaptors participate in transmission of a message from the plasma membrane through a multi-step cascade to a responsive transcription factor – NF-κB being the principal target (Fig.1).

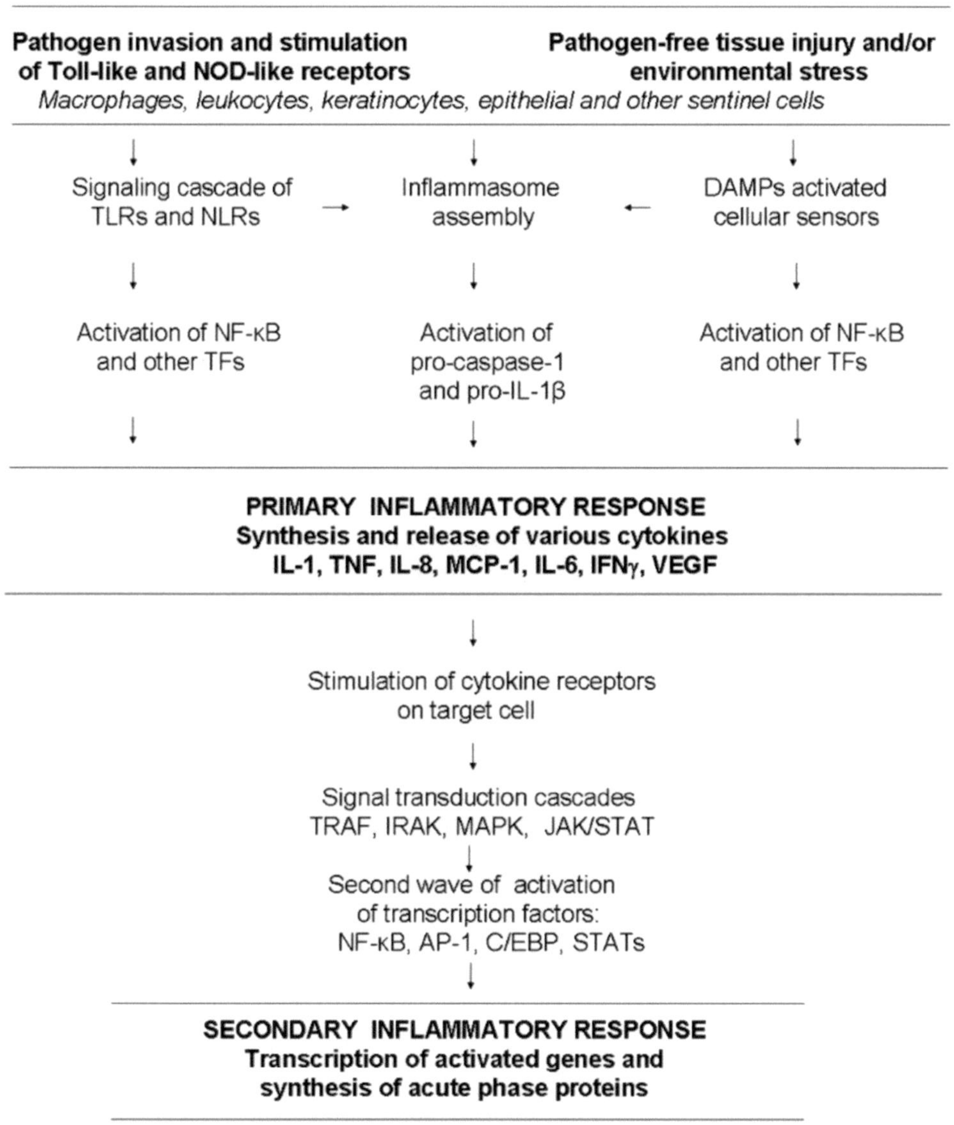

Fig. 1. Scheme of initiation and development of inflammatory response. For abbreviations used and for further detail see the text.

However, some pathogen-derived molecules, such as foreign DNA or RNA, may reach intracellular compartments of infected cells where they are recognized by and bound to NOD-like receptors (**NLRs**) (Akira et al., 2006; Ye & Ting, 2008). The NLRs belong to a large family of cytosolic pattern recognition receptors (34 members in mice, 23 in human) (Jin & Flawell, 2010) that are able to recognize various pathogen associated molecular patterns or danger-associated molecular patterns and thereby initiate the innate immune response against invading pathogens and cellular signals of damage or stress.

These NLRs, multi-domain receptor proteins, are characterized by leucine-reach repeats (LRRs) at the C-terminal region, a central nucleotide binding and oligomerization domain (referred to as NOD domain), toward N-terminal effector domain. From evolutionary point of view it is very interesting that animal NLRs show certain similarities to the products of plant disease-resistant genes (Martinon et al., 2009). Some NLRs act just as receptors while other constitute components of specialized cytosolic structures – **inflammasomes** (Schroder & Tschopp, 2010; Martinon et al., 2009). Certain NLRs interact with the ubiquitin ligase-associated protein SGT1 and HSP90, and this leads to the inhibition of inflammasome activity (Mayor et al. 2007).

In comparison to pathogen induced response the signaling elicited by pathogen-free tissue injury is even more complex and includes various **DAMPs** (damage-associated molecular patterns) such as crystals of uric acid or cholesterol (responsible for symptoms of gout or atherosclerosis) (Rock et al., 2010), fibers of asbestos and grains of silica (accumulated in lungs in asbestosis and silicosis) (Martinon et al., 2009; Rock et al., 2010), chemical irritants such as turpentine oil (Sheikh et al., 2007), deposits of denatured or modified proteins (such as inactivated alpha-1-proteinase inhibitor) (Koj & Guzdek, 1995), or fibrillar amyloid beta peptide found in the brain in Alzheimer disease (Halle et al., 2008). But commonly occurring pathogen-free tissue damage leading to inflammation can be also elicited by extreme temperatures, by hypo- or hyperosmolarity (Shapiro & Dinarello, 1997; Bode et al., 1999), by hypoxia-reoxygenation process (Wenger et al., 1995), UV radiation (Feldmeyer et al., (2007) and accumulation of reactive oxygen species (Bogdan et al., 2000). These signals may - by various means - stimulate cells either through specialized appropriate Toll-like receptors (Takeuchi & Akira, 2010) or certain scavenger receptors, or using other sensitive intracellular surveillance molecules, such as plasma membrane transporters (Schroder and Tchopp, 2010) or activation of MAP kinases (Bode et al., 1999; Chang & Karin, 2001). The use of alternative signaling routes occurs in case of hypoxia which is known to mobilize a specific transcription factor HIF-1 and proline hydroxylases (Zagorska & Dulak 2004; Oliver et al., 2009).

Usually the multi-step signaling cascade activated by pathogen-free tissue injury (or by stress of environmental origin) merges at some stage with the cascade initiated by foreign pathogens resulting in activation of transcription factors, among which the most important is NF-κB (Fig.1). This leads to a prompt transcription of sensitive genes resulting in accumulation of specific mRNAs coding mainly for IL-1β and other cytokines involved in the development of inflammation. It is understood now that translation of some of these mRNAs into active proteins may require an additional signal as it was earlier found in the case of IL-1β (Dinarello, 1996); if this signal is missing, initiation of the inflammatory response may be delayed or entirely aborted.

In order to briefly recapitulate current views on the initiation of inflammatory reaction one should emphasize the importance of signals indicating imminent danger to the cell/organism. Their detection is based on the ability of cells to recognize such signals by a small number of germline-encoded Pattern Recognition Receptors (PRRs). These PRRs are able to discriminate between self and non-self of certain molecular structures that may appear either outside of the cell (e.g. bacterial LPS is bound to Toll-like receptors located on the cell membrane), or are found intracellularly (e.g. foreign DNA or RNA in the cytosol) where they are recognized by NOD-like receptors (NLRs). However, PRRs can be stimulated not only by binding Pathogen Associated Molecular Patterns (**PAMPs**) but also by host own stress and danger signals (**SAMPs and DAMPs**) derived from damaged cells. These signals are recognized by cytosolic, intracellular receptors, among which the most important are NLRs. Moreover, some NLRs are used for the construction of specialized subcellular structures - inflammasomes - serving as the activation platform for the key pro-inflammatory cytokine - IL-1β.

3. The role of inflammasomes

Undoubtedly, IL-1β is the key mediator in the host innate response to infection and the driving force in the development of inflammation. However, since IL-1β is synthesized as a leaderless pro-cytokine it must be processed for secretion and exhibition of biological activity (similar properties are shown also by IL-18 and IL-33) (Dinarello, 1996, 2008, 2010). The proteolytic activation of pro-IL-1β is accomplished by an enzyme initially named ICE (Interleukin-1-converting enzyme) but at present known as caspase-1 belonging to the family of cysteine-aspartyl proteases participating in apoptosis. Caspase-1 is synthesized as zymogen which undergoes autocatalytic processing. Only relatively recently it has been established that efficient activation of pro-caspase-1 and pro-IL-1β takes place in specialized cytoplasmic multiprotein platforms called **inflammasomes** (Dinarello, 2008; Martinon et al., 2009; Schroder & Tschopp, 2010).

As discussed by Martinon et al. (2009), the details of inflammasome structure are only partly revealed but several types of molecules can be distinguished. The best known NLRP3 inflammasome (alternative names - NALP3 or cryopyrin) includes NLRP3 protein which interacts with the **adaptor protein ASC** (apoptosis-associated speck-like protein with a caspase recruitment domain). The resulting complex binds and activates pro-caspase-1 to caspase-1 which in turn is ready to activate pro-IL-1β (Fig.2). It appears that activation of caspase-1 requires zinc and is dependent on pannexin-1, a protein localized upstream in this signaling cascade (Brough et al., 2009).

Assembly and activation of inflammasome can be induced by several factors discussed above, but recent review presented by Martinon et al., (2009) enlarges this list to include various signals of danger and stress (DAMPs or SAMPs). Extracellular ATP represents such a stress signal released locally and recognized by a specific purinergic receptor $P2X_7$ (Ferrari et al., 2006; Lister et al., 2007).

Charles Dinarello was probably first to report that in order to obtain active and mature IL-1β molecules two independent cellular signals are required for effective transcription and translation (Dinarello, 1996). When studying activation of NLRP3 inflammasome Bauernfeind et al., (2009) observed that this process also needs two signals: one provided by the NF-κB cascade is necessary but not sufficient, whereas the second signal is generated by extracellular ATP, or crystal-induced cell damage. Other inducers of inflammasome assembly include such widely different factors as reactive oxygen intermediates, products of lysosomal damage and leakage of potassium from the cell (Martinon et al., 2009; Rock et al., 2010). We know today that the inflammasome may act as a sensor of the oxidative stress by co-operation with thioredoxin (Jin & Flavell, 2010; Zhou et al., 2010). The broad spectrum of modulators of inflammasome assembly and activation confirms the importance of these subcellular structures that are just being recognized as new targets in the anti-inflammatory therapies (Stehlik & Dorfleutner, 2007; Lamkanfi et al., 2009; Dinarello, 2010; Martinon et al., 2010; Rock et al., 2010).

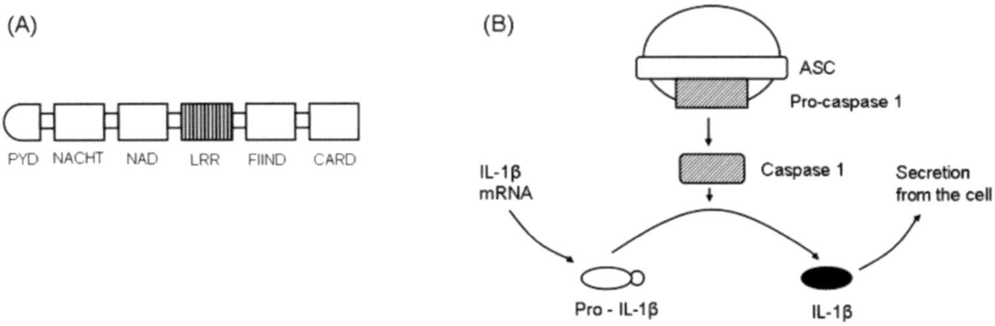

Fig. 2. Principal domains of NLRP1 protein (A) and schematic function of NLRP3 inflammasome (B).

The drawings are based on the data of Agostini et al., (2004); Dinarello, (2008) and Martinon et al. (2009). PYD, pyrin domain; NACHT, central nucleotide binding and oligomerization domain; NAD, NACHT-associated domain; LRR, leucine-rich repeats; FIIND, domain of poorly defined function; CARD, caspase recruitment domain; ASC, apoptosis speck-like protein adjacent to CARD at C-terminal where pro-caspase is initially located.

4. Inflammation control: components and rules

Local inflammation can be transformed within a few hours into a life-threatening generalized inflammatory response and thus the development of mechanisms controlling its course is of prime importance. The list of main players in the field of inflammation development and control is shown in Table 1, but their detailed analysis is beyond the scope of this brief review. The data obtained by techniques of functional genomics indicate that several hundreds of genes participate in the inflammatory response and their coordinated expression is tightly regulated (for references see Koj, 2008; Jura et al., 2008). These genes can be grouped into subsets as coding for various transcription factors, cytokines, chemokines, interferons, cellular growth factors and corresponding receptors, as well as those coding for adhesion molecules and enzymes involved in the production and removal of free radicals, or in modification of newly synthesized polypeptide chains by glycosylation or phosphorylation.

Most of these genes and their products share some striking features concerning the mechanism of biosynthesis and degradation of inflammatory mediators, and especially of cytokines:

- Promoters of these genes often contain multiple binding sites for several transcription factors (TFs): the most important being NF-κB. Its activation can be achieved in several independent signaling cascades, one of them - induced by LPS – being shown in Fig. 3. However, NF-κB is more than just a transcription factor and should be rather regarded as an universal switch in the innate and acquired immune reactions (reviewed in Hoffmann & Baltimore, 2006). Other typical transcription factors used by inflammatory mediators include AP-1, (activator protein-1, usually a hetero-dimer of c-Fos/c-Jun (Hattori et al., 1993)), STAT (signal transducer and activator of transcription known in six isoforms numbered STAT1 - STAT6 (Baumann, 2003; Heinrich et al., 2003; Sehgal, 2008), C/EBP (CAAT enhancer binding protein, occurring in four isoforms (Huang & Liao, 1994) and Elk-1 (Kasza et al., 2010) (for comprehensive list of earlier references see Ray et al., 1990; Koj, 1996, Ruminy et al., 2001). The interactions between the various TFs that compete for binding sites in the promoter regions of various genes are highly complex and regulation of IL-6 expression, described first by Sehgal et al., (1995) and later by van den Berghe et al., (2000), may provide some useful information.

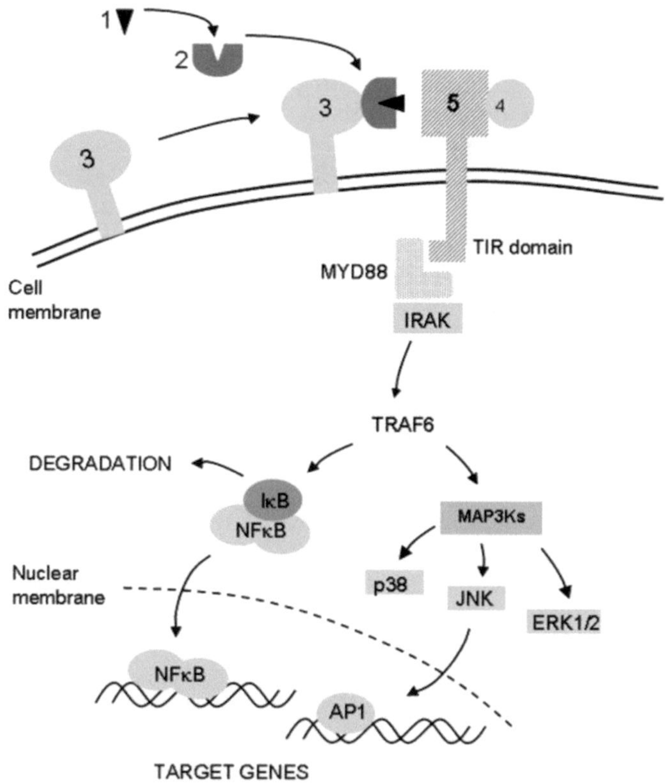

Fig. 3. Simplified scheme of a signaling pathway activated by bacterial endotoxin (LPS).

LPS (1) interacts with LPS-binding protein (2) and with help of plasma membrane receptor CD14 (3) is transferred to Toll-like receptor TLR4 (5) which requires MD2 accessory protein (4). Activation of TLR4 leads to the recruitment of an adaptor protein MyD88 with subsequent involvement of several adaptor or enzymatic proteins (some of them not shown on the scheme): Tollip, IRAK (IL-1R-Associated Kinase) and TRAF (TNF-Receptor Associated Factor). IRAK4 is phosphorylated and activates IRAK1, which in turn interacts with TNF receptor-associated factor 6 (TRAF6) complex causing its oligomerization and activation. Proteins from TRAF6 complex activate IKK and MAP kinases (ERK1/3, JNK, p38). IKK is a complex of two protein kinase subunits, IKKalfa and IKKbeta, and a regulatory subunit IKKgamma (NEMO). Activation of IKK complex leads to phosphorylation of NF-κB inhibitor (IkB) and its degradation, resulting finally in the release of NF-κB and its translocation to the nucleus. AP-1 (Activator protein-1) is another transcription factor activated by this cascade.

- The half-life of mRNAs coding for mediators of inflammation is considerably shorter than that of mRNAs of various housekeeping genes (Sharova et al., 2009). The short-lived mRNAs were found to possess (usually in the 3'untranslated regions) AU-rich elements (ARE) recognized by specific proteins that are able to destabilize mRNA and deliver it to the cellular sites of degradation: **exosomes and/or processing bodies** (P-bodies) (Chen et al., 2001; Garneau et al., 2007; Eulalio et al., 2007). The list of ARE-binding proteins involved in mRNA decay includes tristetraprolin (Stoecklin et al., 2004), AUF-1 and AUF-2, (Lu et al., 2006) TIA-1 and TIAR (Dean et al., 2004), KSRP (Gherzi et al., 2007) and HuR (Dean et al., 2004). This last protein (HuR) acts in a rather unusual way since it stabilizes mRNA and prolongs its life in the cell. On the other hand, macrophage chemotactic protein-induced protein-1 (MCPIP1), studied also in our laboratory (Mizgalska et al,. 2009; Skalniak et al., 2009), is able to degrade mRNAs coding for IL-1β, IL-6 and IL-12p40 (but not for TNFalpha), although it does not require the ARE signal (Matsushita et al., 2009; Mizgalska et al., 2009)
- Finally, the majority of proteins involved in the control of inflammatory response exhibit short half-lives being susceptible to degradation in a proteasome after initial ubiquitination (for references see Evans, 2005).

This variable length of life and a fast turnover of mediators of inflammation, achieved either at the stage of their mRNA or mature protein, permit for elastic control and fine regulation of inflammatory reactions. An additional mechanism used for the tuning of some inflammatory pathways depends on transient phosphorylation of susceptible proteins by kinases from the MAP family (Herlaar & Brown, 1999). According to Chang and Karin (2001) mammals express at least four distinctly regulated groups of mitogen activated protein kinases able to phosphorylate serine-threonine residues: Jun amino-terminal kinases (JNK), p38 proteins in four isoforms, and two groups of extracellular signal-regulated kinases (ERKs). The representatives of all groups participate in regulation of inflammatory mediators, usually in a multi-step cascade reactions. These cascades may stretch from cell membrane receptors to transcription factors in the cell nucleus; moreover, some of MAP kinases fulfill the role of cellular sensors directly responding to chemical and physical stresses (Chang & Karin, 2001). According to Winzen et al (1999) p38 MAP kinase contributes to cytokine- or stress-induced gene expression by stabilizing mRNAs through ARE-targeted mechanism. The central role of p38 MAPK in the early transcriptional responses to various types of stress has been confirmed in the recent studies discussed by Cuenda & Rousseau (2007) and Whitmarsh (2010). However, since disorganized cytokine signal transduction may have disastrous consequences so the action of protein kinases is monitored by protein phosphatases containing SH2 domain (Src homology 2 domain). Still this is not always sufficient and specific proteins (PIAS) inhibiting activated STATs have evolved (Wormald & Hilton, 2003).

Table 1 shows arbitrary assignment of many components: e.g. IL-6 family has not only proinflammatory but also some anti-inflammatory properties depending on the stage of inflammation (Scheller et al., 2011); the IL-1 family includes at least 11 separate proteins; VEGF is usually regarded as vascular endothelial growth factor but at the same time it shows strong pro-inflammatory activity. Leukotriene LTB4 stimulates migration of leukocytes but this effect is inhibited by lipoxin LXB4 (Conti et al., 1991).

5. Resolution of inflammation and termination of acute phase response

After the injury-elicited initiation of inflammatory reaction followed by fully developed inflammatory response the resolution phase is expected. In reality, however, this scheme is not always observed and at least three different results are possible: (a) acute illness with a fatal outcome; (b) prolonged chronic disease; (c) prompt return to health after a period of reconvalescence.

a. When overproduction of proinflammatory mediatiors continues and negative effects of injury prevail, the generalized systemic inflammatory response may exceed the programmed limits of organism defense resulting in death. Such situations occur during the **acute septic shock syndrome** which is extremely resistant to medical treatment and death is caused not only by invading pathogens but often results from the excess of certain cytokines participating in the multiorgan failure (for references see Herzum & Renz, 2008).

b. When invading pathogens, or other injuring factors, continue their action on the organism but a transient equilibrium is achieved, the development of a **chronic inflammatory disease**, such as rheumatoid arthritis, may occur. Taking into account various mechanisms of molecular pathology, chronic inflammatory diseases are being currently divided into two separate groups: **autoimmune** (Zenewicz et al., 2010) and **auto-inflammatory** ones (Kastner et al., 2010). The first group includes rheumatoid arthritis, inflammatory bowel disease (Crohn disease), type 1 diabetes, psoriasis, lupus erythematosus and multiple sclerosis, and is regarded as dysfunction of T-cells. By contrast, the autoinflammatory diseases are caused by dysfunctional macrophages producing excesive amounts of IL-1beta. Typical examples of autoinflammatory diseases are: type 2 diabetes, cryopyrin-associated periodic syndromes (e.g. familial cold autoinflammatory syndrome, Muckle-Wells syndrome) and neonatal onset of multiinflammatory disease. These disorders respond well to the treatment aimed at limiting synthesis and release of IL-1beta (Dinarello, 2010).

c. Full recovery from the acute systemic inflammatory response goes through the **resolution phase** which represents more than just turning off production of proinflammatory mediators proteins and lipids. In fact, the synthesis of a new type of regulatory molecules is often initiated. First, the anti-inflammatory cytokines (listed in Table 1) appear and gain the field by inhibiting synthesis of proinflammatory cytokines. The most important is probably IL-10 family showing pleiotropic immunosuppressive and anti-inflammatory properties (Fickensher et al., 2002). However, as pointed out by Cavaillon (2001) the strict dichotomy of pro- and anti-inflammatory properties is artificial because the biologoical effects depend considerably on the biological context (Scheller et al.). We found that IL-4, IL-13 and IL-10 inhibit synthesis of TNFα and IL-6 in the whole blood stimulated *ex vivo* with LPS, but are ineffective, or even enhance production of IL-6 in cultured HUVEC endothelial cells (Guzdek et al., 2000). The most important anticytokine and antiinflammatory effects are probably exerted by suppressors of cytokine signaling (SOCS) and protein inhibitors of activated STATs (PIAS) (Ferguson & Johnston 2001; Wormald & Hilton, 2005). In Hawiger's laboratory a recombinant variant of cell-penetrating SOCS3 was obtained showing some protective effects in animal models of inflammation (Jo et al., 2005). Among lipid-derived molecules produced in the resolution phase antiinflammatory properties are shown by lipoxins and resolvins (Table 1 and Anderson, 2010). It should be reminded here that in all phases of inflammatory response complex changes in the profile of metabolic regulators occur on many levels - transcription, mRNA stability, translation and posttranslational modification of proteins (Evans, 2005).

The return to biological homeostasis may be facilitated and supported by pharmacological intervention. Traditionally used in therapy low molecular weight antiinflammatory drugs, such as glucocorticoids, salicylates, cyclosporin, pentoxifylline, tenidap, colchicine, statins, specific inhibitors of p38 MAP kinase, and many others, are now being supplemented with natural macromolecular cytokine inhibitors and antagonists (reviewed in Koj, 1998; Dinarello 2010). Particularly promising are various commercially available chimeric antibodies, some soluble cytokine receptors and constructs of designer cytokines non-existing in nature but powerful in action (Scheller & Rose-John, 2006; Dinarello, 2010; Scheller et al., 2011).

Cytokines:	-- Pro-inflammatory: IL-1, TNFα, IFN-γ, VEGF, IL-12, IL-17, IL-18, IL-23, IL-33 -- IL-6 family: IL-6, IL-11, LIF, OSM, CNTF, CT-1 - Anti-inflammatory: IL-4, IL-10, IL-13, IFNalpha, TGFbeta, IL-1Ra, MCPIP1 -- Chemokines: IL-8, MCP-1 -- Cellular growth factors: FGF, EGF, VEGF
Lipid derivatives:	-- glucocorticoids -- prostaglandins (PGE_2), -- leukotrienes (LTB4) -- lipoxins (LXB4) -- resolvins (RvE1 and E2)
Cell Adhesion Molecules - selectins and integrins:	-- VCAM-1, -- ICAM-1 -- E-selectin
Components of complement, clotting and fibrinolysis pathways:	-- more than a dozen proteins (including some clotting factors and plasminogen activators and inhibitors)
Certain intracellular enzymes and plasma acute phase proteins :	-- superoxide dismutases (MnSOD, ZnSOD) -- cyclooxygenases (COX-1 and COX-2) -- protein kinases from the MAP family (p38, ERKs) -- nitric oxide synthase (NOS) -- fibrinogen, CRP, SAA (and a dozen of other APPs)

Table 1. The main players in the field of inflammation development and control

However, apart from those just mentioned well defined autoinflammatory and autoimmune diseases, certain elements of inflammation can be found in various pathological processes, such as atherosclerosis (Libby, 2002) or neurodegenerative disorders (Glass et al., 2010). In this respect participation of liver in the inflammatory response is very important and only recently it has been fully evaluated as the source of various mediators, and especially acute phase proteins that fulfill various functions.

The pioneering and elegant experiments carried out on the perfused rat liver by Miller et al., (1951) demonstrated that all principal proteins present in the plasma of circulating blood derive – with the notable exception of immunoglobulins – from the liver. Since the rat does not respond to injury by increased production of C-reactive protein, Miller's experiments were inconclusive and the origin of CRP remained a mystery until Hurlimann et al., (1966) demonstrated incorporation of radioactive amino acids into immunologically identified CRP after incubation of liver preparations from injured monkeys and rabbits. Today we know that the main acute phase proteins in the rat belong to alpha globulins (historic aspects of APP synthesis have been discussed in detail elsewhere (Kushner, 1982; Gordon & Koj, 1985; Koj, 2008).

6. Molecular mechanisms of induced synthesis of acute phase proteins

The progress in elucidating the mechanisms of liver acute phase response obtained a new impetus when APPs synthesis, studied both *in vivo* and in tissue culture, became a valuable model for molecular biology. After cultured liver cells became routinely used it was possible to conclude that the "Hepatocyte Stimulating Factor" responsible for synthesis of acute phase proteins is a cytokine distinct from interleukin-1 (Baumann et al., 1984) and named interleukin-6 (Gauldie et al., 1987). In subsequent years it was found that IL-6 is the most important member of a large cytokine family sharing common receptor subunit gp130 and showing a high degree of redundancy (Sehgal et al., 1995; Heinrich et al., 2003; Baumann, 2003). This family includes IL-6, IL-11, leukemia inhibitory factor (LIF), oncostatin M (OSM), cardiotrophin-1 (CT-1), cilliary neurotrophic factor (CNTF) and some other cytokines (Scheller et al., 2011). Recently Liang et al., (2009) reported that IL-22, although not belonging to IL-6 family, can induce almost all symptoms of acute phase response in the liver; however, the mechanism of its action is as yet not fully understood.

It should be emphasized here that as a rule several cytokines are involved in the regulation of liver-produced acute phase proteins, and on this ground at least two types of cytokines and corresponding APPs have been distinguished by Baumann and Gauldie (1994). Type 1 cytokines (IL-1 and TNF families) co-operate with type 2 cytokines (IL-6 family) in the induced expression of such proteins as CRP, serum amyloid A, C3 complement or alpha-1-acid glycoprotein, all belonging to type 2 APPs. On the other hand, synthesis of other proteins - human fibrinogen or rat alpha-2-macroglobulin, are stimulated only by cytokines of IL-6 family while the presence of IL-1 or TNF decreases the response. The balance between the signaling pathways induced by two types of cytokines is very delicate as indicated by the experiments of Uhlar & Whitehead (1999). They found that the magnitude of synergistic stimulation of SAA synthesis is influenced not only by cytokine concentrations but also by the order of addition of IL-1 and IL-6 to cultured human hepatoma cells. Table 2 provides examples of different classes of APPs after taking into account stimulation with two types of cytokines.

Positive acute phase proteins show increased levels after treatment with the appropriate cytokine whereas negative APPs are decreased. Class A – increased up to 200-fold; Class B - increased by 2-5 fold, Class C – increased by at least 25 per cent. Class D – decreased by at least 25 per cent. Please note species differences. Type 1 cytokines : IL-1 or TNFa; type 2 cytokines - IL-6 family. Abbreviations: CRP, C-reactive protein; FBG, fibrinogen; C3C, third component of the complement; ALB, albumin; SAA, serum amyloid A; HPT, haptoglobin; CEP, ceruloplasmin; TST, transthyretin (pre-albumin); A2M, alpha-2-macroglobulin; AGP, alpha-1-acid glycoprotein; HPX, haemopexin; TRF, transferrin.

Positive AP-proteins			Negative APPs
Class A	**Class B**	**Class C**	**Class D**
CRP /type 1 (primates, rabbit)	FBG / type 2 (many species)	C3C / type 1 (many species)	ALB / type 1&2 (many species)
SAA / type 1 (man, mouse)	HPT / type2 (man)	CEP / type 1 (many species)	TST / type 1 (many species)
A2M / type 2 (rat)	AGP / type 1 (many species)	HPX / type 2 (many species)	TRF / type 2 (many species)

Table 2. Classification of selected acute phase plasma proteins based on the magnitude of AP-response and type of stimulating cytokine (Koj, 1985a,c).

It should be remembered that many additional factors modulate the cytokine-induced change of APPs synthesis rate, the most important being glucocorticoids that act synergistically with IL-6, especially in the rat (Koj, 1985c; Ruminy et al., 2001).

Synthetic inhibitors of MAP kinases interfere with many signaling pathways (Herlaar & Brown, 1999; Lee et al., 2000). As shown by Westra et al., (2006) inhibition of p38 MAPK in cells of human hepatoma significantly reduced cytokine-induced synthesis of CRP and fibrinogen (but not of SAA). Among other low-molecular weight drugs statins – originally used for inhibition of cholesterol synthesis - were shown to possess broad anti-inflammatory properties (Sparrow et al., 2001) and effectively reduce certain symptoms of acute phase response (Munford, 2001).

A recent report by Patel et al., (2009) indicates that the aryl hydrocarbon receptor (AHR) can repress cytokine-induced synthesis of APPs in mouse liver. A somewhat similar downregulation of the AP-response was reported by Venteclef et al., (2006) for the liver receptor homolog 1 (LRH-1). Overexpression of LRH-1 resulted in the inhibition of IL-1- and IL-6-mediated FBG, SAA, CRP and HPT gene expression. All of the genes inhibited by LRH-1 in response to cytokine stimulation contain functional C/EBP DNA-binding sites within their promoter regions (Venteclef et al., 2006). Since LRH-1 was originally identified as a key player in cholesterol regulatory mechanisms the authors conclude that this liver orphan receptor could be a novel molecular link between cholesterol homeostasis and inflammation. Still another liver receptor, PPAR-α (peroxisome proliferators-activated receptor-alpha), was found to attenuate the IL-6-induced synthesis of APPs (Mansouri et al., 2008). Direct involvement of hepatic PPARα was demonstrated using a liver-restricted expression of PPARα in mice, while as a distal repercussion the decreased expression of adhesion molecules in aorta was observed.

Development of new techniques of the genomics era, such as subtractive hybridization, differential display or microarrays, provided a global approach in the studies of inducible gene expression and synthesis of APPs. Olivier et al., (1999) described a novel set of hepatic mRNAs preferentially expressed during acute inflammation elicited in the rat by turpentine injection. When sequencing 174 selected clones these authors identified 23 already known AP-proteins, 31 proteins known but so far not related to the AP-response, and discovered 36 novel proteins induced in the liver during turpentine-induced inflammation. More recently the Salier's group studied changes in the human liver transcriptome in patients with systemic inflammation (Coulouarn et al., 2004). They found over 150 specific mRNAs expressed in the liver and correlating with the extent of inflammatory processes. This number was increased to over 600 genes in a model system of human hepatoma cells treated with the conditioned medium from endotoxin-stimulated macrophages (Coulouarn et al., 2005). The kinetic analysis of transcription rate and mRNA stability led the authors to a very important conclusion: inflammation-induced mRNAs appear in the cells not in a random fashion but as consecutive transcriptional waves corresponding to functionally related proteins produced in an orderly fashion.

In order to study the effects of low doses of IL-1 and/or IL-6 on human hepatoma cells HepG2 differential display was used in our laboratory (Wegrzyn et al., 2006). We found that out of 88 cDNA species modulated by IL-6 only 38 represented various known genes, 18 clones matched genomic clones in the NCBI data with hypothetical cDNA sequences, and the remaining 32 clones showed no homology with databases. When the cells were stimulated with the mixture of IL-1 and IL-6 only 43 cDNA fragments were amplified suggesting the prevailing negative regulation by IL-1. The identified transcripts modulated by IL-6 alone, or by both cytokines, were found to code for intracellular proteins engaged in general metabolism, protein synthesizing machinery and cellular signaling.

Since macrophages are important for the development of inflammation and the acute phase response, many attempts have been made to discover pathogen-induced changes in these cells using microarrays: in our case we identified IL-1 and IL-6 responsive genes in human monocyte-derived macrophages using Affymetrix microarrays (Jura et al., 2008). A major problem encountered in our experiments aroused from individual variability of basal transcriptome profile among blood donors. However, out of almost 5000 probe sets consistently detected in all array replicates we found more than 200 genes modulated by IL-1 and/or IL-6, among which 34 could be regarded as novel cytokine-responsive genes of various functions. A detailed analysis indicated that 125 transcripts were stimulated by IL-1 and 39 by IL-6, whereas the number of downregulated genes was similar for both cytokines (approximately 30 genes in each group). Among the identified IL-1 responsive genes we found one of particular interest, named ZC3H12A and coding for MCPIP1, which plays a pivotal role in the control of inflammation. Recent experiments indicate that MCPIP1 enhances decay of mRNAs coding for some inflammatory mediators (Mizgalska et al., 2009; Matsushita et al. 2009), but also interferes with NF-κB-dependent signaling pathway (Skalniak et al., 2009; Liang et al., 2009).

Last years brought abundant information on the role of microRNA in the regulation of gene expression - and the field of inflammation is no exception. As reported by Harris and co-workers (2008) miRNA-126 inhibits VCAM-1 expression in HUVEC culture and thus may be considered as a potential drug reducing leukocyte adherence to endothelial cells, and in consequence their migration to the site of injury.

7. Multiple biological functions of acute phase proteins

Acute phase proteins represent the products of a large group of genes conserved during evolution and regulated by numerous cytokines that show considerable redundancy. This indicates the importance of APPs in respect of survival value for the animal organism and explains the origin of accepted paradigm stating that "**the principal function of APPs is their ability to restore homeostasis disturbed by injury and inflammation** (Koj, 1985b)." Recent years brought further support of this idea as indicated by the data presented in Table 3, but only some of the results will be discussed here, starting from proteinase inhibitors.

Function	AP-proteins engaged
1. Inhibition of proteinases	Macroglobulins, serpins, kininogens:- over 20 proteins
2. Blood clotting and fibrinolysis	Fibrinogen, $\alpha_1$proteinase inhibitor, antithrombin III, $\alpha_2$antiplasmin, C1- inactivator, $\alpha_1$glycoprotein, serum amyloid P, C-reactive protein, kininogens
3. Anti-inflammatory properties	Proteinase inhibitors, fibrinopeptides, haptoglobin
4. Removal of pathogens and foreign materials	C3 complement, C-reactive protein, serum amyloid A and P proteins, fibrinogen
5. Modulation of immunological response	Proteinase inhibitors, C-reactive protein, α_2HS-glyco-protein, C3 complement, fibrinogen
6. Transport of various materials	Transferrin, ceruloplasmin, transthyretin, haptoglobin, hemopexin, $\alpha_1$glycoprotein, macroglobulins, albumin

Table 3. Selected examples of homeostatic functions of APPs

Human plasma contains at least ten distinct and well characterized proteins responsible for the inhibition of various serine-, cysteine-, aspartic- and metalloproteinases. The list of inhibitors includes: alpha-2-macrogloblin(A2M), alpha-1-proteinase inhibitor (API), alpha-1-antichymotrypsin (ACT), inter-alpha trypsin inhibitor (ITI), antithrombin III (AT3), C-1-inactivator (C1N), alpha-2-antiplasmin(APL), beta-1-anticollagenase (BAC) and high and low molecular weight kininogens (HMK and LMK, both able to inhibit cysteine proteinases). Among those ten inhibitors the most important are: API and ACT (both being strong acute phase reactants in man), and A2M (a spectacular APP in the rat).

The dynamic equilibrium between the blood or tissue proteinases and their natural inhibitors is drastically disturbed during acute inflammation (Koj et al., 1993). A massive release of proteolytic enzymes from injured tissues and infiltrating leukocytes or macrophages should be promptly neutralized by a range of antiproteases present in body fluids. Since the reaction between proteinases and inhibitors is in most cases irreversible, and the resulting complexes are removed, the enhanced proteolytic activity could seriously deplete the body reserves of these antiproteases. As demonstrated by many authors such situation occurs in certain cases of acute pancreatitis and in septic shock. However, the acute phase response usually facilitates replenishment of proteinase inhibitors due to their enhanced liver synthesis. In human hepatoma cells the expression of API and ACT is stimulated primarily by IL-6 whereas A2M synthesis in man (in distinction to the rat) is enhanced by IFNgamma (Kordula et al., 1992).

The **macroglobulin family of proteinase inhibitors** comprises a large group of proteins characterized by a broad specificity due to the presence of a characteristic bait region whereas irreversible binding of the enzyme requires a labile thiol ester. The entrapped proteinase may show still some activity toward small molecular weight substrates. Synthesis of alpha-2-macroglobulin in the rat is greatly stimulated during inflammation whereas alpha-1 macroglobulin does not change significantly - and these two macroglobulins have different specificity in respect of proteinase inhibition (Tsuji et al., 1994).

The members of **serine proteinase inhibitors named serpins,** show considerable variations in their strict specificity toward the target enzymes. API (initially named antitrypsin) inhibits also leukocyte elastases, whereas ACT blocks leukocytic cathepsin G. A charactertistic structural feature of all serpins is the existence of an exposed peptide loop which in the native form is in the strained position being replaced to a stable configuration by proteolytic attack. Recently it was found that two hormone-transporting proteins - thyroxin-binding globulin and cortisol-binding globulin, belong also to the serpin superfamily. Although they do not show detectable antiprotease activity, their molecules contain a characteristic polypeptide loop easily cleaved by proteinases (Pemberton et al., 1995). After cleavage of cortisol-binding protein by neutrophil elastase a tenfold decrease of affinity for cortisol was observed. In that way cortisol may be delivered preferentially to the inflammation site abounding in serine proteinases of leukocyte origin.

Rats appear to be unique in their ability to produce considerable amounts of **thiostatin - an inhibitor of cysteine proteinases** (known formerly as alpha-1-acute phase globulin, or rat major acute phase globulin). In fact thiostatin is a special type of kininogen releasing biologically active kinins upon treatment with trypsin-like enzymes (Lalmanach et al., 2010). Thiostatin is able to inhibit calpain, papain and cathepsin L.

As already mentioned, plasma proteinase inhibitors may fulfill some additional functions apart from the removal of specific enzymes. Thus it has been shown that macroglobulins bind highly toxic eosinophil cationic proteins, are involved in the transport of cellular growth factors and may reduce the effects of endotoxin-induced shock, but are also able to modulate immunological response: it was reported that API, ACT and A2M inhibit the activity of natural killer cells and reduce the antibody-dependent cell-mediated cytotoxicity (Ades et al., 1982).

Recent years brought abundant information on the role of some APPs in the modulation of immunological response, removal of pathogens or foreign materials and reduced inflammation. Pentraxins are multimeric proteins including "short pentraxins" (CRP and SAP produced in hepatocytes), and "long pentraxins" (PTX3 synthesized in macrophages, fibroblasts and in activated endothelium) (Szyper-Kravitz, 2006; Mantovani et al., 2008). All pentraxins fulfill the function of soluble pattern recognition receptors interacting with certain bacterial pathogens and with surface of apoptotic cells thus playing an important role in the removal of cell debris. Moreover, CRP and SAP bind and activate certain complement components important for the innate immunity. This may have negative effects in some diseases: it is known that during incipient heart infarct human CRP strongly activates complement cascade at the site of ischaemia thus enhancing tissue injury. Pepys and co-workers (2006) recommend to reduce the increased level of newly synthesized CRP by giving to a patient derivatives of phosphatidyl choline, known to be a good competitive ligand for CRP.

Besides pentraxins, mannose-binding lectin (MBL) and apolipoprotein A1 belong to protective molecules (Szyper-Kravitz, 2005). They are produced in hepatocytes but ApoA1 is a negative APP and MBL level is not affected by cytokines. Szyper-Kravitz et al., (2005) suggest that the discussed pentraxins, as well as MBL and ApoA1, are important for autoimmune diseases and thus are often used - along with CRP - as clinical markers of progression of inflammation.

Serum amyloid A (SAA) is a strongly induced and a well known AP-protein in man and mouse but recently Cheng et al., (2008) and He and co-workers (2009) made original observations. According to Cheng TLR2 is a functional receptor for SAA and its stimulation leads to enhanced activity of NF-κB that is accompanied by increased phosphorylation of MAPKs and accelerated degradation of IkBalpha. In this way SAA may affect the course of AP response and some inflammatory diseases. He and co-workers demonstrated that SAA is a potent endogenous inducer of granulocyte colony-stimulating factor (G-CSF) responsible for neutrophilia. This effect of SAA is dependent on Toll-like receptor TLR2.

As indicated by the results of Kramer et al., (2010) some APPs or their proteolytic fragments are involved in the earliest antiviral response in HIV-1 infection. The active components were identified as serum amyloid A and a peptide derived from alpha-1-proteinase inhibitor. Insights gained into the mechanism of action of acute phase reactants against HIV could be exploited for the development of prophylactic vaccine strategies.

The broadest conclusions on the homeostatic potential of APPs derive from the studies of Sander and Trautwein, (2010). They used an original global approach based on the fact that liver AP-response critically depends on gp130 subunit of the membrane-bound receptor of IL-6 family of cytokines, and subsequent interaction of gp130 with STAT3 transcription factor. By creating mice deficient in this receptor the authors blocked induced synthesis of APPs and this strongly increased the mortality of mice in a model of polymicrobial sepsis. Further experiments showed that hepatic gp130-STAT3 interaction was also essential for mobilization and tissue accumulation of myeloid-derived suppressor cells (MDSC), a cell population known from their anti-inflammatory properties in cancer. The authors identified two hepatocyte-produced proteins - serum amyloid A and Cxcl1/KC chemokine - as cooperatively promoting MDSC mobilization. They concluded that gp130 dependent communication between the liver and MDSCs through some APPs controls the inflammatory responses in the infected mice. The discussed results are related to the new function of SAA as an endogenous TLR2 ligand (Cheng et al., 2008).

8. Concluding remarks

Elucidation of molecular events concerning the initiation and development of inflammatory reaction has progressed considerably during the last 10 years. The membrane-bound and cytosolic receptors recognizing pathogen-associated - or stress-associated - molecular patterns deriving either from invading pathogens or from damaged cells, have been identified. These signals generated by stimulated receptors lead to assembly of inflammasomes - molecular platforms activating the main proinflammatory cytokine – interleukin-1. Then IL-1 and other cytokines utilize the multistep signaling cascades to activate the pivotal transcription factor NF-κB subsequently translocated to the nucleus. There, in cooperation with other TFs, NF-κB initiates transcription of hundreds of genes coding for various proteins participating in inflammation. This process is tightly regulated and properly tuned due to cooperation of many different transcription factors and subsequent stabilization or enhanced decay of specific mRNAs in exosomes. Recent studies led to identification of a new multifunctional regulatory protein MCPIP1, which can affect both mRNA stability and NF-κB signaling. Although the inflammatory response may occur in various forms, particularly important for the final outcome is the liver acute phase response regulated mainly by IL-6 family of cytokines. The liver-produced acute phase proteins exhibit multiple functions important for restoring homeostasis disturbed by injury and inflammation. Particularly interesting are new data on APPs classified as proteinase inhibitors from three families (macroglobulins, serpins and thiostatins) and original findings on the role of protective molecules belonging to pentraxins and serum amyloid A protein. These discoveries create chances for new therapeutic strategies concerning the treatment of septic shock syndrome and chronic autoimmune or autoinflammatory diseases.

9. Acknowledgments

This study was supported by Polish Ministry of Science and Higher Education: 336/N-COST/2008/0 and 776/N-COST/2010/0 and by the European Community's Grant: COST action BM0602.

10. References

Ades, E.W., Hinson, A.; Chapuis-Cellier, C. & Arnaud, P. (1982). Modulation of the immune response by plasma protease inhibitors. 1. Alpha-macroglobulin and alpha-1-antitrypsin inhibit natural killing and antibody-dependent cell-mediated cytotoxicity. *Scand. J. Immunol.*15: 109-113.

Agostini, L., Martinon, F., Burns, K., McDermott, M.F., Hawkins, P.N. & Tschopp, J. (2004). NALP3 forms IL-1b-processing inflammasome with increased activity in Muckle-Wells autoinflammatory disorder. *Immunity* 20: 319-325.

Akira, S., Uematsu, S & Takeuchi, O. (2006). Pathogen recognition and innate immunity. *Cell* 124: 783-801.

Anderson, P. (2010). Post-transcriptional regulons coordinate the initiation and resolution of inflammation. *Nature Rev. Immunol.* 10: 24-35.

Bauernfeind, F.G., Horvath, G., Stutz, A., Alnemri, E.S., MacDonald, K., Speert, D., Fernandes-Alnemri, T., Wu, J., Monks, B.G., Fitzgerald, K.A., Hornung, V. & Latz, E. (2009). Cutting edge: NF-κB activating pattern recognition and cytokine receptors license NLRP3 inflammasome activation by regulating NLRP3 expression. *J. Immunol.* 183: 787-791.

Baumann, H., Jahreis, G.P., Sauder, D.N. & Koj, A. (1984). Human keratinocytes and monocytes release factors which regulate the synthesis of major acute phase plasma proteins in hepatic cells from man, rat and mouse. *J. Biol. Chem.* 259: 7331-7342.

Baumann, H. (2003). STAT activation in the acute phase response, In: *Signal Transducers and activators of transcription (STATs)*, P.B. Sehgal, D.E. Levy & T. Hirano (Eds), 465-491, Kluwer Academic Publishers, Dordrecht - Boston – London.

Baumann, H. & Gauldie, J. (1994). The acute phase response. *Immunol. Today* 15: 74-80.

Bode, J.G., Gatsios, P, Ludwig, S, Rapp, U.R., Haussinger, D., Heinrich, P.C. & Graeve, L. (1999). The mitogen activated protein (MAP) kinase p38 and its upstream activator MAP kinase kinase 6 are involved in the activation of signal transducer and activator of transcription by hiperosmolarity. *J. Biol. Chem.* 274: 30222-30227.

Bogdan, C., Roelinghoff, M. & Diefenbach, A. (2000). Reactive oxygen and reactive nitrogen intermediates in innate and specific immunity. *Current Opinion Immunol.* 12: 64-76.

Brentano, F., Schorr, O., Gay, R.E., Gay, S. & Kyburz, D. (2005). RNA released from necrotic synovial fluid cells activates rheumatoid arthritis synovial fibroblasts via Toll-like receptor 3. *Arthritis Rheum.* 52: 2656-65.

Brough, D., Pelegrin, P. & Rothwell, N.J. (2009). Pannexin-1-dependent caspase-1 activation and secretion of IL-1β is regulated by zinc. *Eur. J. Immunol.* 39: 352-358.

Cavaillon, J.M. (2001). Pro- versus anti-inflammatory cytokines: myth or reality. *Cell Mol. Biol.* 47: 695-702.

Chang, L, Karin, M. (2001). Mammalian MAP kinases signaling cascades. *Nature* 410: 37-40.

Chen, C.Y., Gherzi, R., Ong, S.E., Chan, E.L., Raijmakers, R., Pruijn, G.J.M., Stoecklin, G., Moroni, C., Mann, M. & Karin, M. (2001). AU binding proteins recruit the exosome to degrade ARE-containing mRNAs. *Cell* 107: 451-464.

Cheng, N., He, R., Tian, J., Ye, P.P. & Ye, R.D. (2008). Cutting edge: TLR2 is a functional receptor for acute-phase serum amyloid A. *J. Immunol.* 181: 22-26.

Conti, P,. Reale, M., Barbacane, R.C, Panara, R.M. & Bongrazio, M. (1991) Inhibition of leukotriene B4 in neutrophils by lipoxins A4 and B4. *Agents Actions* 32: 85-87.

Coulouarn, C., Lefebvre, G., Derambure, C., Lequerre, T., Scotte, M., Francois, A., Cellier, D., Daveau, M. & Salier, J.P. (2004). Altered gene expression in acute systemic inflammation detected by complete coverage of the human liver transcriptome. *Hepatology* 39: 353-364.

Coulouarn, C., Lefebvre, G., Daveau, R., Letellier, F., Hiron, M., Daveau, M. & Salier, J.P. (2005). Genome-wide response of the human Hep3B hepatoma cells to proinflammatory cytokines, from transcription to translation. *Hepatology* 42: 946-955.

Cuenda, A. & Rousseau S. (2007) p38 MAP kinases pathway regulation, function and role in human diseases. *Biochim. Biophys. Acta* 1773: 1358-1375.

Dean, J.L.E., Sully G., Clark A.R. & Saklatvala, J. (2004) The involvement of AU-rich element binding proteins in p38 mitogen-activated protein kinase pathway-mediated mRNA stabilization. *Cellular Signaling* 16: 1113-1121.

Dinarello, C.A. (1996). Biologic basis for interleukin-1 in disease. *Blood* 87: 2095-2147.

Dinarello, C.A. (2008) Immunological and inflammatory functions of the interleukin-1 family. *Ann. Rev. Immunol.* 27: 519-550.

Dinarello, C.A. (2010). Anti-inflammatory agents: present and future. *Cell* 140: 935-950.

Eulalio, A., Behm-Ansmant, I. & Izaurralde, E. (2007). P-bodies: at the crossroads of post-transcriptional pathways. *Nature Reviews Molec. Cell Biology* 8: 9-22.

Evans, P.C. (2005). Regulation of proinflammatory signaling networks by ubiquitin: identification of novel targets for anti-inflammatory drugs. *Expert Reviews in Molec. Medicine* 7: 1-19.

Fickensher, H., Hor, S., Kuppers, H., Knappe, A., Wittmann, S. & Sticht, H. (2002) The interleukin-10 family of cytokines. *Trends in Immunlogy* 23 (2): 89-96.

Feldmeyer, L., Keller, M., Niklaus, G., Hohl, D., Werner, S. & Beer, H.D. (2007). The inflammasome mediates UVB-induced activation and secretion of interleukin-1beta by keratinocytes. *Current. Biol.* 17: 1140-1145.

Ferguson PR,& Johnston JA (2001) Suppressors of cytokine signalling (SOCS) regulate cytokine and growth factor responses in the immune system. *Mol Asp Immunol* 2 (2) 92-96.

Ferrari, D., Pizzirani, C., Adinolfi, E., Lemoli, R.M., Curti, A., Idzko, M., Panther, E. & DiVirgilio, F. (2006). The $P2X_7$ receptor: a key player in IL-1 processing and release. *J. Immunol.* 176: 3877-3883.

Garneau, N.L., Wilusz, J. & Wilusz, C.J. (2007) The highways and byways of mRNA decay. *Nature Reviews in Molecular Cell Biology* 8: 113-126.

Gauldie, J., Richards, C., Harnish, D., Landsdorf, P. & Baumann H. (1987). Interferon beta-2/B-cell stimulatory factor 2 shares identity with monocyte-derived hepatocyte stimulating factor and regulates the major acute phase protein response in liver cells. *Proc. Natl. Acad. Sci. USA* 84: 7251-7255.

Gherzi, R., Trabucci, M., Ponassi, M., Ruggiero, T., Costa, G., Moroni, C., Chen, C.Y., Khabari, K.S., Andersen, J.S. & Briata, P. (2007) The RNA-binding protein KSRP promotes decay of beta-catenin mRNA and is inactivated by PI3K-AKT signaling. *PLOS Biology* doi: 101371

Glass, C.K., Saijo, K., Winner, B., Marchetto, M.C. & Gage, F.H. (2010). Mechanisms underlying inflammation in neurodegeneration. *Cell* 140: 918-934.

Gordon, A.H., Koj, A. (editors). The acute phase response to injury and infection. Amsterdam-New York-Oxford, Elsevier/North Holland 1985; 1-339.

Guzdek, A, Stalinska, K., Guzik, K. & Koj, A. (2000). Differential responses of hematopoetic and non-hematopoietic cells to antiinflammatory cytokines: IL-4, IL-13, IL-10. *J Physiol Pharmacol* 51 (3): 387-399.

Halle A., Hornung V., Petzold G.C., Stewart, C.R., Monks, B.G., Reinheckel, T., Fitzgerald, K.A., Latz, E., Moore, K.J., Golenbock, D.T. (2008). The NALP3 inflammasome is involved in the innate immune response to amyloid-beta. *Nature Immunology* 9: 857-865.

Harris, T.A., Yamakuchi, M., Ferlito, M., Mendell, J.T. & Lowenstein, C.J. (2008). MicroRNA-126 regulates endothelial expression of vascular cell adhesion molecule 1. *Proc. Natl. Acad. Sci.* 105: 1516-1521.

Hasan, U., Chaffois, C., Gaillard, C., Saulnier, V., Merck, E., Tancredi, S., Guiet, C., Brière, F., Vlach, J., Lebecque, S., Trinchieri, G., & Bates, E.E. (2005). Human TLR10 is a functional receptor, expressed by B cells and plasmacytoid dendritic cells, which activates gene transcription through MyD88. *J. Immunol.* 174: 2942-50.

Hattori, M., Tugores, A., Westwick, J.K., Veloz, L., Leffert, H.L., Karin, M. & Brenner, D.A. (1993). Activation of activating protein-1 during acute phase response. *Am. J. Physiol.* 264: G95-G103.

He, R.L., Zhou, J., Hanson, C.Z., Chen, J., Cheng, N. & Ye, R.D. (2009). Serum amyloid A induces G-CSF expression and neutrophilia via Toll-like receptor 2. *Blood* 113:429-437.

Heinrich, P.C., Behrmann, I., Haan, S., Hermanns, H.M., Mueller-Newen, G. & Schaper, F. (2003). Principles of interleukin-6-type cytokine signalling and its regulation. *Biochem. J.* 374: 1-20.

Herlaar, E. & Brown, Z. (1999). p38 MAPK signaling cascades in inflammatory disease. *Molecular Medicine Today* 5: 439-447.

Herzum, I. & Renz, H. (2008). Inflammatory markers in SIRS, sepsis and septic shock. *Current Medicinal Chemistry* 15: 581-587.

Hoffmann, O. & Baltimore, D. (2006). Circuitry of nuclear factor kappaB signaling. *Immunol. Reviews* 210: 171-186.

Huang, JH & Liao, W.S.L. (1994). Induction of the mouse serum amyloid A3 gene by cytokines requires both C/EBP family proteins and a novel constitutive nuclear factor. *Molecular and Cellular Biology* 14: 4475-4484.

Hurlimann, J., Thorbecke, G.J. & Hochwald, G.M. (1966). The liver as the site of C-reactive protein formation. *J. Exp. Med.* 123: 365-378.

Jin, C. & Flavell, R.A. (2010). Inflammasome activation. The missing link: how the inflammasome senses oxidative stress. *Immunol Cell Biol* 88: 510-512.

Jo, D., Liu, D., Yao, S., Collins, R.D. & Hawiger, J. (2005). Intracellular protein therapy with SOCS3 inhibits inflammation and apoptosis. *Nature Medicine* 11: 892-898.

Jura, J., Wegrzyn, P., Korostynski, M., Guzik, K., Oczko-Wojciechowska, M., Jarzab, M., Kowalska, M., Piechota, M., Przewlocki, P. & Koj, A. (2008). Identification of interleukin-1 and interleukin-6-responsive genes in human monocyte-derived macrophages using microarrays. *Biochim. Biophys. Acta* 1779, 383-389.

Kastner, D.L., Aksentijevich, I. & Goldbach-Mansky R. (2010). Autoinflammatory disease reloaded: a clinical perspective. *Cell*, 140: 784-790.

Kasza, A., Wyrzykowska, P., Horwacik, I., Tymoszuk, P., Mizgalska, D., Palmer, K., Rokita, H., Sharrocks, A.D. & Jura, J. (2010). Transcription factors Elk-1 and SRF are engaged in IL-1-dependent regulation of ZC3H12A expression. *BMC Molec. Biology* 11:14.

Kawai, T. & Akira, S. (2010). The role of pattern-recognition receptors in innate immunity: update on Toll-like receptors. *Nat Immunol.* 11: 373-84.

Koj, A. (1985a). Definition and classification of acute phase proteins. In Gordon AH and Koj A Eds. *The Acute Phase Response to Injury and Infection*, Amsterdam-New York – Oxford, Elsevier/North Holland 1985; 139-144.

Koj, A. (1985b). Biological functions of acute phase proteins. Ibid 145-160.

Koj, A. (1985c). Regulation of synthesis of acute phase proteins. Ibid. 205-220.

Koj, A., Korzus, E., Baumann, H., Nakamura T. & Travis, J. (1993). Regulation of synthesis of some proteinase inhibitors in human hepatoma HepG2 cells by cytokines, hepatocyte growth factor and retinoic acid . *Biol. Chem. Hoppe-Seyler* 374: 193-201.

Koj, A. & Guzdek, A. (1995). Modified proteins as possible signals in the acute phase response. *Ann. NY Acad. Sci.* 762: 108-119.

Koj, A. (1996). Initiation of acute phase response and synthesis of cytokines *Biochim. Biophys. Acta* 1317:84-94.

Koj, A. (1998). Termination of acute phase response: role of some cytokines and anti-inflammatory drugs *Gen. Pharmacol.* 31: 9-18.

Koj, A. (2008). From the obscure and mysterious acute phase response to Toll-like receptors and the cytokine network. *Current Immunol. Reviews* 4: 199-214.

Kordula, T., Rose-John, S., Heinrich, P.C. & Koj, A. (1992). Interferon gamma regulates alpha-2-macroglobulin and alpha-1-antichymotrypsin expression at the pretranslational level in HepG2 cells. *Folia Histochem. Cytobiol.* 30: 147-150.

Kramer, H.B., Lavender, K.J., Quin, L., Stacey, A.R., Liu, M.K.P., diGleria, K., Simmons, A., Gasper-Smith, N., Haynes, B.F., McMichael, A.J., Borrow, P. & Kessler, B.M. (2010). Elevation of intact and proteolytic fragments of acute phase proteins constitutes the earliest systemic antiviral response in HIV-1 infection. *PLOS Pathogens* 6: e1000893.

Kushner, I. (1982). The phenomenon of the acute phase response. *Ann. N Y Acad. Sci.* 389: 39-48.

Lalmanach, G., Naudin, C., Lecaille, F. & Fritz, H. (2010). Kininogens: more than cysteine protease inhibitors and kinin precursors. *Biochimie*, 92: 1568-1579.

Lamkanfi, M., Mueller, J.L., Vitari, A.C., Misaghi, S., Fedorova, A., Deshayes, K., Lee, W.P., Hoffman H.M. & Dixit, V.M. (2009). Glyburide inhibits the cryopyrin/Nalp3 inflammasome. *J. Cell Biol.* 187: 61-70.

Lee, J.C., Kumar, S., Griswold, D.E., Underwood, D.C., Votta, B.J. & Adams, J.L. (2000). Inhibition of p38 MAP kinase as a therapeutic strategy. *Immunopharmacology* 47: 185-201.

Liang, S.C., Nickerson-Nutter, C., Pittman, D.D., Carrier, Y., Goodwin, D.G., Shields, K.M., Lambert, A.J., Schelling, S.H., Medley, Q.G., Ma, H.L.; Dunussi-Joannopoulos, K. & Fouser, L.A. (2010). IL-22 induces an acute phase response. *J. Immunology* 185: 5531-5538.

Liang, J.; Saad, Y.; Lei, T.; Wang, J.; Qi, D.; Yang, Q.; Kolattukudy, P.E. & Fu, M. (2009). MCP-induced protein 1 deubiquitinates TRAF proteins and negatively regulates JNK and NF-κB signaling. *J. Exp. Med.* DOI: 10.1084/jem.20092641.

Libby, P. (2002). Inflammation in atherosclerosis. *Nature* 420: 868-874.

Lister, M.F., Sharkey, J., Sawatzky, D.A., Hodgkiss, J.P., Davidson, D.J., Rossi, A.G. & Finlayson, K. (2007). The role of the purinergic $P2X_7$ receptor in inflammation. *J. Inflam.* 4: 5 doi: 10.1186/1476.

Lu, J.Y., Sadri, W. & Schneider, R.J. (2006) Endotoxin shock in AUF1 knockout mice mediated by failure to degrade proinflammatory cytokine mRNAs. *Genes Dev.* 20: 3174-3184.

Mansouri, RM., Bauge, E. Staels, H. & Gervois, P. (2008). Systemic and distal repercussions of liver specific peroxisome proliferator activated receptor alpha control of the acute phase response. *Endocrinology* 149: 3215-3223.

Mantovani, A., Garlanda, C., Doni, A. & Bottazzi, B. (2008). Pentraxins in innate immunity: from C-reactive protein to the long pentraxin PTX3. *J. Clin. Immunol.* 28: 1-13.

Martinon, F., Mayor, A. & Tschopp, J. (2009). The inflammasomes: guardians of the body. *Ann. Rev. Immunol.* 27: 229-265.

Matsushita, K., Takeuchi, O., Standley, D.M., Kumagai, Y., Kawagoe, T., Miyake, T., Satoh, T., Kato, H., Tsujimura, T., Nakamura, H. & Akira, S. (2009). Zc3h12a is an RNase essential for controlling immune responses by regulating mRNA decay. *Nature* 458: 1185-1190.

Mayor, A., Matinon, F., de Smedt, T., Petrilli, V. & Tschopp, J. (2007). A crucial function of SGT1 and HSP90 in inflammasome activity links mammalian and plant innate immune responses. *Nature Immunol* 8: 497-503.

Medzhitov, R., Preston-Hurlburt, P. & Jameway, C.A. (1997). A human homologue of the Drosophila Toll protein signals activation of adaptive immunity. *Nature* 388: 394-397.

Medzhitov, R. (2010). Inflammation 2010: New adventures of an old flame. *Cell* 140: 771-776.

Miller, L.L., Bly, C.G., Watson, M.L. & Bale, W.F. (1951). The dominant role of the liver in plasma protein synthesis. *J Exp. Med.* 94: 431-453.

Mizgalska, D., Wegrzyn, P., Murzyn, K., Kasza, A., Koj, A. & Jura, J. (2009). Interleukin-1 inducible MCPIP protein has structural and functional properties of RNase and participates in degradation of IL-1β mRNA *FEBS J.* 276, 7386-7399.

Munford, R.S. (2001). Statins and the acute phase response. *N. Engl. J. Med.* 344: 2016-2018.

Nathan, C. (2002). Points of control in inflammation. *Nature* 420: 846-852.

Oliver, K.M., Taylor, C.T. & Cummins, E.P. (2009). Regulation of NF-κB signaling during inflammation: the role of hydroxylases. *Arthritis Res. Ther.* 11: 215-223.

Olivier, E., Soury, E., Risler, J.L., Smith, F., Schneider, K., Lochner K., Jouzeau, J.Y., Fey, G.H. & Salier, J.P. (1999). A novel set of hepatic mRNAs preferentially expressed during an acute inflammation in rat represents mostly intracellular proteins. *Genomics* 57: 352-364.

O'Neill, L.A.J. & Bowie, A.G. (2007). The family of five: TIR-domain-containing adaptors in Toll-like receptor signaling. *Nature Reviews Immunology* 7: 353-364.

Ospelt, C. & Gay, S. (2009). TLRs and chronic inflammation. *Biochem Cell Biol.* 42: 495-505.

Patel, R.D., Murray, I.A., Flaveny, C.A., Kusnadi, A. & Perdew, G.H. (2009). AH receptor represses acute-phase response gene expression without binding to its cognate response element. *Laboratory Investigations* 89: 695-707.

Pemberton, P.A., Wong, D.T., Gibson, H.L., Kiefer, M.C., Fitzpatrick, P.A., Sager, R. & Barr, P.J. (1995). The tumor suppressor maspin does not undergo the stressed to relaxed transition or inhibit trypsin-like serine proteases. Evidence that maspin is not a protease inhibitory serpin. *J. Biol. Chem.* 270: 15832-7.

Pepys, M.B.; Hirschfield, G.M.; Tennent, G.A; Galllimore, J.R; Kahan, M.C., Bellotti, V., Hawkins PM, Myers, R.M. Smith, MD, Polara A,, Cobb A.J.A. Ley SV, Aquilina JA., Robinson CV, Sharif I, Gray GA, Sabin CA, Jenvey MC, Kolstoe SE,Thompson D. & Wood, S.P. (2006). Targeting C-reactive protein for the treatment of cardiovascular disease. *Nature* 440:1217-21.

Ray, A., LaForge, K.S., & Sehgal, P.B. (1990). On the mechanism for the efficient repression of the interleukin-6 promoter by glucocorticoids: Enhancer, TATA box and RNA start site (Inr motif) occlusion. *Mol. Cell Biol.* 10: 5736-5746.

Rock, K.L., Latz, E., Ontiveros, F., & Kono, H. (2010). The sterile inflammatory response. *Ann. Rev. Immunol.* 28: 321-342.

Ruminy, P., Gangneux, C., Claeyssens, S., Scotte, M., Daveau, M. & Salier, J.P. (2001). Gene transcription in hepatocytes during the acute phase of a systemic inflammation: from transcription factors to target genes. *Inflammation Research* 50: 383-390.

Sander, L.E., Sackett, S.D., Dierssen, U., Beraza, N., Linke, R.P., Mueller, M., Blander, J.M., Tacke, F. & Trautwein, C. (2010). Hepatic acute phase proteins control innate immune responses during infection by promoting myeloid-derived suppressor cell function. *J. Exp. Med.* 207: 1453-1464.

Scheller, J. & Rose-John, S. (2006). Interleukin-6 and its receptor: from bench to bedside. *Med. Microbiol. Immunol.* 195: 175-183.

Scheller, J., Chalaris, A., Schmidt-Arras, D. & Rose-John, S. (2011). The pro- and anti-inflammatory properties of the cytokine interleukin-6. *Biochim. Biophys. Acta* 1813: 878-888.

Schroder, K. & Tschopp, J. (2010). The inflammasomes. *Cell* 140: 821-832.

Sehgal, P.B., Wang, L., Rayanade R., Pan, H.& Margulies, L. (1995). Interleukin-6 type cytokines. *Ann N Y Acad Sci*, 762: 1-14.

Sehgal, P.B. (2008). Paradigm shifts in the cell biology of STAT signaling. *Seminars in Cell and Developmental Biology* 13: 329-340.

Shapiro, L. & Dinarello, C.A. (1997). Hyperosmotic stress as a stimulant for proinflammatory cytokine production. *Exp. Cell Research* 23: 1354-362.

Sharova, L.V., Sharov, A.A. Nedorezov, T., Piao, Y., Shaik, N. & Ko, M.S.H. (2009). Database for mRNA half-life of 19977 genes obtained by DNA microarray analysis of pluripotent and differentiating mouse embryonic stem cells. *DNA Research* 16: 45-58.

Sheikh, N., Dudas, J. & Ramadori, G. (2007). Changes of gene expression of iron regulatory proteins during turpentine oil-induced acute phase response in the rat. *Lab. Invest.* 87: 713-725.

Skalniak, L., Mizgalska, D., Zarebski, A., Wyrzykowska, P., Koj, A. & Jura, J. (2009). Regulatory feedback loop between NF-κB and MCP-1-induced protein 1-RNase. *FEBS J.* 276: 5892-5905.

Sparrow, C.P., Burton, C.A., Hernandez, M., Mundt, S., Hassing, H., Patel, S., Rosa, R., Hermanowski-Vosatka, A., Wang, P.R., Zhang, D., Peterson, L., Detmers, P.A., Chao, Y.S. & Wright, S.D. (2001). Simvastatin has anti-inflammatory and antiatherosclerotic activities independent of plasma cholesterol lowering. *Arteriosclerosis, Thrombosis and Vascular Biology* 21: 115-121.

Stehlik, C., & Dorfleutner, A. (2007). COPs and POPs: modulators of inflammasome activity. *J. Immunol.* 179: 7993-7998.

Stoecklin, G., Stubbs, T., Kedersha N., Wax, S., Rigby, W.F., Blackwell, T.K. & Anderson, B. (2004). MK-2 induced tristetraprolin: 14-3-3 complexes prevent stress granules association and ARE-mRNA decay. *EMBO J.* 23: 1313-1324.

Szyper-Kravitz, M., Pitashny, M. & Shoenfeld, Y. (2005). Protective molecules - C-reactive protein (CRP), serum amyloid P (SAP), pentraxin3 (PTX3), mannose-binding lectin (MBL), and apolipoprotein A1 (ApoA1), and their autoantibodies: prevalence and clinical significance in autoimmunity. *J. Clin. Immunol.* 25: 582-591.

Takeuchi O. & Akira S. (2010). Pattern recognition receptors and inflammation. *Cell* 140: 805-820.

Tillett, W.S. & Francis, T. (1930). Serological reactions in pneumonia with a non-protein somatic fraction of pneumococcus. *J. Exp. Med.* 73: 173-182.

Tsuji, A., Akamatsu, T., Nagamune, H. & Matsuda, Y. (1994). Identification of targeting proteinase for rat alpha-1-macroglobulin in vivo. Mast cell tryptase is a major component of the alpha-1-macroglobulin-proteinase complex endocytosed into rat liver lysosomes. *Biochem. J.* 298: 79-85.

Uhlar, C.M. & Whitehead, A.S. (1999). The kinetics and magnitude of the synergistic activation of the serum amyloid A promoter by IL-1β and IL-6 is determined by the order of cytokine addition. *Scand. J. Immunol.* 49: 399-404.

Van den Berghe, W., Vermeulen, L., de Wilde, G., de Bosscher K., Boone, E. & Haegeman, G. (2000). Signal transduction by tumor necrosis factor and gene regulation of the inflammatory cytokine interleukin-6. *Biochem Pharmacol.* 60: 1185-1195.

Venteclef, N., Smith, J.C., Goodwin, B. & Delerive P. (2006) Liver receptor homolog 1 is a negative regulator of the hepatic acute phase response. *Molecular and Cellular Biology* 26: 6799-6807.

Wenger, R.H., Rolfs, A., Marti, H.H., Bauer, C., Gassman, M. (1995). Hypoxia, a novel inducer of acute phase gene expression in a human hepatoma cell line. *J Biol. Chem.* 270: 27865-27870.

Węgrzyn, P., Jura, J., Kupiec, T., Piekoszewski, W., Władyka, B., Zarebski, A. & Koj, A. (2006). A search for genes modulated by interleukin-6 alone or with interleukin-

1beta in HepG2 cells using differential display analysis. *Biochim. Biophys. Acta* 1762: 319-328.

Whitmarsh A.J. (2010) A central role for p38 MAPK in the early transcriptional response to stress. *BMC Biology* 8:47 doi:10.1186/1741-7007-8-47.

Winzen, R., Kracht., M, Ritter, B., Wilhelm, A., Chen, C.Y., Shyu, A.B., Muller, M., Resch, K. & Holtmann, H. (1999) The p38 MAP kinase pathway signals for cytokine-induced mRNA stabilization via MAP-kinase activated protein kinase-2 and an AU-rich region-targeted mechanism. *EMBO J.* 18: 4969-4980

Westra, J., Bizet, J., Doornbos-van der Meer, B., van Rijswijk, M.H. & Limburg, P.C. (2006). Differential influence of p38 mitogen activated protein kinase (MAPK) inhibition on acute phase protein synthesis in human hepatoma cell lines. *Ann. Rheum. Dis.* 65: 929-935.

Wormald, S. & Hilton, D.J. (2004). Inhibitors of cytokine signal transduction. *J. Biol. Chem.* 279: 821-824.

Ye, Z. & Ting, J.P.Y. (2008). NLR, the nucleotide-binding domain leucine rich repeat containing gene family. *Current Opinion Immunol.* 20: 3-9.

Zagorska, A. & Dulak, J. (2004). HIF-1: the known and unknown of hypoxia sensing. *Acta Biochim. Pol.* 51: 563-585.

Zenewicz, L.A., Abraham, C., Flavell, R.A. & Cho, J.H. (2010). Unravelling the genetics of autoimmunity. *Cell* 140: 791-797.

Zhou, R., Tardivel, A., Thorens, B., Choi, I. & Tschopp, J. (2010). Thioredoxin-interacting protein links oxidative stress to inflammasome activation. *Nature Immunol.* 11: 136-140.

IL-22 Induces an Acute-Phase Response Associated to a Cohort of Acute Phase Proteins and Antimicrobial Peptides as Players of Homeostasis

Francisco Veas and Gregor Dubois
Comparative Molecular Immuno-Physiopathology Lab. UMR-MD3
Faculty of Pharmacy, University Montpellier 1, Montpellier
France

1. Introduction

Upon different external *stimuli* including bacteria and virus infection, and internal *stimuli* including both self-damaged products from trauma, burn injury, surgery, cancer mediated inflammatory disorders, exhausting exercises, child delivery and stroke as well as different immune diseases, an organism need to react in order to continuously preserve an equilibrated thermodynamic state, namely homeostasis. This process is highly conserved in living beings. The absence of this global state generates pathological processes and ultimately, the death.

1.1 Acute phase response

In mammals, a complex network of intercellular and intracellular signaling participates to the maintain of homeostasis after stimulus by recognizing non-self elements in the body, involving pro-inflammatory processes, including cytokines, cytokine modulators, and hormones associated to a number of systemic changes referred as the acute-phase response (APR). Moreover, APR occuring quickly after *stimuli*, is a transient modulation of physiological process favoring innate defense of organisms during this early phase of physiological perturbed situation or illnesses (infection or trauma) involving modulation of production, mostly by the liver, of some blood proteins namely acute phase proteins (APP) to resolve the local inflammation, repair the injured tissue, and re-establish homeostasis. Thus, both pro- and anti-inflammatory responses are initiated almost at the same time, with a little delay of anti-inflammatory responses and concomitantly signals act synergistically (Adib-Conquy & Cavaillon, 2009).
Inflammation is key in homeostatic processes elicited by microbial components or by tissue damage products. The outcomes, **either tissue repair or persistent inflammatory damage and degeneration**, strongly depend of the local cell death profile and its associated molecules as well as on the features of infiltrating antigen cell presenting cells. Monocytes, platelets and endothelial cells participate in vascular inflammation that regulates the

humoral innate immunity and participates in homeostatic processes by activating, for example, anti-inflammatory regulators.
The acute-phase response is resolved as soon as stimulation disappears. These APR regulation is due to the expression of inflammation regulators including IL-10, SOCS, soluble receptors of inflammatory cytokines (IL-1ra) as well as due to short span of APP and their mRNA half-lives. In cases where inflammation becomes deregulated, the acute-phase response become chronic, and local inflammation potentially becomes systemic.
Not only pathogenic, but also, in a lesser extent, non-pathogenic microorganisms harbor the highly conserved non-self molecules which are critical for their survival or for their pathogenicity. During infectious processes cells, including macrophages respond to exogenous danger signals induced by the pathogens associated molecular patterns (PAMPs) or Microbe-associated molecular patterns (MAMPs) that are not found as a part of eukaryotic cells. This response is amplified by endogenous mediators released and by co-factors or concomitant stressful events, and molecular mechanisms involved in the vicious circle destruction-reconstruction of vessels and tissues, act through injury-associated signals known as Damage-Associated Molecular Patterns (**DAMPS or Alarmins)** and **acute phase proteins**.
Among PAMPs, Gram-negative and Gram-positive bacteria respectively express at their surface LPS and peptidoglycan as well as lipotechoic acid. In addition, molecules found in microorganisms include mannose (almost absent in humans), bacterial unmethylated CpG DNA, bacterial flagellin, the amino acid *N*-formyl-methionine found in bacterial proteins, double-stranded and single-stranded RNA from viruses, and glucans, mannans, and zymosan from fungal cell walls. More than 1 000 recognition elements have been identified and designated by soluble pattern-recognition receptors.
Damage-associated molecular patterns (**DAMPs**) or **alarmins**, are released by stressed cells and act as endogenous danger signals promoting and enhancing the inflammatory response. The following molecules: **S100A8** and **S100A9** participate in migration and cytoskeletal metabolism. Cell damage or activation of phagocytes triggers their release into the extracellular space where they become danger signals that activate immune cells and vascular endothelium. S100A8 and S100A9 seem to interact with RAGE4 and TLRs (Vogl et al., 2007); the nuclear, high mobility group box-1 (**HMGB1**) protein that is not characterized by having pro-inflammatory activity but it binds LPS, DNA or IL-1β and induces signaling pathways leading to NF-κB activation thereby enhancing inflammatory pathways; and Serum amyloid A (**SAA**) released by **necrotic cells** are the major DAMPs increased in serum of **several inflammatory diseases**, including cancer, sepsis, atherosclerosis, and arthritis. Several receptors appear to mediate the effect of SAA, including FPRL1, RAGE, TLR2 and TLR4. The downstream signaling pathways triggered by SAA include ERK and p38 activation induces chemotactic for neutrophils and the production of proinflammatory cytokines and NO(He et al., 2009; Sandri et al., 2008). DAMPs activate innate immune response through pattern recognition receptors (PRRs) (Bianchi, 2007) such as Receptor for advanced glycation end products (RAGE) found in endothelial cells and macrophages and activate MAPkinase-dependent inflammation upon interaction with one of the following factors HMGB1, S100 proteins and β-amyloids (van Beijnum et al., 2008). Some DAMPs engage TLRs to induce and amplify the inflammatory response. **TLR2** and **TLR4** signaling have been shown to mediate NF-κB activation initiated by HMGB1 (Park et al., 2006), S100A8 (Vogl et al., 2007) and SAA (He et al., 2009; Sandri et al., 2008). Different signaling

pathways are involved that may cross-talk at several levels, but all culminate in the activation of NF-κB.

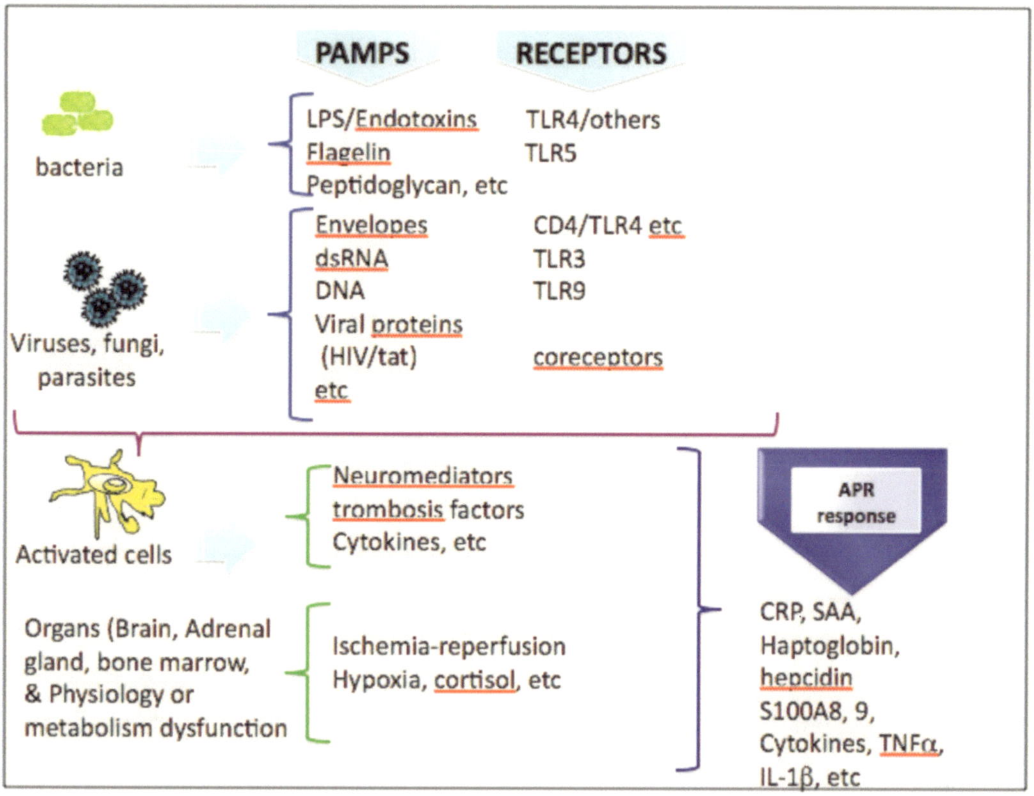

Fig. 1. PAMPS as inducers of the APR.

2. Organs involved in the APR

Organs involved in the APR include: **brain**, (involved in fever, anorexia, somnolence and increased synthesis of CRH and ACTH); **liver**, (increased amounts of metallothionein and antioxidants and which re-orchestrates its pattern of plasma protein synthesis); **bone marrow**, (erythropoiesis is suppressed and thrombocytosis induced, and loss of bone substance occurs; **the adrenal gland**, (cortisol production is enhanced by both direct and indirect stimulation); **muscle**, (decreased protein synthesis and proteolysis may occur); and **fat cells**, (alterations in lipid metabolism)(Kushner, 1993).

2.1 Acute phase proteins

A change of approximately 25% in plasma concentration has been suggested as the definition of acute phase proteins (APP, (Morley & Kushner, 1982)). Changes in plasma protein concentrations mainly depend of their synthesis by liver cells in response to circulating inflammation-associated cytokines.

CRP present at high concentrations in a patient with pneumonia allowed its discovery in 1930. CRP is one of the major APP, which increase in response to sudden homoeostatic disequilibrium. More generally, during the acute-phase response, circulating levels of plasma proteins increase (positive APPs) or decrease (negative APPs).

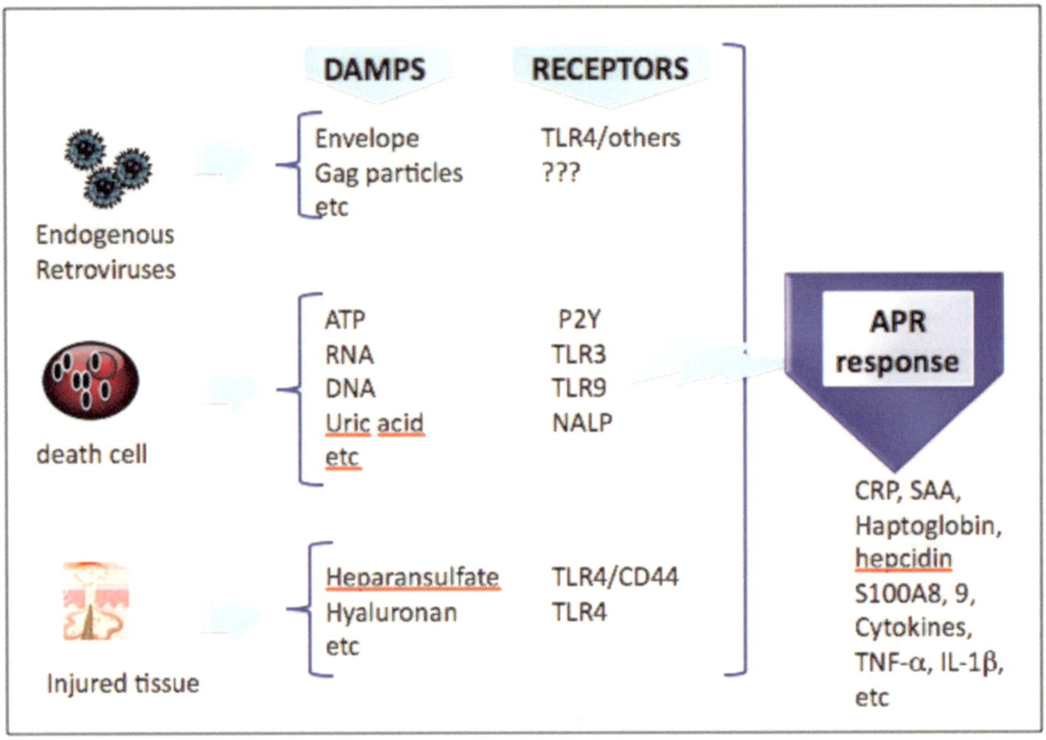

Fig. 2. DAMPs as inducers of the APR

Thus, upon stimuli, amount changes of different proteins are observed. In normal situations, the major positive APP, CRP and SAA, are present in only very low amounts, but they are able to rapidly increase by around of 1000-fold upon infection for example. In a similar situation, haptoglobin, α-acid glycoprotein, α_1-protease inhibitor, α-antichymotrypsin and fibrinogen, increase about 2–5-fold. Whereas, only a modest elevation, of about 50%, is exhibited by both, ceruloplasmin and the complement components C3 and C4. In contrast, the negative APPs, such as albumin, transferrin, transthyretin, α_2 HS glycoprotein, α-fetoprotein, insulin-like growth factor-1 (IGF-1) and coagulation factor XII, typically decrease during the acute-phase response.

Even if not possible for all APP, most of them have been classified in functional categories as illustrated here with some examples: **Antiproteases**: α_1-protease inhibitor, α_1-antichymotrypsin, pancreatic secretory trypsin inhibitor and inter-a-trypsin inhibitors; **Molecules of coagulation and fibrinolysis**: plasminogen, tissue plasminogen activator (tPA), urokinase, protein S, vitronectin and plasminogen activator inhibitor 1 (PAI-1); **Complement molecules**: complement factors C3, C4, C9, C-1 inhibitor, C4b-binding protein, factor B, and mannose-binding lectin (MBL); **Transport proteins**: ceruloplasmin, haptoglobin and hemopexin. This is the case of the major APP, CRP, SAA, a1-acid glycoprotein, fibronectin, angiotensinogen, ferritin and beta2-glycoprotein I. It is to be noteworthy that the expression level of APP could be specie-dependent, such as APP in alpha-macroglobulin that is highly expressed in rat but not in humans (Gabay & Kushner, 1999).

Certain APPs are involved in the regulation of the inflammatory response. These include secreted phospholipase A2 (pLA2), lipopolysaccharide (LPS)-binding protein, and interleukin 1 receptor antagonist (IL-1Ra) (Gabay et al., 1997). In response to the non-self antigen exposure, a healthy host must rapidly interact with it to initiate an antigen-non-specific recognition *via* innate immunity mechanisms controlling and maintaining homeostasis. This response helps **the organism not only to eliminate microbes and/or** preventing infection, but also eliminates all defective self-molecules.

Most of the APP play a protective role, such as haptoglobin (Cid et al., 1993),Thus, for example, hemopexin exhibits an anti-oxydant activity as well as certain anti-proteases including α1-antichymotrypsin suppresses superoxide anion production, vitronectin inhibits cell lysis complement-mediated (Kilpatrick et al., 1992). Among the main acute phase proteins, two of them are hyper-reactive, the C-reactive protein (CRP) and the mannose-binding lectin (MBL) that act as soluble pattern-recognition receptors. The CRP binds to membrane phospholipids of microorganisms such as phosphorylcholine from bacteria and phosphatidylethenolamine from fungus. It allows binding of microorganism to phagocytes, and activates the classical complement pathway (Ahmed et al., 1996; Cermak et al., 1993; Jiang et al., 2006). Most of the effects of the other main acute-phase protein in humans, the serum amyloid A (SAA), are still unknown. SAA rapidly bind to high-density lipoprotein and influence cholesterol metabolism during inflammatory states. SAA mainly induces lymphocytes and phagocytic cells adhesion and chemotaxis may increase the oxidation of low-density lipoproteins (Banka et al., 1995; Berliner et al., 1995; Malle & De Beer, 1996)

Mostly, these molecules play a role of scavenger proteins by transporting microorganism up to cells (mainly macrophages) in charge of the non-self evacuation. Beta2-glycoprotein I (Agar et al., 2011), also known under the name of Apolipoprotein H (ApoH) is one of the acute phase proteins exhibiting the most striking scavenger properties, strikingly is able to catch early apoptotic cells in a Ca2+-independent manner(d'Angeac et al., 2005). This protein traps every kind of pathogenic microorganisms, including parasites (examples: *Leishmania donovani, Plasmodium falciparum,* etc), Gram + or Gram - bacteria (*Escherichia coli, Salmonella, Listeria monocytogenes, Staphylococcus aureus,* etc) and RNA or DNA enveloped or non-enveloped viruses (Hepatitis B, Hantaviruses, HIV, Rotaviruses, and others viruses) (Godoy et al., 2009; Stefas et al., 1997; Stefas et al., 2001). In addition, products of the complement pathways, in turn, promote inflammation; chemoattract phagocytes to the infected zone, also attach microbes to phagocytes, and finally induce cytolysis of infected cells.

During the acute-phase response, in addition to plasma proteins changes induced by or associated to pro-inflammatory cytokines, other kinds of changes are observed, such as those associated with neuroendocrine, including somnolence (may reduce energy requirements), anorexia, fever, etc. that are related with an increased secretion of corticotrophin-releasing hormone (CRH), adrenocorticotrophic hormone (ACTH), cortisol and arginine, vasopressin, insulin serum levels and decreased insulin-like growth factor 1 (IGF-1). Haematopoietic changes include the anaemia of chronic disease, leucocytosis and thrombocytosis. Metabolic changes include, loss of muscle with decreased nitrogen, gluconeogenesis, increased leptin, osteoporosis and cachexia. Intrahepatic changes include increased synthesis of metallothionein, inducible nitric oxide synthase (iNOS), a haeme oxygenase (HO), manganese superoxide dismutase (mSOD), hepatocyte growth factor activator (HGFa), glutathione and tissue inhibitor of metalloproteinase 1 (TIMP-1). In addition, changes in lipid metabolism occur, including increased hepatic lipogenesis, lipolysis in adipose tissue, decreased lipoprotein lipase activity in muscle and adipose tissue, increased plasma levels of triglycerides. Fever may stimulate chemotaxis, cytokine production, complement-mediated opsonization, and T-cell function. Increased hepatic production of the antioxidant agents, haeme oxygenase and manganese superoxide dismutase may be required for the limitation of oxidant mediated-tissue injury. Hypercortisolaemia can modulate the immune and inflammatory responses and play a major role in the maintenance of haemodynamic stability in patients with severe illness.(Gabay & Kushner, 1999).

Lipids produced in excess circulate and are also used as nutrients by immune cells from inflammation to rebuild their damaged membranes. A lipid excess that could enhance inflammatory processes. Some of these circulating lipoproteins, such as leptin, are able to bind LPS and decrease its inflammatory effects, moreover, may play a direct or indirect a role in host defense against different microbial agents such as the scavenger role of Apoliproprotein H.

As for inflammatory processes, the APR is beneficial for the host when this response happens in within very short kinetics. In contrast, a persistence of the acute-phase response due to chronic stimulation, in chronic diseases, metabolic disturbances strongly inducing a loss of skeletal muscles, adipose tissue and osteoporosis, frequently leads to cachexia. This persistence associating cytokines activity with the acute-phase response could become fatal, as observed in septic shock.

In some patients with chronic inflammatory conditions, chronically cleaved SAA could induce amyloidosis with deleterious consequences forming plaques in brain that could enhance neurological diseases, such as Alzheimer disease.

3. APR and Antimicrobial activities

Thus, cells receiving PAMPS and/or DAMPS (or alarmins) *stimuli* through corresponding molecular interactions, will, in turn, initiate APR by modulating the expression of pro-inflammatory cytokines and APP. Some of these APPs exhibit antimicrobial activities similarly to antimicrobial peptides (AMP).

Gene-encoded anti-microbial peptides (AMPs) are widespread in nature, as they are synthesized by microorganisms as well as by multicellular organisms from both the vegetal and the animal kingdoms. These naturally occurring AMPs form a first line of host defense against pathogens and are involved in innate immunity. Depending on their tissue distribution, AMPs ensure either a systemic or a local protection of the organism against environmental pathogens. They are classified into three major groups: (i) peptides with an alpha-helical conformation (insect cecropins, magainins, etc.), (ii) cyclic and open-ended cyclic peptides with pairs of cysteine residues (defensins, protegrin, etc.), and (iii) peptides with an over-representation of some amino acids (proline rich, histidine rich, etc.). Most AMPs display hydrophobic and cationic properties, have a molecular mass below 25-30 kDa, and adopt an amphipathic structure (alpha-helix, beta-hairpin-like beta-sheet, beta-sheet, or alpha-helix/beta-sheet mixed structures) that is believed to be essential to their anti-microbial action. Interestingly, in recent years, a series of novel AMPs have been discovered as processed forms of large proteins. Despite the extreme diversity in their primary and secondary structures, all natural AMPs have the in vitro particularity to affect a large number of microorganisms (bacteria, fungi, yeast, virus, etc.) with identical or complementary activity spectra. This review focuses on AMPs forming alpha-helices, beta-hairpin-like beta-sheets, beta-sheets, or alpha-helix/beta-sheet mixed structures from invertebrate and vertebrate origins. These molecules show some promise for therapeutic use (Bulet et al., 2004).

AMP are cationic small proteins involved in host innate immune defense by mainly binding negatively charged (acidic) phospholipids (Fig. 3), even other different mechanism remain to be elucidated. The presence of cholesterol and the absence of acidic phospholipids in normal human cells avoid that AMP could attack the self cells.

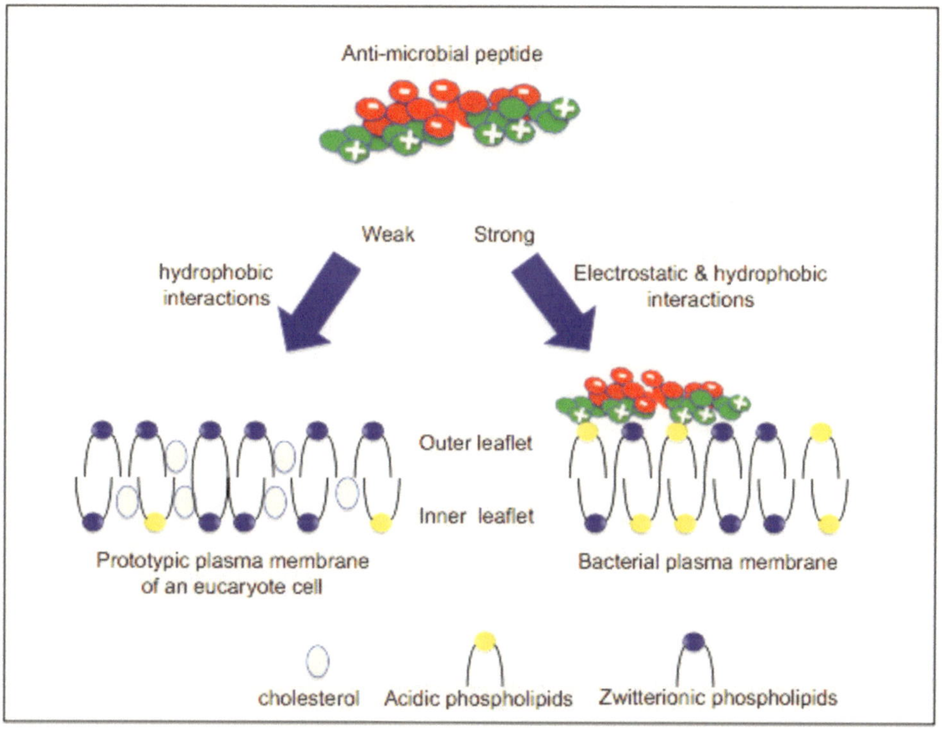

Fig. 3. Antimicrobial peptide activity on membranes from eukaryote and prokaryotes cells.

AMPs are highly conserved in within organism's evolution, thus they are present from bacteria, amoebas up to Humans. In vertebrates, they are abundant in mucosal tissues (eyes, mouth, genitourinary, skin, lung, trachea), some patrol cells (neutrophils, platelets, etc), intestinal tract (duodenum). In humans, Paneth cells are an important source, that mainly secrets alpha-defensins, when stimulated by bacterial PAMPs (lipopolysaccharide, muramyl dipeptide and lipid A). In addition to defensins, these cells secrete lysozyme and phospholipase A2 that also exhibit an antimicrobial activity. These secretory molecules show a broad anti-infectious spectrum of agents, (bacteria, fungi and viruses) protecting the gut as a gastrointestinal innate barrier.

Then, upon bacteria killing by AMP, bacteria release inflammatory mediators (LPS, LTA), that will induce the cell (monocytes, macrophage) responses, adherence of PMN and chemotaxis, histamine degranulation of mast cells, fibroblast growth as well as the induction of adherence, apoptosis of viral- or bacteria-infected host cells, inhibition of fibrin clot lysis (to limit bacterial spread) and inhibition of proteases (to limit tissue injury). If inflammation becomes chronic AMP will participate in both T cell recruitment as well as enhancement of monocyte chemotaxis and macrophage response.

A rich literature has reported results directly or indirectly demonstrating the efficiency of AMP. Mice carrying a genetically engineered metalloproteinase deficiency showed an increased susceptibility to bacterial infection generating an absence of soluble α-defensins to protect mice against bacteria due to the absence of their extracellular cleavage and activation (Wilson et al., 1999). In a mouse model of septicemia, LL-37 binds to and neutralizes LPS and protects against endotoxic shock (Bals et al., 1999). Histatins protect from periodontal disease by inhibiting the *B. gingivalis* protease (Nishikata et al., 1991).

Due the efficiency against microbes the use of AMP, some AMP have been extracted from species different of those where effects are needed. This is the case of dermaseptin (DS), a 34 amino acid residue cationic peptide isolated from *Phyllomedusa sauvagii* skin, has been incubated *in vitro* with promastigotes of *Leishmania mexicana*. Immunocytochemical, and electron microscopic observations have shown that the amphipathic peptide generates disrupt the lipid bilayer leading of the surface membrane and death of the parasite (Hernandez et al., 1992).

Hepcidin (gene name, *HAMP*), an IL-6-inducible acute phase protein that also exhibit antimicrobial properties, is the key negative regulator of iron metabolism. Liver is the primary source of *HAMP* synthesis, but it is also produced by other tissues such as kidney or heart and is found in body fluids such as urine or cerebrospinal fluid. Hepcidin is a stress-inducible peptide of the biliary epithelia. In the bile, hepcidin help to protect against bacterial infections (Strnad et al., 2011).

Studies in transgenic mice confirmed that **C-reactive protein** is protective against microbial pathogens thru its *in vitro* ability to bind microbes, activating the complement classical and alternative pathways as well as FcγRII (Szalai, 2002).

SAA is the major acute phase protein in man and most mammals. Recently, it was demonstrated that SAA binds to many Gram-negative bacteria including *Escherichia coli* and *Pseudomonas aeruginosa* through outer membrane protein A (OmpA) family members. At normal concentrations of SAA, the SAA-*E coli* opsonization increase, both the rate of neutrophils with bacteria as well as the number of bacteria. The amount of neutrophil reactive oxygen intermediate production and phagocytosis by both neutrophils and IL-10 and TNFa-producers macrophages are enhanced in a SAA-dependent manner (Shah et al., 2006).

CRP have both properties to induce proinflammatory cytokines and tissues factor and anti-inflammatory for example inhibiting superoxide anions secretion by neutrophils as well as inducing IL-1ra synthesis by PBMC. Serum amyloid A consists rapidly bind to high-density lipoprotein and influence cholesterol metabolism during inflammatory states (Banka et al., 1995). SAA could contribute to the inflammatory state by inducing chemotaxis and adhesion (Malle & De Beer, 1996).

4. Cytokines and acute phase response

A complex network of intercellular signaling involving cytokines, cytokine modulators and hormones regulates the acute-phase response (APR). Inflammation-associated cytokines, produced by both cell in the inflammatory site circulating immune cells, induce changes in expression of APP by liver cells. Liver is one of the primary organs required for the

constitutive production of blood proteins and one of the major sources of acute-phase proteins. Thus, liver in uncontrolled local tissue inflammation processes produce, IL-6 and other family members, TNF-α, and IL-1β leading the production of these acute-phase proteins, mainly SAA, fibrinogen, CRP that are indicative of an APR.
APR participate at a very early stage after stimulus by recognizing non-self elements in the body, **quickly after infection**, preceding both the complete activation and the setting up of immune responses. Also, the acute-phase response is resolved as soon as stimulation disappears. These APR regulation is due to the expression of inflammation regulators including IL-10, SOCS, soluble receptors of inflammatory cytokines (IL-1ra) as well as due to short span of APP and their mRNA half-lives.
Activated immune cells including monocytes and lymphocytes release pro-inflammatory cytokines to stimulate hepatocytes; subsequently induce synthesis and secretion of acute phase proteins. Tumor necrosis factor-alpha (TNF-alpha), interleukin-1 beta (IL-1beta), and interleukin-6 (IL-6) following their pattern-recognition receptors (PRRs) bind pathogen associated molecular patterns (PAMPs). IL-22 is a more recently discovered cytokine that is also produced by liver cells.

5. IL-22 expression and functions

A study on HepG2 hepatocellular carcinoma-derived cell line allowed to identify an IL-22–dependent induction of APP gene expression (Dumoutier et al., 2000). Wolk et al. subsequently reported increased levels of circulating SAA as a consequence of IL-22 addition (Wolk et al., 2004).
Interleukin-22 (IL-22), a cytokine from the IL-10 family but exhibit low homology with IL-10, produced by several immune cell subsets, mainly including (IL-6, TNFa)-stimulated Th-22 that will produce the largest amounts (37 up to 65% of the total depending on the tissue) in the absence of IL-17 production, IL-12-stimulted or activated (CD3) Th-1/Tbet+ (35%), (IL-1b, IL-6, TGFb, IL-23)-stimulated Th-17/RORgt+ (10%) that in addition will produce IL-17A&F IL-21 and IL-28. Innate lymphocytes NK22/NKp44+ (Duhen et al., 2009; Eyerich et al., 2009; Trifari et al., 2009) and NK cells (Wolk & Sabat, 2006) and γδ T and LTi-like cells that are IL-22 producers (Zenewicz et al., 2008). Other T cell subset have been shown an IL-22 production such as the T8 /Tc22 in atopic dermatitis (Nograles et al., 2009) and in psoriasis where also Tc17-Il-17A production was associated (Res et al., 2010).
It has been demonstrated that IL-22 does not act on immune cells as compared with other T or NK cells secreted cytokines. Direct effects of IL-22 are restricted to non-hematopoietic cells carrying IL-22 receptors that are expressed on the surface of only epithelial cells and some fibroblasts in a large variety of organs, including parenchymal tissue of the gut, lung, skin, and liver.
The expression of the IL-22R1 chain determines cells and organs exhibiting an IL-22 target profile (Boniface et al., 2005). Thus, the main IL-22R1 and IL-10R2 expressers are epithelial and fibroblast cells (Wolk et al., 2004; Wolk et al., 2005) excluding to the immune monocytoid or lymphoid cells and they are carriers of both IL-22R and IL-10R2 (Kotenko, 2002; Langer et al., 2004; Pestka et al., 2004; Sabat et al., 2007)
Depending on local inflammatory processes in its targeted tissues, this cytokine is quickly over-expressed in its source cells and exhibit three main documented activities (Fig 4): (i) **antimicrobial** by inducing AMPs (SAA, A-antitrypsin, haptoglobin, hepcidin, S100A7, S100A8 S100A9, β-Def-1 & 2, RegIII β, γ, etc), (ii) **tissue-damage protection** *via* induction of

APR (IL-6, TNFa, CXCL1, S100A7, S100A8 S100A9, β-Def-1 & 2, IL-20, etc) and (iii) **tissue repair and remodeling** by enhancing expression of MMP-1,2 as well as Muc-1, 3 10, 13 and some survival genes (Bcl-2, Bcl-X_L).

Thus, a localized production of IL-22 in the liver seems to promote hepatocyte survival and proliferation, but could primes the liver to be more susceptible to tumor development without significantly affecting liver inflammation (Park et al., 2011). Damaged cultured keratinocytes become repaired after IL-22-dependent remodeling (Eyerich et al., 2009). AAT that has been reported as a potential biomarker for hepatitis B in diagnosis (Tan et al., 2011). IL-22 contributes to regenerate tissues following liver surgery (Ren et al., 2010) or alcool-cirrhotic damages (Ki et al., 2010).

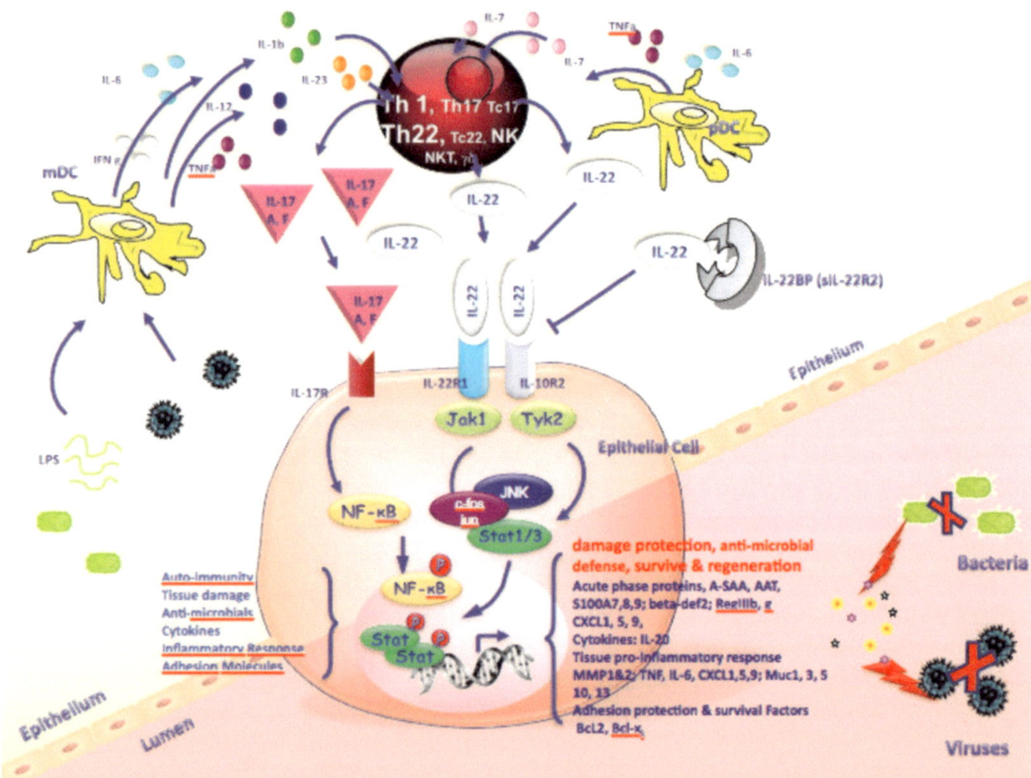

Fig. 4. Mucosal innate protection and tissue damage, the double game of IL-17 & IL-22 cytokines is determined by the local environment situation. Main IL-22 pathways playing a pivotal role in the protection of mucosal tissues against intracellular and extracellular infectious agents such as extracellular bacterias or sexually transmitted viruses. In vivo or ex vivo data these localized anti-infectious activities could involve several possible pathways including both different mode of action of anti-microbials and the infectious pathways used by pathogens. In addition IL-22 will play an important role in both tissue damage protection through APP induction and regeneration.

In the aim to understand the factors that impede immune responses to persistent viruses is essential in designing therapies for HIV infection, Pellegrini *et al* (Pellegrini et al., 2011) have

done a study on mice infected with LCMV clone-13 that exhibit persistent high-level viremia and a dysfunctional immune response. Interleukin-7, a cytokine that is critical for immune development and homeostasis, was used here to promote immunity toward clone-13, enabling elucidation of the inhibitory pathways underlying impaired antiviral immune response. IL-7 downregulated the critical repressor of cytokine signaling, Socs3, resulting in amplified cytokine production, increased T cell effector function and numbers, and viral clearance. Additionally, IL-7 promoted production of IL-22 that abrogated liver pathology.
Recently an improvement intestinal inflammation in a mouse model of ulcerative colitis by IL-22 was mediated by enhanced mucus production has been reported. A local gene delivery was used to inhibit IL-22 activity through overexpression of IL-22-binding protein. Treatment with IL-22-binding protein suppressed goblet cell restitution (reparation) during the recovery phase (Sugimoto et al., 2008).
Aging is characterized by a progressive alteration of **homeostatic** mechanisms modulated by environmental and genetic factors. It is associated with a pro-inflammatory status. Cytokine dysregulation is believed to play a key role in the proposed remodeling of the immune-inflammatory responses accompanying old age. Centenarians displayed significantly higher circulating IL-22 levels compared to control population (Basile et al., 2011). This pro-inflammatory condition is probably not only protective against infections, but also it contributes to a better predisposition to preserve homeostasis, thus promoting the longevity of these subjects.
Once the IL-22 expression is set up, the biological activity of this cytokine will be mainly regulated by two factors: (i) the expression level of its appropriated receptor, IL-22R1 on its target epithelial cells (Li et al., 2004; Xie et al., 2000) and (ii) the expression level and localization of the soluble IL-22 binding protein (IL-22 BP) (Dumoutier et al., 2001).

6. IL-22 induces expression of an acute-phase response

Liang et al assessed effects of IL-22 in mice (Liang et al., 2010). By utilizing adenoviral-mediated delivery of IL-22 and systemic administration of IL-22 protein, we observed that IL-22 modulates factors involved in coagulation, including fibrinogen levels and platelet numbers, and cellular constituents of blood, such as neutrophil and RBC counts. Thus, IL-22 induces effects on systemic biochemical, cellular, and physiological parameters as well as thymic atrophy, body weight loss, and renal proximal tubule metabolic activity. These cellular and physiological parameters are indicative of a proper APR (Gabay & Kushner, 1999) in systemic inflammatory state. AdIL-22 mouse infection induces sustained high levels of circulating SAA and fibrinogen respectively on days 3, 7, and 14 and on Days 1 3, and 7 in blood. These observations demonstrated that exposure IL-22 for 2 wk resulted in the modulation of acute-phase proteins of the acute phase response (Liang et al., 2010).
Following the interaction between IL-22 and its receptors, several observations report that IL-22 induces **APP, anti-microbial peptides gene expression**, cytokines, chemokines, and matrix metalloproteinases (Boniface et al., 2005), from **skin, gut, lung, or liver** epithelial **cells**. IL-22 modulates local inflammation, through **mucosal barrier integrity** and generating a protective inflammatory response against mucosal entry pathogens including viruses (Misse et al., 2007)and extracellular bacteria (Aujla & Kolls, 2009; Zheng et al., 2008).
The majority of IL-22 effects are benefic or **protective** (gut, vagina, lungs, liver) for the host, but in some situations of chronic inflammation, it has been reported that this cytokine could have **pathogenic** effects (skin, joints) including in noninfectious inflammatory disease states.

In rheumatoid arthritis, IL-22 play an inflammatory role, may result in bone damage (Geboes et al., 2009). Thus, IL-22 alone has been reported to be able to induce skin hyperplasia and epidermal wound healing (Boniface et al., 2005; Eyerich et al., 2009). The effect of IL-22 signaling will depend on the local cellular situation. Surprisingly, it has been shown *T. trichiura* colonization of the intestine may reduce symptomatic colitis by promoting goblet cell hyperplasia and mucus production through Th2 cytokines and IL-22 (Broadhurst et al., 2010).

7. IL-22 induces antimicrobial responses is depending of the "niche" circumstances

Zheng et al. reported that *in vivo* IL-22 induced the anti-microbial peptides **named the RegIII** proteins in intestinal epithelial cells. An intestinal infection *Citrobacter rodentium* in IL-22-deficient mice induced death (Zheng et al., 2008). Moreover IL-22 in intestine is differentially generated by a subset of NK cells, NKp46+(Satoh-Takayama et al., 2008). Aujla et al. reported that in a mouse model IL-22 upregulated the expression of lipocalin 2 in lung tissue and increased the transepithelial resistance to bacteria, and consequently, and here also the IL-22 neutralization during pulmonary *Klebsiella pneumoniae* infection death of these animals is observed (Aujla & Kolls, 2009). During pulmonary *K. pneumoniae* infection, it seems that both IL-22 and IL-17A cytokines produced by T cells were necessary for the host defense. Whereas for intestinal infection with *C. rodentium*, IL-22 was produced earlier than IL-17A and this latter was dispensable. Also, independently of IL-17, IL-22 can protect against *Salmonella enteritica* that induces systemic infections (Schulz et al., 2008), due to IL-22 increased levels upon intraperitoneal mice contamination (Siegemund et al., 2009). In contrast, multi-microbial sepsis can be avoided by inhibiting IL-22 with IL-22BP-Fc 4 h before sepsis induction leading to enhanced accumulation of neutrophils and mononuclear phagocytes and a reduced bacterial load at the site of infection. In addition, IL-22 blockade led to an enhanced bacterial clearance in liver and kidney and reduced kidney injury. These results imply an important proinflammatory role of IL-22 during septic peritonitis, contributing to bacterial spread and organ failure(Weber et al., 2007). IL-22 therefore, appears to play an important role in the regulation of inflammatory processes *in vivo*.
Analysis of Th1, Th2, and Th17 cytokine responses in cultured PBMCs from individuals of a cohort of subjects infected with *Leishmania donovani* having developed a visceral disease Kala Azar (KA) or having been protected against KA showed that IL-17 and IL-22 were strongly and independently associated with protection against KA. These results suggest that, along with Th1 cytokines, IL-17 and IL-22 play complementary roles in human protection against KA, and that a defect in Th17 induction may increase the risk of KA(Pitta et al., 2009). However mechanisms of protection in this case remain unclear.
Some clinical reports on *Candida albicans* state that IL-22 is associated to the presence of IL-22 (Liu et al., 2009), and some established correlations tend to show that IL-22 could play a role in controlling this infection (Puel et al., 2010). In animal models the role of IL-22 seems related to IL-17 environment (De Luca et al., 2010), IL-22 will show positive effects if IL-17RA is deficient but in an IL-17-independent manner. Another report from mouse model studies on *C. albicans* state that IL-17 and IL-23 but not IL-22 and IL-12 are required (Kagami et al., 2010).
These contradictory results must be taken into account, because would IL-17 and IL-22 certainly do not exhibit the same behavior in humans and in mouse, consequently,

physiopathological observations in animal models do not allow to extract conclusions extendable to humans.
IL-22 could synergize with other cytokines such as IL-7, a cytokine that is critical for immune development and homeostasis, to protect mouse organs from pathogenic effects of a LCMV (clone-13). Mice infected with have persistent high-level viremia and a dysfunctional immune response. IL-7 was used to promote immunity toward clone-13, enabling elucidation of the inhibitory pathways underlying impaired antiviral immune response. Mechanistically, IL-7 downregulated a critical repressor of cytokine signaling, Socs3, resulting in amplified cytokine production, increased T cell effector function and viral clearance. IL-7 enhanced thymic output to expand the naive T cell pool, including T cells that were not LCMV specific. Additionally, IL-7 promoted production of cytoprotective IL-22 that abrogated liver pathology (Pellegrini et al., 2011). This example is not far from the observations reporting that the IL-22 expression was increased in the presence in viral hepatitis C cases but didn't show in vitro models a direct effect on HCV (Dambacher et al., 2008). In contrast, IL-22 alone could be considered to treat Theiler's virus-induced encephalomyelitis, a mouse infection characterized in susceptible animals by chronic inflammation and demyelination (Levillayer et al., 2007).
Means to avoid the HIV mucosal entry is a crucial objectives to fight against this viral dissemination. The earliest responses to acute HIV-1 infection (AHI) will be due to the action of the mucosal epithelial cells, macrophages and DCs, NK cells as well as antimicrobial factors such as beta-defensins, activated complement. We have shown that natural constitutive higher IL-22 levels of transcripts and proteins are found in repeatedly HIV-1-exposed, uninfected individuals (ESN) as compared with "normal healthy individuals at an approximative ratio 3/1. These higher quantities of one of the major innate inducer protection systems permit an absence of infection in ESN. IL-22 induces A-SAA that, in turn, will agonistically bind to formyl peptide cell receptor (FPR) and therefore induce indirect down modulation of CCR5 in the same immature myeloid dendritic cells, which consequently will drastically reduce HIV-1 infection (Misse et al., 2007). In addition, IL-22-mediated antiviral effects include the stimulation of the production of beta-defensins 2 and 3 by ectocervix epithelial cells as well (F. Veas, M. Clerici, unpublished observations). Some of these individuals could exhibit other complementary HIV protection systems such as APOBEC, or anti-CCR5 IgA antibodies (Miyazawa et al., 2009), as well as the over expression of CCL28 in ESN that helps massive migration of anti-viral IgA secretory B cells up to mucosal tissues (Castelletti et al., 2007).
It has been recently reported that in HIV infected persons, an induction of acute phase protein serum amyloid A (A-SAA) occurred as early as 5-7 days prior to the first detection of plasma viral RNA, considerably prior to any elevation in systemic cytokine levels. Furthermore, a proteolytic fragment of alpha-1-antitrypsin (AAT), was observed in plasma coincident with viremia. Both A-SAA and AAT fragment have anti-viral activity *in vitro* and quantitation of their plasma levels indicated that circulating concentrations are likely to be within the range of their inhibitory activity (Kramer et al., 2010).
IL-22 is a potent inducer of AAT and MMP then mucosal or topic treatments could be beneficial to avoid the HIV mucosal entry and therefore can be crucial to fight against this viral dissemination.
High systemic levels of IL-10, CRP and IL-22 in HIV-1C-infected Indian patients were associated with low viral replication *in vitro*. Whereas using healthy-donor PBMC *in vitro*, these isolates exhibited a high replication capacity.in *In vitro*, pretreatment of virus cultures

with IL-10 and CRP resulted in a significant reduction of virus production, whereas IL-22, which lacks action on immune cells appears to mediate its anti-HIV effect through interaction with both IL-10 and CRP, and its own protective effect on mucosal membranes (Arias et al., 2010).

Insights gained into the mechanism of action of acute-phase reactants and other innate molecules against HIV and how they are induced could be exploited for the future development of more efficient prophylactic vaccine strategies.

8. Conclusion

APR has major consequences during a local inflammation process with systemic consequences to maintain the whole organism homeostasis. The continuous discovery of new mediators/receptors of this response allow to more precisely tunes the knowledge about subtle necessary equilibrium to understand diseases set up to propose new possible therapeutic approaches. The double game of inflammatory processes to destroy the non-self and repair the self clearly is not ease to delimitate and this knowledge is a tremendous and pivotal challenge for a well adapted personalized medicine.

Moreover, data are mostly harvested from animal models that do not reflect physiopathological patterns that are generated in humans with their own kinetics. Nevertheless, today animal models are absolutely necessary, but observations need to be improved with more adapted reagents particularly for the *in vivo* real time observations of the physiopathological evolution and conditions.

Another imperious need is to assess functional concentrations of mediators/receptors such as IL-22 that are present in healthy individuals resisting to diseases such as infections, in a way to measure over the time their concentrations and understand their signification in terms of their homeostatic values in relation with complex networks

9. Acknowledgement

We are indebted to support from the Institut de Recherche pour le Développement, the University Montpellier 1 and the Région Languedoc-Roussillon, France.

10. References

Adib-Conquy, M. & Cavaillon, J. M. (2009). Compensatory anti-inflammatory response syndrome. *Thrombosis and haemostasis* Vol.101, No.1, pp.36-47.

Agar, C., de Groot, P. G., Morgelin, M., Monk, S. D., van Os, G. M., Levels, J. H., de Laat, B., Urbanus, R. T., Herwald, H., van der Poll, T. & Meijers, J. C. (2011). {beta}2-glycoprotein I: a novel component of innate immunity. *Blood.*

Ahmed, N., Thorley, R., Xia, D., Samols, D. & Webster, R. O. (1996). Transgenic mice expressing rabbit C-reactive protein exhibit diminished chemotactic factor-induced alveolitis. *American journal of respiratory and critical care medicine* Vol.153, No.3, pp.1141-1147.

Arias, J. F., Nishihara, R., Bala, M. & Ikuta, K. (2010). High systemic levels of interleukin-10, interleukin-22 and C-reactive protein in Indian patients are associated with low in vitro replication of HIV-1 subtype C viruses. *Retrovirology* Vol.7, pp.15.

Aujla, S. J. & Kolls, J. K. (2009). IL-22: a critical mediator in mucosal host defense. *Journal of molecular medicine* Vol.87, No.5, pp.451-454.

Bals, R., Weiner, D. J., Moscioni, A. D., Meegalla, R. L. & Wilson, J. M. (1999). Augmentation of innate host defense by expression of a cathelicidin antimicrobial peptide. *Infection and immunity* Vol.67, No.11, pp.6084-6089.

Banka, C. L., Yuan, T., de Beer, M. C., Kindy, M., Curtiss, L. K. & de Beer, F. C. (1995). Serum amyloid A (SAA): influence on HDL-mediated cellular cholesterol efflux. *Journal of lipid research* Vol.36, No.5, pp.1058-1065.

Basile, G., Paffumi, I., D'Angelo, A. G., Figliomeni, P., Cucinotta, M. D., Pace, E., Ferraro, M., Saitta, S., Lasco, A. & Gangemi, S. (2011). Healthy centenarians show high levels of circulating interleukin-22 (IL-22). *Archives of gerontology and geriatrics.*

Berliner, J. A., Navab, M., Fogelman, A. M., Frank, J. S., Demer, L. L., Edwards, P. A., Watson, A. D. & Lusis, A. J. (1995). Atherosclerosis: basic mechanisms. Oxidation, inflammation, and genetics. *Circulation* Vol.91, No.9, pp.2488-2496.

Bianchi, M. E. (2007). DAMPs, PAMPs and alarmins: all we need to know about danger. *Journal of leukocyte biology* Vol.81, No.1, pp.1-5.

Boniface, K., Bernard, F. X., Garcia, M., Gurney, A. L., Lecron, J. C. & Morel, F. (2005). IL-22 inhibits epidermal differentiation and induces proinflammatory gene expression and migration of human keratinocytes. *Journal of immunology* Vol.174, No.6, pp.3695-3702.

Broadhurst, M. J., Leung, J. M., Kashyap, V., McCune, J. M., Mahadevan, U., McKerrow, J. H. & Loke, P. (2010). IL-22+ CD4+ T cells are associated with therapeutic trichuris trichiura infection in an ulcerative colitis patient. *Science translational medicine* Vol.2, No.60, pp.60ra88.

Bulet, P., Stocklin, R. & Menin, L. (2004). Anti-microbial peptides: from invertebrates to vertebrates. *Immunological reviews* Vol.198, pp.169-184.

Castelletti, E., Lo Caputo, S., Kuhn, L., Borelli, M., Gajardo, J., Sinkala, M., Trabattoni, D., Kankasa, C., Lauri, E., Clivio, A., *et al.* (2007). The mucosae-associated epithelial chemokine (MEC/CCL28) modulates immunity in HIV infection. *PloS one* Vol.2, No.10, pp.e969.

Cermak, J., Key, N. S., Bach, R. R., Balla, J., Jacob, H. S. & Vercellotti, G. M. (1993). C-reactive protein induces human peripheral blood monocytes to synthesize tissue factor. *Blood* Vol.82, No.2, pp.513-520.

Cid, M. C., Grant, D. S., Hoffman, G. S., Auerbach, R., Fauci, A. S. & Kleinman, H. K. (1993). Identification of haptoglobin as an angiogenic factor in sera from patients with systemic vasculitis. *The Journal of clinical investigation* Vol.91, No.3, pp.977-985.

d'Angeac, A. D., Stefas, I., Duperray, C., Rucheton, M., Graafland, H., Montero, J. L. & Chicheportiche, R. (2005). Oxidation and biotinylation of beta 2 glycoprotein I glycan chains induce an increase in its affinity for anionic phospholipids similar to that obtained by the addition of anti-beta 2 glycoprotein I or anti-cardiolipin antibodies. *Journal of Immunological Methods* Vol.300, No.1-2, pp.160-178.

Dambacher, J., Beigel, F., Zitzmann, K., Heeg, M. H., Goke, B., Diepolder, H. M., Auernhammer, C. J. & Brand, S. (2008). The role of interleukin-22 in hepatitis C virus infection. *Cytokine* Vol.41, No.3, pp.209-216.

De Luca, A., Zelante, T., D'Angelo, C., Zagarella, S., Fallarino, F., Spreca, A., Iannitti, R. G., Bonifazi, P., Renauld, J. C., Bistoni, F., *et al.* (2010). IL-22 defines a novel immune pathway of antifungal resistance. *Mucosal immunology* Vol.3, No.4, pp.361-373.

Duhen, T., Geiger, R., Jarrossay, D., Lanzavecchia, A. & Sallusto, F. (2009). Production of interleukin 22 but not interleukin 17 by a subset of human skin-homing memory T cells. *Nature immunology* Vol.10, No.8, pp.857-863.

Dumoutier, L., Lejeune, D., Colau, D. & Renauld, J. C. (2001). Cloning and characterization of IL-22 binding protein, a natural antagonist of IL-10-related T cell-derived inducible factor/IL-22. *Journal of immunology* Vol.166, No.12, pp.7090-7095.

Dumoutier, L., Van Roost, E., Ameye, G., Michaux, L. & Renauld, J. C. (2000). IL-TIF/IL-22: genomic organization and mapping of the human and mouse genes. *Genes and immunity* Vol.1, No.8, pp.488-494.

Eyerich, S., Eyerich, K., Pennino, D., Carbone, T., Nasorri, F., Pallotta, S., Cianfarani, F., Odorisio, T., Traidl-Hoffmann, C., Behrendt, H., *et al.* (2009). Th22 cells represent a distinct human T cell subset involved in epidermal immunity and remodeling. *The Journal of clinical investigation* Vol.119, No.12, pp.3573-3585.

Gabay, C. & Kushner, I. (1999). Acute-phase proteins and other systemic responses to inflammation. *The New England journal of medicine* Vol.340, No.6, pp.448-454.

Gabay, C., Smith, M. F., Eidlen, D. & Arend, W. P. (1997). Interleukin 1 receptor antagonist (IL-1Ra) is an acute-phase protein. *The Journal of clinical investigation* Vol.99, No.12, pp.2930-2940.

Geboes, L., Dumoutier, L., Kelchtermans, H., Schurgers, E., Mitera, T., Renauld, J. C. & Matthys, P. (2009). Proinflammatory role of the Th17 cytokine interleukin-22 in collagen-induced arthritis in C57BL/6 mice. *Arthritis and rheumatism* Vol.60, No.2, pp.390-395.

Godoy, P., Marsac, D., Stefas, E., Ferrer, P., Tischler, N. D., Pino, K., Ramdohr, P., Vial, P., Valenzuela, P. D., Ferres, M., *et al.* (2009). Andes virus antigens are shed in urine of patients with acute hantavirus cardiopulmonary syndrome. *Journal of Virology* Vol.83, No.10, pp.5046-5055.

He, R. L., Zhou, J., Hanson, C. Z., Chen, J., Cheng, N. & Ye, R. D. (2009). Serum amyloid A induces G-CSF expression and neutrophilia via Toll-like receptor 2. *Blood* Vol.113, No.2, pp.429-437.

Hernandez, C., Mor, A., Dagger, F., Nicolas, P., Hernandez, A., Benedetti, E. L. & Dunia, I. (1992). Functional and structural damage in Leishmania mexicana exposed to the cationic peptide dermaseptin. *European journal of cell biology* Vol.59, No.2, pp.414-424.

Jiang, S., Xia, D. & Samols, D. (2006). Expression of rabbit C-reactive protein in transgenic mice inhibits development of antigen-induced arthritis. *Scandinavian journal of rheumatology* Vol.35, No.5, pp.351-355.

Kagami, S., Rizzo, H. L., Kurtz, S. E., Miller, L. S. & Blauvelt, A. (2010). IL-23 and IL-17A, but not IL-12 and IL-22, are required for optimal skin host defense against Candida albicans. *Journal of immunology* Vol.185, No.9, pp.5453-5462.

Ki, S. H., Park, O., Zheng, M., Morales-Ibanez, O., Kolls, J. K., Bataller, R. & Gao, B. (2010). Interleukin-22 treatment ameliorates alcoholic liver injury in a murine model of chronic-binge ethanol feeding: role of signal transducer and activator of transcription 3. *Hepatology* Vol.52, No.4, pp.1291-1300.

Kilpatrick, L., McCawley, L., Nachiappan, V., Greer, W., Majumdar, S., Korchak, H. M. & Douglas, S. D. (1992). Alpha-1-antichymotrypsin inhibits the NADPH oxidase-enzyme complex in phorbol ester-stimulated neutrophil membranes. *Journal of immunology* Vol.149, No.9, pp.3059-3065.

Kotenko, S. V. (2002). The family of IL-10-related cytokines and their receptors: related, but to what extent? *Cytokine & growth factor reviews* Vol.13, No.3, pp.223-240.

Kramer, H. B., Lavender, K. J., Qin, L., Stacey, A. R., Liu, M. K., di Gleria, K., Simmons, A., Gasper-Smith, N., Haynes, B. F., McMichael, A. J., *et al.* (2010). Elevation of intact and proteolytic fragments of acute phase proteins constitutes the earliest systemic antiviral response in HIV-1 infection. *PLoS pathogens* Vol.6, No.5, pp.e1000893.

Kushner, I. (1993). Regulation of the acute phase response by cytokines. *Perspectives in biology and medicine* Vol.36, No.4, pp.611-622.

Langer, J. A., Cutrone, E. C. & Kotenko, S. (2004). The Class II cytokine receptor (CRF2) family: overview and patterns of receptor-ligand interactions. *Cytokine & growth factor reviews* Vol.15, No.1, pp.33-48.

Levillayer, F., Mas, M., Levi-Acobas, F., Brahic, M. & Bureau, J. F. (2007). Interleukin 22 is a candidate gene for Tmevp3, a locus controlling Theiler's virus-induced neurological diseases. *Genetics* Vol.176, No.3, pp.1835-1844.

Li, J., Tomkinson, K. N., Tan, X. Y., Wu, P., Yan, G., Spaulding, V., Deng, B., Annis-Freeman, B., Heveron, K., Zollner, R., *et al.* (2004). Temporal associations between interleukin 22 and the extracellular domains of IL-22R and IL-10R2. *International immunopharmacology* Vol.4, No.5, pp.693-708.

Liang, S. C., Nickerson-Nutter, C., Pittman, D. D., Carrier, Y., Goodwin, D. G., Shields, K. M., Lambert, A. J., Schelling, S. H., Medley, Q. G., Ma, H. L., *et al.* (2010). IL-22 induces an acute-phase response. *Journal of immunology* Vol.185, No.9, pp.5531-5538.

Liu, Y., Yang, B., Zhou, M., Li, L., Zhou, H., Zhang, J., Chen, H. & Wu, C. (2009). Memory IL-22-producing CD4+ T cells specific for Candida albicans are present in humans. *European Journal of Immunology* Vol.39, No.6, pp.1472-1479.

Malle, E. & De Beer, F. C. (1996). Human serum amyloid A (SAA) protein: a prominent acute-phase reactant for clinical practice. *European journal of clinical investigation* Vol.26, No.6, pp.427-435.

Misse, D., Yssel, H., Trabattoni, D., Oblet, C., Lo Caputo, S., Mazzotta, F., Pene, J., Gonzalez, J. P., Clerici, M. & Veas, F. (2007). IL-22 participates in an innate anti-HIV-1 host-resistance network through acute-phase protein induction. *Journal of immunology* Vol.178, No.1, pp.407-415.

Miyazawa, M., Lopalco, L., Mazzotta, F., Lo Caputo, S., Veas, F. & Clerici, M. (2009). The 'immunologic advantage' of HIV-exposed seronegative individuals. *AIDS* Vol.23, No.2, pp.161-175.

Morley, J. J. & Kushner, I. (1982). Serum C-reactive protein levels in disease. *Annals of the New York Academy of Sciences* Vol.389, pp.406-418.

Nishikata, M., Kanehira, T., Oh, H., Tani, H., Tazaki, M. & Kuboki, Y. (1991). Salivary histatin as an inhibitor of a protease produced by the oral bacterium Bacteroides gingivalis. *Biochemical and biophysical research communications* Vol.174, No.2, pp.625-630.

Nograles, K. E., Zaba, L. C., Shemer, A., Fuentes-Duculan, J., Cardinale, I., Kikuchi, T., Ramon, M., Bergman, R., Krueger, J. G. & Guttman-Yassky, E. (2009). IL-22-

producing "T22" T cells account for upregulated IL-22 in atopic dermatitis despite reduced IL-17-producing TH17 T cells. *The Journal of allergy and clinical immunology* Vol.123, No.6, pp.1244-1252 e1242.

Park, J. S., Gamboni-Robertson, F., He, Q., Svetkauskaite, D., Kim, J. Y., Strassheim, D., Sohn, J. W., Yamada, S., Maruyama, I., Banerjee, A., *et al.* (2006). High mobility group box 1 protein interacts with multiple Toll-like receptors. *American journal of physiology Cell physiology* Vol.290, No.3, pp.C917-924.

Park, O., Wang, H., Weng, H., Feigenbaum, L., Li, H., Yin, S., Ki, S. H., Yoo, S. H., Dooley, S., Wang, F. S., *et al.* (2011). In vivo consequences of liver-specific interleukin-22 expression in mice: Implications for human liver disease progression. *Hepatology* Vol.54, No.1, pp.252-261.

Pellegrini, M., Calzascia, T., Toe, J. G., Preston, S. P., Lin, A. E., Elford, A. R., Shahinian, A., Lang, P. A., Lang, K. S., Morre, M., *et al.* (2011). IL-7 engages multiple mechanisms to overcome chronic viral infection and limit organ pathology. *Cell* Vol.144, No.4, pp.601-613.

Pestka, S., Krause, C. D., Sarkar, D., Walter, M. R., Shi, Y. & Fisher, P. B. (2004). Interleukin-10 and related cytokines and receptors. *Annual review of immunology* Vol.22, pp.929-979.

Pitta, M. G., Romano, A., Cabantous, S., Henri, S., Hammad, A., Kouriba, B., Argiro, L., el Kheir, M., Bucheton, B., Mary, C., *et al.* (2009). IL-17 and IL-22 are associated with protection against human kala azar caused by Leishmania donovani. *The Journal of Clinical Investigation* Vol.119, No.8, pp.2379-2387.

Puel, A., Doffinger, R., Natividad, A., Chrabieh, M., Barcenas-Morales, G., Picard, C., Cobat, A., Ouachee-Chardin, M., Toulon, A., Bustamante, J., *et al.* (2010). Autoantibodies against IL-17A, IL-17F, and IL-22 in patients with chronic mucocutaneous candidiasis and autoimmune polyendocrine syndrome type I. *The Journal of experimental medicine* Vol.207, No.2, pp.291-297.

Ren, X., Hu, B. & Colletti, L. M. (2010). IL-22 is involved in liver regeneration after hepatectomy. *American journal of physiology Gastrointestinal and liver physiology* Vol.298, No.1, pp.G74-80.

Res, P. C., Piskin, G., de Boer, O. J., van der Loos, C. M., Teeling, P., Bos, J. D. & Teunissen, M. B. (2010). Overrepresentation of IL-17A and IL-22 producing CD8 T cells in lesional skin suggests their involvement in the pathogenesis of psoriasis. *PloS one* Vol.5, No.11, pp.e14108.

Sabat, R., Wallace, E., Endesfelder, S. & Wolk, K. (2007). IL-19 and IL-20: two novel cytokines with importance in inflammatory diseases. *Expert opinion on therapeutic targets* Vol.11, No.5, pp.601-612.

Sandri, S., Rodriguez, D., Gomes, E., Monteiro, H. P., Russo, M. & Campa, A. (2008). Is serum amyloid A an endogenous TLR4 agonist? *Journal of leukocyte biology* Vol.83, No.5, pp.1174-1180.

Satoh-Takayama, N., Vosshenrich, C. A., Lesjean-Pottier, S., Sawa, S., Lochner, M., Rattis, F., Mention, J. J., Thiam, K., Cerf-Bensussan, N., Mandelboim, O., *et al.* (2008). Microbial flora drives interleukin 22 production in intestinal NKp46+ cells that provide innate mucosal immune defense. *Immunity* Vol.29, No.6, pp.958-970.

Schulz, S. M., Kohler, G., Schutze, N., Knauer, J., Straubinger, R. K., Chackerian, A. A., Witte, E., Wolk, K., Sabat, R., Iwakura, Y., *et al.* (2008). Protective immunity to systemic infection with attenuated Salmonella enterica serovar enteritidis in the absence of IL-12 is associated with IL-23-dependent IL-22, but not IL-17. *Journal of immunology* Vol.181, No.11, pp.7891-7901.

Shah, C., Hari-Dass, R. & Raynes, J. G. (2006). Serum amyloid A is an innate immune opsonin for Gram-negative bacteria. *Blood* Vol.108, No.5, pp.1751-1757.

Siegemund, S., Schutze, N., Schulz, S., Wolk, K., Nasilowska, K., Straubinger, R. K., Sabat, R. & Alber, G. (2009). Differential IL-23 requirement for IL-22 and IL-17A production during innate immunity against Salmonella enterica serovar Enteritidis. *International immunology* Vol.21, No.5, pp.555-565.

Stefas, E., Rucheton, M., Graafland, H., Moynier, M., Sompeyrac, C., Bahraoui, E. M. & Veas, F. (1997). Human plasmatic apolipoprotein H binds human immunodeficiency virus type 1 and type 2 proteins. *AIDS Research and Human Retroviruses* Vol.13, No.1, pp.97-104.

Stefas, I., Rucheton, M., D'Angeac, A. D., Morel-Baccard, C., Seigneurin, J. M., Zarski, J. P., Martin, M., Cerutti, M., Bossy, J. P., Misse, D., *et al.* (2001). Hepatitis B virus Dane particles bind to human plasma apolipoprotein H. *Hepatology* Vol.33, No.1, pp.207-217.

Strnad, P., Schwarz, P., Rasenack, M. C., Kucukoglu, O., Habib, R. I., Heuberger, D., Ehehalt, R., Muller, M. W., Stiehl, A., Adler, G. & Kulaksiz, H. (2011). Hepcidin is an antibacterial, stress-inducible peptide of the biliary system. *PloS one* Vol.6, No.1, pp.e16454.

Sugimoto, K., Ogawa, A., Mizoguchi, E., Shimomura, Y., Andoh, A., Bhan, A. K., Blumberg, R. S., Xavier, R. J. & Mizoguchi, A. (2008). IL-22 ameliorates intestinal inflammation in a mouse model of ulcerative colitis. *The Journal of Clinical Investigation* Vol.118, No.2, pp.534-544.

Szalai, A. J. (2002). The antimicrobial activity of C-reactive protein. *Microbes and infection / Institut Pasteur* Vol.4, No.2, pp.201-205.

Tan, X. F., Wu, S. S., Li, S. P., Chen, Z. & Chen, F. (2011). Alpha-1 antitrypsin is a potential biomarker for hepatitis B. *Virology journal* Vol.8, pp.274.

Trifari, S., Kaplan, C. D., Tran, E. H., Crellin, N. K. & Spits, H. (2009). Identification of a human helper T cell population that has abundant production of interleukin 22 and is distinct from T(H)-17, T(H)1 and T(H)2 cells. *Nature immunology* Vol.10, No.8, pp.864-871.

van Beijnum, J. R., Buurman, W. A. & Griffioen, A. W. (2008). Convergence and amplification of toll-like receptor (TLR) and receptor for advanced glycation end products (RAGE) signaling pathways via high mobility group B1 (HMGB1). *Angiogenesis* Vol.11, No.1, pp.91-99.

Vogl, T., Tenbrock, K., Ludwig, S., Leukert, N., Ehrhardt, C., van Zoelen, M. A., Nacken, W., Foell, D., van der Poll, T., Sorg, C. & Roth, J. (2007). Mrp8 and Mrp14 are endogenous activators of Toll-like receptor 4, promoting lethal, endotoxin-induced shock. *Nature medicine* Vol.13, No.9, pp.1042-1049.

Weber, G. F., Schlautkotter, S., Kaiser-Moore, S., Altmayr, F., Holzmann, B. & Weighardt, H. (2007). Inhibition of interleukin-22 attenuates bacterial load and organ failure during acute polymicrobial sepsis. *Infection and immunity* Vol.75, No.4, pp.1690-1697.

Wilson, C. L., Ouellette, A. J., Satchell, D. P., Ayabe, T., Lopez-Boado, Y. S., Stratman, J. L., Hultgren, S. J., Matrisian, L. M. & Parks, W. C. (1999). Regulation of intestinal alpha-defensin activation by the metalloproteinase matrilysin in innate host defense. *Science* Vol.286, No.5437, pp.113-117.

Wolk, K., Kunz, S., Witte, E., Friedrich, M., Asadullah, K. & Sabat, R. (2004). IL-22 increases the innate immunity of tissues. *Immunity* Vol.21, No.2, pp.241-254.

Wolk, K. & Sabat, R. (2006). Interleukin-22: a novel T- and NK-cell derived cytokine that regulates the biology of tissue cells. *Cytokine & growth factor reviews* Vol.17, No.5, pp.367-380.

Wolk, K., Witte, E., Reineke, U., Witte, K., Friedrich, M., Sterry, W., Asadullah, K., Volk, H. D. & Sabat, R. (2005). Is there an interaction between interleukin-10 and interleukin-22? *Genes and immunity* Vol.6, No.1, pp.8-18.

Xie, M. H., Aggarwal, S., Ho, W. H., Foster, J., Zhang, Z., Stinson, J., Wood, W. I., Goddard, A. D. & Gurney, A. L. (2000). Interleukin (IL)-22, a novel human cytokine that signals through the interferon receptor-related proteins CRF2-4 and IL-22R. *The Journal of biological chemistry* Vol.275, No.40, pp.31335-31339.

Zenewicz, L. A., Yancopoulos, G. D., Valenzuela, D. M., Murphy, A. J., Stevens, S. & Flavell, R. A. (2008). Innate and adaptive interleukin-22 protects mice from inflammatory bowel disease. *Immunity* Vol.29, No.6, pp.947-957.

Zheng, Y., Valdez, P. A., Danilenko, D. M., Hu, Y., Sa, S. M., Gong, Q., Abbas, A. R., Modrusan, Z., Ghilardi, N., de Sauvage, F. J. & Ouyang, W. (2008). Interleukin-22 mediates early host defense against attaching and effacing bacterial pathogens. *Nature medicine* Vol.14, No.3, pp.282-289.

5

Hemostatic Soluble Plasma Proteins During Acute-Phase Response and Chronic Inflammation

Irina I. Patalakh
Palladin Institute of Biochemistry of the NAS of Ukraine, Kyiv Ukraine

1. Introduction

Coagulation and inflammation are the interdependent processes attributed to the host defence response to injuries. A synchronized activity of both pathways represents an essential prerequisite for restitution of host homeostasis after ultimate disturbances of the latter. Crosstalk between coagulation and inflammation is considered to inherit from primitive coagulation systems similar to invertebrates. For instance, in Horseshoe "crabs" (*Limulus*) coagulogen, a clotting protein with the bactericidal function, and coagulation-related serine proteases are both located in circulating hemolymph cells (hemocytes) and are capable of simultaneously protecting against injury, as well as to isolate pathogens within cysts (Tanaka et al., 2009). In humans, the complement system as a part of innate immunity remains closely related to the hemostasis system (Markiewski et al., 2007). The organizations of these two systems demonstrate several similarities of both structural and functional features. Both systems are organized into proteolytic cascades; serine proteases of the chymotrypsin family are the components of the latter. Proteases of each system are, in their molecular structure, glycoproteins, which have a highly conservative catalytic site composed of serine, histidine, and aspartic amino acid residues. These proteases exist in the form of inactive zymogens and are subsequently activated by upstream, active proteases. Proteins of the complement and hemostasis systems are mostly synthesized in the liver by hepatocytes, besides being additionally produced during an acute-phase response stimulated by common inflammatory mediators. The biological role of the complement system is mentioned here in order to note that the above-mentioned similarities represent a forcible argument in favour of the common origin of both immunity and hemostasis phenomena. The complement system has been described in detail recently (Castellheim et al., 2009; Markiewski et al., 2007) and will not be further discussed here. Though, it is worthwhile to mention that the blood hemostasis system in humans, hypothetically, has been evolved progressively from the archaic innate immunity organization, diverging to certain narrow-specific pathways, which are responsible for the coagulation control.
Hemostasis in humans is organized as closely interrelated enzyme cascade systems: (i) fibrin clotting system (coagulation); (ii) multilevel system for preventing uncontrolled fibrin formation (anticoagulation); and (iii) system for limiting the amount of cross-linked fibrin (fibrinolysis). Together, coagulation, anticoagulation and fibrinolysis are associated into a

self-regulated and highly organized molecular machine that provides either acceleration or reduction of blood hemostasis process (Spronk et al., 2003). Accurate regulation of the coagulation rate is an effective mechanism, preventing circulatory disorders. This regulatory mechanism is known to be a part of the acute phase of the inflammatory reaction which provides rapid restoration of physiological homeostasis.

Hemostasis is closely linked to innate immunity and inflammation through particular regulatory coupling like protein C system (Fig. 1). Cooperation between hemostasis and innate immunity facilitates injury recognition, vessel wall reparation, and prevention of excessive bleeding without causing thrombosis. These processes are mediated by a balance of cellular surface components, cell-derived factors, and soluble plasma proteins (SPPs). After interruption of the vascular integrity, concentrations of some hemostatic SPPs (HSPPs) change in a manner typical of those of acute-phase proteins (APPs). In agreement with definition of APPs (Kushner & Rzewnicki, 1994; Morley & Kushner, 1982), at least several HSPPs including fibrinogen, plasminogen, and PAI-1 should also be classified as APPs, since: (i) the intensity of synthesis of these HSPPs dramatically changes (by more than 50%) during pathological processes (ii) HSPPs synthesis in hepatocytes during the acute-phase response are regulated by inflammatory-associated cytokines; (iii) due to chronic stimulation by inflammatory mediators, HSPPs may persist in circulation and participate in the formation of a "semantically paradoxical chronic acute-phase response" (Gabay & Kushner, 2001). The above-indicated similarities between inflammation and hemostasis determine their unidirectional changes. These changes involve pro-coagulant activities of inflammatory processes, as well as the pro-inflammatory efficacy of the hemostatic molecular machine.

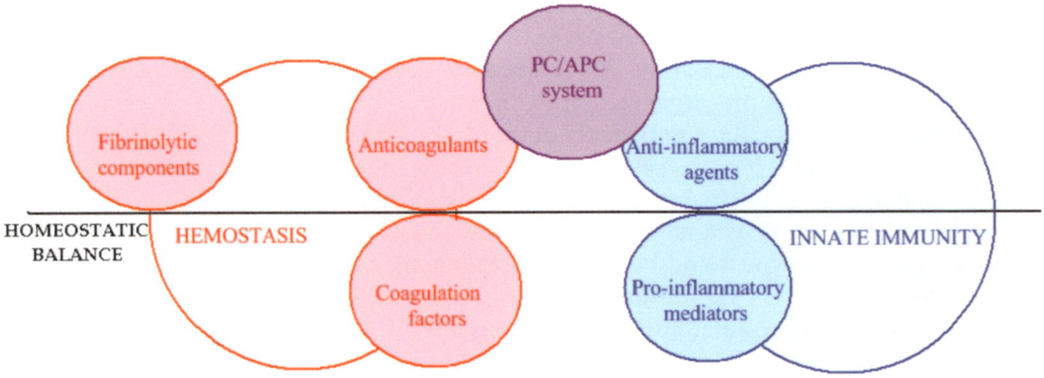

Fig. 1. Schematic representation of the protein C-dependent cross-point between hemostatic and inflammatory pathways. Diagram illustrates a putative regulatory mechanism, maintaining homeostasis within physiological limits. Both pathways are balanced by the PC/APC (protein C/activated protein C) system, directly by attenuation of production of thrombin as a pro-inflammatory and pro-coagulant agent, or indirectly, by controlling NF-kB-dependent anti-inflammatory pathways through EPCRs (endothelial protein C receptors) and PARs (protease-activated receptors) at the surface of the target cells. See the text for discussion in detail.

The capacity of inflammatory mediators to regulate hemostasis, as well as some aspects of the coagulation ability to affect inflammatory events have been extensively reviewed (Butenas et al., 2009; Danese et al., 2010; Esmon, 2005; Jennewein et al., 2011; Levi et al., 2004; Medcalf, 2007). Reciprocal regulation of gene expression is the most important mechanism, by which inflammatory and hemostatic pathways interact with each other. The role of cell surface receptors in providing APP-associated signalling has been recently elucidated (Busso et al., 2008; Guitton et al., 2011). The role of the increased HSPPs in the regulation of hemostasis and inflammation pathways under pathophysiological conditions, however, remains less clear. The molecular mechanisms, responsible for the influence of inflammation upon hemostasis and *vice versa*, remain largely unknown. We would like to review here the most important post-translational events, which might perturb HSPPs structure and functions, as well as those influencing measurable levels of HSPPs during inflammation.

2. Cooperation of inflammatory and hemostatic pathways during acute phase response

In normal conditions, HSPPs are presented by a soluble fibrous protein, fibrinogen, abundant serine protease zymogens (inactive enzymatic precursors), and minute amounts of active proteases, as well as by non-enzymatic cofactors and protease inhibitors (Table 1).

Precursor conversion	HSPP identification	The basic function in hemostasis	Proteolytic activation	Expression during the acute-phase response
Clotting factors				
Fibrinogen (Fg) → fibrin (Fn)	a fibrous (structural) protein	substrate for polymerization to fibrin that is important in tissue repair	by thrombin	increase, 1,5-4,0-fold
Prothrombin (II) → thrombin (IIa)	trypsin-like serine protease (endopeptidase)	the conversion of Fg to Fn leading to the formation of a fibrin clot	by prothrombinase	no change or weak increase
Factor V (V) → activated factor V (Va)	ceruloplasmin-like binding protein	as a cofactor for Xa participates in thrombin activation, not enzymatically active	by thrombin	ND
Factor VII (VII) → activated factor VIIa (VIIa)	serine protease (endopeptidase)	the catalytic component of the extrinsic tenase, activates IX to IXa and X to Xa	by thrombin, IXa, Xa, XIIa	ND
Factor VIII (VIII) → activated factor VIIIa (VIIIa)	ceruloplasmin-like binding protein	cofactor for IXa in conversion of X to Xa, receptor for IXa and X, not enzymatically active	by thrombin	increase
Factor IX (IX) → activated factor IXa (IXa)	serine protease (endopeptidase)	the enzyme component of the intrinsic tenase, activates X to Xa	by XIa or TF-VIIa/PL-Ca^{2+}	ND
Factor X (X) → activated factor Xa	serine protease (endopeptidase)	the enzyme component of the prothrombinase is	by IXa-VIIIa/PL-Ca^{2+},	ND

Precursor conversion	HSPP identification	The basic function in hemostasis	Proteolytic activation	Expression during the acute-phase response
(Xa)		responsible for rapid thrombin activation	TF-VIIa/PL-Ca^{2+}	
Factor XI (X) → activated factor XIa(XIa)	serine protease (endopeptidase)	the conversion of IX to IXa within the intrinsic pathway	by surface bound α-XIIa	ND
Factor XII (XII) → activated factor XII (α-XIIa)	serine protease (endopeptidase)	initiation of the intrinsic coagulation pathway *via* conversion XI to XIa	by kallikrein	decrease
Factor α-XIIa (α-XIIa) → factor β-XIIa (β-XIIa)	serine protease (endopeptidase)	solution phase activation of kallikrein, factor VII and the complement cascade	by kallikrein	decrease
Factor XIII (XIII) → activated factor XIIIa (XIIIa)	transglutami-nase (transpeptidase)	stabilization of the fibrin clot *via* cross linking the α and γ-chains of Fn, α_2-PI, V, vWF	by thrombin	ND
Anticoagulants				
Tissue factor pathway inhibitor (TFPI)	Kunitz-type protease inhibitor	reverse inhibition of Xa and IIa, then TF-VIIa independently from Ca^{2+}	-	decrease
Antithrombin (AT)	serpin	Inhibition of VIIa, IXa, Xa and XIa, kallikrein, plasmin, IIa	-	decrease
Protein C (PC)→ Activated protein C (APC)	trypsin-like serine protease (endopeptidase)	inactivation of Va and VIIIa, that inhibits the prothrombinase and tenase and, finally, IIa	by α-throm-bin/throm-bomodulin, by Xa or IIa without Ca^{2+}	no change or decrease
Protein S (PS)	binding protein	as cofactor for APC	-	increase
Fibrinolytic proteins				
Tissue-type plasminogen activator, single chain form (sc-tPA) → active two-chain form (tc-tPA)	serine protease (endopeptidase)	the main endothelium-derived activator of the fibrinolytic system, converts Pg to Pm	by plasmin	decrease or weak increase
Glu-plasminogen (Glu-Pg) → plasmin (Pm)	serine protease (endopeptidase)	responsible for the fibrin clot digestion	by t-PA, u-PA, elastase, XIIa	increase, 2-3- fold
Urokinase-type plasminogen activator, single chain (sc-uPA)	serine protease (endopeptidase)	activator of the Pg conversion to Pm	-	increase
Proteinase inhibitors				
α_1-Antitrypsin or alpha 1-proteinase	serpin	protects tissues from proteolytic enzymes,	-	increase

Precursor conversion	HSPP identification	The basic function in hemostasis	Proteolytic activation	Expression during the acute-phase response
inhibitor (α_1-PI)		inhibits IIa and APC		
α_2-macroglobulin (α_2-M)	broad-range protease inhibitor	inhibits IIa, APC Pm, kallikrein, a remover of plasma enzymes	-	increase, about 100-fold
α_2-antiplasmin (α_2 – plasmin inhibitor) (α_2 -PI)	serpin	inhibitor of Pm, forms covalent complexes interfered with the binding of Pg(Pm) to Fn	-	ND
Thrombin activable fibrinolytic inhibitor (TAFI) → activated form (TAFIa)	carboxypepti-dase	inhibitor of fibrinolysis, removes Pg-binding sites on Fn	by thrombin, plasmin, trypsin	ND
Plasminogen activator inhibitor of type 1 (PAI-1)	serpin	the major inhibitor of tPA that regulates the fibrinolysis by attenuation of Pm production	-	increase
Plasminogen activator inhibitor of type2 (PAI-2)	serpin	inhibitor of urokinase as well as tPA	-	ND
Plasminogen activator inhibitor of type3 (PAI-3 or PCI)	serpin	the major inhibitor of APC as well as tPA and urokinase	-	ND

Table 1. The main characteristics of hemostatic soluble plasma proteins (HSPPs)

Physiological anticoagulants are also available to suppress appropriate clotting factors. Some of the clotting factors (like thrombin or factor V) can promote both coagulation and anticoagulation; thus, these factors are called Janus-faced proteins.

A hemostatic response to the activating signal is manifested by a series of transformations of proenzymes to activated enzymes in a cascade-like manner. The formation of thrombin at the final stage of the coagulation cascade is aimed at conversion of soluble fibrinogen into insoluble fibrin, the non-cellular matrix of blood thrombus. The thrombus formation is considerably accelerated due to accumulation of tissue factor (TF) at the sites of vascular endothelial damage. Tissue factor, a membrane-bound glycoprotein, is considered the common physiologic trigger of both hemostasis and inflammation pathways. Under normal conditions, none cells, which contact with the bloodstream, express TF. An injury, as the initial triggering signal, starts up the TF expression and the externalization at the surface ofinflammatory cells (primarily, monocytes) and vascular wall cells (endothelial or smooth muscle cells). Immediately upon exposure to the bloodstream, TF contacts with activated coagulation factor VIIa (VIIa), whose trace amounts (about 1 % of total inactive enzyme precursor, coagulation factor VII) are conventionally present in circulation. The formation of macromolecular complex TF-VIIa is a crucial event that initiates the first stage of the coagulation process, initiation phase. Alongside with that TF initiates local inflammatory reaction.

2.1 Initiation phase of the coagulation process

Tissue factor-VIIa complexes, newly appeared on the boundary between blood flow and the vessel wall, begin to bind plasma-derived coagulation factor VII to produce additionally factor VIIa. Thus, TF acts as a cofactor in the factor VII/VIIa autoactivation process (Fig. 2). Membrane-bound TF/VIIa complexes also interact with small amounts of coagulation factor X (X) and coagulation factor IX (IX). Activated factors X (Xa) and IX (IXa) start up prothrombin (coagulation factor II) conversion to thrombin (IIa). This first cycle of restricted thrombin production is limited by two plasma-derived inhibitors, tissue factor pathway inhibitor (TFPI) and antithrombin (AT). The former one neutralizes factor Xa when forms a quaternary structure with TF-VIIa-Xa. As well, AT upon binding to heparan sulphate/heparin, rapidly inactivates free factors Xa, IXa, and thrombin, initially accumulated at the site of vascular injury. So, TF-VIIa itself is incapable to generate substantial amounts of thrombin during the initiation phase. However, the TF-dependent cycle of thrombin production can overcome inhibition by TFPI and AT, when TF is maintained at a sufficiently high level (Tanaka et al., 2009). Blood-borne forms of TF (soluble sTF or TF-positive microparticles) shed from disrupted cell membranes of different origin presumably can be an additional driver of the increased TF-initiated thrombin production (Sommeijer et al., 2006). Apparently, cell-exposed and blood-borne TF can promote transduction of inflammatory signals *via* cellular protease-activated receptors (PARs). For example, sTF-mediated inflammation in animal models might develop *via* platelet PAR-4 signalling, while TF-proteases complexes (TF-VIIa and TF-VIIa-Xa) induce the activity of signalling pathways in vascular cells *via* PAR-1 and PAR-2 (Busso et al., 2008; Rao & Pendurthi, 2005; Riewald & Ruf, 2001). Being a mediator of both inflammatory and hemostatic pathways, TF integrates different extra cellular signals and cellular responses, thus participating in the development of a host acute-phase response (Fig. 2). As an extremely potent triggering molecule, TF is capable of translating injury signals into activation of the coagulation cascade, sustaining thrombin initiation, and promoting its propagation.

2.2 Propagation phase of the coagulation process

Trace amounts of thrombin promote formation of a IXa-VIIIa-Ca^{2+}-phospholipid assembly (tenase complex) or a Xa-Va-Ca^{2+}-phospholipid assembly (prothrombinase complex) *via* feedback activation of non-enzymatic cofactors VIII (VIIIa) and V (Va) after their binding to negatively charged phospholipids (phosphatidylinositol and phosphatidylserine) on the surface of activated platelets in the presence of calcium ions. Thrombin also activates factor XI (XIa), which additionally stimulates the tenase complex. Tenase-produced prothrombinase complexes lead to the explosive generation of thrombin, which ultimately leads to generation of a fibrin clot. During an episode of TF-initiated coagulation, tenase and prothrombinase complexes are generated in concentrations that might be sufficient to maintain the TF-independent procoagulant response as long, as the reactants are available. From this moment, normal coagulation may become fully independent of TF (Butenas et al., 2009). The propagation phase can continue and prolong the acute-phase response, where driving of thrombin generation is a requisite for an adequate bleeding prevention *via* more fibrin deposition. By binding to PARs, thrombin activates platelets, endothelial cells, and immune cells. As a result, cytokines and chemokines are additionally expressed, as well as certain HSPP secretion is intensified, leukocyte and platelet recruitment to inflammatory *foci* increases, and fibrin deposition is accumulated. These events considerably enhance local

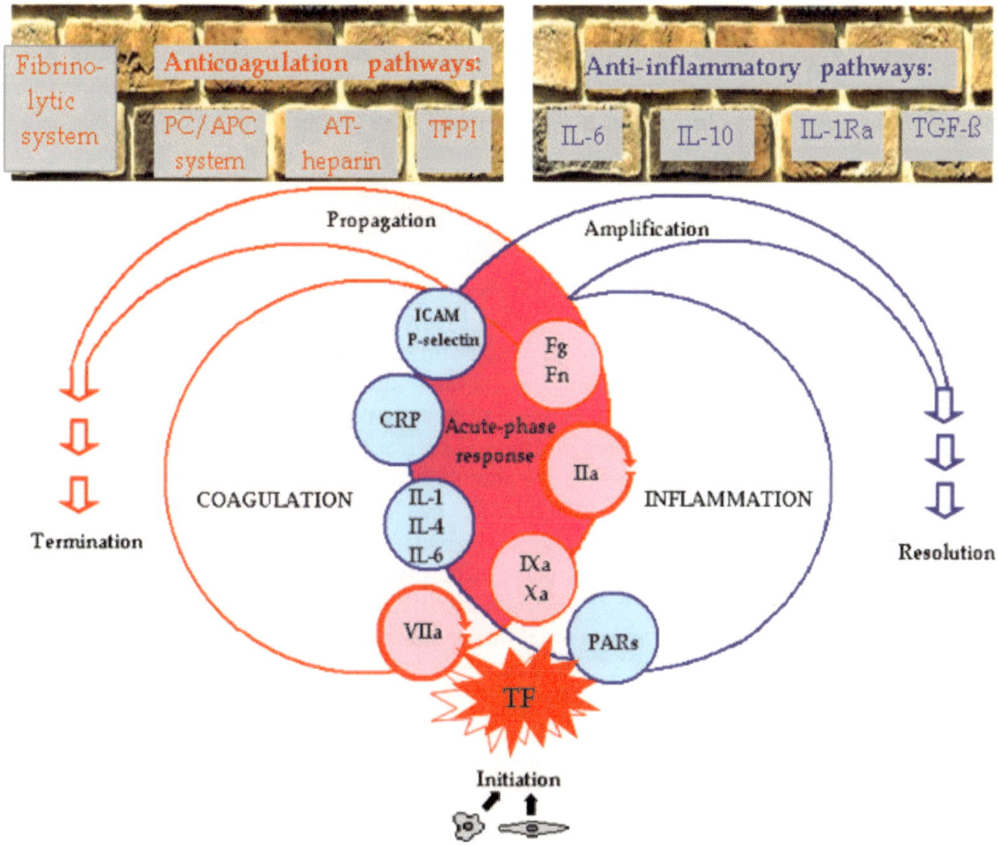

Fig. 2. Schematic representation of the regulatory crosstalk between hemostasis and inflammation in response to exposed TF (coagulation factors and cytokines are all present in circulating plasma whereas TF is the only cell surface glycoprotein shown here). The interconnection of coagulation and inflammation pathways is an essential prerequisite for host homeostasis restitution after injury. Coagulation factors (as shown here with pink circles) and inflammatory mediators (blue circles) promote both coagulation and inflammation through complex and reciprocal interactions, thereby sustaining the acute phase response. At least, two clotting factors, factor VIIa and thrombin, contribute in pro-inflammatory action of coagulation system through positive feed-back autoactivation mechanism (closed-loop arrows). Red curved arrow represents propagation phase of coagulation, blue curved arrow represents amplification of inflammation. In proportion to increasing levels of clotting and inflammatory APP, anticoagulation and anti-inflammation processes are activated. The limiting action of the anticoagulant and fibrinolytic systems on coagulation as well as anti-inflammatory mechanism of inflammation attenuation is depicted by brick-built barrier. Abbreviations: IIa, VIIa, IXa, Xa and XIa indicate activated coagulation factors; Fg, fibrinogen; Fn, fibrin; TF, tissue factor; PARs, protease-activated receptors; IL, interleukin; CRP, C-reactive protein; ICAM, intercellular adhesion molecule-1; PC/APC, protein C/activated protein C; AT, antithrombin; TFPI, tissue factor pathway inhibitor; IL-1Ra, interleukin-1 receptor antagonist; TGF-ß, transforming growth factor beta.

inflammation and coagulation. Furthermore, the formation of thrombi in the microvasculature provides a mechanical barrier that blocks spreading of inflammatory/coagulation mediators into the circulation. Such limited clotting restricts thrombus propagation and prevents from acute local inflammation turning into systemic complications. An anti-clotting molecular process induced by several physiological anticoagulants and fibrinolytic agents is designated for regulation of an adequate clot size and formation of an effective thrombus. Two hemostatic pathways, anticoagulation and fibrinolysis, both are responsible for coagulation termination (Fig. 2).

2.3 Termination phase of the coagulation process

After bleeding is arrested, and the injured vessel is repaired, coagulation attenuation begins to dominate over its propagation due to accumulation of inhibitors of blood clotting. Natural clotting inhibitors are orchestrated through successive induction of three major anticoagulant-dependent pathways: tissue factor pathway inhibitor-, heparin/antithrombin- and the protein C-dependent pathways. A tissue factor pathway inhibitor (TFPI), as was mentioned above, is a most effective inhibitor of coagulation at the initiation phase. This inhibitor specifically blocks the TF-VIIa-Xa complex after trace factor Xa has been formed (Spronk et al., 2003). Antithrombin (AT) is a direct protease inhibitor, which attenuates accumulation of coagulation factors IXa, Xa, and IIa during the propagation phase. Heparin-like glycosaminoglycans accelerate the rate of inactivation of these clotting factors by AT. The protein C system provides multi-directional attenuation of thrombin procoagulant activity and this terminates coagulation. Thrombomodulin (TM), a endothelial cell membrane-associated protein, is capable of to tackling excessive thrombin, thus changing its specific enzyme activity. Within the thrombin-thrombomodulin complex, thrombin looses its affinity to fibrinogen or cellular PARs. Instead this, it possesses an ability to convert precursor protein C (PC) into an anticoagulant enzyme, activated protein C (APC). Activated protein C interrupts thrombin propagation *via* limited proteolysis of cofactors Va and VIIIa. Cofactor protein S and platelet membrane phospholipids provide manifold acceleration of the APC activity. Endothelial protein C receptors (EPCR) enhance the thrombin-thrombomodulin affinity to PC. In such a way the protein C system down-regulates the coagulation cascade to moderate the explosive trend of thrombin production. Its anticoagulant competence enhances, due to the modulation of the thrombin activity through two mechanisms, inhibition of prothrombin converting into thrombin and promotion of thrombin inversion from a procoagulant enzyme into an anticoagulant one. Inhibition of thrombin formation can also reduce thrombin's pro-inflammatory activities (Sarangi et al., 2010).

In a complementary mode with respect to anticoagulation, the surplus clots are dissolved by proteases of the fibrinolytic system. Activation of intravascular fibrinolysis is controlled through enhancing synthesis and secretion of tissue plasminogen activator (tPA) by endothelial cells during fibrin clotting. Tissue plasminogen activator is released into the clot and binds in the clot volume with fibrin(ogen) and plasminogen (Pg). The formation of ternary Fn-tPA-Pg complex extremely effectively accelerates Pg converting into the serine protease plasmin (Pm). Plasmin cleaves fibrin into soluble fragments, the so called fibrin degradation products (FDPs). The rate and extent of local delivery of tPA during the clot formation is important for enhancing the process of fibrinolysis (Schrauwen et al., 1994). To avoid excessive clot digestion, which can affect bleeding, the activity of fibrinolytic system is down-regulated by numerous plasma- and cell-derived inhibitors (Meltzer et al., 2010). These are (i) plasminogen activator inhibitor of type 1 (PAI-1) that highly specifically inactivates tPA, (ii) α_2-antiplasmin, primary Pm inhibitor that prevents Pm-dependent non-specific proteolysis due to effective neutralization of Pm, and (iii) thrombin activable fibrinolytic inhibitor (TAFI) that down-regulates the cofactor activity of fibrin during activation of plasminogen and, thereby, suppresses fibrinolysis.

The activities of both coagulation and fibrinolytic cascades are normally latent but have the potential to be accelerated in an extremely acute manner during inflammation. The coagulation and fibrinolysis pathways have to follow each other, retaining a delicate physiological balance preventing thrombosis and bleeding. Activation of the coagulation cascade leads to increases in the plasma levels of coagulation factors VIIa, Xa, and thrombin, which are pro-inflammatory factors contributing to the acute-phase response (Fig. 2). In addition, fibrin deposition and fibrin degradation products, FDPs, enhance inflammation. Coagulation factors elicit inflammation *via* affecting a number of blood/vascular cells through protease-activated receptor (PAR)-mediated pathways up-regulating the expression of numerous APPs (tumour necrosis factor-alpha, interleukins, adhesion molecules, and growth factors) (Chua, 2005). At least fibrin, thrombin, and coagulation factor Xa, all are important cell-signalling effector molecules that are responsible for receptor triggering. When PARs are activated constantly (e.g., under the action of repeated stimuli), the acute-phase response can be inverted into a chronic one. Therefore, the inflammatory consequence caused by coagulation should be abolished within a necessary time intervals; otherwise it could be enormous. Resolution of the acute-phase response requires down-regulation of inflammatory/procoagulant APPs expression. In particular, IL-4, IL-10, TGF- ß are anti-inflammatory agents that inhibit the production of numerous inflammatory cytokines, including TNF-α, IL-1ß, IL-6, IL-8, and, finally, IL-10 itself (de Waal et al., 1991; Walley et al., 1996). In fact, human blood monocytes are known to produce both pro- and anti-inflammatory cytokines. During resolution, monocytes and macrophages considerably increase production of the latter above the former, thereby preventing prolongation or escalation of an early inflammatory response (Fig. 2). The concentration of cytokine-induced procoagulants is reciprocally decreased; thus, vascular homeostasis is restored.

A failure of the control of these processes causes incorrect inflammation termination or even its propagation. Such an inconsistency leads to deregulation of hemostasis, which, in turn, might force the further leap of inflammatory responses. Under pathological conditions, cytokines are released by immune regulatory cells in sites of the local inflammatory response. This process may be acute but limited in time (reverting to the normal homeostatic state) or persistent (resulting in chronic activation of coagulation and fibrinolysis). Initially acting within the frame of the adaptive defence system, inflammation and hemostasis might develop from a local response to a systemic host reaction. Escalation of inflammation can induce endothelial dysfunction subsequently activating the coagulation cascade, and *vice versa* – hypercoagulation follows amplification of inflammation (Levi et al., 2004)

Under these conditions mutual activation of coagulation and fibrinolysis might follow to potentially exhausting consumptive coagulopathy and disseminated intravascular coagulation. A detrimental inflammatory response resulting from coupling of procoagulant and pro-inflammatory stimuli might cause thrombophilia, and, furthermore, provoke the thrombotic events. In such a way, inflammation/coagulation interaction drastically increases a risk of thrombus formation implicated in the pathogenesis of several diseases in humans. On the one hand, these are thrombophilias, atherosclerosis, and other cardio-vascular pathologies, as well as intercurrent illnesses (like trauma and cancer) or surgery. On the other hand, these are acute/chronic inflammatory diseases, including sepsis, inflammatory bowel disease, and lung and heart inflammation (Fig. 3).

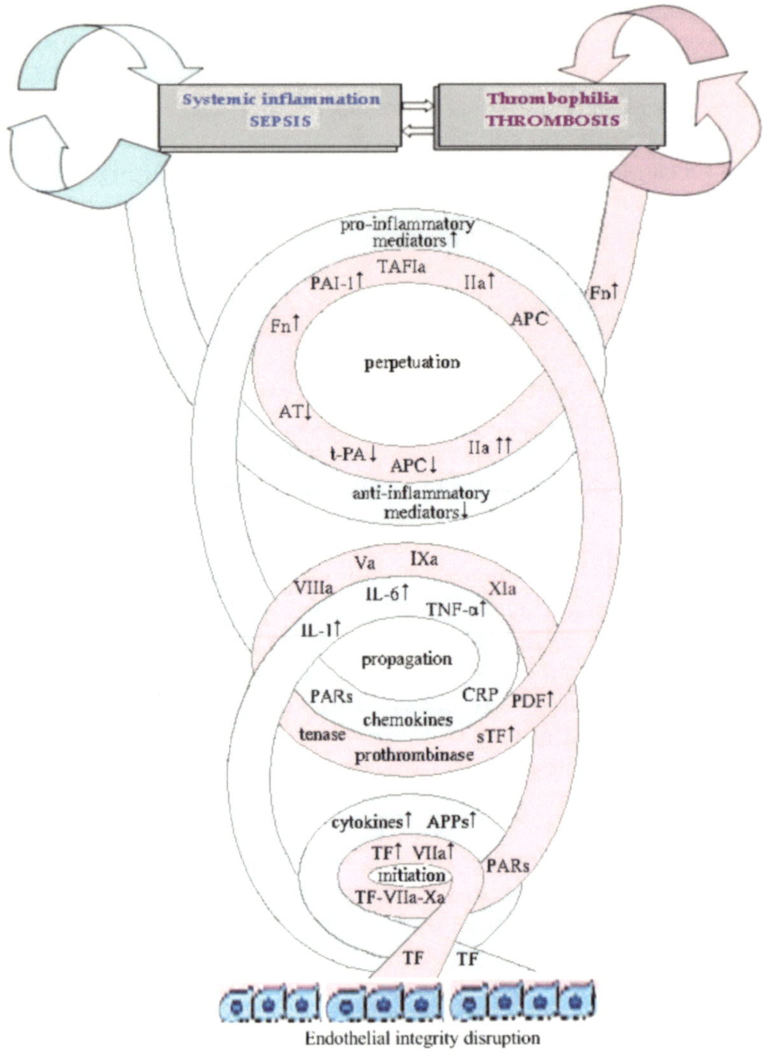

Fig. 3. A simplified hypothetic model of pathophysiological interactions between inflammatory and hemostatic APPs. Each spiral turn represents a potentially vicious cycle driven by excessive concentrations of some components (this is shown as arrows up) and/or insufficient concentrations of other components (as arrows down). Amplification of HSPP activation during an initiation phase is exerted through interaction with the components of the innate immune system, which, in turn, prolongs inflammation during the propagation phase. As a result, both processes, coagulation and inflammation, can come into perpetuation phase. These complex interactions can lead to life-threatening complications, such as thrombosis or sepsis. Refer to the text for discussion in detail.

Abbreviations: IIa, VIIa, IXa, Xa, and XIa indicate activated coagulation factors; Va and VIIIa - non enzymatic cofactors; Fn, fibrin; TF, tissue factor; sTF, blood-borne (soluble) forms of tissue factor; PARs, protease-activated receptors; IL, interleukin; CRP, C-reactive protein; TNF–α, tumour necrosis factor alpha; tPA, tissue activator of plasminogen; APC, activated protein C; AT, antithrombin; PAI-1, plasminogen activator inhibitor of type 1; TAFI, thrombin activable fibrinolytic inhibitor.

3. Pro-inflammatory environment sustains coagulation

Recently, a clear association of high APP levels with a human procoagulant phenotype and impaired fibrinolysis were found in some studies. Indeed, a certain relationship is believed between the plasma levels of C-reactive protein (CRP) and some HSPPs. C-reactive protein is at present used as a sensitive biomarker of acute and chronic inflammation. This is the only APP that correctly displays the severity of vascular pathologies: from an endothelium-derived focal inflammatory response to a hard coronary lesion (Calabrò et al., 2009; Willerson & Ridker, 2004). CRP levels are now detected using a high-sensitivity assay (hsCRP); these indices are found to be an accurate predictor of cardiovascular disease (CVD) (de Ferranti & Rifai, 2007).

The procoagulant function of the C-reactive protein is still debated (MacCallum, 2005), but there is some evidence proving that CRP is associated with the metabolism of HSPP. In *ex vivo* experiments on cell systems, CRP was found to induce expression of inflammatory cytokines or TF in monocytes (Cermak et al., 1993), of thrombomodulin and von Willebrand factor (vWF) in human umbilical vein endothelial cells (HUVECs) (Blann & Lip, 2003), and of PAI-1 in human arterial endothelial cells (HAECs) (Chen et al., 2008; Devaraj et al., 2003). Close correlation of the CRP amount with increasing fibrinogen levels was found in patients with acute ischemic stroke (Tamam et al., 2005). The CRP expression reflects not only to be a predictor but rather an active mediator of atherothrombotic events, as was reported for *in vivo* CRP-dependent induction of TF in blood monocytes (Sardo et al., 2008). Increased levels of hsCRP are associated with such CVD, as severe unstable angina, myocardial infarction, stroke, and peripheral arterial disease (de Ferranti & Rifai, 2007). The causative role of CRP in thrombogenesis is at present believed doubtful, but its active participation is supported by some results described earlier. One of the small group evaluation reports revealed that activation of coagulation and fibrinolysis induced by recombinant CRP infusion provoked increases in the levels of prothrombin F1+2 and D-dimer, as well as in the vWF and PAI-1 concentrations (Bisoendial et al., 2005). CRP also attenuated the fibrinolytic capacity, by inhibiting the tPA activity and stimulating PAI-1. An increased ECLT (euglobulin clot lysis time) and, hence, a decreased fibrinolytic capacity in the blood plasma obtained from volunteers with high CRP levels were found (Zouaoui Boudjeltia et al., 2004). These data confirm a conclusion on down-regulation of fibrinolysis during the enhanced inflammatory response indicated by CRP.

The studies that elucidate the inhibitory role of cytokines in fibrinolysis are not limited to that of CRP. A multifunctional cytokine, IL-1, was shown to stimulate up-regulation of specific mRNA expression of urokinase-type plasminogen activator (u-PA) (Wojta et al., 1994). IL-1 also increased accumulation of PAI-1 in cardiac microvascular endothelial cells (Okada et al., 1998) and also controlled expression of PAI-1 and u-PA in human astrocytes (Kasza et al., 2002). Production of PAI-1 protein in human adult cardiac myocytes was found to be increased up to two times by interleukin-1α and tumour necrosis factor-α (TNF-α) and up to five times by transforming growth factor-ß (TGF- ß) and oncostatin M. However, t-PA production in human cardiac myocytes did not change after cytokine treatment (Macfelda et al., 2002). By contrast, IL-1 and tissue necrosis factor alpha inhibited t-PA in HUVEC (Bevilacqua et al., 1986).

During severe inflammation, the function of fibrinolysis can be impaired. The same is true with respect to anticoagulant pathways. It was recently documented that an increase in serum CRP level in dogs was accompanied by lowering of the AT concentration (Cheng et al., 2009). Under inflammation conditions, the AT plasma level can decreased due to impaired synthesis (like other negative APPs) or due to protein degradation by elastase produced by activated neutrophils (Viles-Gonzalez et al., 2005). In addition, AT might be consumed proportionally to inhibition of the target proteases or removed from circulation after binding to fluid-phase complement attack complexes within the complement cascade (Esmon, 2005). Another natural anticoagulant, TFPI, seems to be incapable of regulating an enhanced thrombin amount during severe inflammation, since a low endogenous concentration of the anticoagulant does not increase (Bastarache et al., 2008). It would be noted that TFPI concentrations do not follow the development of disseminated intravascular coagulation and cannot prevent hypercoagulation (Wiinberg et al., 2008). TFPI is expressed primarily in the microvessels; thus, it might only nominally participate in hemostasis balancing in the larger vessels. Apparently, this pathway only slightly contributes to the coagulation/inflammation cross-over (DelGiudice & White, 2009). The PC anticoagulant system is more extensively present in the vascular network (Viles-Gonzalez et al., 2005). This system plays a pivotal role in hemostasis, shutting down coagulation and promoting fibrinolysis. These events might fail because of the presence of some vulnerable components. Down-regulation of membrane TM and EPCR by endotoxin, IL-1b, and TNF-α has been noted elsewhere (Esmon, 2005). The disappearance of TM from the endothelial cell surface impairs the process of activation of protein C. Not only the amount of APC but also its anticoagulant activity might be decreased under pathological conditions. Protein S, when forming an inactive complex with complement protein C4b (C4BP), thereby looses its ability to promote APC (Dahlback, 1991). Additionally, soluble forms of TM and EPCR can appear during inflammation in the blood flow. They may bind APC without potentiation of its activity or, moreover, even might inhibit APC anticoagulant function. sEPCRs have been found to block binding of protein C and APC to phospholipids and to alter the active site of APC (Liaw et al., 2000).

Tissue factor, in addition to its procoagulant function, has been recently identified as a key secondary inflammatory mediator that markedly accelerates the feedback intensification of coagulation and inflammation pathways. Its concentration in circulation dramatically increases when the endothelium is disrupted and the blood begins to contact with extra vascular cells. In addition, inflammatory mediators many times increase the tissue factor protein amount and activity through stimulation of expression of this protein and through increasing the number of TF-positive microparticles as a consequence of paracrine and autocrine activity of the inflammatory cells (Esmon, 2005). It should be noted that TNF-α and IL-1ß are produced by lymphocytes and macrophages during vascular inflammation, and these events can also enhance the expression of the TF. The TF expression can be stimulated by several inflammatory mediators, namely TNF-α, IL-1, IL-6, activated complement, and immune complexes (DelGiudice & White, 2009). Activated T cells increase both TF expression and activity *via* paracrine stimulation of endothelial cells (Monaco et al., 2002). LPS-stimulated monocytes enhance intracellular transport of increased amounts of TF to the cell surface as well as the shedding of TF-containing microparticles (Egorina et al., 2005). Subsequently, soluble TF indirectly promotes inflammation by stimulation of thrombin production and by involvement of platelets *via* thrombin-activated PAR-dependent signalling. In PAR-4-deficient mice, recombinant sTF did not induce inflammation but was able to activate thrombin production, demonstrating, in such a way, the necessity of thrombin-sensitive platelets for sTF-mediated inflammation (Busso et al., 2008). Activation of platelets leads to release, from their α-granules, of a cocktail of chemokines and cytokines including IL-8, platelet factor–4 (PF4), and macrophage inflammatory protein–1a (MIP-1a) and to the expression of platelet surface adhesion molecules including P-selectin and CD40-ligand (CD40L). Platelet-derived CD40L is able to induce TF on the cell surface of endothelial cells and also of monocytes (Lindmark et al., 2000). Apparently, interaction between TF and flowing blood prolongs activation of the coagulation cascade through additional thrombin generation, which, in turn, might potentiate the formation of a platelet-rich thrombus. As was found recently, the inflammatory response involves activation not only of blood-borne cells (leukocytes and platelets), but also of the cells derived from the vascular wall (endothelial and smooth muscle cells, etc.). Binary TF-VIIa and ternary TF-VIIa-Xa complexes can also modulate inflammation *via* protease-activated receptor 2 (PAR 2) cleaving (Ahamed et al., 2006). Some vascular-bed specificities influence the TF-dependent mechanism of modulation of the acute response. In particular, vessel wall- derived TF forces mainly arterial thrombogenesis, since instable or ruptured atherosclerotic plaques are characterized by a high concentration of TF in both cellular and acellular regions. At the same time, soluble TF contributes mainly to venous thrombosis and microvascular thrombosis (Owens & Mackman, 2010). Nevertheless, circulating TF was found to be associated with the increased blood thrombogenicity in patients with unstable angina and chronic coronary artery disease (Corti et al., 2003). TF causes progression of coagulation within initial stages of disseminated intravascular coagulation (DIC) (Wiinberg et al., 2008). In animal models, TF was shown to participate in generalization of deep vein thrombosis (DVT) (Himber et al., 2003). Some reports indicate that myocardial inflammation and cardiomyocytes injuring enhance expression of TF, thereby increasing local formation of thrombin (Erlich et al., 2000; Luther et al., 2000).

Coagulation factor Xa was found to increase induction of endothelial TF and E-selectin by all the pro-inflammatory cytokines (e.g. TNF, IL-1ß, and CD40L). TF, in turn, initiates a new wave of factor Xa production after the formation of the TF-VIIa complex and activation of zymogens of factors IX and X. Binding of TF-VIIa to PAR-2 also results in up-regulation of the inflammatory responses in macrophages and neutrophils (Cunningham et al., 1999). A synergistic pattern of activity of factor Xa and inflammatory cytokines, resulting in both re-activation of coagulation cascade and augmentation of inflammatory mediators, is a good illustration of the apparent positive feedback mechanism, by which enhanced coagulation maintains pro-inflammatory environment and *vice versa* (Hezi-Yamit et al., 2005) .

4. Hypercoagulation and impaired fibrinolysis perpetuate inflammation

The above-mentioned facts proved the capacity of the inflammatory factors to regulate coagulation and fibrinolysis. A converse molecular mechanism, by which hemostasis stimulates inflammation is at present less obvious but undergoes increasing investigations. Fibrinogen, the precursor of fibrin, is considered a rapid and sensitive marker of both coagulation and the acute-phase response, while its synthesis is enhanced during early inflammatory reactions. Fibrinogen contributes to coagulation being a terminal substrate in plasma clotting, which is cleaved specifically by thrombin. By splitting fibrinopeptide A and fibrinopeptide B from fibrinogen thrombin forms fibrin-monomers are spontaneously polymerized producing fibrin. Fibrin, in turn, provides plasma clotting, platelet aggregation and wound healing or thrombus formation. In addition, fibrin(ogen) participates in activation of vascular cells and regulation of the inflammatory response. Pro-inflammatory effects of fibrin(ogen) manifest itself after the abnormal fibrin deposition; this affects the vascular bed and enhances primarily local and, then, systemic inflammation through expression of the pro-inflammatory mediators. In fact, fibrin(ogen) increases the mRNA levels and induces synthesis of inflammatory cytokines IL-6 and TNF-alpha in human peripheral blood mononuclear cells (PBMCs) (Jensen et al., 2007), of IL-8 in HUVEC (Qi et al., 1997), and of transcription factor NF-kB in mononuclear phagocytes (Sitrin et al., 1998). Fg can manifest a pro-inflammatory action independently of its clotting function due to the existence of a high-affinity integrin binding site or multiple low-affinity binding sites, which interact with inflammatory competent cells. In particular, induction of cytokines IL-1β, IL-6, TNF-α has been found to be associated with fibrin binding to integrin receptors Mac-1 (CD11b/CD18) in monocytes (Trezzini et al., 1991). Cytokine secretion is suggested to be directly triggered by the process of Fg polymerization to Fn. The activity of thrombin that increases in Fg-deficient mice after LPS administration does not correlate with the levels of inflammatory mediators produced by bone marrow-derived macrophages and duration of their action. Both thrombin and Fg acting separately or in combination exert no effect on the cytokine production. It was concluded that up-regulation of secretion results in conformation changes of the Fg molecular structure during its conversion into Fn (Cruz-Topete et al., 2006). Some recently obtained data supported this conclusion. Molecular determinants of fibrin(ogen)-mediated pro-inflammatory activity were found to be localized in a γ-chain. These determinants can enhance the inflammatory cell recruitment and activation *via* interaction with integrin receptors Mac-1. Several specific sequences (all are attributed to the fibrinogen γ-chain) were found to participate in the interaction of fibrinogen with leucocytes. There are γ190-202, γ377-395, and γ383-395 sequences (the latter is localized within the γ-chain of the D nodule), which are capable of affecting leukocyte adhesion, their migration, or cytokine expression (Jennewein et al., 2011). In addition to Mac-1, leukocyte integrin receptors $\alpha_M\beta_2$ (but not platelet receptors $\alpha_{IIb}\beta_3$) may be involved in the progression of inflammatory disease (Flick et al., 2004; Flick et al., 2007). The core recognition motif, γ-chain residues 383–395, was suggested to determine the affinity of Fg and Fn to $\alpha_M\beta_2$. Obviously, soluble Fg has cryptic $\alpha_M\beta_2$ binding sites, which are inaccessible for integrin $\alpha_M\beta_2$ binding. Structural conformation changes during Fg immobilization or conversion of the latter into Fn permit Fg/Fn binding to integrin and provide local leukocyte activation. Being non-diffusible component fibrin deposition attaches to site of injury, marking spatial and temporal coverage for inflammatory cell targeting. Indeed, one might speculate that fibrin-mediated activation of $\alpha_M\beta_2$ in macrophages and neutrophils represents a possible mechanism of the inflammatory response amplification during hypercoagulation. As a result, NF-kB-dependent intracellular signaling, which is triggered by fibrin interaction with $\alpha_M\beta_2$, leads to a vicious cycle of cell recruitment, adhesion, degranulation, generalization of oxidative responses and release of inflammatory mediators (Flick et al., 2004; Flick et al., 2007).

The involvement of fibrinogen in coagulation, as well as that of fibrin in the fibrinolytic process, is accompanied by generation of the various fibrin(ogen) degradation products, FDPs. These small and large fragments can exert an independent regulatory effect on the inflammatory process. In particular, fibrinopeptides A and B, the products of Fg conversion into Fn, are suggested to show a pro-inflammatory action on leucocytes functioning as chemoattractants. In contrast, the peptide Bβ15-42 which is generated by plasmin cleavage of fibrin, can mediate powerful anti-inflammatory effects. FDPs, which are formed after Fg(Fn) digestion by plasmin, also seem to modulate inflammation (Jennewein et al., 2011). Fg, Fn and FDPs were shown to induce intensification of CRP production in vascular smooth muscle cells. Herein, FDPs have the most prominent pro-inflammatory potency, as compared to that of fibrin(ogen) (Guo et al., 2009).

It is interesting that plasmin(ogen) also generates degradation products during activation of fibrinolysis. These are either the first three, or the first four kringle domains (K1-3, K1-4) or only kringle domain 5 (K5). Angiostatin, a proteolytic fragment that contains K1-4, acts as a powerful anti-inflammatory modulator. In particular, angiostatin demonstrated a lowering adhesiveness of leukocytes to extracellular matrix proteins and the endothelium. Interaction of the angiostatin kringle domain K4 with integrin receptor Mac-1 down-regulates transcriptional factor NF-kB, whereby attenuates NF-kB-related expression of neutrophil-derived tissue factor (Chavakis et al., 2005). The kringle domain K5 has been found to restrict the neutrophil chemotactic activity (Perri et al., 2007). Obviously, impaired fibrinolysis looses this anti-inflammatory action.

The formation of fibrin deposition is a direct consequence of increased thrombin production. A pro-inflammatory action of thrombin is realized by two interdependent ways: (i) by direct promotion of hypercoagulation accompanied by the pro-inflammatory effects described above; (ii) by stimulation of vascular and blood-borne cells and their further involvement in the inflammatory response. Being a powerful signal molecule, thrombin interacts specifically with PAR-1, PAR-2, or PAR-3 and activates the signaling pathways in endothelial cells, platelets, mononuclear cells, and fibroblasts. Thrombin-induced intracellular pathways up-regulate the expression of several cytokines and growth factors, as well as the secretion of intercellular adhesion molecule-1 (ICAM-1) and vascular cell adhesion molecule-1 (VCAM-1) (Levi & Poll, 2008). Thrombin is a key protease-agonist, which controls the platelet involvement in the formation of thrombi by stimulation of platelet aggregation, granule secretion, and additional recruitment in the inflammatory process. In an *in vitro* endothelial-cell-monolayer model, thrombin was shown to affect PAR-1-mediated signalling in a concentration-dependent manner. Low thrombin concentrations (20–40 pM) results in endothelial barrier protection, whereas high thrombin concentrations (> 80 pM) lead to disruption of this barrier (Feistritzer & Riewald, 2005). When activated protein C occupies PAR-1, thrombin can realise disruptive effects through activation of PAR-4; this effect requires a higher concentration of thrombin (Bae et al., 2007). Upon binding to thrombomodulin, thrombin inverts its coagulant and inflammatory functions into anticoagulant and anti-inflammatory ones. TM competes effectively with procoagulant substrates (fibrinogen, V, VIII, and PARs) for the same exosite-1 of thrombin but inhibits activation of the coagulation cascades. Moreover, a thrombin-TM complexation down-regulates inflammation/coagulation-pathways *via* a feedback inhibition mechanism, while, at the same time, it initializes protein C-dependent anticoagulant pathway *via* PC activation (Bae et al., 2007). APC, in addition to its anticoagulant function, acts as a pleiotropic agent with anti-inflammatory, profibrinolytic, and cytoprotective effects. After its activation, APC dissociates from the thrombin-TM complex and comes into plasma, where it acts as anticoagulant and profibrinolytic agent, or binds to cell membrane EPCR and regulates intracellular inflammatory pathways. APC is now considered as a signaling molecule that possesses an ability to selectively regulate cytokine production during the inflammatory response. On the one hand, APC down-regulates the production of such pro-inflammatory cytokines, as TNF-α, IL-1ß, IL-6, and IL-8 in monocytes (Stephenson et al., 2006). On the other hand, APC up-regulates anti-inflammatory IL-10 that can reduce the protein concentration and activity of TF, as it was found after treatment of LPS-stimulated monocytes with recombinant APC, rAPC (Toltl et al., 2008). NF-kB-mediated signal transduction events are modulated directly by APC interaction with EPCR on the plasma membrane of endothelial cells and mononuclears. APC-EPCR inhibits NF-kB nuclear translocation, which then results in inhibition of downstream NF-kB-regulated genes, e.g., ICAM-1, VCAM-1, and E-selectin in endothelial cells or TF in mononuclear cells (Joyce et al., 2001; White et al., 2000). APC has recently been reported to impair TNF signaling in vascular endothelial cells by preclusion of phosphorylation of NF-κB p65 and, thereby, by attenuating expression of cell adhesion molecules (including VCAM-1) (Guitton et al., 2011). At the same time, APC does not affect neutrophil respiratory bursts, phagocytic activity, and expression of monocyte adhesion molecules (Stephenson et al., 2006). In fact, APC does not seem to suppress the innate defensive mechanisms. As a consequence, the action of inflammatory cytokines and oxidative agents sharply reduce the efficiency of TM in PC activation and promote pro-inflammatory efficiency of thrombin.

5. Phenotypic variability of hemostasis during acute and chronic inflammation

Abnormal exposure of the procoagulant and pro-inflammatory agents contributes to sustaining of both local and systemic procoagulant/inflammatory potentials. Prolonged activation of inflammatory cells promotes the production of large amounts of inflammatory mediators by downstream-cells affecting not only *via* an autocrine mechanism, but also in a paracrine manner. The duration and amplitude of a cytokine-mediated systemic inflammation signal, upon reaching the liver, determine the probable pattern of HSPPs additionally produced during the acute inflammatory response. The HSPP level is known to be up-regulated by various pro-inflammatory cytokines similarly to other acute phase proteins, i.e., at the transcriptional and post-transcriptional levels. Genetic factors *per se* may contribute in different manners to a total variability of the HSPP systemic levels: cover about 50% variation in the fibrinogen level or 30% in factor VII plasma level, but exert a negligible effect on the plasma level of t-PA (neither that of antigen nor of its activity) (Voetsch & Loscalzo, 2004). Activated protein C, that breaks thrombus generation through regulation of both coagulation and fibrinolysis apparently is not additionally expressed during the acute-host response. There is some evidence that cytokine-dependent down-regulation of protein C synthesis occurs (Yamamoto et al., 1999); this allows one to classify this agent rather as a negative acute-phase protein. In case, lowering of the plasma protein C level is observed in some diseases, which are attended with inflammation (Danese et al., 2010). Another fact, which is a stronger proof, is that cytokines decrease the capacity of the endothelium to activate protein C precursor in activated protein C because they are able to down-regulate the amount of endothelial membrane-bound thrombomodulin (Esmon, 2004). Alternatively, some authors hypothesize that plasma pool of precursor PC can rapidly decline because of enhanced APC consumption after counteracting with plasma inhibitors (Danese et al., 2010; Patalakh et al., 2009). It is obvious, that in pathological states, the relative proportions of HSPPs significantly vary depending on either driving or suppression of their production by inflammation. Changes in the plasma protein ratio can lead to disproportion between procoagulant and anticoagulant patterns under different pathophysiological conditions. Activated proteases are rapidly cleared from circulation and this determines only a crude assessment of their production. That is why their plasma levels do not always respond "in unison" upon systemic inflammation.

5.1 Transcriptional regulation of HSPP production during inflammation

Unlike CRP (type-1 acute phase protein) up-regulated by synergistic action of IL-6 and IL-1beta, most hemostatic proteases (type-2 acute phase proteins) require IL-6 alone for maximal induction of their synthesis (Trautwein et al., 1994). IL-6 is a key effector that effectively promotes the coagulation pathway, not only by up-regulation of expression of some procoagulant factors (such as TF, fibrinogen, and factor VIII) but also by down-regulation of synthesis of some anticoagulants (such as antithrombin and protein S) (Hou et al., 2008). Cytokine IL-6 is suggested to act as a common inductor for several vascular acute-phase proteins (CRP, α- and β- chains of Fg, Pg, α_2-macroglobulin, and PAI-1). Under transcriptional control by the cytokine IL-6, their circulating levels increase *via* cooperative up-regulation of the corresponding gene promoter activity. The congruence of the HSPP gene responses to IL-6 is provided by an IL-6- responsive element (IL6-RE) that is required for maximal stimulation of the promoter activity by IL-6 (Bannach et al., 2004). Interestingly, IL-6-REs were identified in human CRP and α_2-macroglobulin genes, as well as in two genes responsible for synthesis of fibrinogen α- and ß-chains. The same IL-6-REs is located in the region identified as a cytokine-response region of murine Pg and human PAI-1(Bannach et al., 2004; Loppnow & Libby, 1990). More than one IL-6-RE can exist in the promoter region required for the full responsiveness to IL- 6. Two macroglobulin promoters, e.g., have two functionally cooperated REs, which provide the full IL-6 response of the gene (Trautwein et al., 1994). It was assumed that any small differences in the amount or sequence homology of IL-6-REs in the HSPP genes can vary their inducibility by IL-6 (Hattory et al., 1990). Likewise, distinct transcription factors help to transduce the inflammation signal from cytokine to IL-6-RE in a cell- and/or tissue-specific manner. Such mechanisms might allow differential regulation of HSPPs gene expression induced by IL-6. IL-6-dependent regulatory machine is a good example for demonstration how the overall expression of a single plasma protease gene can be controlled by the inflammatory signal that begins in the extracellular milieu and terminates at separate sites on the promoter region of the gene.

Not only IL-6, but a number of cytokines, alone or in a combination, may also influence HSPP synthesis. TNF-α and other inflammatory agents are known to markedly suppress fibrinolysis, mainly *via* stimulation of PAI-1 and down-regulation of t-PA expression. The transcriptional and post-transcriptional regulation of the fibrinolytic system by inflammatory signals was recently reviewed in detail (Medcalf, 2007). Simultaneously acting cytokines can exert additive, inhibitory, or synergistic effects on the HSPP production. TNF-α and IL-1 provide mutual down-regulation of the mRNA for murine protein C. These cytokines are able to control gene expression independently or in combination with IL-6 (Yamamoto et al., 1999), whereas IL-6-mediated induction of Fg synthesis was partially inhibited by IL-1 or TNF-α (Mackiewicz et al., 1991). Various environmental factors and individual features of the patient (including age, body mass index, levels of plasma triglycerides and atherosclerotic transformation of the vessel wall) influence the cytokine-regulated levels of HSPP. For instance, shear stress can up-regulate cytokine-induced expression of t-PA, TGF-ß1, and ICAM-I genes at the transcriptional level (Kawai et al., 1996). These additional influences modify local or systemic inflammatory responses depending on the host phenotype (Lowry, 2009).

5.2 Alterations of the HSPP plasma levels caused by post-transcriptional and post-translational events

Marked alterations in the plasma HSPP levels following an acute-phase stimulus are determined not only by transcriptional regulation but also by post-transcriptional and post-

translational mechanisms. The latter were found for such classic APPs, as serum amyloid A (SAA), complement factors B, and C3 (Jiang et al., 1995). It was reported that the α_2-macroglobulin gene transcription rate might increase (up to nine-fold) during the acute inflammatory response, while its protein plasma concentrations can rise much more significantly (to 100-fold) (Hattory et al., 1990). The other study demonstrated that aortic endothelial cells decreased production and secretion of t-PA after incubation with CRP without any alteration of the tPA mRNA level, thus underlying a suggestion that CRP-mediated tPA inhibition is a posttranscriptional event (Singh et al., 2005). In contrast, post-transcriptional regulation should not play a substantial role in monocyte-derived production of fibrinogen α-chain or α-1 protease inhibitor (α -PI) proteins (Jiang et al., 1995).
Despite the HSPPs are largely regulated by transcriptional control, they still strongly require the post-transcriptional regulation (including co-translational and post-translational modification) to confer their optimal functionality. They should form the disulfide bonds to get native conformation as well as should be carboxylated, hydroxylated, phosphorylated, sulfated or glycosylated to achieve a specific function. In particular, the main coagulation factors II, VII, IX, X and protein C (all are the vitamin K-dependent proteins) are processed through further post-translational modification to become biologically active. Prior to secretion into the blood they should be modified by a vitamin K-dependent gamma-glutamyl carboxylase, getting in such a way, an amount of negatively charged γ-carboxyglutamic acid (Gla) residues. Gla-residues have a chelating activity oriented to Ca^{2+}-cations (Table 2). They are orchestrated in the "Gla domain" to participate in the Ca^{2+}-dependent binding of parent protein to cell membrane or macromolecular complexes.
Similarly to most secretory proteins, HSPPs are enriched by disulfide bonds (Table 2). Before secretion, they undergo oxidative maturation that leads to binding of the appropriate pairs of cystein residues. The disulfide bonds are formed in the rough endoplasmic reticulum, since this process requires an oxidative environment. These functional groups are well-known as playing an important role in protein folding (by stabilizing the tertiary and quaternary structure). Furthermore, disulfide bonds can be responsible for intra- and intermolecular reorganization or even proteins aggregation. In the few last years, a number of studies on functional disulfides have highlighted their two important functions, namely catalytic and allosteric (Chen & Hogg, 2006; Manukyan et al., 2008; Popescu et al., 2010).
In addition to carboxylation and formation of disulfide bonds, a series of post-translational modifications occurs to attach N- or O-linked glycans to secreted proteins (Table 2). Several N-linked glycosylation sites are well-known to be an attributive feature of HSPPs, which are glycoproteins. N-glycosylation has been recently discovered to be a crucial event in the regulation of the glycoprotein structure and function. *Via* promotion or inhibition of intra- and intermolecular binding, glycans can regulate protein folding, cell adhesion and aggregation. Glycosylation can also modulate the activity of plasma membrane receptors at the surface of the vascular endothelial cells, platelets, and leukocytes influencing in such a way intracellular signal transduction systems, which are responsible for homeostasis in circulation (Skropeta, 2009). Probably, a degree of initial core glycosylation might affect the efficiency of protein's γ–carboxylation in endoplasmic reticulum before secretion (McClure et al., 1992).
There are available data, suggesting that glycosylation is higher in proteins synthesized during the acute-phase responses. *In vitro* studies with isolated hepatocytes and hepatoma cell lines proved that inflammatory cytokines regulate changes in glycosylation independently of the rate of synthesis of the APP (Van Dijk & Mackiewicz, 1995). Variations

Protein	Percent carbo-hydrate (w/w)	number of modified residue			
		Glycosylation	Disulfide bond	Hydroxylation, phosphorylation or sulfation	Carboxylation
fII		3 N-linked	10 (+2 predicted)	none	10 Gla residues
fV	~25%	5 N-linked (+21 predicted)	6 (+1 predicted)	1 phosphothreonine 1 phosphoserine 7 sulfotyrosine	none
fVII	13%	2 O-linked 2 N-linked	12	one β-hydroxyaspartate	10 Gla residues
fVIII		1 N-linked (+21predicted)	7 (+1 predicted)	6 sulfotyrosine	none
fIX	17%	4 O-linked 2 N-linked	11	one β-hydroxyaspartate 2 phosphoserine 1 sulfotyrosine	12 Gla residues
fX	15 %	2 O-linked 2 N-linked	12	one β-hydroxyaspartate	11 Gla residues
fXI	5%	5 N-linked	18	2 phosphorilated	none
fXII	17%	7 O-linked 2 N-linked	20	none	none
Glu-Pg	~2%	2 O-linked 1 N-linked	24	1 phosphoserine	none
tPA		1 O-linked 3 N-linked	17	none	none
TFPI		2 N-linked 3 O-linked	9	none	none
AT	9%	4 N-linked	3	1 phosphoserine	none
PC	23 %	4 N-linked	12	one β-hydroxyaspartate	9 Gla residues
α_2 -PI	14%	4 N-linked	1	1 sulfotyrosine	none
PAI-1		2 N-linked (+1 predicted)	none	none	none
TAFI		5 N-linked	3	none	none

(Data based on Protein Knowledgebase UniProtKB)

Table 2. Post-translational modifications of the major hemostasis soluble plasma proteins

in different glycoforms of APP in circulation most likely result from alterations in oligosaccharide branching, increased sialylation, and decreased galactosylation (Gabay & Kushner, 1999). The replacement of individual N-glycans by other ones exerts very specific and diverse effects on the protein structure and/or function. Human hemostatic proteins, coagulation factor IX and protein C, which both are the vitamin K-dependent proteins synthesized and secreted by hepatocytes, vary extensively in their glycosylation levels. Coagulant factor IX has two N-glycosylation sites and is characterised by significantly more heterogeneity of N-glycan structures than anticoagulant protein C. PC has four N-glycosylation sites, Q97, Q248, Q313, and Q329; the latter has an unusual consensus sequence, Asn-X-Cys. Desialylation of PC and factor IX was shown to result in a two-threefold increase in the anticoagulant activity of protein C and in a loss of the coagulant activity of factor IX (Gil et al., 2009; Grinnell et al., 1991). Alterations in the glycosylation pattern have been suggested to be specific in certain diseases (An et al., 2009; Ohtsubo & Marth, 2006). Nevertheless, it remains unclear whether inflammation signals control processing of coagulation proenzymes or not. Well-documented inflammation impact on glycosylation of classic APPs allows researchers to suggest such a control. The most important mechanism, through which the inflammatory environment is able to alter the enzyme activity and/or substrate specificity in local environments or in a systemic disease are modifications of the glycan moiety or heterogeneity. Experiments with glycoprotein deglycosylation showed that the removal of distinct glycan or total deglycosylation usually leads to remarkable reduction of the protein binding and enzymatic activity. However, at least two examples have been recently elucidated (Skropeta, 2009), where the enzyme activity increased upon deglycosylation of HSPPs. In particular, removal of the two of four existing glycosylation sites in the human protein C molecule resulted in a two–threefold increase in the anticoagulant activity of APC due to an enhanced affinity of thrombin, the natural activator of PC. Interestingly, two fibrinolytic proteins, tPA and its specific substrate, Pg, interact more or less effectively depending on the peculiarities of attached glycans. Indeed, tPA can exist as two glycoforms, type I with three N-glycosylated sites and type II with two N-glycans. Plasminogen also exists in two glycoforms; type 1 has both N- and O-linked glycans, while type 2 has only an O-linked glycan. The combination of type II tPA with type 2 plasminogen induced a twofold more intense conversion of plasminogen to plasmin compared to interaction of more heavily glycosylated type I tPA with type 1 Pg. Changes in the microheterogenity and unique structure of glycans are now known to be ensued from folding of the glycoprotein early form during post-translation processing in the secretory pathway. Glycosylation is an enzymatic process regulated by distinct glycosyltransferases in the endoplasmic reticulum, which modulate unfolded glycoproteins prior to trafficking to the Golgi apparatus. Unexpectedly, one experiment demonstrated that an alterated O-glycosylation pathway affects the N-glycosylated coagulation proteins in NAcT-1-deficient mice. In particular, the deficiency of a polypeptide GalNAc transferase (ppGalNAcT) contributed to shifting of O-glycan repertoire by other glycosyltransferases, as well as affected blood coagulation resulting in prolongation of the activated partial thromboplastin time, APTT, and bleeding time. These abnormalities were accompanied by mild or moderate decreases in the circulating levels of factors V, VII, VIII, IX, X, and XII, whereas the level of von Willebrand factor tended to raise (Tenno et al., 2007). The reported results might be interpreted as a consequence of pleuotropic effects of O-glycosylation that contribute to regulation of HSPP expression and/or turnover (primarily secretion and clearance). Additionally, alterations in the degree of branching and of levels of sialylation, fucosylation, and mannosylation can dramatically change the glycoprotein turnover. Although our information about glycan-mediated pathophysiological mechanisms is still very limited, their impact on the enzyme secretion, stability, and activity and on molecular trafficking and clearance allows researchers to suggest that glycosylation plays a special role in the phenotypical variability of hemostatic and inflammatory proteins in circulation. Apparently, the acute-phase response generates a characteristic protein profile by alteration of synthesis, secretion, and clearance of protein reflected in their final concentrations. The actual level of plasma proteins under pathological conditions is also determined by changes in their stability, post-secretion proteolysis, functional activity, and accessibility for interaction.

Marked alterations in the plasma protein levels are probably paralleled by modifications of their disulphide bonds. The role of disulfides in regulation of the functional activity of HSPPs was subjected to intense research. A direct influence of inflammatory conditions on the structure or functions of plasma proteins is an intriguing question. Recently, we demonstrated that the concentration of DTNBA-active polypeptides produced in the course of the reaction of plasma and serum proteins with 5,5'-dithiobis(2-nitrobenzoic acid), was noticeable increased in patients with stable *angina pectoris* compared to healthy subjects. *In vitro* blood coagulation was accompanied by a six-fold drop of the SS-containing components and 2,5-fold elevation of SH-containing polypeptides in patients, whereas mild changes were documented in control subjects. In addition, positive correlation of the plasma level of SH-containing polypeptides with concentrations of CRP and low-density lipoproteins was observed. Based on our findings, we can speculate that hypercoagulation in sclerotized vessels can enhance inflammation by promoting the development of oxidative stress. Activated, and thereby, partially degraded HSPPs, after their more open conformation has been obtained, can exhibit earlier buried disulphide bridges, which can serve as pro-oxidant derivates during thiol-disulfide exchange (Patalakh et al., 2008). Earlier, in the study of Procyk and colleagues (1992), it was found that thrombin looses its ability to cleave Fg in a calcium-free medium under non-denaturing conditions after reduction of several disulfide bonds in α- and γ-chains of fibrinogen. The loss of thrombin clottability was suggested to result from perturbation of carboxy-terminal polymerization sites in the fibrinogen γ-chain. It is interesting that tPA converted Pg into Pm more effectively on the surface of non-clottable (partially reduced) Fg rather than on untreated Fg (Procyk et al., 1992). These data confirm the statement on the ability of disrupted disulfide bonds to modulate the functional activity of major HSPPs *via* conformational changes. Newly obtained data suggest that particular SS-bonds are involved in regulation of HSPP functions *via* reduction or oxidation. Most hemostasis-related proteins probably contain these functionally active allosteric disulfide bonds; among them, there are TF, Fg, Pg(Pm), tPA, uPA, an uPA receptor, vitronectin, glycoprotein 1bα, $ß_3$ subunit of $\alpha_{IIb}ß_3$ integrin, and thrombomodulin (Chen & Hogg, 2006). We hypothesized that at least one common sensitive element in the protein structures of the plasma pattern might facilitate the adequate integrated response of the hemostasis system to an inflammatory impact. Redox-mediated signals, which are generated in plasma during inflammation, might control hemostasis pathways *via* such a sensitive element in protein structures. And *vice versa*, exposed disulfide bonds through one-electron reduction can generate active intermediates transmitting pro-inflammatory or pro-oxidant extracellular signals to cell receptors and, thus, can induce production of more APPs and HSPPs, especially *via* the MAPK-mediated pathway (Forman et al., 2004; Rees et al., 2008).

Although HSPPs are synthesised and secreted principally in hepatocytes (Ruminy et al., 2001) other cell types can be additionally involved. For example, vascular endothelial cells represent an almost exclusive source of such a fibrinolytic component, as tPA produced by the endothelium in both physiological and pathophysiological states. Another fibrinolytic component, PAI-1, has additional sites of synthesis, such as vascular endothelial cells, leukocytes, adipocytes, and platelets, but this occurs predominantly after their activation at inflammatory *foci*. Synthesis of protein C, which mainly occurs in the liver, was also identified in the kidneys, lungs, brain, and male reproductive tissue. Therefore, a systemic or local inflammatory signal is able to recruit more than one cells source of HSPP. Aggregated platelets, activated leukocytes, and cells presented in the vascular wall release cytokines thereby altering local HSPP secretion. Impairment of total HSPP production because of disorders of the liver functions during systemic inflammation can be accompanied by increased protein consumption or by a decrease in the hepatic clearance for individual proteins. Perpetuation of inflammation in patients suffering from sepsis is known to depress the activity of Pg or α_2-plasmin inhibitor (α_2-PI) rather because of a low synthetic function of the liver but not consumption coagulopathy (Asakura et al., 2001). In contrast, increased consumption is the main reason for suppression of the plasma level of such enzymatically active proteases, as APC, thrombin, Pm, and tPA. In turn, depletion of the pool of proteases results in ineffective consumption and clearance of their substrates. Additionally to the protein expression, this mechanism can participate in elevation of such hemostatic APPs as factors VIIIa and Va, Fg, Fn, and Pg (Baklaja & Pešic, 2008). Finally, the rate of secretion and/or clearance processes of plasma proteins should be markedly distinct from the rate of their synthesis. Respectively, the half-life time of involved factors is shortened or prolonged.

It is obvious that the plasma levels of naturally active (e.g., tPA) or *in situ* activated hemostatic proteases (e.g., thrombin or APC) fluctuate during inflammation rather due to stimulation of secretion, reactivity, and clearance than due to the respective gene expression in the cells. The above-mentioned regulatory mechanisms can affect significantly the HSPP kinetic profile with either a rise or a decline of their plasma levels. According to the study of Jern and colleagues (Jern et al., 1999), there is no correlation between the net release rate of total t-PA and plasma levels of either total or active tPA. These authors also suggested that the local endothelial release rate, rather than the systemic plasma level of t-PA, determines the plasma fibrinolytic potential destined to clot digestion *in situ*. The assay-measured plasma concentration of tPA insufficiently displays this local discrete increment. Moreover, while cytokine-induced PAI-I secretion increases, tPA secretion alternatively decreases (as after CRP-regulated secretion) or remains unchanged. Platelets have a large PAI-1 storage pool within secretory α-granules (about 90 % of the plasma level). After platelet activation, PAI-1 is released from α-granules along with other coagulation proteins, adhesion molecules, integrins, growth factors, and inflammatory modulators. Such a pro-inflammatory milieu facilitates the recruitment of additional platelet and inflammatory cells encouraging generate and amplify inflammation signals. Tissue plasminogen activator is secreted from the intracellular storage compartment after stimulation of PARs on the surface of endothelial cells. There are two pathways involved in tPA secretion from endothelial cells, constitutive and regulated secretion. Rates of the constitutive tPA release is differentiated markedly by the genotype; however, genetic variation most likely is not reflected in the circulating plasma t-PA levels. It was reported that CRP impaired the release of tPA *via* Fc-γ receptors but did not affect tPA mRNA (Devaraj et al., 2005). Stimulation of endothelial cells with IL-1ß or TNF-α did not change their ability to produce tPA (Jern et al., 1999). Shear stress can modulate the cytokine effects by enhancing t-PA secretion and attenuating the PAI-1 release (Kawai et al., 1996).

Probably, the recovery of the tPA plasma pool in proportion to excessive consumption by PAI-1 is rapid but transient, since the augmented local tPA secretion is limited by the rate of its synthesis. Because of the fact that the tPA-PAI-1 complex is usually cleared at a lower rate than free tPA, this can lead to the appearance of a disproportion between the antigen and activity values. Notably, activated protein C is suggested to compete with tPA for PAI-1 complexation. The importance of APC-PAI-1 *in vivo* association is still disputable because the PAI-1 reactivity with respect to APC is very low in a purified system. Nevertheless, it was demonstrated that vitronectin, a pro-inflammatory protein, enhances the reactivity of PAI-1 with APC about 300 times (Rezaie, 2001).

In a study with patients suffering from chronic cardiac failure (CCF) and stable *angina pectoris* (SAP) we found an abnormality of the ratios between the plasma levels of t-PA, PC, and PAI-1 (Patalakh et al, 2009; Patalakh et al, 2007). An insufficiency of PC and t-PA proteins was accompanied by increase in the PAI-1 concentration and activity in the blood plasma of patients with high intravascular inflammation (hs-CRP levels were 12,95±1,81 and 6,83±1,48 mg/ml for SAP and CCF, respectively). We believe that these changes are a manifestation of reduction of the blood fibrinolytic potential. Using a regression analytical procedure, we simulated a potential profibrinolytic effect of endogenous PC as association of its plasma level with PAI-1 attenuation. The effect became apparent within a close-cut range of the PAI-1 concentrations and descended at low (<0,8 nM) or high (>3 nM) PAI concentrations. It was also predicted that the profibrinolytic function of APC during CCF duration might be realized under conditions where the precursor PC concentration did not decrease below 50-60 nM.

Some evidence do exist that the plasma levels of PC are associated with the systemic inflammatory response to trauma, infection, resuscitated cardiac arrest, non-stable *angina pectoris*, etc. It seems that most cardio-vascular diseases during their severe inflammation stage are complicated by a transient PC deficiency. The nature of this failure is not completely clear. We suppose that the PAI-1 inhibitory activity is involved into PC plasma pool depletion during acute inflammation. It seems that phenotypic PC alterations reflect different aspects of the APC turnover, up-regulated by inflammation stimuli. It seems that conversion of PC into APC, forced by the increasing thrombin production, can lead to rapid consumption of PC since APC undergoes action of the abundant amount of serine protease inhibitors, accumulated in the blood during the acute-phase response. PAI-1 is the most up-regulated inhibitor of APC during acute inflammation. Activated platelets additionally produce PAI-1 during coagulation and thrombus formation. Particularly due to vitronectin activation PAI-1 should contribute significantly to the acquired protein C deficiency. Only when present in physiological concentrations, APC can deplete PAI-1 and, thus, promote the involvement of t-PA in fibrinolysis. Due to severe or prolonged conversion of PC into APC, the plasma pool of PC may be exhausted. As a result, further generation of activated protein C will be disturbed. The retarded turnover of protein C ($t_{1/2}$~ 8 hours) and an extremely short clotting time (about 2-3 min) might cause depression of the protein C pathway and, consequently, uncontrolled promotion of the thrombin pathway. As a result APC loses its crucial role in the regulation of hemostasis and inflammation. While coagulation and inflammation are escalated, anticoagulant and fibrinolytic blood potentials are dropped. The described progression of events might provoke inflammatory and thrombogenic diseases in a manner we illustrate in figure 3.

6. Conclusion

Recent advances in our understanding of the nature of critical factors, linking hypercoagulation with both acute and chronic inflammation are rather promising. Nevertheless, we only can propose some speculations predicting the balance disruption between procoagulant and anticoagulant components under conditions of abnormal hemostasis, as well as consequences of their ratio abnormality on inflammation duration. The problem is complicated by the existence of poorly predictable mechanisms of most urgent thrombotic events that are happened rather "now" and "here". A transient deficiency or acute inactivation of common hemostatic soluble plasma proteins, affecting hemostasis and inflammation by a mutual regulatory mechanism, was suggested as a key pathogenic factor of such life-threatening complications. Post-translational HSPPs modifications reviewed here could be considered as crucial phenomenon impacted by the inflammatory process. Apparently, inflammation-associated variations in the structure and function of hemostatic proteins can influence their catalytic efficiency and measurable plasma levels. These changes should be taken into account in indication of pathological hemostasis. The recent knowledge on regulatory crosstalk between hemostatic system components and the inflammatory system allows discovering new therapeutic targets to be developed. This new approach could not only change the traditional paradigm of clotting factor substitution therapy, but also anti-inflammatory therapies. Activated protein C is expected to be an attractive therapeutic target with prominent anticoagulant, profibrinolytic, and anti-inflammatory properties, which can simultaneously regulate both inflammation and coagulation. Nevertheless, the results of several clinical trials with recombinant APC or modified rAPC were found to be rather disappointing. Indeed, the peculiarities of the protein structure, attributed to regulatory components with pleiotropic action such as APC, may play a pivotal role in providing clinical benefit of designed protein variants. Hemostasis is a thorough "molecular machine", which can not readily be improved. To understand and to reconstruct perturbed functions of this machinery should be a prominent goal for both basic and clinical research studies.

7. Acknowledgment

The author is thankful to Professor Stanislaw A. Kudinov, Dept. of Enzyme Chemistry and Biochemistry (Palladin Institute of Biochemistry of the NAS of Ukraine) for initiating the idea of this review. The author would like also thank Professor Francisco Veas for advice and for critically reading the manuscript. We acknowledge the financial support from the Anisimov Property Management LTD (Ukraine) and from Sergey Davydov, businessman.

8. References

Ahamed J., Versteeg H.H., Kerver M., Chen V.M., Mueller B.M., Hogg P.J. & Ruf W. (2006). Disulfide isomerization switches tissue factor from coagulation to cell signaling. *Proc. Nat.l Acad. Sci. USA*. Vol. 103, No. 38, pp. 13932-13937.

An H.J., Kronewitter S.R., de Leoz M.L. & Lebrilla C.B. (2009). Glycomics and disease markers. *Curr. Opin. Chem. Biol.*, Vol.13, No (5-6), pp. 601-607.

Asakura H., Ontachi Y., Mizutani T., Kato M., Ito, T., Saito M., Morishita E., Yamazaki M., Suga Y., Miyamoto K.-I. & Nakao S. (2001). Depressed plasma activity of plasminogen or [alpha]2 plasmin inhibitor is not due to consumption coagulopathy in septic patients with disseminated intravascular coagulation. *Blood Coagulation & Fibrinolysis,* Vol.12, Issue 4, pp. 275-281.

Bae J.S., Yang L., Manithody C.& Rezaie A.R. (2007). The ligand occupancy of endothelial protein C receptor switches the PAR-1-dependent signaling specificity of thrombin from a permeability-enhancing to a barrier-protective response in endothelial cells. *Blood,* Vol.110, No.12, pp. 3909–3916.

Baklaja R., M. C. Pešic M. C. & Czarnecki J. (2008). *Hemostasis and hemorrhagic disorders.* Fermentation-Biotec GmbH, ISBN - 978-3-00-025826-8, 337 p.

Bannach F.G., Guttierez-Fernandez A., Parmer R.J. & Miles L.A. (2004). Interleukin-6-induced plasminogen gene expression in murine hepatocytes is mediated by transcription factor CCAAT/enhancer binding protein ß (C/EBPß). *J. Thromb. Haemost.,* 2004, Vol. 2, No.12, pp. 2205–2212.

Bastarache J.A., Wang L., Wang Z., Albertine K.H., Matthay M.A.& Ware L.B. (2008). Intra-alveolar tissue factor pathway inhibitor is not sufficient to block tissue factor procoagulant activity. *Am. J. Physiol. Lung Cell Mol. Physiol.,* Vol. 294, No.5, pp. L874 - L881.

Bevilacqua M.P., Pober J.S., Majeau G.R., Fiers W., Cotran R.S. & Gimbrone M.A.Jr. (1986). Recombinant TNF induces procoagulant activity in cultured human vascular endothelium: characterization and comparison with the actions of IL-1. *Proc. Natl. Acad. Sci. U S A.* , Vol. 83, No.12, pp.4533– 4537.

Bisoendial R.J., Kastelein J.J., Levels J.H., Zwaginga J.J., van den Bogaard B., Reitsma P.H., Meijers J.C., Hartman D., Levi M. & Stroes ES. (2005). Activation of inflammation and coagulation after infusion of C-reactive protein in humans. *Circ Res.,* Vol. 96, No. 7, pp. 714-716.

Blann A.D. & Lip G.Y. (2003). Effects of CRP on the release of von Willebrand factor, E-selectin, thrombomodulin and intercellular adhesion molecule-1 from HUVEC. *Blood Coagul. Fibrinolysis,* Vol. 14, No. 4, pp. 335–340.

Busso N., Chobaz-Péclat V., Hamilton J., Spee P., Wagtmann N. & So A. (2008). Essential role of platelet activation *via* protease activated receptor 4 in tissue factor-initiated inflammation. *Arthritis Res. Ther.,* Vol. 10, No.2, R42.

Butenas S., Orfeo T. & Mann K.G. (2009). Tissue Factor in Coagulation: Which? Where? When? *Arterioscler. Thromb. Vasc. Biol.,* Vol. 29, No.12, pp. 1989-1996.

Calabrò P., Golia E. & Yeh E.T. (2009). CRP and the risk of atherosclerotic events. *Semin. Immunopathol.,* Vol. 31, No.1, pp. 79-94.

Castellheim A., Brekke O.L., Espevik T., Harboe M. & Mollnes T.E. (2009). Innate immune responses to danger signals in systemic inflammatory response syndrome and sepsis. *Scand. J. Immunol.,* Vol. 69, No. 6, pp.479-491.

Cermak J., Key N.S., Bach R.R., Balla J., Jacob H.S. & Vercellotti G.M. (1993). CRP induces human peripheral blood monocytes to synthesize tissue factor. *Blood,* Vol. 82, pp. 513–520.

Chavakis T., Athanasopoulos A., Rhee J.S., Orlova V., Schmidt-Wöll T., Bierhaus A., May A.E., Celik I., Nawroth P.P. & Preissner K.T. (2005). Angiostatin is a novel anti-inflammatory factor by inhibiting leukocyte recruitment. *Blood,* Vol.105, No. 3, pp. 1036-1043.

Chen C., Nan B., Lin P. & Yao Q. (2008). C-reactive protein increases plasminogen activator inhibitor-1 expression in human endothelial cells. *Thrombosis Research*, Vol. 122, No. 1, pp. 125-133.

Chen V.M. & Hogg P.J. (2006). Allosteric disulfide bonds in thrombosis and thrombolysis. *J. Thromb. Haemost.* Vol. 4, No. 12, pp. 2533-2541.

Cheng T., Mathews K. A., Abrams-Ogg A.C.G. & Wood R. D. (2009). Relationship between assays of inflammation and coagulation: A novel interpretation of the canine activated clotting time. *The Canadian Journal of Veterinary Research.*, Vol. 73, No. 2, pp. 97–102.

Chua A.J. (2005). Tissue factor mediates inflammation. *Archives of Biochemistry and Biophysics*, Vol. 440, No. 2, pp. 123-132.

Corti R., Fuster V. & Badimon J.J. (2003). Pathogenetic concepts of acute coronary syndromes. *J. Am. Coll. Cardiol.*, Vol. 41, No. 4 , pp. 7S-14S.

Cruz-Topete D., Iwaki T., Ploplis V.A.& Castellino F.J. (2006). Delayed inflammatory responses to endotoxin in fibrinogen-deficient mice. *The Journal of Pathology*, Vol. 210, No. 3, pp. 325–333

Cunningham M.A., Romas P., Hutchinson P., Holdsworth S. R. & Tipping P.G. (1999). Tissue factor and factor VIIa receptor/ligand interactions induce proinflammatory effects in macrophages. *Blood*, Vol. 94, No.10, pp. 3413 - 3420.

Dahlback B. (1991). Protein S and C4b-binding protein: components involved in the regulation of the protein C anticoagulant system. *Thromb. Haemost.*, Vol. 66, No. 1, pp. 49-61.

Danese S., Vetrano S., Zhang L., Poplis V.A. & Castellino F.J. (2010). The protein C pathway in tissue inflammation and injury: pathogenic role and therapeutic implications. *Blood*, Vol. 115, No. 6, pp. 1121–1130.

de Ferranti S.D., & Rifai N. (2007). C-reactive protein: a nontraditional serum marker of cardiovascular risk. *Cardiovasc. Pathol.*, Vol. 16, No. 1, pp. 14-21.

de Waal M.R., Abrams J., Bennett B., Figdor C.G., & de Vries J.E. (1991). Interleukin 10(IL-10) inhibits cytokine synthesis by human monocytes: an autoregulatory role of IL-10 produced by monocytes. *J. Exp. Med.*, Vol.174, No.5, pp. 1209–1220.

DelGiudice L.A. & White G.A. (2009). The role of tissue factor and tissue factor pathway inhibitor in health and disease states. *J. Vet. Emerg. Crit. Care* (San Antonio), Vol. 19. No. 1, pp. 23-29.

Devaraj S., Du Clos T.W. & Jialal I. (2005). Binding and internalization of CRP by Fc gamma receptors on human aortic endothelial cells mediates biological effects. *Arterioscler. Thromb. Vasc. Biol.*, Vol.25, No.7, pp. 1359–1363.

Devaraj S., Xu D.Y. & , Jialal I. (2003). C-reactive protein increases plasminogen activator inhibitor-1 expression and activity in human aortic endothelial cells: implications for the metabolic syndrome and atherothrombosis. *Circulation*, Vol. 107, No.3, pp. 398–404.

Egorina E.M., Sovershaev M.A., Bjorkoy G., Gruber F.X., Olsen J.O., Parhami-Seren B., Mann K.G. & Osterud B. (2005). Intracellular and surface distribution of monocyte tissue factor: application to intersubject variability. *Arterioscler. Thromb. Vasc. Biol.*, Vol. 25, No. 7, pp. 1493-1498.

Erlich J.H., Boyle E.M., Labriola J., Kovacich J.C., Santucci R.A., Fearns C., Morgan E.N., Yun W., Luther T., Kojikawa O., Martin T.R., Pohlman T.H., Verrier E.D. & Mackman N.

(2000). Inhibition of the tissue factor-thrombin pathway limits infarct size after myocardial ischemia-reperfusion injury by reducing inflammation. *Am. J. Pathol.*, Vol. 157, No. 6, pp. 1849–1862.

Esmon C.T. (2004). Crosstalk between inflammation and thrombosis. *Maturitas*, Vol. 47, No. 4, pp. 305-314.

Esmon C.T. (2005). The interactions between inflammation and coagulation. *Br. J. Haematol.*, Vol. 131, No. 4, pp. 417-430.

Feistritzer C.& Riewald M. (2005). Endothelial barrier protection by activated protein C through PAR1-dependent sphingosine 1-phosphate receptor-1 crossactivation. *Blood*, Vol.105, No.8, pp. 3178–3184.

Flick M.J., Du X. & Degen J.L. (2004). Fibrin(ogen)-$\alpha_M\beta_2$ interactions regulate leukocyte function and innate immunity in vivo. *Exp. Biol. Med.*, Vol. 229, pp. 1105–1110.

Flick M.J., LaJeunesse C.M., Talmage K.E., Witte D.P., Palumbo J.S., Pinkerton M.D., Thornton S. & Degen J.L. (2007). Fibrin(ogen) exacerbates inflammatory joint disease through a mechanism linked to the integrin alphaMbeta2 binding motif. *J. Clin. Invest.*, Vol. 117, No.11, pp. 3224-3235.

Forman H.J., Fukuto J.M.& Torres M. (2004). Redox signaling: thiol chemistry defines which reactive oxygen and nitrogen species can act as second messengers. *Am. J. Physiol. Cell Physiol.*, Vol.287, No.2, pp. C246-C256.

Gabay C. & Kushner I. (2001). Acute-phase proteins. Encyclopedia of Life Sciences. Available from: onlinelibrary.wiley.com/doi/ 10.1038/npg.els.0000497/pdf.

Gabay C. & Kushner I.(1999). Acute-phase proteins and other systemic responses to inflammation. *N. Engl. J. Med.*, Vol. 340, No.6, pp. 448 - 454.

Gil G.C., Velander W.H. & Van Cott K.E. (2009). N-glycosylation microheterogeneity and site occupancy of an Asn-X-Cys sequon in plasma-derived and recombinant protein C. *Proteomics.*, Vol. 9, No.9, pp. 2555-2567.

Grinnell B.W., Walls J.D. & Gerlitz B. (1991). Glycosylation of human protein C affects its secretion, processing, functional activities, and activation by thrombin. *J. Biol. Chem.*, Vol. 266, No. 15, pp. 9778-9785.

Guitton C., Cottereau A., Gérard N., Quillard T., Chauveau A., Devallière J., Tonnerre P. & Charreau B. (2011). Protective cross talk between activated protein C and TNF signaling in vascular endothelial cells: implication of EPCR, noncanonical NF-κB, and ERK1/2 MAP kinases. *Am. J. Physiol. Cell Physiol.*, Vol. 300, No. 4, pp. C833-C842.

Guo F., Liu J., Wang C., Liu N. & Lu P. (2009). Fibrinogen, fibrin, and FDP induce C-reactive protein generation in rat vascular smooth muscle cells: Pro-inflammatory effect on atherosclerosis. *Biochemical and Biophysical Research Communications*, Volume 390, Issue 3, pp. 942-946.

Hattory M., Abraham L.J., Northemmann W. & Fey G.H. (1990). Acute-phase reaction induces a specific complex between hepatic uclear proteins and the interleukin 6 response element of the rat a2-macroglobulin gene. *Proc. Natl. Acad. Sci. USA*, Vol. 87, No. 6,pp. 2364-2368.

Hezi-Yamit A., Wong P.W., Bien-Ly N., Komuves L.G., Prasad K.S.S., Phillips D.R. & Sinha U. (2005). Synergistic induction of tissue factor by coagulation factor Xa and TNF: Evidence for involvement of negative regulatory signaling cascades. *PNAS*, Vol. 102, No. 34, pp. 12077–12082.

Himber J., Wohlgensinger C., Roux S., Damico L.A., Fallon J.T., Kirchhofer D., Nemerson Y., Riederer M.A. (2003). Inhibition of tissue factor limits the growth of venous thrombus in the rabbit. *J.Thromb. Haemost.*, Vol. 1, No. 5, pp. 889–895.

Hou T., Tieu B.C., Ray S., Recinos 3d A., Cui R., Tilton R.G. & Brasier A.R. (2008). Roles of IL-6-gp130 signaling in vascular inflammation. *Current Cardiology Reviews*, Vol. 4, No.3, pp. 179-192.

Jennewein C., Tran N., Paulus P., Ellinghaus P., Eble J.A.& Zacharowski K. (2011). Novel aspects of fibrin(ogen) fragments in the course of inflammation. *Molecular medicine* (Cambridge, Mass.). (In press).

Jensen T., Kierulf P., Sandset P.M., Klingenberg O., Joø G.B., Godal H.C. & Skjønsberg O.H. (2007). Fibrinogen and fibrin induce synthesis of proinflammatory cytokines from isolated peripheral blood mononuclear cells. *Thromb. Haemost.*, Vol. 97 No.5, pp. 822-829.

Jern C., Ladenvall P., Wall U. & Jern S. (1999). Gene polymorphism of t-PA is associated with forearm vascular release rate of t-PA. *Arterioscler. Thromb. Vasc. Biol.*, Vol. 19, No. 2, pp. 454–459.

Jiang S.-L., Samols D., Rzewnicki D., Macintyre S.S., Greber I., Sipe J. & Kushne I. (1995). Kinetic modeling and mathematical analysis indicate that acute phase gene expression in Hep 3B cells is regulated by both transcriptional and posttranscriptional mechanisms. *J. Clin. Invest.*, Vol. 95, No.3, pp. 1253-1261.

Joyce D.E., Gelbert L., Ciaccia A., DeHoff B.& Grinnell B.W. (2001). Gene expression profile of antithrombotic protein C defines new mechanisms modulating inflammation and apoptosis. *J.Biol.Chem.*, Vol. 276, No.14, pp. 11199-1203.

Kasza A., Kiss D.L., Gopalan S., Xu W., Rydel R.E., Koj A. & Kordula T. (2002). Mechanism of plasminogen activator inhibitor-1 regulation by oncostatin M and interleukin-1 in human astrocytes. *Journal of Neurochemistry*, Vol. 83, No.3, pp. 696–703.

Kawai Y., Matsumoto Y., Watanabe K., Yamamoto H., Satoh K., Murata M., Handa M. & Ikeda Y. (1996). Hemodynamic forces modulate the effects of cytokines on fibrinolytic activity of endothelial cells. *Blood,* Vol. 87, No. 6, pp. 2314-2321.

Kushner I. & Rzewnicki D.L. (1994). The acute phase response: General aspects. *Bailliére' s Clinical Rheumatology,* Vol. 8, No. 3, pp. 513-530.

Levi M. & Poll T. (2008). The role of natural anticoagulants in the pathogenesis and management of systemic activation of coagulation and inflammation in critically ill patients. *Semin. Thromb. Hemost.*, Vol. 34, No.5, pp. 459-468.

Levi M., van der Poll T. & Buller H.R. (2004). Bidirectional relation between inflammation and coagulation. *Circulation*, Vol. 109, No.22, pp. 2698–2704.

Liaw P.C., Neuenschwander P.F., Smirnov M.D. & Esmon C.T. (2000). Mechanisms by which soluble endothelial cell protein C receptor modulates protein C and activated protein C function. *J. Biol. Chem.*, Vol. 275, No.8, pp. 5447-5452.

Lindmark E., Tenno T.& Siegbahn A. (2000). Role of platelet P-selectin and CD40 ligand in the induction of monocytic tissue factor expression. *Arterioscler. Thromb. Vasc. Biol.*, Vol. 20, No. 10, pp. 2322-2328.

Loppnow H. & Libby P. (1990). Proliferating or interleukin 1-activated human vascular smooth muscle cells secrete copious interleukin 6. *J. Clin. Invest.*, Vol. 85, No.3, pp. 731–738.

Lowry S.F. (2009). The evolution of an inflammatory response. *Surg. Infect. (Larchmt)*, Vol. 10, No. 5, pp. 419-425.

Luther T., Dittert D.D., Kotzsch M., Erlich J., Albrecht S., Mackman N. & Muller M. (2000). Functional implications of tissue factor localization to cell-cell contacts in myocardium. *J. Pathol.*, Vol. 192, No. 1, pp. 121–130.

MacCallum P.K. (2005). Markers of hemostasis and systemic inflammation in heart disease and atherosclerosis in smokers. *Proc. Am. Thorac. Soc.*, Vol. 2, No.1, pp. 34-43.

Macfelda K., Weiss T. W., Kaun C., Breuss J.M., Kapeller B., Zorn G., Oberndorfer U., Voegele-Kadletz M., Huber-Beckmann R., Ullrich R., Binder B. R., Losert U. M., Maurer G., Pacher R., Huber K. & Wojta J. (2002). Plasminogen activator inhibitor 1 expression is regulated by the inflammatory mediators interleukin-1α, tumor necrosis factor-α, transforming growth factor-ß and oncostatin M in human cardiac myocytes. *J. Mol. Cell. Cardiol.*, Vol. 34, No. 12, pp. 1681-1691.

Mackiewicz A., Speroff T., Ganapathi M.K. & Kushner I. (1991). Effects of cytokine combinations on acute phase protein production in two human hepatoma cell lines. *J. Immunol.*, Vol.146, No.9, pp. 3032-3037.

Manukyan D., von Bruehl M.L., Massberg S. & Engelmann B. (2008). Protein disulfide isomerase as a trigger for tissue factor-dependent fibrin generation. *Thromb. Res.*, No. 122, Suppl. 1, pp. S19-22.

Markiewski M.M., Nilsson B., Ekdahl K.N., Mollnes T.E. & Lambris J.D. (2007). Complement and coagulation: strangers or partners in crime? *Trends Immunol.* Vol. 28, No.4, pp. 184-192.

McClure D.B., Walls J.D. & Grinnell B.W. (1992). Post-translational processing events in the secretion pathway of human protein C, a complex vitamin K-dependent antithrombotic factor. *J. Biol. Chem.*, Vol. 267, No.27, pp. 19710-19717.

Medcalf R.L. (2007). Fibrinolysis, inflammation, and regulation of the plasminogen activating system. *J.Thromb. Haemost.*, Vol. 5, Suppl 1, pp. 132–142.

Meltzer M.E., Doggen C. J. M., de Groot P. G., Rosendaal F. R. & Lisman T. (2010). Plasma levels of fibrinolytic proteins and the risk of myocardial infarction in men *Blood.*, Vol.116, No.4, pp. 529-536.

Monaco C., Andreakos E., Young S., Feldmann M. & Paleolog E. (2002). T cell-mediated signaling to vascular endothelium: induction of cytokines, chemokines, and tissue factor. *J. Leukoc. Biol.*, Vol. 71, No. 4, pp. 659–668.

Morley J.J. & Kushner I. (1982) Serum C-reactive protein levels in disease. *Annals of the New York Academy of Sciences*, Vol. 389, pp. 406–418.

Ohtsubo K. & Marth J.D. (2006). Glycosylation in Cellular Mechanisms of Health and Disease. *Cell*, Vol. 126, No. 5, pp. 855-867.

Okada H., Woodcock-Mitchell J., Mitchell J., Sakamoto T., Marutsuka K., Sobel B.E. & Fujii S. (1998). Induction of plasminogen activator inhibitor type 1 and type 1 collagen expression in rat cardiac microvascular endothelial cells by interleukin-1 and its dependence on oxygen-centered free radicals. *Circulation.*, Vol. 97, No. 21, pp. 2175-2182.

Owens A.P. 3rd & Mackman N. (2010). Tissue factor and thrombosis: The clot starts here. *Thromb. Haemost.*, Vol. 104, No. 3, pp. 432-439.

Patalakh I.I., Lutai M.I., Gavrilenko T.I., Lomanovsky O.N., Kornilina Ye.M., Shkrabak M.A. & Kudinov S.A. (2007) Activity of the fibrinolytic system in patients with stable *angina pectoris* with signs of inflammation. *Laboratory diagnostics* (Ukraine), Vol. 4, No. 42, pp. 14 -19.

Patalakh I.I., Ryabenko D.V., Kornilina E.M. & Kudinov S.A. (2009). Protein C in regulation of blood plasma fibrinolytic potential in patients with chronic heart failure. *Circulation and haemostasis* (Ukraine), Vol. 3-4, pp. 93-101.

Patalakh I.I., Urvant L.P., Yevstratova I.N., Drobotko T.F.& Lomakovsky O.M. (2008). Plasma protein thiol/disulfides: the role in atherogenesis. *Laboratory diagnostics* (Ukraine), Vol. 4, No. 46, pp. 11-19.

Perri S. R., Martineau D., François M., Lejeune L., Bisson L., Durocher Y. & Galipeau J. (2007). Plasminogen Kringle 5 blocks tumor progression by antiangiogenic and proinflammatory pathways. *Molecular Cancer Therapeutics*, Vol. 6, No. 2, pp. 441–449.

Popescu N.I., Lupu C. & Lupu F. (2010) Role of PDI in regulating tissue factor: FVIIa activity. *Thromb. Res.*, Vol. 125, Suppl 1, pp. S38-41.

Procyk R., Medved L., Engelke K.J., Kudryk B.& Blombäck B. (1992). Nonclottable fibrin obtained from partially reduced fibrinogen: characterization and tissue plasminogen activator stimulation. *Biochemistry*, Vol. 31, No. 8, pp. 2273–2278.

Qi J., Goralnick S.& Kreutzer D.L. (1997). Fibrin regulation of interleukin-8 gene expression in human vascular endothelial cells. *Blood*, Vol., No.90, pp. 3595-3602.

Rao L.V.& Pendurthi U.R. (2005). Tissue factor-factor VIIa signaling. *Arterioscler. Thromb. Vasc. Biol.*, Vol. 25, No. 1, pp. 47-56.

Rees M.D., Kennett E.C., Whitelock J.M.& Davies M.J. (2008). Oxidative damage to extracellular matrix and its role in human pathologies. *Free Radic. Biol. Med.*, Vol. 44, No.12, pp. 1973-2001.

Rezaie A.R. (2001). Vitronectin functions as a cofactor for rapid inhibition of activated protein C by plasminogen activator inhibitor-1. *J. Biol. Chem.*, Vol. 276, No. 19, pp. 15567-15570.

Riewald M. & Ruf W. (2001). Mechanistic coupling of protease signaling and initiation of coagulation by tissue factor. *Proc. Natl. Acad. Sci. U S A.*, Vol. 98, No. 14, pp. 7742-7747.

Ruminy P., Gangneux C., Claeyssens S., Scotte M., Daveau M. & Salier J.P. (2001). Gene transcription in hepatocytes during the acute phase of a systemic inflammation: from transcription factors to target genes. *Inflamm. Res..*, Vol. 50, No. 8, pp. 383-390.

Sarangi P.P., Lee H.W., Kim M. Activated protein C action in inflammation. (2010). *Br. J. Haematol.* , Vol.148, No. 6, pp. 817-33.

Sardo M.A., Campo S., Mandraffino G, Saitta C., Bonaiuto A., Castaldo M., Cinquegrani M., Pizzimenti G. & Saitta A. (2008). Tissue factor and monocyte chemoattractant protein-1 expression in hypertensive individuals with normal or increased carotid intima-media wall thickness. *Clin. Chem.*, Vol. 54, No. 5, pp. 814-823.

Schrauwen Y., de Vries R.E.M., Kooistra T. & Emeis J.J. (1994). Acute release of tissue-type plasminogen activator (t-PA) from the endothelium; regulatory mechanisms and therapeutic target. *Fibrinolysis*, Vol. 8, Suppl. 2, pp. 8 –12.

Singh U., Devaraj S. & Jialal I. (2005). C-reactive protein decreases tissue plasminogen activator activity in human aortic endothelial cells: evidence that protein is a procoagulant. *Arterioscler. Thromb. Vasc. Biol.*, Vol. 25, No. 10, pp. 2216-2221.

Sitrin R.G., Pan, P.M., Srikanth, S.& Todd, R.F., 3rd. (1998). Fibrinogen activates NF-kappa B transcription factors in mononuclear phagocytes. *J. Immunol., Vol.*161, No.3, pp. 1462-1470.

Skropeta D. (2009). The effect of individual N-glycans on enzyme activity. *Bioorg. Med. Chem.*, Vol.17, No.7, pp. 2645–2653.

Sommeijer D.W., Hansen H.R., van Oerle R., Hamulyak K., van Zanten A.P., Meesters E., Spronk H.M. & ten Cate H. (2006). Soluble tissue factor is a candidate marker for progression of microvascular disease in patients with Type 2 diabetes. *J. Thromb. Haemost.*, Vol. 4, No. 3, pp. 574-580.

Spronk H.M.H., Govers-Riemslag J.W.P. & Cate H. (2003). The blood coagulation system as a molecular machine. *BioEssays,* Vol. 25, No. 12, pp. 1220–1228.

Stephenson D.A, Toltl., L.J., Beaudin S., & Liaw P. C. (2006). Modulation of monocyte function by activated protein C, a natural anticoagulant. *J. Immunol.,* Vol. 177, No.4, pp. 2115–2122.

Tamam Y., Iltumur K. & Apak I. (2005). Assesment of acute phase proteins in acute ischemic stroke. *J. Exp. Med.*, Vol. 206, No. 2, pp. 91-98.

Tanaka K.A., Key N. S. & Levy J. H. (2009). Blood coagulation: hemostasis and thrombin regulation. *Anesth. Analg.*, Vol. 108., No. 5, pp. 1433–1446.

Tenno M., Ohtsubo K., Hagen F.K., Ditto D., Zarbock A., Schaerli P., von Andrian U.H., Ley K., Le D., Tabak L.A. & Marth J.D. (2007). Initiation of protein O glycosylation by the polypeptide GalNAcT-1 in vascular biology and humoral immunity. *Mol. Cell Biol.*, Vol. 27, No. 24, pp. 8783-8796.

Toltl L.J., Beaudin S. & Liaw P.C. (2008). Activated protein C up-regulates IL-10 and inhibits tissue factor in blood monocytes. *J. Immunol.*, Vol. 181, No. 3, pp. 2165-2173.

Trautwein C., Böker K. & Manns M.P. (1994). Hepatocyte and immune system: acute phase reaction as a contribution to early defence mechanisms. *Gut,* Vol. 35, No. 9, pp. 1163-1166.

Trezzini C., Schüepp B., Maly F.E. & Jungi T.W. (1991). Evidence that exposure to fibrinogen or to antibodies directed against Mac-1 (CD11b/CD18; CR3) modulates human monocyte effector functions. *Br. J. Haematol.*, Vol. 77, No. 1, pp. 16-24.

Van Dijk W. & Mackiewicz A. (1995). Interleukin-6-type cytokine-induced changes in acute phase protein glycosylation. *Ann. N. Y. Acad. Sci..,* Vol. 762, pp. 319-330.

Viles-Gonzalez J.F., Fuster V. & Badimon J.J. (2005). Thrombin/inflammation paradigms: a closer look at arterial and venous thrombosis. *Am. Heart J.,* No. 149, pp. (1 Suppl): S19-S31.

Voetsch B. & Loscalzo J. (2004). Genetic determinants of arterial thrombosis. *Arterioscler. Thromb. Vasc. Biol.*, Vol. 24, No. 2, pp. 216-229.

Walley K.R., Lukacs N.W., Standiford T.J., Strieter R.M. & Kunkel S.L. (1996). Balance of inflammatory cytokines related to severity and mortality of murine sepsis. *Infect. Immun.,* Vol. 64, No. 11, pp. 4733–4738.

White B., Schmidt M., Murphy C., Livingstone W., O'Toole D., Lawler M., O'Neill L., Kelleher D., Schwarz H. P. & Smith O. P. (2000). Activated protein C inhibits lipopolysaccharide-induced nuclear translocation of nuclear factor kB (NF-kB) and tumour necrosis factor α (TNF-α) production in the THP-1 monocytic cell line. *Br. J. Haematol.*, Vol. 110, Issue 1, pp. 130–134.

Wiinberg B., Jensen A.L., Johansson P.I., Rozanski E., Tranholm M.& Kristensen A.T. (2008). Thromboelastographic evaluation of hemostatic function in dogs with disseminated intravascular coagulation. *J.Vet. Intern. Med.*, Vol. 22, No. 2, pp. 357–365.

Willerson J.T.& Ridker P.M. (2004). Inflammation as a cardiovascular risk factor. *Circulation*, Vol.109, 21 Suppl1 II-2-II-10.

Wojta J., Zoellner H., Gallicchio M., Filonzi E.L., Hamilton J.A. & McGrath K. (1994). Interferon-alpha 2 counteracts interleukin-1 alpha-stimulated expression of urokinase-type plasminogen activator in human foreskin microvascular endothelial cells in vitro. *Lymphokine Cytokine Res.*, Vol. 13, No. 2, pp. 133-138.

Yamamoto K., Shimokawa T., Kojima T., Loskutoff D. J. & Saito H. (1999). Regulation of murine protein C gene expression *in vivo*: effects of tumor necrosis factor-alpha, interleukin-1, and transforming growth factor-beta. *Thrombosis and Haemostasis*, Vol. 82, No. 4, pp. 1207-1379.

Zouaoui Boudjeltia K., Piagnerelli M., Brohee D., Guillaume M., Cauchie P., Vincent J.L., Remacle C., Bouckaert Y. & Vanhaeverbeek M. (2004). Relationship between CRP and hypofibrinolysis: Is this a possible mechanism to explain the association between CRP and outcome in critically ill patients? *Thromb. J.*, Vol. 2, No. 1, pp. 7–12.

6

Brain Barriers and the Acute-Phase Response

Fernanda Marques, Margarida Correia-Neves,
João Carlos Sousa, Nuno Sousa and Joana Almeida Palha
Life and Health Sciences Research Institute (ICVS)
School of Health Sciences, University of Minho, Campus Gualtar, Braga
ICVS/3B's - PT Government Associate Laboratory, Braga/Guimarães
Portugal

1. Introduction

Recent findings on the brain response to peripheral inflammation have broadened our knowledge on the acute phase response. Notably, such advances may lead to the characterization of acute phase proteins in body fluids other than the blood. Among these, and of particular interest, is the cerebrospinal fluid (CSF) that fills the brain ventricles, the subarachnoid space and the spinal cord.

Acute phase response is a term used to describe, mostly, the liver response to an inflammatory insult, a process that, among other effects, ultimately results in changes in the plasma concentrations of various proteins. The triggers of liver response include the inflammatory insult and the molecules produced by multiple cell types, from inflammatory cells (e.g. neutrophils and macrophages), to endothelial and liver cells. As a consequence, the liver synthesizes a number of so-termed acute phase proteins that are classified, depending on whether their expression is increased or decreased, as positive or negative acute phase response proteins, respectively. Among the positive acute phase proteins are binding proteins, opsonins (e.g. C-reactive protein) and iron-related proteins [e.g. hepcidin (HAMP), ceruloplasmin, lipocalin 2 (LCN2) and ferritin]. The negative acute phase proteins also include binding proteins (e.g. albumin, transthyretin, retinol-binding protein), as well as iron-related proteins (e.g. transferrin). Nonetheless, acute phase response is not a process restricted to the liver. Throughout the years, acute phase proteins expression has also been found altered at the barriers of the brain. Most of these findings originated from work on the brain parenchyma response to inflammation (Quan et al., 1998; Nadeau & Rivest, 1999); however, surprisingly, only recently were the barriers of the brain specifically considered in the overall response to peripheral inflammation. In this chapter we will address the contribution of the barriers of the brain in the acute-phase response to peripheral inflammatory stimuli.

2. The barriers of the brain

For a long time the brain was considered isolated from the immune system and unable to mount an immune response when challenged by invading pathogens. This immune-privileged view of the brain was based on multiple observations: allografts survive longer in the central nervous system (CNS) than in other organs (Fuchs & Bullard, 1988); the CNS lacks both lymphatic vessels and constitutive expression of major histocompatibility complex class I and II molecules on parenchymal cells (Perry, 1998) and, lastly, the CNS was thought to be devoid of classical antigen-presenting cells, such as dendritic cells (Matyszak & Perry, 1996). The assumption of an immune-privileged system was further supported by the discovery of two barriers that confer invaluable protection to the brain: the blood-brain barrier (BBB) and the blood-CSF barrier (BCSFB) (reviewed by Abbott, 2005). While these barriers protect the brain from the fluctuations of blood components that are direct triggers of neuronal function (e.g. amino acids that function as neurotransmitters), it is now clear that they are much more than obstacles to the passage of molecules and cells into and out of the brain. Throughout this chapter we will highlight how both barriers actively participate in brain homeostasis. We will also explore the interplay between the immune and the central nervous systems in physiological and immune-challenged conditions.

2.1 The blood-brain barrier

The BBB is formed by the tight junctions between the endothelial cells of the capillaries that irrigate the brain parenchyma. Additionally, on a larger organizational level, the basal lamina, astrocytic end-feets, pericytes and neurons that surround the central BBB core, altogether make the neurovascular unit (Fig. 1A).

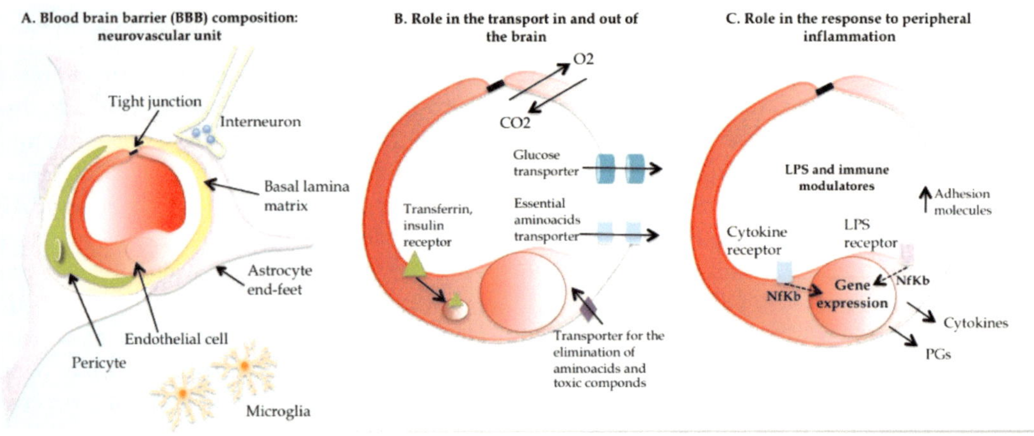

Fig. 1. Neurovascular unit composition, function and role in the response to peripheral inflammation. A. The blood-brain barrier (BBB) is formed by the tight junctions that connect the endothelial cells of the capillaries that irrigate the brain parenchyma. Together with the basal lamina, pericytes, and astrocytic end-feet it forms the neurovascular unit. B. The endothelial cells of the BBB have a crucial role in the transport of ions and solutes into and out of the brain. Some substances diffuse freely into and out of the brain parenchyma (O_2 and CO_2), others such as nutrients need specific transporters, while molecules such as insulin, leptin and transferrin are transported by receptor-mediated endocytosis. Similarly, there are also transporters in the abluminal side of the endothelial cells described to participate in the removal of brain derived metabolites. Panel C depicts some of the pathways activated in the BBB in response to peripheral inflammation.

With the exception of small lipophilic molecules, such as O_2 and CO_2 that freely diffuse across endothelial cells depending on their concentration gradient, the passage of blood-born molecules through the BBB requires the presence of specific transporter or receptor systems. Nutrients, like glucose and amino acids enter the brain through specific transporters, while molecules such as insulin, leptin and transferrin are transported by receptor-mediated endocytosis (Pardridge et al., 1985; Zhang & Pardridge, 2001). Conversely, similar mechanisms constitute a way out of the brain for molecules produced by the brain metabolism, *via* transporters and receptors located in the "brain side" of the endothelial cell (Fig. 1B). However, unlike the longer established mechanisms for the transfer of nutrients and molecules, the physiological passage of immune cells into the brain has not been shown until very recently. Specifically, it has been demonstrated that T cells are able to breach both the BBB and the BCSFB to perform immune surveillance of the CNS (Engelhardt & Coisne, 2011). More so, in pathological situations, including auto-immune brain disorders such as multiple sclerosis, the brain barriers become "leaky" leading to a drastic increase in the infiltration of immune cells into the brain (Engelhardt, 2006).

The brain barriers are needed; the neural milieu must be protected from the drastic concentration changes in blood molecules such as nutrients and ions. Nonetheless, the brain must also be able to rapidly respond to changes, since many of the humoral regulation centers are located within the brain. For these reasons, two brain regions lack the BBB: the circumventricular organs and the choroid plexus (CP). The CP will be addressed below, but we will first briefly describe the circumventricular organs. These brain regions, composed of the area postrema, median eminence, pineal gland, subfornical organ and lamina terminalis, are specialized neuroendocrine sites characterized by their small size and capillary irrigation (fenestration). They can either secrete or constitute sites of action for a variety of different hormones, neurotransmitters and cytokines, for which circumventricular organs are classified as either secretory or sensory, respectively. Compared to other brain regions, except the CP, the circumventricular organs are unique in that they allow exchanges with the periphery. These exchanges are due to the permeability of the endothelium; nonetheless, circumventricular organs do not form an open door into the brain parenchyma given the presence of tight junctions between the tanycytes, the specialized ependymal cells that surround them (Brightman & Kadota, 1992).

2.2 The blood-cerebrospinal fluid barrier

The CP is rapidly and actively exposed to any alteration in the blood milieu. It is formed by a monolayer of epithelial cells that originate from the ependymal cells that line the brain ventricles (two lateral ventricles, and the third and fourth ventricles). The CP's stroma is highly vascularised and populated by multiple cell types, from fibroblast to macrophages and lymphocytes or neutrophils, in proportions that reflect peripheral conditions (Emerich et al., 2005). The presence of tight junctions in the apical side of the CP's epithelial cells forms a barrier between the stroma and the CSF that is aptly termed the blood-CSF barrier (BCSFB) (Fig. 2A). Similarly to the BBB, the BCSFB prevents the paracellular passage of molecules and cells from the blood; however, in this case, into to the CSF. Of note, blood flow in the CP's stroma is up to 10 times higher that of the other brain regions (Johanson et al., 2011). Again, resembling the BBB, the BCSFB also contains transporters and receptors; specifically, their presence in the basolateral and apical sides of the cell membrane allows the controlled passage of molecules in and out of the brain. In particular, the apical side of the epithelial cells faces the CSF and contains numerous villosities, which increase the surface contact area between the blood and the CSF.

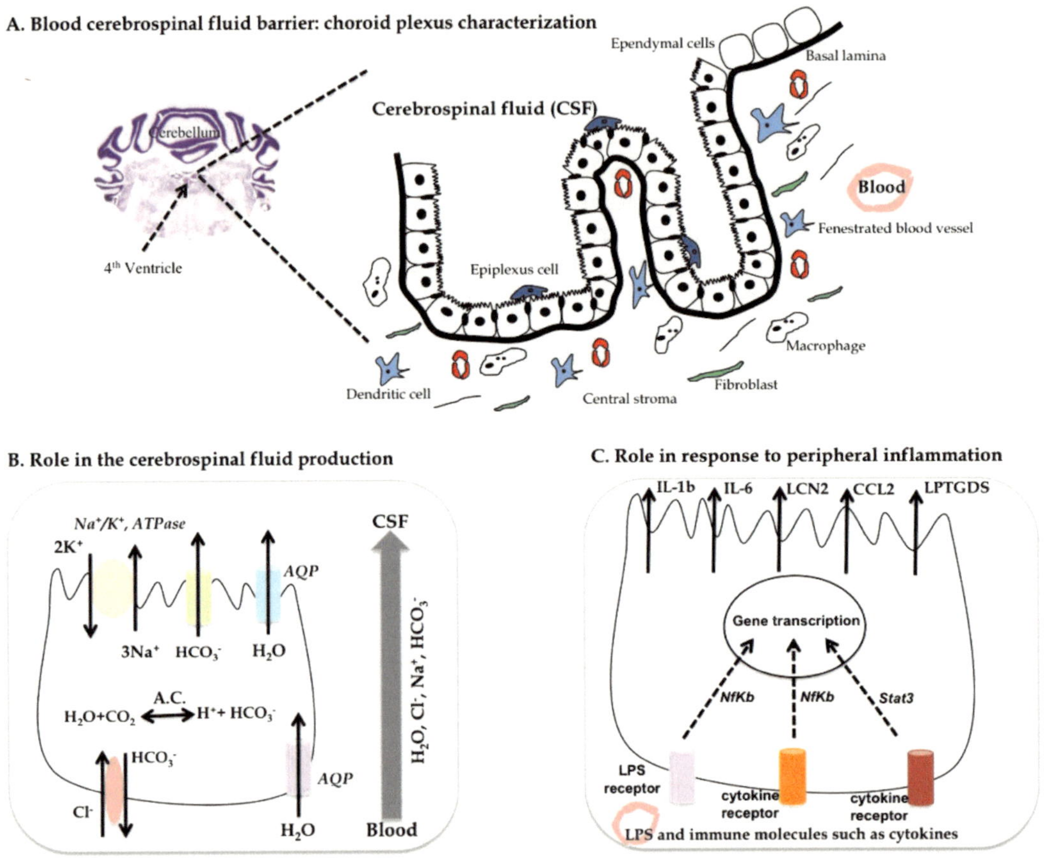

Fig. 2. Blood-cerebrospinal fluid barrier composition, function and role in the response to peripheral inflammation. A. The choroid plexus (CP) is formed by a monolayer of epithelial cells originating in the ependymal cells that line the brain ventricles, forming a closed structure - the stroma. The stroma is a connective tissue rich in fenestrated blood vessels and contains various cells types, such as macrophages, dendritic cells and fibroblasts. The CP epithelial cells are juxtaposed due to the apical localization of the tight junctions. While the apical side contacts with the cerebrospinal fluid (CSF), the basolateral side faces the fenestrated blood vessels. B. Choroid plexus has the required enzymes, transporters and channels to allow the passage of ions and water needed for the production of the CSF. Panel C. depicts aspects of the CP response to peripheral inflammation. In such conditions, lypopolysacharide (LPS) and immune modulators present in the blood (e.g. IL1-β and IL-6), activate the basolateral side of the CP epithelial cells. In response, the CP transcriptome is altered resulting in the production of several proteins, some of which are then secreted into the CSF.

The CP's main function is the production of CSF, which fills the ventricles, the subarachnoid space and the spinal cord (Speake et al., 2001), ensuring an optimal environment for the CNS cells. In the adult human's CNS there are about 150 mL of circulating CSF that are renewed approximately four times daily (Wright, 1978). The CSF is a clear, slightly viscous fluid that surrounds the CNS and exchanges with the brain interstitial fluid. Given its circulation and exposure it participates in the delivery of nutrients into the brain and also in the removal of waste products generated within the brain. On the other hand, the CSF itself contains few cells and has a protein concentration about 10 times lower than that of the blood (Segal, 2001). The CP generates most of the CSF; the remainder 10-30% is of extrachoroidal origin, mostly from metabolism of the brain parenchyma and from the BBB (Johanson, 2008). Of notice, the CP in itself contributes to the composition of the CSF by secreting several carrier proteins and growth factors (reviewed by Chodobski & Szmydynger-Chodobska, 2001). The high number of mitochondria present in the CP indicates its secretory activity. Additionally, the choroidal CSF secretion relies on the active production of an osmotic gradient that is mainly driven by carbonic anhydrase and Na^+/K^+ ATPase, and supported by the abundant expression of water channels (aquaporins) on the apical and basaloteral sides (Fig. 2B).

While the CSF system is expected to reflect brain homeostasis, recent evidence has revealed that it also reflects challenges induced in the periphery, including during response to peripheral inflammation which will next be discussed in detail.

3. Acute phase response

The term "acute phase" is associated with alterations in the liver transcription profile that, in response to an acute inflammatory stimulus, is reflected in the concentration of several plasma proteins. Several cells of the immune system also similarly contribute to changes in the concentration of plasma proteins, notably by secreting several cytokines and other immune-modulators that then act on many organ systems, including the CNS. The brain barriers are critical sites for cytokine signal transduction and for the initiation of the brain responses to peripheral inflammation. Circulating cytokines can act on the brain *via* various mechanisms that include: (i) fast transmission pathways, involving primary afferent neurons of the vagus nerve, innervating the site of inflammation; (ii) direct entry into the brain through the BBB or BCSFB *via* a saturable transport mechanism (cytokines are hydrophilic small proteins and are not expected to cross the BBB in the absence of a transport system); (iii) interactions within the circumventricular organs (reviewed by Hosoi et al., 2002); (iv) binding to receptors at the BBB (Gaillard, 1998) or BCSFB that activate intracellular mechanisms leading to the formation of short-lived substances, such as prostaglandins (PGs) and nitric oxide. These substances may diffuse across the brain barriers and play a role in the modulation of behavior and other brain disturbances observed during inflammatory states (for reviews, see Saper & Breder 1992, 1994; Dantzer, 2001; Dantzer et al., 2008). Binding to the brain barriers receptors may also activate the production of new cytokines through the activation of transcription factors. This mechanism triggers the synthesis and secretion of cytokines and/or chemokines or other immune mediators by the barriers themselves (Marques et al., 2009b; Verma et al., 2006) (Fig. 1C and 2C).

The subject on whether peripheral inflammation triggers inflammation within the brain has raised the interest of investigators. Of notice, while studying particular events and molecules within the brain parenchyma, several groups have observed staining for various immune-mediators in the brain barriers; among these are tumor necrosis factor-alpha (TNF-a) and interleukin 1-beta (IL1-β) in both CP and BBB endothelial cells (Marques et al., 2007; Nadeau & Rivest 1999; Quan et al., 1999). In addition, "acute phase proteins" can be differently expressed in a tissue-specific manner in response to acute peripheral inflammation. For instance, while peripheral inflammation with the Gram negative bacterial cell wall component lypopolysacharide (LPS) (Dickson et al., 1986; Marques et al., 2007) results in decreased expression of the gene encoding for transthyretin in the liver (Birch & Schreiber, 1986), it does not influence its expression in the CP. This differential response possibly reflects tissue-specific transcription factors regulation (Costa et al., 1990; Yan et al., 1990), while other signal transduction pathways may also be involved.

Despite all evidence on the barriers themselves as a site of homeostasis in response to peripheral stimulus, only recently have they been considered as a whole in mediating or participating in the response to peripheral inflammation. This will be next discussed in detail for the BCSFB, with particular emphasis on the *de novo* synthesizes of cytokines and of short-lived substances such as PGs. A special attention will be given to the CP, and particularly to its epithelial cells, because alterations in the CP response will ultimately be reflected in the composition of the CSF, which will impact on the brain parenchyma. A final note will be given to the CP as a neuroendocrine organ, given the strong evidence suggesting its participation in regional brain iron homeostasis, which is a novel concept.

3.1 The choroid plexus response to acute peripheral inflammation: triggers, mediators and effectors

The CP is ideally equipped to respond to peripheral stimulus and to communicate with the CNS since it is extremely well vascularised and because it produces most of the CSF. In addition, it possesses molecules important for leukocyte adhesion such as, lymphocyte selectin (L-selectin), intercellular adhesion molecule 1 (ICAM-1) and vascular cell adhesion molecule 1 (VCAM-1) that are found expressed at low levels in CP epithelial cells and can be up-regulated during inflammation (Endo et al., 1998; Wolburg et al., 1999). As such, the CP is suggested to be one of the first places for cell entry into the brain during inflammatory disease (Reboldi et al., 2009), which will also condition the CSF cell content.

A recent study characterized the complete CP transcriptome in the context of peripheral inflammation induced by a single intraperitoneal injection of LPS (Marques et al., 2009b). These results can be accessed in the GEOdatabase (GSE23714). In this work the kinetic CP transcriptome alterations were evaluated at 1, 3, 6, 12, 24 and 72 h after LPS injection. Interestingly, similarly to the liver, the CP showed a rapid and transient response. Specifically, the CP displayed a response to LPS that peaked between 3 to 6 h after LPS administration and rapidly returned to baseline after 72 h. During this response, the expression of a large number of genes encodes for chemokines (such as chemokine C-C motif ligands 2, 3, 4, 7, 9, 11 and 19 and chemokine C-X-C motif ligands 1, 2, 9, 10, 13 and 16), cytokines (such as IL-1β, IL6 and TNF-α), adhesion molecules (Icam-1, selectin platelet and selection endothelial cell), acute phase proteins (serum amyloid A3, serum amyloid A1 and LCN2), and transporters (amino acid transporters) was altered (Marques et al., 2009b). Interestingly, several well-described pathways recognized to have diverse roles in the regulation of the immune system were also found altered in these conditions. Among these roles, we found the activation of the toll-like receptors (TLRs) and interleukin receptors leading to the subsequent activation of: (i) the transcription factor nuclear factor kappa B (NF-kβ), which regulates the transcription of pro-inflammatory cytokines including TNF-α, IL-1β and IL6; (ii) members of the mitogen-activated proteins kinase family (MAPK), notably p38 and JUN N-terminal kinase (JNK); (iii) the JAK/STAT signalling pathway, and (iv) the transcription factors known as interferon regulatory factors (IRFs) (Miyamoto et al., 1988). Termination of the CP response may be, at least in part, a consequence of the negative feedback inhibition of STAT signalling by SOCS/CIS (Naka et al., 2005), as some of the genes encoding for proteins in this pathway are up-regulated after LPS administration. A similar mechanism has been described in the BBB (Laflamme et al., 1999; Laflamme & Rivest 1999; Lebel et al., 2000). Finally, of notice, the glucocorticoid receptor signalling pathway was also found altered, which is of interest given the role of the hypothalamus/pituitary/adrenal axis in the interplay between the immune and the central nervous systems in sickness behaviour.

Two interesting aspects should be taken into account: the blood-born molecules that trigger the CP response and the impact of the response itself. In this regard, particularly relevant are the molecules secreted into the CSF that ultimately reach and modulate responses within the brain parenchyma. With respect to triggers of the CP response, possible candidate molecules of interest are those that in response to an acute inflammatory stimulus have an increase in their blood concentration. Agents such as LPS, but also intrinsic immune modulators such as cytokines and chemokines, are potential triggers given that, for several of these (e.g. IL-1β, IL-6 and TNF-α), the CP has receptors in the basolateral side of the epithelial cells (Marques et al., 2011). Accordingly, *in vitro* studies of primary cultures of rat CP epithelial cells exposed on the basolateral side (blood side *in vivo*) to LPS, or to serum collected from rats 3 and 6 h after LPS injection (Marques et al., 2009b), clearly showed that the CP response can be triggered by LPS directly and/or by blood-borne molecules. For example, while both LPS and serum from LPS-injected rats induced the expression of *Il1β*, *Il6*, and *Cxcl1* in *in vitro* CP cultures, only the serum from LPS-injected rats had an effect on the expression of the transcription factor interferon regulatory factor 1 (*Irf1*). Of note, *in vitro* studies are a complement of the *in vivo* work since they permit a dissection of what is the real contribution of the CP epithelial cells; in *in vivo* studies the complete CP is usually studied, including not only the contribution of epithelial cells but also of all other cells present in the CP stroma. Among these are macrophages, dendritic cells (Hanly & Petito, 1998; Ling et al., 1998; McMenamin, 1999) and fibroblasts. Epiplexus cells may also contribute, this time by interacting on the apical surface of the epithelial cells where they are found (Emerich et al., 2005; Ling et al., 1998). All of these cells, particularly macrophages, are able to produce immune modulators that can activate receptors in the basolateral membrane of the CP epithelial cells, ultimately contributing to the overall CP and brain response to inflammation.

Our initial work on the mouse CP response to peripheral inflammation, focused on proteins highly expressed and secreted by the CP. Of notice, we observed an increase in the prostaglandin D2 synthase (PTGDS) at 6, 12 and 24 h after peripheral acute injection of LPS, which returned to basal levels at 72 h (Marques et al., 2007) This was accompanied by increased CSF PTGDS concentration (Marques et al., 2007); in agreement with the kinetic profile of increased CSF concentration previously reported in rats after intraperitoneal injection of LPS (Ishizaka et al., 2001). PTGDS catalyzes the isomeration of prostaglandin H2 (PGH2) to produce prostaglandin D2 (PGD2), the major prostanoid in the CNS. Prostaglandin D2 can be transformed into multiple different prostaglandins, which themselves, can display anti- or pro-inflammatory properties. Among this is the conversion of PGD2 into the bioactive cyclopentenone-type prostaglandins of the J2-series such as 15-deoxy-$\Delta^{12,14}$-prostaglandin J2 (15d-PGJ2). By repressing the expression of genes encoding for inflammatory mediators (e.g. TNF-α) 15-dPGJ2 can be considered anti-inflammatory; however it has also been described to have pro-inflammatory through induction of cyclooxygenase 2 (COX-2) (Harris et al., 2002). In the context of the present discussion, the observation that endothelial cells with increased endogenous PGD2 levels downregulate the expression of VCAM-1 (Negoro et al., 2005) is of interest since it may contribute to the resolution of inflammation.

The first step of prostaglandin synthesis occurs through the action of COX-1 or COX-2 on arachidonic acid (AA), originating PGH2, which depending on the enzyme can be next transformed into multiple different prostaglandins. The COX-1 enzyme is ubiquitously expressed, while the COX-2 is mainly involved in inflammatory processes and therefore of particular relevance in the brain response to inflammation. Several studies have shown an increase in COX-2 expression in the BBB endothelial cells after central or systemic injection of endotoxin or cytokines (Cao et al., 1996; Laflamme et al., 1999). Additionally, the development of selective COX-2 inhibitors further suggests an important role for this cyclooxygenase in the BBB in response to acute inflammation; specifically, its inhibition lead to a decrease in the expression of tight junctions proteins in the endothelial cells of the barrier (Germann et al., 2008). In accordance, it has also been shown that COX-2 null-mice exhibit an increase in LPS-induced BBB disruption, mediated by an increase in matrix metalloproteinases 9 and 3 activities (Choi et al., 2010). These results further support the hypothesis that COX-2 may mediate the neuroinflammatory response, especially in maintaining the integrity of the neurovascular unit (Choi et al., 2010). Finally, cyclooxygenases can differentially modulate leukocyte recruitment into the inflamed brain (Choi et al., 2010). Interestingly, neither COX-1 nor COX-2 expression is altered in the CP transcriptome (that includes the epithelial cells of the BCSFB) in response to peripheral inflammation (Marques et al., 2009b). Altogether, these observations indicate that the BBB and BCSFB responses to inflammation may be different regarding the activation of pathways needed to maintain barrier integrity. Still, any alteration in the permeability properties may render the brain parenchyma more susceptible to noxious molecules and to the infiltration of immune cells. Reflecting the aspect of barrier integrity, it has been shown that a single LPS injection induces down-regulation in the transcripts of tight junction proteins and an increase in those encoding for extracellular matrix remodelling proteins such as metalloproteinases (Marques et al., 2009b).

In summary, the CP displays the adequate anatomical (at the interface between the blood and the CSF) and functional (membrane receptors, signal transduction pathways and secretory) setting to participate in the immune system-brain interplay. The relevance of such occurrence will depend on whether it is reflected in the CSF composition, as is the case for IL-6, CCL-2, PTGDS and LCN2 (Fig. 2C).

3.2 Iron modulation at the brain barriers is part of the acute phase response

While signalling in and out of the brain is currently accepted to occur at the brain barriers, evidence is accumulating on their participation in specific homeostatic circuitries. Particularly interesting is the possibility that the brain barriers participate on regulating brain iron homeostasis, which is relevant in neurodegenerative disorders where accumulation of iron has been reported.

As referred before, the kinetic response of the CP to peripheral inflammation resembles the liver acute phase response, in terms of duration and gene/pathways activation (Marques et al., 2009b). Remarkably, results from our studies show that, in response to inflammation, the CP seems to be a specific site for iron homeostasis. Specifically, it induces the *de novo* synthesis of major iron modulators that are not normally expressed and/or are expressed in very low levels, such as HAMP (hepcidin) and LCN2. Notably, these genes follow expression kinetics greatly similar to those of the liver (Ceciliani et al., 2002; Gabay & Kushner 1999). A striking observation was that of the altered expression of LCN2. This protein is not present at the brain barriers in basal conditions, however its expression and secretion increase dramatically in response to a single injection of LPS in the periphery (Marques et al., 2008). LCN2 is an iron-related protein that was first described as an effective defence strategy for the body to control the growth of pathogens; by binding to iron-loaded siderophores, the iron chelators secreted by pathogens (Flo et al., 2004). Additionally, LCN2 was traditionally viewed as a liver acute phase protein (Liu & Nilsen-Hamilton, 1995; Sunil et al., 2007), which was also produced by neutrophils, lung, spleen and uterus (Kjeldsen et al., 2000). However, from our work, LCN2 is now also known to be an acute phase protein in the endothelial cells of the BBB and in epithelial cells of the BCSFB (Marques et al., 2008) Namely, *Lcn2* mRNA levels are up regulated as early as 1 h after peripheral inflammation, returning to basal levels after 72 h; in accordance, it is present in the CSF during the first 24 h post-stimuli, while undetectable in basal conditions (Marques et al., 2008). These observations suggested that LCN2 could be part of the host-innate immune response to infection at the barriers of the brain and in the CSF. These findings prompted us to further investigate the CP as a site of brain regional iron homeostasis, as will be next discussed.

During an immune response iron metabolism is tightly regulated. This regulation is crucial since iron is an essential element for the body homeostasis. Iron deficiency or excess can lead, respectively, to pathological conditions such as anemia or hemochromatosis. Furthermore, since no mechanism other than bleeding and cell renovation is known for iron excretion, the body maintains a tight iron regulation, although the mechanisms involved in this regulation have only recently been partially characterized. In particular, the liver was identified as the regulatory site for iron homeostasis through the synthesis and secretion of HAMP (Krause et al., 2000). Regulation of iron availability is made by the enterocytes, which determine the quantity of dietary iron that is absorbed. When iron stores are high, iron absorption is blocked; when low, iron absorption increases. This is controlled by the availability of ferroportin (the only iron exporter described), at the basolateral side of the enterocyte, which is regulated by HAMP (Krause et al., 2000). Circulating HAMP binds ferroportin on the surface of enterocytes, leading to its internalization and degradation, and blocking iron absorption into the bloodstream (Nemeth et al., 2004a). Under physiological conditions the level of HAMP is regulated by body iron requirements; however, HAMP expression can be modulated by pro-inflammatory cytokines such as IL-6 and IL-1β during inflammatory response. This represents a host defence mechanism: by decreasing serum iron levels the host decreases iron availability for invading bacteria (Ganz, 2007). It follows that other cells of the body, specifically cells of the immune system, are equipped with the machinery capable of regulating iron homeostasis through the regulation of several iron-related genes and proteins (Porto & De Sousa, 2007). This is significant given the immune cells protective function and role in combating microorganisms. Still, the complete mechanism beyond HAMP regulation is far from fully understood.

The novel concept of regional iron homeostasis regulation, in the context of inflammation, adds another level of complexity to iron homeostasis. If confirmed, local brain iron homeostasis at the barriers might explain why diseases of iron accumulation in the periphery seem to spare the brain (Pientrangel, 2010). In the CP, ferroportin is localized in the apical side of the epithelial cells (Wu et al., 2004) and, in response to peripheral administration of LPS, the CP triggers a transient transcription of the HAMP encoding gene, which may result in inhibition of iron release into the CSF and the brain parenchyma.

In addition, the expression of several other iron-related genes, such as ferritins and ceruloplasmin, are also induced by the inflammatory stimulus. Finally, it should be noted that the stimulation of the *Hamp* gene is triggered not only directly by LPS but also by molecules whose expression increases in the blood in response to inflammation. An example of these is IL-6 (Marques et al., 2009a), a cytokine previously shown to regulate *Hamp* expression in the liver, upon interaction with the cognate cellular receptor, and through the STAT3 signalling transduction pathway (Kemna et al., 2005; Nemeth et al., 2003; Nemeth et al., 2004b). The same mechanism seems to be operational in the CP; primary cultures of rat CP epithelial cells when stimulated, in the basolateral side, with LPS or with IL-6, respond by inducing the expression of *Hamp*. The activation of the IL-6-mediated signalling transduction pathway was also observed *in vivo* when mice were acutely injected with LPS. In this case, increased phosphorylation of STAT3 was observed in the CP (Marques et al., 2009a). Of interest, *Hamp* expression was not induced when LPS or IL-6 were applied to the apical membrane of the CP epithelial cells, indicating that the receptors for LPS and IL-6 may be located in the basolateral (facing the blood) membrane.

Another well described pathway mediating *Hamp* expression is that of the SMAD4 complex. Members of this complex were initially discovered from observations that patients with mutations in hemochromatosis (*Hfe*), transferrin receptor type 2 (*Tfr2*), or hemochromatosis type 2 (juvenile) (*Hjv*) genes display iron deposition similar and consistent with elevated iron absorption, suggesting that these molecules may contribute to the regulation of *Hamp* expression. Interestingly, all of these molecules belong to the bone morphogenetic protein (BMP) signalling complex, which constitutes the most powerful mechanism known to activate *Hamp* transcription through SMAD4 activation (Verga Falzacappa et al., 2008). In support of these observations, TFR2 and the IL-6-mediated pathways seem to cross talk, at least in peripheral organs. Resembling its effect on HAMP regulation via the STAT3 signalling transduction pathway, IL-6 also functions as a stimuli in the SMAD4-mediated response. Wang et al. (2005) reported that the liver-specific disruption of *Smad4* results in a markedly decreased *Hamp* expression when stimulated with IL-6. Similarly, a recent study using human hepatocyte cell cultures showed that mutations in the BMP-response element strongly hamper *Hamp* activation in response to IL-6 (Verga Falzacappa et al., 2008). In our CP transcriptome characterization study, no alterations were found in the expression levels of *Hfe* or *Hjv*; however, the expression of *Tfr2* and of *Smad4* was strongly increased after LPS stimulation (Marques et al., 2009a).

Although in-depth studies are necessary to fully characterize the CP's regulation of iron homeostasis, altogether a mechanism is coming into view. In response to peripheral inflammation, the CP, by secreting HAMP, may trigger the internalization of ferroportin, therefore preventing iron release into the CSF. Concomitantly, it secretes into the CSF other iron-related proteins, such as LCN2 and ceruloplasmin that, by themselves further restrict iron availability for potentially invading microorganisms.

The novel role here proposed for the CP-CSF barrier in regulating iron metabolism may also be present in diseases of the CNS in which iron accumulates or has been described to mediate neuronal toxicity. Among these are Alzheimer's disease and multiple sclerosis. Of interest, even though in different severity scales, both have underlying inflammatory processes.

4. Conclusion and future perspectives

In the present chapter our goal was to highlight evidence that brain barriers participate in the communication of inflammatory stimuli into the brain. A few aspects, which were not specifically addressed, deserve a final mention, particularly that of neurogenesis and of multiple (or chronical) exposures to acute inflammatory stimuli/events. By modulating the composition of the CSF, or of the interstitial fluid of the brain, inflammatory stimuli induced in the periphery will influence neuronal function and processes such as neurogenesis. In this respect, in adults, LPS has been shown to alter the proliferative and migration profile of brain progenitor cells in the hippocampus (Fujioka & Akema, 2010). Notably, several of the proteins whose concentration is altered in the CSF in response to acute inflammation are recognized as modulators of adult neurogenesis. Future studies will certainly bring us novel clues on the role of neurogenesis as well as its alteration under inflammatory conditions. Also, while the focus of this book is the acute response, it should be mentioned that throughout lifespan, individuals are exposed to several independent acute inflammatory events. It is still unknown how repeated exposure to inflammation may predispose to diseases of the CNS, and how are the barriers of the brain compromised or participants in such response. Nonetheless, it is now known that the response of the CP to repeated prolonged inflammatory stimuli is less drastic and broad than that of a single acute exposure (Marques et al, 2009c). Future studies should further elucidate on how the brain barriers' attenuate and/or mediate any deleterious effects to normal brain functioning.

5. Acknowledgement

The work referenced here was supported by grants from Fundação para a Ciência e a Tecnologia FCT/FEDER (POCTI/SAU-NEU/56618/2004; PTDC/SAU-NEU/105180/2008), and by the DANA Foundation, USA. Fernanda Marques is the recipient of posdoctoral fellowship from FCT (Portugal).
We are grateful to Dr. Nadine Santos for critically reviewing this manuscript.

6. References

Abbott, N. J. (2005). Dynamics of CNS barriers: evolution, differentiation, and modulation. *Cellular and Molecular Neurobiology*, Vol.25, No.1, pp. 5-23

Birch, H. E. & Schreiber, G. (1986). Transcriptional regulation of plasma protein synthesis during inflammation. *Journal of Biological Chemistry*, Vol.261, No.18, pp. 8077-8080

Brightman, M. W. & Kadota, Y. (1992). Nonpermeable and permeable vessels of the brain. *NIDA Research Monograph*, Vol.120, pp. 87-107

Cao, C.; Matsumura, K.; Yamagata, K. & Watanabe, Y. (1996). Endothelial cells of the rat brain vasculature express cyclooxygenase-2 mRNA in response to systemic interleukin-1 beta: a possible site of prostaglandin synthesis responsible for fever. *Brain Research*, Vol.733, No.2, pp. 263-272

Ceciliani, F.; Giordano, A. & Spagnolo, V. (2002). The systemic reaction during inflammation: the acute-phase proteins. *Protein & Peptide Letters*, Vol.9, No.3, pp. 211-223

Chodobski, A. & Szmydynger-Chodobska, J. (2001). Choroid plexus: target for polypeptides and site of their synthesis. *Microscopy Research and Technique*, Vol.52, No.1, pp. 65-82

Choi, S. H.; Aid, S.; Choi, U. & Bosetti, F. (2010). Cyclooxygenases-1 and -2 differentially modulate leukocyte recruitment into the inflamed brain. *Pharmacogenomics Journal*, Vol.10, No.5, pp. 448-457, ISSN 1473-1150

Costa, R. H.; Van Dyke, T. A.; Yan, C.; Kuo, F. & Darnell, J. E., Jr. (1990). Similarities in transthyretin gene expression and differences in transcription factors: liver and yolk sac compared to choroid plexus. *Proceedings of the National Academy of Sciences*, Vol.87, No.17, pp. 6589-6593, ISSN 0027-8424

Dantzer, R. (2001). Cytokine-induced sickness behavior: mechanisms and implications. *Annals of the New York Academy of Sciences*, Vol.933, pp. 222-234

Dantzer, R.; O'Connor, J. C.; Freund, G. G.; Johnson, R. W. & Kelley, K. W. (2008). From inflammation to sickness and depression: when the immune system subjugates the brain. *Nature Reviews Neuroscience*, Vol.9, No.1, pp. 46-56

Dickson, P. W.; Aldred, A. R.; Marley, P. D.; Bannister, D. & Schreiber, G. (1986). Rat choroid plexus specializes in the synthesis and the secretion of transthyretin (prealbumin). Regulation of transthyretin synthesis in choroid plexus is independent from that in liver. *Journal of Biological Chemistry*, Vol.261, No.8, pp. 3475-3478

Emerich, D. F.; Skinner, S. J.; Borlongan, C. V.; Vasconcellos, A. V. & Thanos, C. G. (2005). The choroid plexus in the rise, fall and repair of the brain. *Bioessays*, Vol.27, No.3, pp. 262-274

Endo, H.; Sasaki, K.; Tonosaki, A. & Kayama, T. (1998). Three-dimensional and ultrastructural ICAM-1 distribution in the choroid plexus, arachnoid membrane and dural sinus of inflammatory rats induced by LPS injection in the lateral ventricles. *Brain Research*, Vol.793, No.1-2, pp. 297-301

Engelhardt, B. (2006). Regulation of immune cell entry into the central nervous system. *Results & Problems in Cell Differentiation*, Vol.43, pp. 259-280

Engelhardt, B. & Coisne, C. (2011). Fluids and barriers of the CNS establish immune privilege by confining immune surveillance to a two-walled castle moat surrounding the CNS castle. *Fluids and Barriers of the CNS*, Vol.8, No.1, pp. 4, ISSN 2045-8118

Flo, T. H.; Smith, K. D.; Sato, S.; Rodriguez, D. J.; Holmes, M. A.; Strong, R. K.; Akira, S. & Aderem, A. (2004). Lipocalin 2 mediates an innate immune response to bacterial infection by sequestrating iron. *Nature*, Vol.432, No.7019, pp. 917-921

Fuchs, H. E. & Bullard, D. E. (1988). Immunology of transplantation in the central nervous system. *Applied Neurophysiology*, Vol.51, No.6, pp. 278-296

Fujioka, H. & Akema, T. (2010). Lipopolysaccharide acutely inhibits proliferation of neural precursor cells in the dentate gyrus in adult rats. *Brain Research*, Vol.1352, pp.35-42

Funk, C. D. (2001). Prostaglandins and leukotrienes: advances in eicosanoid biology. *Science*, Vol.294, No.5548, pp. 1871-1875, ISSN 0036-8075

Furuyashiki, T. & Narumiya, S. (2009). Roles of prostaglandin E receptors in stress responses. *Current Opinion in Pharmacology*, Vol.9, No.1, pp. 31-38, ISSN 1471-4892

Gabay, C. & Kushner, I. (1999). Acute-phase proteins and other systemic responses to inflammation. *New England Journal of Medicine*, Vol.340, No.6, pp. 448-454

Gaillard, R. C. (1998). Cytokines in the neuroendocrine system. *International Reviews of Immunology*, Vol.17, No.1-4, pp. 181-216

Ganz, T. (2007). Molecular control of iron transport. *Journal of the American Society of Nephrology*, Vol.18, No.2, pp. 394-400

Germann, B.; Neuhaus, W.; Hofer-Warbinek, R. & Noe, C. R. (2008). Applying blood-brain barrier in vitro models to study the influence of drugs on endothelial cells-effects of selected COX-inhibitors. *Pharmazie*, Vol.63, No.4, pp. 303-307, ISSN 0031-7144

Hanly, A. & Petito, C. K. (1998). HLA-DR-positive dendritic cells of the normal human choroid plexus: a potential reservoir of HIV in the central nervous system. *Human Pathology*, Vol.29, No.1, pp. 88-93

Harris, S. G.; Padilla, J.; Koumas, L.; Ray, D. & Phipps, R. P. (2002).Prostaglandins as modulators of immunity. *Trends Immunology*, Vol.23, pp. 144–150

Hosoi, T.; Okuma, Y. & Nomura, Y. (2002). The mechanisms of immune-to-brain communication in inflammation as a drug target. *Current Drug Targets - Inflammation & Allergy*, Vol.1, No.3, pp. 257-262

Ishizaka, M.; Ohe, Y.; Senbongi, T.; Wakabayashi, K. & Ishikawa, K. (2001). Inflammatory stimuli increase prostaglandin D synthase levels in cerebrospinal fluid of rats. *Neuroreport*, Vol.12, No.6, pp. 1161-1165,

Johanson, C. E.; Duncan, J. A., 3rd; Klinge, P. M.; Brinker, T.; Stopa, E. G. & Silverberg, G. D. (2008). Multiplicity of cerebrospinal fluid functions: New challenges in health and disease. *Cerebrospinal Fluid Research*, Vol.5, pp. 10, ISSN 1743-8454

Johanson, C. E.; Stopa, E. G. & McMillan, P. N. (2011). The blood-cerebrospinal fluid barrier: structure and functional significance. *Methods in Molecular Biology*, Vol.686, pp. 101-131, ISSN 1940-6029

Kemna, E.; Pickkers, P.; Nemeth, E.; van der Hoeven, H. & Swinkels, D. (2005). Time-course analysis of hepcidin, serum iron, and plasma cytokine levels in humans injected with LPS. *Blood*, Vol.106, No.5, pp. 1864-1866

Kjeldsen, L.; Cowland, J. B. & Borregaard, N. (2000). Human neutrophil gelatinase-associated lipocalin and homologous proteins in rat and mouse. *Biochimica et Biophysica Acta*, Vol.1482, No.1-2, pp. 272-283, ISSN 0006-3002

Krause, A.; Neitz, S.; Magert, H. J.; Schulz, A.; Forssmann, W. G.; Schulz-Knappe, P. & Adermann, K. (2000). LEAP-1, a novel highly disulfide-bonded human peptide, exhibits antimicrobial activity. *FEBS Letters*, Vol.480, No.2-3, pp. 147-150

Laflamme, N.; Lacroix, S. & Rivest, S. (1999). An essential role of interleukin-1beta in mediating NF-kappaB activity and COX-2 transcription in cells of the blood-brain barrier in response to a systemic and localized inflammation but not during endotoxemia. *Journal of Neuroscience*, Vol.19, No.24, pp. 10923-10930

Laflamme, N. & Rivest, S. (1999). Effects of systemic immunogenic insults and circulating proinflammatory cytokines on the transcription of the inhibitory factor kappaB alpha within specific cellular populations of the rat brain. *Journal of Neurochemistry*, Vol.73, No.1, pp. 309-321

Lebel, E.; Vallieres, L. & Rivest, S. (2000). Selective involvement of interleukin-6 in the transcriptional activation of the suppressor of cytokine signaling-3 in the brain during systemic immune challenges. *Endocrinology*, Vol.141, No.10, pp. 3749-3763

Ling, E. A.; Kaur, C. & Lu, J. (1998). Origin, nature, and some functional considerations of intraventricular macrophages, with special reference to the epiplexus cells. *Microscopy Research and Technique*, Vol.41, No.1, pp. 43-56

Liu, Q. & Nilsen-Hamilton, M. (1995). Identification of a new acute phase protein. *Journal of Biological Chemistry*, Vol.270, No.38, pp. 22565-22570

Marques, F.; Falcao, A. M.; Sousa, J. C.; Coppola, G.; Geschwind, D.; Sousa, N.; Correia-Neves, M. & Palha, J. A. (2009a). Altered iron metabolism is part of the choroid plexus response to peripheral inflammation. *Endocrinology*, Vol.150, No.6, pp. 2822-2828, ISSN 1945-7170

Marques, F.; Rodrigues, A. J.; Sousa, J. C.; Coppola, G.; Geschwind, D. H.; Sousa, N.; Correia-Neves, M. & Palha, J. A. (2008). Lipocalin 2 is a choroid plexus acute-phase protein. *Journal of Cerebral Blood Flow & Metabolism*, Vol.28, No.3, pp. 450-455,

Marques, F.; Sousa, J. C.; Coppola, G.; Falcao, A. M.; Rodrigues, A. J.; Geschwind, D. H.; Sousa, N.; Correia-Neves, M. & Palha, J. A. (2009b). Kinetic profile of the transcriptome changes induced in the choroid plexus by peripheral inflammation. *Journal of Cerebral Blood Flow & Metabolism*, Vol.29, No.5, pp. 921-932

Marques, F.; Sousa, J. C.; Coppola, G.; Gao, F.; Puga, R.; Brentani, H.; Geschwind, D. H.; Sousa, N.; Correia-Neves, M. & Palha, J. A. (2011). Transcriptome signature of the adult mouse choroid plexus. *Fluids and Barriers of the CNS*, Vol.8, No.1, pp. 10, ISSN 2045-8118

Marques, F.; Sousa, J. C.; Coppola, G.; Geschwind, D. H.; Sousa, N.; Palha, J. A. & Correia-Neves, M. (2009c). The choroid plexus response to a repeated peripheral inflammatory stimulus. *BMC Neuroscience*, Vol.10, pp. 135, ISSN 1471-2202

Marques, F.; Sousa, J. C.; Correia-Neves, M.; Oliveira, P.; Sousa, N. & Palha, J. A. (2007). The choroid plexus response to peripheral inflammatory stimulus. *Neuroscience*, Vol.144, No.2, pp. 424-430

Matyszak, M. K. & Perry, V. H. (1996). The potential role of dendritic cells in immune-mediated inflammatory diseases in the central nervous system. *Neuroscience*, Vol.74, No.2, pp. 599-608

McMenamin, P. G. (1999). Distribution and phenotype of dendritic cells and resident tISSNue macrophages in the dura mater, leptomeninges, and choroid plexus of the rat brain as demonstrated in wholemount preparations. *Journal of Comparative Neurology*, Vol.405, No.4, pp. 553-562

Miyamoto, M.; Fujita, T.; Kimura, Y.; Maruyama, M.; Harada, H.; Sudo, Y.; Miyata, T. & Taniguchi, T. (1988). Regulated expression of a gene encoding a nuclear factor, IRF-1, that specifically binds to IFN-beta gene regulatory elements. *Cell*, Vol.54, No.6, pp. 903-913

Nadeau, S. & Rivest, S. (1999). Regulation of the gene encoding tumor necrosis factor alpha (TNF-alpha) in the rat brain and pituitary in response in different models of systemic immune challenge. *Journal of Neuropathology & Experimental Neurology*, Vol.58, No.1, pp. 61-77

Naka, T.; Fujimoto, M.; Tsutsui, H. & Yoshimura, A. (2005). Negative regulation of cytokine and TLR signalings by SOCS and others. *Advances in Immunology*, Vol.87, pp. 61-122

Negoro, H.; Shin, W. S.; Hakamada-Taguchi, R.; Eguchi, N.; Urade, Y.; Goto, A.; Toyo-Oka, T.; Fujita, T.; Omata, M. & Uehara, Y. (2005). Endogenous prostaglandin D(2) synthesis decreases vascular cell adhesion molecule-1 expression in human umbilical vein endothelial cells. *Life Sciences*, Vol.78, pp. 22–29

Nemeth, E.; Rivera, S.; Gabayan, V.; Keller, C.; Taudorf, S.; Pedersen, B. K. & Ganz, T. (2004a). IL-6 mediates hypoferremia of inflammation by inducing the synthesis of the iron regulatory hormone hepcidin. *Journal of Clinical Investigation*, Vol.113, No.9, pp. 1271-1276

Nemeth, E.; Tuttle, M. S.; Powelson, J.; Vaughn, M. B.; Donovan, A.; Ward, D. M.; Ganz, T. & Kaplan, J. (2004b). Hepcidin regulates cellular iron efflux by binding to ferroportin and inducing its internalization. *Science*, Vol.306, No.5704, pp. 2090-2093

Nemeth, E.; Valore, E. V.; Territo, M.; Schiller, G.; Lichtenstein, A. & Ganz, T. (2003). Hepcidin, a putative mediator of anemia of inflammation, is a type II acute-phase protein. *Blood*, Vol.101, No.7, pp. 2461-2463

Pardridge, W. M.; Eisenberg, J. & Yang, J. (1985). Human blood-brain barrier insulin receptor. *Journal of Neurochemistry*, Vol.44, No.6, pp. 1771-1778

Perry, V. H. (1998). A revised view of the central nervous system microenvironment and major histocompatibility complex class II antigen presentation. *Journal of Neuroimmunology*, Vol.90, No.2, pp. 113-121

Pientrangelo, A. (2010). Hereditary hemochromatosis: pathogenesis, diagnosis, and treatment. *Gastroenterology*, Vol.139, No.2, pp. 393-408

Porto, G. & De Sousa, M. (2007). Iron overload and immunity. *World Journal of Gastroenterology*, Vol.13, No.35, pp. 4707-4715

Quan, N.; Stern, E. L.; Whiteside, M. B. & Herkenham, M. (1999). Induction of pro-inflammatory cytokine mRNAs in the brain after peripheral injection of subseptic doses of lipopolysaccharide in the rat. *Journal of Neuroimmunology*, Vol.93, No.1-2, pp. 72-80

Quan, N.; Whiteside, M. & Herkenham, M. (1998). Time course and localization patterns of interleukin-1beta messenger RNA expression in brain and pituitary after peripheral administration of lipopolysaccharide. *Neuroscience*, Vol.83, No.1, pp. 281-293

Reboldi, A.; Coisne, C.; Baumjohann, D.; Benvenuto, F.; Bottinelli, D.; Lira, S.; Uccelli, A.; Lanzavecchia, A.; Engelhardt, B. & Sallusto, F. (2009). C-C chemokine receptor 6-regulated entry of T(H)-17 cells into the CNS through the choroid plexus is required for the initiation of EAE. *Nature Immunology*, pp. 514-523

Saper, C. B. & Breder, C. D. (1992). Endogenous pyrogens in the CNS: role in the febrile response. *Progress in Brain Research*, Vol.93, pp. 419-428; discussion 428-419, ISSN 0079-6123

Saper, C. B. & Breder, C. D. (1994). The neurologic basis of fever. *New England Journal of Medicine*, Vol.330, No.26, pp. 1880-1886, ISSN 0028-4793

Segal, M. B. (2001). Transport of nutrients across the choroid plexus. *Microscopy Research and Technique*, Vol.52, No.1, pp. 38-48

Speake, T.; Whitwell, C.; Kajita, H.; Majid, A. & Brown, P. D. (2001). Mechanisms of CSF secretion by the choroid plexus. *Microscopy Research and Technique*, Vol.52, No.1, pp. 49-59

Sunil, V. R.; Patel, K. J.; Nilsen-Hamilton, M.; Heck, D. E.; Laskin, J. D. & Laskin, D. L. (2007). Acute endotoxemia is associated with upregulation of lipocalin 24p3/Lcn2 in lung and liver. *Experimental and Molecular Pathology*, pp. 177-187

Verga Falzacappa, M. V.; Casanovas, G.; Hentze, M. W. & Muckenthaler, M. U. (2008). A bone morphogenetic protein (BMP)-responsive element in the hepcidin promoter controls HFE2-mediated hepatic hepcidin expression and its response to IL-6 in cultured cells. *The Journal of Molecular Medicine*, pp. 531-540

Verma, S.; Nakaoke, R.; Dohgu, S. & Banks, W. A. (2006). Release of cytokines by brain endothelial cells: A polarized response to lipopolysaccharide. *Brain, Behavior, and Immunity*, Vol.20, No.5, pp. 449-455, ISSN 0889-1591

Wang, R. H.; Li, C.; Xu, X.; Zheng, Y.; Xiao, C.; Zerfas, P.; Cooperman, S.; Eckhaus, M.; Rouault, T.; Mishra, L. & Deng, C. X. (2005). A role of SMAD4 in iron metabolism through the positive regulation of hepcidin expression. Cell Metabolism, Vol.2, No.6, pp. 399-409

Wolburg, K.; Gerhardt, H.; Schulz, M.; Wolburg, H. & Engelhardt, B. (1999). Ultrastructural localization of adhesion molecules in the healthy and inflamed choroid plexus of the mouse. *Cell and TISSNue Research*, Vol.296, No.2, pp. 259-269

Wright, E. M. (1978). Transport processes in the formation of the cerebrospinal fluid. *Reviews of Physiology, Biochemistry & Pharmacology*, Vol.83, pp. 3-34

Wu, L. J.; Leenders, A. G.; Cooperman, S.; Meyron-Holtz, E.; Smith, S.; Land, W.; Tsai, R. Y.; Berger, U. V.; Sheng, Z. H. & Rouault, T. A. (2004). Expression of the iron transporter ferroportin in synaptic vesicles and the blood-brain barrier. *Brain Research*, Vol.1001, No.1-2, pp. 108-117

Yan, C.; Costa, R. H.; Darnell, J. E., Jr.; Chen, J. D. & Van Dyke, T. A. (1990). Distinct positive and negative elements control the limited hepatocyte and choroid plexus expression of transthyretin in transgenic mice. *Embo Journal*, Vol.9, No.3, pp. 869-878

Zhang, Y. & Pardridge, W. M. (2001). Rapid transferrin efflux from brain to blood across the blood-brain barrier. *Journal of Neurochemistry*, Vol.76, No.5, pp. 1597-1600

7

Acute Phase Proteins: Ferritin and Ferritin Isoforms

Alida Maria Koorts and Margaretha Viljoen
University of Pretoria
South Africa

1. Introduction

Ferritin is a positive acute phase reactant, exhibiting increased levels in blood during the acute phase response. Nevertheless, the precise role of ferritin as an acute phase reactant remains to be clarified. As for other acute phase proteins, ferritin is produced and secreted by hepatocytes. However, ferritin is also produced and secreted by other cell types, including macrophages and cancer cells. Many isoforms of ferritin (isoferritins) are found in the body, depending on the H-subunit to L-subunit ratio in the ferritin protein shell. The subunit composition of ferritin molecules is a major determinant of the functional properties of the ferritin isoforms. Expression of ferritin and its subunits is governed by the amount of metabolically available iron, the presence of oxidative stress and both pro- and anti-inflammatory cytokines. Ferritin as an acute phase reactant is well known for its intracellular iron sequestration and storage abilities during immune activation (Weiss & Goodnough, 2005). This function is of high importance for protection of the body against microbial proliferation, oxidative damage, inflammation and cancer. Although the regulation of iron appears to be a primary function of ferritin in both normal conditions and during the acute phase response, other functions, beyond the control of iron bio-availability, have also been described. Although more investigations are required in order to clarify the precise role of ferritin as an acute phase reactant, this chapter shows a synopsis on the present knowledge on ferritin during the acute phase response. In the first part of this chapter (2-4), the processes of iron sequestration, storage and release by the ferritin molecule, the significance of the presence of isoferritins, and the regulation of the expression of ferritin by iron are described. In the next section (5) changes with diseases, and possible significance of extracellular (plasma) ferritin is discussed. In the last section (6-11) the differential up-regulation of H-subunit rich ferritins during the acute phase response, the importance of H-subunit rich ferritins in the withholding of iron by the macrophage, as well as its role in immune modulation, its pro-apoptotic and anti-apoptotic activities, and variations in cancer are addressed.

2. The ferritin molecule: Sequestration, storage and release of iron

The major functions of intracellular ferritin are the sequestration, storage and release of cellular iron. Body iron can be present as either the highly toxic Fe^{2+}-ions or as harmless, insoluble Fe^{3+}-ions. Ferritin detoxifies Fe^{2+}-ions by converting them to the insoluble Fe^{3+}-

ions. Ferritin can accumulate up to 4500 iron atoms as a ferrihydrite mineral in a hollow protein shell and releases these iron atoms when there is an increase in the cell's need for bio-available iron. The ferritin molecule consists of an outer three-dimensional protein shell with a diameter of 12-13 nm enclosing an inner cavity with a diameter of 7-8 nm. In this inner cavity, ferritin is capable of sequestering variable amounts of Fe^{3+}-atoms as a ferrihydrite mineral. The ferritin protein shell consists of 24 protein subunits of two types, the H-subunit and the L-subunit. These ferritin subunits perform different functions in the multi-step mineralization process of iron. Fe^{2+}-ions enter the ferritin cavity through channels in the protein shell facilitated by the presence of local iron binding sites. Upon entering the shell the Fe^{2+}-ions are oxidized followed by hydrolysis, nucleation and iron core growth. Oxidation of the Fe^{2+}-ions is an obligatory first step and is governed by the H-subunit's ferroxidase center which enzymatically oxidizes Fe^{2+}-ions to Fe^{3+}-ions. The subsequent hydrolysis and nucleation of the generated Fe^{3+}-compound is brought about by the L-subunit. The highly mobile Fe^{3+}-monomers are directed to the inner cavity and properly placed on the protein shell/mineral interface by the L-subunit resulting in the formation of a ferrihydrite mineral core (Figure 1) (Chasteen, 1998; Harrison & Arosio, 1996).

Two mechanisms are proposed for the release of iron from ferritin. Iron can be either released from the intact ferritin molecule or released upon the degradation of the ferritin molecule (Aisen, 1991; Deiss, 1983). Two processes are chemically feasible for removing iron from the intact ferritin molecule. The first process involves the reduction of Fe^{3+}-ions to Fe^{2+}-ions followed by chelation of Fe^{2+}-ions, and the second process the direct chelation of Fe^{3+}-ions (Gálvez *et al.*, 2005; Harrison & Arosio, 1996; Liu *et al.*, 2003). The release of iron from ferritin by these processes is aided by reductants and iron chelators. Reductants and chelators gain access to the interior of the ferritin molecule through three-fold channels in the protein shell. It is suggested that the channels of the ferritin protein shell are dynamic and control the access of reductants and chelators, since reductants and chelators too large to pass through the channels can under certain conditions gain access to the interior of the ferritin molecule (Liu *et al.*, 2003). Chaotropes can increase the access of reductants and chelators to the interior of ferritin by influencing the gating of the channel (Gálvez *et al.*, 2005; Liu *et al.*, 2003). Various reductants and chelators, including physiological and toxicological substances, can release iron from ferritin (Agrawal *et al.*, 2001; Gálvez *et al.*, 2005; Hynes & Coinceanainn, 2002; Sánchez *et al.*, 2005). The hydrous ferric oxide cores can be reduced by one electron per iron atom accompanied by an uptake of two protons per electron from the surrounding medium (Watt *et al.*, 1985). This is then followed by the chelation of Fe^{2+}-ions and the transport to sites where Fe^{2+}-ions are needed (Joshi & Clauberg, 1988; Watt *et al.*, 1985). Effective reducing agents for the release of iron from ferritin include flavins, cysteine, glutathione, ascorbic acid and superoxide (Ponka *et al.*, 1998). This mechanism for the release of iron from the intact ferritin molecule can provide the cell with iron for metabolic processes. However, the released iron may lead to the generation of free radicals that may damage the ferritin molecule itself (Rosseau & Puntarulo, 2009).

In addition to the release of iron from the intact ferritin molecule iron can also be released upon the degradation of the ferritin molecule. Two mechanisms are known to be involved in the degradation of cytosolic ferritin, i.e., the 20S proteasome enzymatic system in the cytosol, and proteolytic enzymes in the lysosomes. The proteolytic enzymes in the lysosomes appear to be of greater importance than the cytosolic proteasome enzymatic system for the degradation of ferritin and the subsequent release of iron (Kidane *et al.*, 2006; Zhang *et al.*, 2010). Specific iron chelators determine the route of ferritin degradation (De Domenico *et al.*, 2009a). Depending on the type of cell, the iron status and whether ferritin is degraded free in the cytosol or within a lysosome, different amounts of iron are made available for metabolic processes. Degradation of ferritin in the cytosol results in the complete release of the iron from ferritin, whereas degradation of ferritin in the confinements of a lysosome can result in the entrapment of ferritin iron (Wixom *et al.*, 1980). Cytosolic degradation may therefore be the major iron turnover mechanism providing the cell with easily accessible iron for shunting into metabolic pathways, while degradation within membrane-encapsulated secondary lysosomes, with subsequent haemosiderin formation, may prevent the uncontrolled release of iron and may become prominent when there is iron overload (Harrison & Arosio, 1996; Wixom *et al.*, 1980). Nevertheless, degradation of ferritin in lysosomes can also produce soluble iron, although these larger masses of ferritin/haemosiderin may require more time for the release of their iron contents. The iron so released would then be translocated back to the cytosol for reutilization in metabolic processes or for sequestration by ferritin (Deiss, 1983; Ponka *et al.*, 1998; Radisky & Kaplan, 1998). It seems as if the release of iron from lysosomes depends on the magnitude of aggregate formation and the subsequent deposition of iron as haemosiderin.

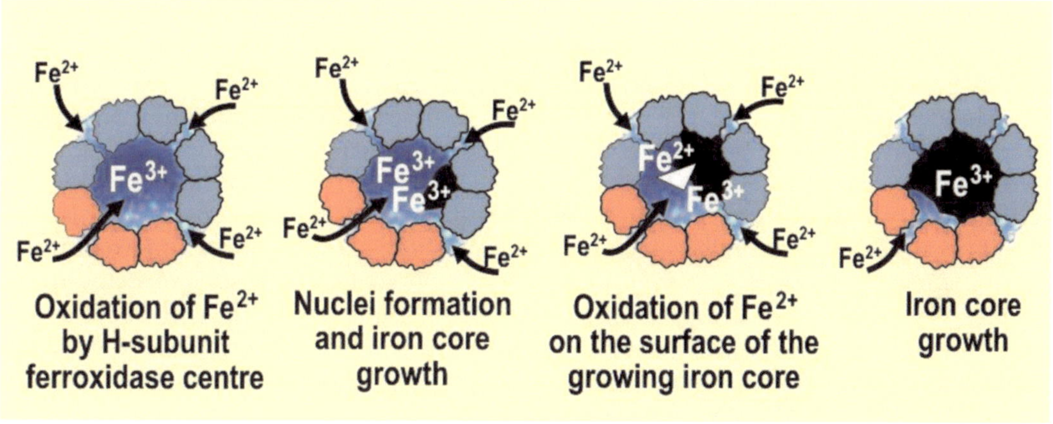

Fig. 1. An animated presentation of ferritin molecules with eight subunits - five L-subunits in blue, and three H-subunits in red to show the mineralization process of iron by the ferritin protein shell. Oxidation of Fe^{2+} is performed by the ferroxidase centre of the H-subunit. This is followed by nuclei formation and iron core growth facilitated by L-subunits. Once the iron core reaches a sufficient size oxidation of Fe^{2+} can take place on the surface of the iron core.

3. The ferritin molecule: Isoferritins

The multiple forms of ferritin have their molecular basis in the ratio of the two types of subunits, the H-subunit and the L-subunit. The ferritin protein shell can exist as heteropolymers of various combinations of these two types of subunits - a phenomenon that gives rise to the existence of isoferritins (Chiancone & Stefanini, 1984). As the roles of the H-subunit and L-subunit in the mineralization process differ, the subunit composition of ferritin will influence the metabolic properties of the assembled ferritin molecules (Harrison & Arosio, 1996; Levi *et al.*, 1994). H-subunit rich ferritins have been shown to accumulate and release iron faster than do L-subunit rich ferritins (Arosio *et al.*, 1991; Chiancone & Stefanini, 1984; Wagstaff *et al.*, 1982; Worwood, 1990), and it is suggested that the H-subunit rich ferritins permit more dynamic intracellular traffic of iron (Chiancone & Stefanini, 1984; Speyer & Fielding, 1979). L-subunit rich ferritins apparently contain higher iron amounts than the H-subunit rich ferritins (Bomford *et al.*, 1981; Chiancone & Stefanini, 1984), and there are indications that the L-subunit rich ferritins predominate in cell types that play a role in iron storage (Boyd *et al.*, 1985; Chiancone & Stefanini, 1984; Coccia *et al.*, 1992; Powell *et al.*, 1975). It would further appear that a specific subunit composition may support iron storage, and that iron loading would increase the expression of the L-subunit upon which these L-subunit rich ferritins will sequester the bulk of the iron surplus (Bomford *et al.*, 1981; Invernizzi *et al.*, 1990). In general, L-subunit rich ferritins contain 1 500 iron atoms or more, whereas H-subunit rich ferritins contain less than a 1 000 iron atoms (Harrison & Arosio, 1996). In situations of iron overload it may be advantageous to the cell to synthesize L-subunit rich ferritins, since these ferritins are not only able to store higher iron amounts, but can also retain iron more firmly and turn over iron more slowly than their H-subunit rich counterparts (White & Munro, 1988). The assumed role that the L-subunit rich ferritins play in the sequestration of the surplus iron during iron overload is underlined by the fact that their concentration in liver, serum and cultured cells is related to iron levels, whereas the H-subunit rich ferritins appear either to be non-affected (in liver) or negatively affected (in serum) by increases in iron concentrations (Ruggeri *et al.*, 1984). Furthermore, upon iron supplementation of patients with functional iron deficiency in the presence of tissue iron overload there would appear to be a proportionately greater change in L-subunit rich ferritins than in H-subunit rich ferritins (Ruggeri *et al.*, 1984). Due to the H-subunit rich ferritin's more dynamic ability of iron uptake and release it would appear to be largely found in cells having high iron requirements for metabolic activities and a non-existent role in iron storage (Cazzola *et al.*, 1983). Cells with a high content of H-subunit rich ferritins include erythroid cells, heart cells, pancreatic cells, kidney cells, lymphocytes and monocytes (Jones *et al.*, 1983; Worwood, 1982), whereas the L-subunit rich ferritins are found predominantly in liver and spleen – organs associated with long-term iron storage (Powell *et al.*, 1975; Worwood, 1982). The H- to L-subunit ratio of a specific type of cell does, however, not remain constant and the proportion of the H- and L-subunits present in the ferritin shell changes during differentiation and in various pathological states (Arosio *et al.*, 1976; Boyd *et al.*, 1985; Ponka *et al.*, 1998; Theil, 1990).

4. The ferritin molecule: iron-dependent regulation of the expression of the H-subunit and L-subunit

Metabolically available iron is a major determinant of the regulation of ferritin expression. In order to accomplish a finely tuned system of ferritin expression as a function of the size of the metabolically available iron pool (the labile iron pool) the ferritin gene structure contains sequences that sense the size of the labile iron pool (Harford *et al.*, 1994). The 5′-untranslated region (5′-UTR) of both the H- and L-subunit mRNA contains a highly conserved 28-base sequence known as the iron-responsive element (IRE) sensitive to the metabolically active available iron (Worwood, 1990). The IREs are comprised of cis-acting nucleotide sequences.

These nucleotide sequences form stem-loop structures that contain a six-membered loop with the sequence CAGUGN (Ponka *et al.*, 1998). These stem-loop structures are recognized by trans-acting cytosolic RNA-binding proteins required for the coordinated expression of the H- and L-subunits (Theil, 1990). These cytosolic RNA-binding proteins, iron-responsive protein 1 (IRP1) and iron-responsive protein 2 (IRP2), cause a decrease in H- and L-subunit mRNA translation by binding to the stem-loop structures of the 5′-UTR of the respective mRNAs. IRP1 and IRP2 mediate the translational efficiency by obscuring the subsequent binding of the 43S translation pre-initiation complex needed for the initiation of translation (Rogers *et al.*, 1994). Although both the H-subunit and the L-subunit mRNA of ferritin contain an IRE, the IREs are regulated differentially. The IRE of the L-subunit mRNA was shown to be the primary responder to iron in hypoxic conditions, but this differential sensitivity is lost in normoxic conditions (Sammarco *et al.*, 2008). IRP1 and IRP2 both sense and homeostatically control the metabolically available iron. For IRP1 this is accomplished by the existence of two conformationally distinct forms. IRP1 is a 90 kD iron-sulphur cluster protein. When iron is abundant it exists as a cytosolic aconitase. When iron is scarce it assumes an open configuration associated with the loss of iron atoms from the iron-sulphur cluster and the subsequent binding to the IRE stem-loop structure, acting as a repressor of ferritin translation (Torti & Torti, 2002). In contrast, the 105 kD IRP2 protein is regulated by degradation: IRP2 protein is abundant in iron scarcity, but is degraded rapidly in iron excess through targeting of a unique 73 amino acid sequence and subsequent oxidation and ubiquitination (Meyron-Holtz *et al.*, 1999; Torti & Torti, 2002,). This response of ferritin synthesis to the size of the metabolically available pool of iron endows the cell with an exceptionally rapid mechanism for increasing ferritin synthesis upon iron influx. Iron influx increases the labile iron pool and, *via* binding to IRP1 and IRP2, causes a rapid increase in ferritin translation. This rapid response is achieved by a shift of stored mRNA from the ribonucleoprotein (RNP) fraction to polysomes (translational shift) (White & Munro, 1988). The ferritin response to iron influx can thus be viewed as a protective rapid response system, allowing immediate formation of additional ferritin in which to store the surplus iron (Truty *et al.*, 2001). Although the H-subunit and L-subunit mRNA shift from the RNP fraction to polysomes to the same extent (White & Munro, 1988), the transcription of the L-subunit gene is preferentially stimulated by an increase in metabolically available iron (Worwood, 1990) resulting in an increase in the ratio of L-subunit to H-subunit mRNA, which appears first in the RNP fraction and later in the polysomes (White & Munro, 1988). This increase in the L-subunit to H-subunit mRNA ratio in the polysomes accounts for the change in the ratio of L-subunit to H-subunit protein synthesis following iron administration (White & Munro, 1988). Coordinated translational control and differential transcriptional control thus exist between these two genes (White & Munro, 1988).

5. Extracellular ferritin

Most of the synthesized ferritin remains within the cell where it sequesters and releases iron in order to maintain intracellular iron homeostasis. Besides the presence of ferritin in the cytosol of the cell, ferritin is also found in smaller quantities in the plasma. It is suggested that ferritin may enter the circulation either *via* secretion of ferritin by cells or through the release of ferritin from damaged cells (Worwood, 1990). Both mechanisms probably contribute to plasma levels. Ferritin destined for intracellular iron homeostasis is synthesized on free polyribosomes, whereas a small amount of ferritin may be synthesized on the rough endoplasmic reticulum for secretion into the plasma (Covell & Worwood, 1984; Cragg *et al.*, 1981). The range of plasma ferritin in the normal adult varies between 15-300 μg/l (Covell & Worwood, 1984; Worwood, 1990), and consists mainly of glycosylated L-subunit rich ferritins containing insignificant amounts of iron, even in conditions of iron overload (Covell & Worwood, 1984; Cragg *et al.*, 1981; Jacobs & Worwood, 1975; Ponka *et al.*, 1998). For instance, while the iron content of ferritin in the liver and spleen could be more than 0.2 μg Fe/μg protein in conditions of iron overload, the iron content of plasma ferritin may still be as low as 0.02-0.07 μg Fe/μg protein (Worwood *et al.*, 1976). Although the function of plasma ferritin is, as yet not completely clear, it is now known that extracellular ferritin can act as iron delivery system for ferritin receptor-mediated endocytosis by cells (Kalgaonkar & Lonnerdal, 2009; Leimberg *et al.*, 2008; Sibile *et al.*, 1988). Extracellular ferritin has further been implicated in functions such as immune modulation, the regulation of myelopoiesis, as well as in the regulation of blood vessel formation, and modulation of bradykinin release and others (De Domenico *et al.*, 2009b; Parthasara *et al.*, 2002).

The concentration of ferritin in plasma is a function of the rate of secretion or release from cells and the clearance by other cells (Hershko & Konijn, 1984). The major cell type responsible for the clearance of plasma ferritins is the hepatocyte. A specific receptor for both glycosylated and non-glycosylated ferritin has been demonstrated on the hepatocyte membrane (Hershko & Konijn, 1984). These receptors bind both the H-subunit and the L-subunit of ferritin (Halliday *et al.*, 1979). However, a significant difference is indicated between the rates of clearance for the non-glycosylated ferritin of tissues, and the glycosylated plasma ferritin (Hershko & Konijn, 1984). These differences in clearance may result in a significantly longer half-life for the glycosylated, secreted ferritins in the circulation compared to that of the non-glycosylated tissue ferritins (Bellotti *et al.*, 1987; Halliday *et al.*, 1979; Hershko & Konijn, 1984; Worwood, 1990). The scavenger receptor (receptors that bind various ligands) SCARA5, has recently been identified as a cell surface receptor that preferentially binds to L-subunit rich ferritins followed by internalization (Li *et al.*, 2009). The clearance of ferritin may, however, also be influenced by the interaction between ferritin and other plasma components such as plasma proteins, ferritin-immune complexes and ferritin auto-antibodies. Of particular interest is the fact that α-2-macroglobulin has been identified as a ferritin binding protein (Massover, 1994). Alpha-2-macroglobulin-binding is known to augment the clearance of substances from the circulation.

Under normal conditions a quantitative relationship exists between the level of plasma ferritin and the amount of storage iron (Cazzola & Ascari, 1986). In conditions of iron overload there is generally an increase in the expression of intracellular L-subunit rich ferritins, paralleled by an increase in these ferritins in the plasma (Halliday & Powell, 1979). Although the specific cellular origin of plasma ferritin is not known (Torti & Torti, 1994), various experiments indicated a large contribution made by the reticulo-endothelial cells. An increase in plasma ferritin levels is known to occur in parallel with the increase in reticulo-endothelial cell ferritin after an increase in reticulo-endothelial cell iron during phagocytosis of non-viable red blood cells (Finch *et al.*, 1984; Jacobs & Worwood, 1975). However, elevated plasma ferritin levels are also seen in patients with parenchymal iron overload whose reticulo-endothelial cells are virtually devoid of iron (Finch *et al.*, 1984).

Serum ferritin levels are determined in the clinic as part of iron studies and low ferritin levels in anaemic patients are generally considered indicative of iron deficiency anaemia

(Guyatt *et al.*, 1990). However, to use ferritin as a measure of body iron in the presence of inflammatory conditions woud lead to erroneous underestimation of the degree of iron deficiency. The reason for this is probably that although iron is a major trigger for the synthesis of ferritin, cytokines would appear to take over the central role in the regulation of ferritin synthesis during inflammatory conditions (Feelders *et al.*, 1998). The cytokines involved in stimulation of ferritin synthesis are mainly of a pro-inflammatory nature and it is known that pro-inflammatory cytokine activity forms an integral part of the acute phase response. For the detection of iron deficiency in the presence of inflammation, several ways of correcting measured ferritin levels for the effect of inflammation have been suggested, amongst others by the World Health Organization (WHO, 2004 & 2007). Inflammation may, however, be present at subclinical levels, yet influence the ferritin levels. In a meta-analysis, examining the adjustment of plasma ferritin concentrations to compensate for the effects of subclinical inflammation in the assessment of iron deficiency, Thurnham *et al.* (Thurnham *et al.*, 2010) found the simultaneous measurement of C-reactive protein and α_1-acidic glycoprotein to be a good estimate of the full effect of inflammation for the correction of ferritin levels.

Plasma ferritin concentration is affected by a number of factors other than the amount of storage iron and inflammatory activity. Other conditions known to influence plasma ferritin levels include tissue necrosis, damage to ferritin-rich tissue, infections, neoplastic disease, increased red blood cell turnover, malnutrition as in anorexia nervosa and surgery (Cazzola & Ascari, 1986; Hershko & Konijn, 1984; Kennedy *et al.*, 2004; Rubin *et al.*, 1984; Torti & Torti, 1994; Worwood, 1982). When any of these conditions are present, the relationship between plasma ferritin concentration and amount of storage iron no longer holds. With tissue necrosis, as in hepatocellular injury, the increase in plasma ferritin is, for instance, due to the release of ferritin from the damaged cells, since the increase in ferritin is dependent on both the magnitude of cellular damage and liver iron stores (Halliday & Powell, 1979). Furthermore, an increase in non-glycosylated, iron-rich ferritins has been reported upon tissue damage, which is indicative of the release of ferritin from damaged tissue, rather than an increase due to active secretion (Cragg *et al.*, 1981).

Neoplastic diseases are in general accompanied by raised levels of ferritin in the plasma. It is suggested that the increase in plasma ferritin may be related to an increased production of ferritin by the malignant cells. In leukemia the normal concentration of ferritin in circulating leukocytes is increased up to six-fold in acute myeloblastic leukemia, more than twenty-fold in acute myelomonocytic leukemia, and two- to three-fold in chronic granulocytic leukemia (Jacobs & Worwood, 1975). In the presence of various solid tumours, including tumours of the breast, pancreas and liver, an increase of H-subunit rich ferritins was shown in the cells of the tumours, as well as an increase in plasma ferritin. In addition, the plasma ferritins reflected the increase in H-subunit rich ferritins of the tumours. Therefore the tumours seem to produce and secrete these H-subunit rich ferritins (Kew *et al.*, 1978; Niitsu *et al.*, 1984). This assumption, that the raised ferritin levels seen in a number of malignancies are the result of secretion from the malignant cells, does, however, not exclude the possibility of a further augmentation of plasma ferritin levels through cancer-related cytokine activity.

Raised levels of plasma ferritin have also been reported for Still's disease - a systemic inflammatory disorder (Evenson *et al.*, 2007), the haemophagocytic syndrome - a disorder strongly associated with autoimmunity (Sekigawa *et al.*, 2001), and in patients at risk for coronary artery disease and myocardial infarction (De Godoy *et al.*, 2007). Low serum levels of ferritin were seen in neurological disorders such as neuroferritinopathy - a disorder of the basal ganglia, (Levi *et al.*, 2005), in restless legs syndrome (Kotagal & Silber, 2004), and in neurally-mediated syncopy in children and adolescents (Jarjour & Jarjour, 2008). Plasma ferritin in these conditions would therefore not be a good indicator of iron stores.

Ferritin levels have, on occasion, been described as a biomarker for a number of pathologies (Goswami *et al.*, 2009). Suggestions are that raised levels of ferritin can be used as biomarker for pathological conditions such as artherosclerosis, certain types of cancer, diabetes mellitus 2, a number of pregnancy complications, foetal growth restriction and others (Goswami *et al.*, 2009; Hou *et al.*, 2000). Although increases in serum ferritin due to inherited disorders, such as haemochromatosis, porphyria, hereditary hyperferritinaemia-cataract syndrome (Kato & Niitsu, 2002), and certain neurological diseases can occur, increases are generally not disease specific. The value of a raised ferritin level as differential diagnostic marker is therefore relatively limited as it is feasible to assume that the increased levels would predominantly be secondary to activities such as altered iron metabolism, oxidative stress, inflammatory processes and, in a small number of conditions, abnormal synthesis or clearance. Nevertheless, the determination of ferritin levels has been reported to have a role in the assessment of disease progression in conditions such as cancer, liver failure, acquired iron overload, multiple trauma, after organ transplantation, in acute and chronic inflammatory conditions and other (Wang *et al.*, 2010). In addition to the identification of iron deficiency in otherwise normal individuals, and of iron overload, ferritin levels thus appear to be of clinical value in the assessment of prognosis and disease progression of certain disorders. Abnormal ferritin levels in the absence of abnormal total body iron may warrant further investigation. Although the value of ferritin as a reflection of body iron stores may be compromised during the acute phase response, the potential exists for ferritin as indicator of disease progression.

6. Acute phase response, inflammatory response and ferritin

The acute phase response is a systemic reaction to local or systemic infection, tissue damage, cancer and in general, immune disturbances. It is a non-specific, early defense system (Cray *et al.*, 2009), and can therefore be seen as part of the innate immune system. The acute phase response is induced in the liver and also in various other tissues, and consists of both intracellular and extracellular acute phase proteins (Tilg *et al.*, 1997). The inflammatory response, with the associated production of cytokines, forms an integral part of the acute phase response. Cytokines, both pro-inflammatory and anti-inflammatory, take part in the regulation of the production of the acute phase proteins, and mediate an increase in the so-called positive acute phase proteins and a decrease in the so-called negative acute phase proteins. Cytokines shown to modulate the production of acute phase proteins include the pro-inflammatory cytokines interleukin-1β (Il-1β) and interleukin-6 (Il-6), (Ramadori & Christ, 1999), and the anti-inflammatory cytokine interleukin-10 (Il-10) (El Kasmi *et al.*, 2006). Up or down transcriptional regulation provides the necessary control for the synthesis of the acute phase proteins. One of the transcription factors involved in the synthesis of the acute phase proteins, signal transducer and activator of transcription 3 (stat3), originally named acute phase response factor (APRF), regulates the response to both pro- and anti-inflammatory cytokines (Desiderio & Yoo, 2003; Turkson & Jove, 2000). Ferritin is considered a positive acute phase protein and is up-regulated intracellularly in many cell types, and extracellularly, in the plasma as a result of an increase in cellular secretion. An important role for ferritin during the acute phase response is to restrict the availability of iron by sequestration into the cavity of the ferritin protein shell. Furthermore, ferritin can modulate many immune functions, play a role in pro-apoptotic and anti-apoptotic pathways, and is implicated in the pathology of cancer.

Oxygen radicals, i.e., molecules containing unpaired electrons are generated in large amounts during infectious and inflammatory conditions (Di Virgilio, 2004). They react with proteins, lipids and nucleic acids, resulting in degradation of the phagocytosed material in the confinements of the phagosome in the neutrophil and macrophage. However, large amounts of these toxic metabolites leak to the fluids and tissues in the area of the inflammatory reaction and by reacting with cellular constituents can result in substantial damage (Closa & Folch-Puy, 2004; Liu & Pope, 2004). Iron, due to its role in Fenton-type chemistry, can result in exacerbation of oxygen radical production. Such an increase in unwanted oxygen radical production due to toxic amounts of iron can be seen in chronic inflammatory conditions. An increase in the iron content in the synovium is, for instance, present in rheumatoid arthritis (Giordano *et al.*, 1991), and a significant correlation exists between thiobarbituric acid-reactive material (lipid peroxidation product), the amount of iron in the synovial fluid, and the inflammatory activity of the disease (Rowley *et al.*, 1984). Furthermore, when anaemic rheumatoid arthritis patients receive iron supplementation, lipid peroxidation is stimulated resulting in worsening of the synovial inflammation (Blake *et al.*, 1985).

In general, a reduction in the bio-availability of iron will offer protection against cell injury by hydroxyl radicals that are generated from neutrophil- and macrophage-derived superoxides (Rogers *et al.*, 1990). Iron sequestration by cells in the zone of inflammation may therefore provide protection against the free radical assault (Rogers *et al.*, 1994). This role of host cell protection against an increase in the free radical onslaught is consistent with observations that a reduction in ferritin sensitizes cells to pro-oxidant cytotoxicity, and that overexpression of ferritin reduces reactive oxidant species (ROS) in cells challenged by oxidants and by implication reduces the oxidative toxicity (Torti & Torti, 1994). Macrophages, although contributing to the production of ROS, can also provide protection against it by reducing the available iron.

The restriction of bio-available iron during infections and inflammation controls the production of reactive oxygen species. In addition, with-holding of bio-available iron from micro-organisms can restrict their proliferation and spreading during infections. Most micro-organisms need a substantial amount of iron to ensure their survival and are endowed with various mechanisms and molecules to obtain iron from host ferroproteins such as haemoglobin, ferritin and transferrin (Ganz, 2009). For infections, such as tuberculosis, increased macrophage iron is associated with more severe infections with worse outcomes (Boelaert *et al.*, 2007). Whereas, supplementing with iron can result in susceptibilty to malaria infections in areas with endemic malaria (Prentice, 2008). In order to suppress the growth of the pathogen the host responds by sequestering iron as evidenced by increased ferritin expression in the chronic phase of trypanosomiasis (Stijlemans *et al.*, 2008).

7. Differential up-regulation of H-subunit rich ferritins during the acute phase response

The overexpression of either the H- or the L- subunit is known to protect against oxidative stress (Orino *et al.*, 2001). Nevertheless, the H-subunit rich ferritins have been shown to offer better protection than L-subunit rich ferritins. L-subunit rich ferritins predominate in cell types that play a role in the storage of iron (Boyd *et al.*, 1985; Chiancone & Stefanini, 1984;

Powell *et al.*, 1975), and there are indications that L-subunit rich ferritins contain more iron than those ferritins rich in H-subunits (Bomford *et al.*, 1981; Chiancone & Stefanini, 1984). However, rapid sequestration of iron is called for in inflammation to protect cells against the unwanted accumulation of reactive oxygen species that could damage various cellular components. H-subunit rich ferritins have been shown to accumulate and release iron faster than L-subunit rich ferritins (Arosio *et al.*, 1991; Chiancone & Stefanini, 1984; Wagstaff *et al.*, 1982; Worwood, 1990), and it is suggested that the H-subunit rich ferritins permit a more dynamic intracellular traffic of iron than L-subunit rich ferritins (Chiancone & Stefanini, 1984; Speyer & Fielding, 1979). It is generally assumed that H-subunit rich ferritins are also responsible for the rapid sequestration of iron in situations where iron can contribute to damage to the cell (Arosio & Levi, 2002), and that an increase in the expression of the H-subunit rich ferritins protects the cell against oxidative stress by attenuating the production of hydroxyl radicals by the Fenton reaction (Cozzi *et al.*, 2000; Zhao *et al.*, 2006). The induction of H-subunit rich ferritins *in vivo* results in a phenotype of tissue-specific iron depletion. H-subunit rich ferritins can act as a potent regulator of iron metabolism in tissues and these effects can dominate normal iron homeostatic mechanisms (Wilkinson *et al.*, 2006). However, cells can limit the accumulation of H-subunits by differentially secreting H-subunits in variance with L-subunits. Such a mechanism could play a significant role in regulating the amount of cytosolic H-subunit rich ferritin and might protect the cell against unwarranted rapid sequestration of iron by H-subunit rich ferritins (Goralska *et al.*, 2003).

Cytokines, central mediators of the inflammatory activity of the acute phase response, have been shown to up-regulate the expression of ferritin (Konijn & Hershko, 1977; Piñero *et al.*, 2000). Pro-inflammatory cytokines reported to have the ability to induce ferritin expression include Il-1α, Il-1β, Il-2, Il-6, tumour necrosis factor-α (TNF-α), and interferon-γ (IFN-γ) (Miller *et al.*, 1991; Pang *et al.*, 1996; Rogers *et al.*, 1990; Rogers, 1996; Stites *et al.*, 1999; Torti & Torti, 2002). These cytokines modulate ferritin expression by both transcriptional and translational mechanisms (Piñero *et al.*, 2000), but largely by an increase in the rate of transcription of the ferritin genes (Miller *et al.*, 1991; Torti & Torti, 2002). Furthermore, cytokines differentially regulate the expression of the ferritin subunits, and it is mostly the H-subunit of ferritin that is increased by cytokine induction at variance with the L-subunit (Miller *et al.*, 1991; Pang *et al.*, 1996; Rogers, 1996; Stites *et al.*, 1999; Torti & Torti, 2002).

Cytokines can also up-regulate the expression of ferritin by stimulating the production of reactive oxygen species. Pro-inflammatory cytokines increase the production of reactive oxygen species in various ways (Gougerot-Pocidalo *et al.*, 2002; Yang *et al.*, 2007). Furthermore, free oxygen radicals can, in turn, mediate signal transduction pathways that induce cytokine production and anti-oxidants have been shown to inhibit this transcriptional increase in the production of inflammatory cytokines (Ali *et al.*, 1999; Blackwell *et al.*, 1996; Dröge, 2002; Kosmidou *et al.*, 2002; Tapia *et al.*, 2003). An increase in oxidative stress is known to result in the transcriptional up-regulation of ferritin. This is part of a cellular anti-oxidant response induced by pro-oxidants to provide protection against reactive oxygen species. Induction of transcription is governed by the anti-oxidant responsive element (ARE) present in the ferritin genes upstream to the transcription initiation site. The H-subunit and the L-subunit genes both contain AREs, but at different positions upstream from the transcription initiation site and more importantly these AREs are regulated differentially (Hintze & Theil, 2005; Iwasaki & MacKenzie, 2006; Torti & Torti, 1994). Damage to mitochondria with the consequent increase in iron-mediated reactive oxygen radical accumulation resulted in the preferential transcription of the H-subunit of ferritin governed by the ARE of the H-subunit's gene (MacKenzie *et al.*, 2008). In addition, oxidants can also up-regulate the expresion of ferritin through their influence on IRP1 (Cairo *et al.*, 1996; Orino *et al.*, 2001; Tsuji *et al.*, 2000), and by releasing iron from cellular proteins (Cairo *et al.*, 1995).

8. The macrophage, iron metabolism and H-subunit rich ferritins during the acute phase response

The macrophage is central to the decrease in plasma iron that is associated with immune activation. This hypoferraemic state is predominantly orchestrated by cytokines. Various iron homeostatic processes are affected by these cytokines with the combined actions resulting in entrapment of iron in the macrophage and a decrease in serum iron. This process is known as the iron transfer block (Weiss & Goodnough, 2005). The so-called iron transfer block is generally associated with chronic inflammatory conditions. Inflammation, mediated by cytokines, produces a shift in iron handling by the macrophage in favour of iron storage, in time leading to hypoferraemia (Alvarez-Hernández *et al.*, 1989; Fahmy & Young, 1993; Worwood, 1990), haemosiderosis of the macrophage (Finch *et al.*, 1984; Lipschitz *et al.*, 1971; Worwood, 1990), and the anaemia of chronic disease (Weiss & Goodnough, 2005). The latter is, however, only partly due to a decrease in iron available for haemotopoiesis as factors such as suppression of the proliferation of erythroid progenitor cells, a decrease in the synthesis of erythropoietin, a decrease in the sensitivity of erythroblasts to erythropoietin and a decrease in the red blood cell life span, contribute (Weiss & Goodnough, 2005). Ferritin plays a major part in the establishment and maintenance of an iron transfer block and thus in the hypoferraemic state of the inflammatory reaction. TNF-α, Il-1β, Il-6 and Il-10 have all been shown to directly stimulate the transcription and translation of ferritin (Ludwiczek *et al.*, 2003; Weiss & Goodnough, 2005). Activation of macrophages by cytokines such as, TNF-α and Il-1, results in the slower release of iron compared to non-stimulated macrophages, thus supporting the proposed role of cytokines in ferritin-mediated iron sequestration by macrophages (Alvarez-Hernández *et al.*, 1986; Savarino *et al.*, 1999). However, other iron homeostasis proteins also contribute to the reduction in serum iron. Most proteins involved in the acquisition, storage and release of iron are influenced, to different extents and at different time-points during the inflammatory reaction, by cytokines. With an inflammatory reaction the cytokine Il-6 has, for instance, been shown to stimulate the hepatic expression of the acute phase protein hepcidin. Hepcidin, in turn, inhibits duodenal absorption of iron by down-regulating ferroportin expression thus reducing serum iron (Ganz, 2004). IFN-γ, by increasing the expression of the divalent metal transporter 1, has been shown to stimulate the uptake of ferrous iron by macrophages. Not only pro-inflammatory, but also anti-inflammatory cytokines are involved in the establishment of an iron transfer block. It has, for instance, been shown that Il-4 and Il-10 can up-regulate transferrin receptor expression, resulting in an increase in transferrin receptor-mediated uptake of iron by the macrophage (Ludwiczek *et al.*, 2003; Weiss & Goodnough, 2005). Furthermore, an increase in the phagocytosis and degradation of senescent erythrocytes is known to occur with an inflammatory reaction. This process is directly up-regulated by TNF-α stimulation as a result of the increase in the expression of C3bi (CD11b/CD18) receptors responsible for the recognition and uptake of damaged erythrocytes. In addition, TNF-α can indirectly up-regulate this process by damaging circulating erythrocytes. These damaged erythrocytes are then phagocytosed upon binding to C3bi (CD11b/CD18) receptors followed by degradation (Ludwiczek *et al.*, 2003; Weiss &

Goodnough, 2005). Not only is haemoglobin iron obtained by degradation of red blood cells, but free plasma haemoglobin is taken up by the haemoglobin scavenger receptor, CD163. Il-10 and Il-6 contribute to macrophage haemoglobin acquisition by stimulating the expression of the haemoglobin scavenger receptor, CD163 (Ludwiczek *et al.*, 2003). INF-γ, down-regulates the expression of ferroportin, the major transmembrane protein responsible for the release of macrophage iron, thus inhibiting iron export from macrophages (Ludwiczek *et al.*, 2003), a process that is also affected by hepcidin (Deicher & Hörl, 2006). Down-regulation of ferroportin occurs only later in the inflammatory response after the onset of hypoferraemia. It is therefore suggested that the down-regulation of ferroportin is not responsible for the development of the iron transfer block, but that it plays a major role in the maintenance of the iron transfer block (Ludwiczek *et al.*, 2003). Many of the pro-inflammatory mediated effects on iron homeostasis are counterbalanced by anti-inflammatory cytokines such as IL-4 and IL-13 (Ludwiczek *et al.*, 2003).

The abnormal retention of iron by the macrophage, due to an increase of ferritin synthesis, has long been seen as a non-specific acute phase reactant of inflammation (Konijn & Hershko, 1977; Worwood, 1990). The increase in ferritin synthesis occurs prior to the reduction of serum iron levels and is considered to result in a diversion of iron from the intracellular labile iron pool to ferritin, and subsequently to haemosiderin (Alvarez-Hernández *et al.*, 1986; Fillet *et al.*, 1989; Jurado, 1997; Torrance *et al.*, 1978; Worwood, 1990). The increase in ferritin expression by the macrophage mostly influences the early phase of iron release. In normal conditions two-thirds of the iron entering the macrophage/reticulo-endothelial system (RES) is released during this phase, but an increase in ferritin expression can result in a decrease in the release of iron during this phase to only 10% of the iron entering the macrophage/RES (Fillet *et al.*, 1974; Torrance *et al.*, 1978). However, the slow release phase of iron from the macrophage is also influenced and can result in a situation where 33% of the iron is still present in storage form in the macrophage/RES after 60 days (Noyes *et al.*, 1960). Furthermore, once the macrophage and other macrophage-like cells have been activated, as occurs during inflammation, these cells express increased levels of transferrin receptors (Fahmy & Young, 1993), and are therefore able to acquire increased amounts of iron by endocytosis of the iron-transferrin-transferrin receptor complex. The increase in iron uptake via this route will contribute to the high magnitude of iron sequestration and to the ensuing haemosiderosis of macrophages and other macrophage-like cells. These iron-withholding mechanisms are implemented as a defense strategy in order to deplete biologically active iron in the zone of inflammation or, once the inflammatory response cannot be contained, systemically (Fuchs *et al.*, 1993).

Haemosiderin formation can also aid in protection against iron toxicity. Haemosiderin is derived from ferritin as a result of degradation of the ferritin protein shell in secondary lysosomes (Finch *et al.*, 1984; Fischbach *et al.*, 1971; Ford *et al.*, 1984). Evidence for this is found in observations that haemosiderin contains various amounts of degraded ferritin, as well as aggregated dense particles of irregular shape with diameters ranging from 10-75 Å, which ultrastructurally resemble iron cores (Ringeling *et al.*, 1989, Wixom *et al.*, 1980), and that haemosiderin granules are recognised by anti-ferritin antibodies (Harrison & Arosio, 1996). Ferritin is frequently found in secondary lysosomes and autophagosomes of normal cells, such as hepatocytes and macrophages, but its quantity in these organelles increases greatly after loading with iron (Richter, 1978) - demonstrating the protective function of haemosiderin formation against the toxicity of iron. Ferritin finds its way into lysosomes by autophagocytosis and/or fusion of ferritin clusters with the lysosomal membrane. Autophagocytosis is responsible for the turnover of cellular constituents including cellular proteins and involves the formation of autophagic vacuoles by invagination of intracytoplasmic membranes enclosing a relatively large volume of cytoplasm, together with various cellular constituents (Wixom *et al.*, 1980). The autophagic vacuole receives digestive enzymes by fusion with a primary or secondary lysosome and becomes an autophagosome (Wixom *et al.*, 1980). Within this lysosomal organelle the ferritin protein shell is degraded by the action of lysosomal proteases (Richter, 1984). It is suggested that the polymerization of ferritin (formation of oligomers of ferritin), which results in a change in solubility, heat stability and surface charge, may predispose ferritin to incorporation into lysosomes and transformation into haemosiderin (Chiancone & Stefanini, 1984; Ringeling *et al.*, 1989). Only once the ferritin protein shell has been modified, most probably by denaturation, resulting in the formation of insoluble ferritin molecules, does proteolytic decomposition of the ferritin protein shell by lysosomal enzymes take place (Richter, 1984). However, not all ferritin molecules in these lysosomal organelles are susceptible to the action of lysosomal proteases. Degradation of the ferritin protein shell results in the exposure of the iron oxyhydroxide mineral cores followed by aggregation of these oxyhydroxide particles and the formation of insoluble masses of iron oxyhydroxide (haemosiderin) (Fischbach *et al.*, 1971; Richter, 1978; Weir *et al.*, 1985). Although the main purpose of the formation of haemosiderin would appear to be protection against iron overload, these larger masses of ferritin/haemosiderin can, at a much slower rate, also release iron. This iron is then translocated back to the cytosol for reutilization in metabolic processes or for sequestration by ferritin (Deiss, 1983; Ponka *et al.*, 1998; Radisky & Kaplan, 1998). Haemosiderin is, however, not necessarily the end product as massive quantities of iron oxyhydroxide (haemosiderin) from these secondary lysosomes, can accumulate to form cytoplasmic organelles known as siderosomes (Richter, 1978). The haemosiderin-containing siderosomes can thus be regarded as the end-product of secondary lysosome action in which the wall of the original secondary lysosome now encapsulates the digested ferritin iron cores (Harrison & Arosio, 1996; Wixom *et al.*, 1980) – although clusters of electron-dense material without membranes or only partially enclosed membranes can also occur (Deiss, 1983; Harrison & Arosio, 1996; Iancu, 1982). Within siderosomes, ferritin can be identified as individual particles, in clusters, in paracrystalline hexagonal arrays, or in circular arrangements (Iancu, 1992). In cells with marked iron overload, solitary siderosomes seem to fuse and to form larger bodies described as "compound siderosomes" (Iancu, 1992).

The formation of haemosiderin in reticulo-endothelial cells and other macrophage-like cells is influenced by inflammatory and infectious conditions. Macrophages subjected to increased oxidative stress also degrade ferritin faster than macrophages not challenged with an increase in the production of reactive oxygen species (Mehlhase *et al.*, 2005). It is therefore, suggested that during inflammatory and infectious conditions the proportion of poorly accessible (non-chelatable) iron associated with ferritin similarly increases, suggesting a pathway from non-ferritin iron to loosely associated ferritin iron to a well-sequestered non-chelatable form existing as haemosiderin (Fahmy & Young, 1993). Cytokines such as TNF-α and IFN-γ may be responsible for these effects during inflammatory and infectious conditions. These cytokines may increase lysosomal activity resulting in increased degradation of intracellular ferritin, leading to the formation of haemosiderin, from which iron would be less easily liberated for subsequent extracellular release (Alvarez-Hernández *et al.*, 1989). *In vitro* incubation of cells with either TNF-α or

IFN-γ increases the expression of ferritin H-subunit mRNA, but not L-subunit mRNA (Fahmy & Young, 1993). Such a differential regulation of ferritin subunit expression might result in increased amounts of haemosiderin formation, since H-subunit rich ferritins are more susceptible to lysosomal degradation.

H-subunit rich ferritins have indeed been shown to play a role in the iron redistribution during inflammation, and also in the iron redistribution of the acute phase response. It has, as mentioned before, been reported that H-subunit rich ferritins turnover more rapidly than L-subunit rich ferritins (Boyd *et al.*, 1985; Truty *et al.*, 2001; Worwood, 1982). Haemosiderin, which contains the degraded ferritin molecules as a result of the lysosomal breakdown of ferritin, shows the predominance of denatured subunits to be of the H-subunit type (Miyazaki *et al.*, 2002; Ruggeri *et al.*, 1992). A mechanism may therefore exist for preferentially directing ferritins rich in the H-subunit into lysosomes which would result in the formation of haemosiderin containing a high proportion of denatured H-subunits. It is already known that a too great proportion of H-subunits in the ferritin protein shell results in ferritin aggregation (Harrison & Arosio, 1996). This may be due to the inadequacy of the ferritin protein shell to retain the formed Fe^{3+}-ions resulting in the loss of Fe^{3+}-ions and hydrolysis of Fe^{3+}-ions on the outside of the ferritin molecule (Harrison & Arosio, 1996), which may be the signal for ferritin to be incorporated into lysosomes. Once inside the lysosome the presence of a large number of H-subunits in the ferritin protein shell increases the chances of degradation (Bomford *et al.*, 1981), since H-subunit rich ferritins, during denaturing conditions, are less stable than L-subunit rich ferritins (Kim *et al.*, 2001; Miyazaki *et al.*, 2002). The salt-bridge present in the L-subunit appears to be important for the differences in stabilities between H-subunit rich ferritins and L-subunit rich ferritins (Arosio *et al.*, 1991). Futhermore, H-subunit rich ferritins are more susceptible to proteolysis due to less ordered secondary structures (Bomford *et al.*, 1981). In particular the loop L becomes more exposed and/or less immobilized when the proportion of H-subunits increases and therefore more accessible to lysosomal enzymes (Chiancone & Stefanini, 1984).

9. Immune modulation by secreted H-subunit rich ferritins

Many functions attributed to H-subunit rich ferritins point to a role for these isoferritins in immune modulation, including pro-inflammatory and anti-inflammatory activities. H-subunit rich ferritins are present in most biologic fluids, but not, or only in low concentrations, in plasma (Morikawa *et al.*, 1995). The ferritin present in plasma is mostly L-subunit rich. However, during certain disease states the concentration of H-subunit rich ferritin is increased. At present it would appear that the H-subunit rich ferritins are derived mostly from monocytes and macrophages as indicated by the secretion of H-subunit rich ferritins from many monocyte-macrophage cell lines, as well as by monocytes from blood and bone marrow (Broxmeyer *et al.*, 1984). In a recent study it was shown that murine serum ferritin is mainly secreted by macrophages through a non-classical secretion process involving secretory lysosomes and not the endoplasmic reticulum (Cohen *et al.*, 2010). The release of H-subunit rich ferritins from monocytes appears to be controlled by T-cell subsets, where T-helper cells enhance the release and T-suppressor cells suppress the release (Worwood, 1990). These effects are most probably brought about by cytokines, since pro-inflammatory cytokines are known to induce the secretion of ferritin as part of the acute phase response. The secretion of ferritin was shown to be stimulated by cytokines in a primary human hepatocyte culture where IL-1α and Il-6 induced a transient secretion of ferritin at 24 hours, followed by a decline to baseline, while TNF-α treatment resulted in a sustained increase in ferritin secretion (Torti & Torti, 2002).

H-subunit rich ferritins can suppress various functions of immune cells. H-subunit rich ferritins can, for instance, exert inhibitory effects on E-rosette formation of T- lymphocytes (CD2 is the surface molecule on T-lymphocytes which facilitates binding to sheep erythrocytes and the formation of so-called E-rosettes), suppress the *in vitro* responses of lymphocytes to various mitogens including PHA and con A, inhibit the mixed-lymphocyte reaction, inhibit delayed-type hypersensitivity responses, block the access to T-lymphocytes by various regulatory factors by occupying the surface of the cells (Hie-won *et al.*, 1984; Worwood, 1990), and decrease leukocyte migration (Worwood, 1990).

Receptors for H-subunit rich ferritins have been found on various T-cell lines, CD4 and CD8 T-lymphocytes and on CD19 B-lymphocytes, and the expression of H-subunit rich ferritin binding sites on these cells appears to be closely and positively linked to their activation and proliferation status (Meyron-Holtz *et al.*, 1994; Morikawa *et al.*, 1995). It would therefore appear that H-subunit rich ferritins may perhaps act as feedback inhibitors of activation of peripheral blood cells. Quiescent circulating lymphocytes, reticulocytes, erythrocytes, and monocytes show little expression of the H-subunit rich ferritin receptor, but PHA-stimulated lymphocytes, erythropoietin-induced burst forming unit (BFU) cells, and differentiated macrophages have all been shown to express above average levels of the receptor (Halliday *et al.*, 1994), which may result in these cells being more susceptible to inhibition by H-subunit rich ferritins. Increased binding of H-subunit rich ferritins to peripheral lymphocytes have also been shown to occur in patients with malignant disorders and the magnitude of H-subunit rich ferritin binding to lymphocytes was shown to be related to the stage of the malignant process (Ciriello *et al.*, 1987). It is postulated that two receptor systems exist for the binding and execution of H-subunit rich ferritin's effects. The first receptor system internalizes the bound ferritin. This system is similar to the receptor system operating in erythroid precursors. Developing erythroid cells in the bone marrow are often found in close proximity to a central "mother" reticulo-endothelial cell which supplies ferritin to these developing red blood cell precursors (Deiss, 1983; Jacobs *et al.*, 1984). This process, known as rhopheocytosis, is a highly regulated pathway for iron assimilation by erythroid progenitor cells (Gelvan *et al.*, 1996; Konijn *et al.*, 1994; Meyron-Holtz *et al.*, 1994). However, a regulatory effect on cell proliferation and maturation occurs, whereas in erythroid precursors such a regulatory effect has not been observed (Meyron-Holtz *et al.*, 1994; Meyron-Holtz *et al.*, 1999). The second receptor system, with a Kd three orders of magnitude lower, does not result in the internalization of the bound ferritin (Meyron-Holtz *et al.*, 1994; Meyron-Holtz *et al.*, 1999). This suggests a mechanism for the regulation of cellular proliferation and maturation by ferritin not involving iron or the sequestration of iron.

Three specific receptors involving binding and internalization of H-subunit rich ferritins have been identified recently. The first involves a receptor identical to TIM-2 (member of the T-cell immunoglobulin and mucin-domain gene family) that specifically binds extracellular H-subunit rich ferritins followed by the internalization of H-subunit rich ferritins, and is expressed in B-cells and in non-haematopoietic organs such as the liver and kidney. Internalization of the H-subunit rich ferritins resulted in immunosuppression by inhibiting T-cell activation (Knickelbein *et al.*, 2006). The second receptor that binds H-subunit rich ferritins is transferrin receptor 1. The binding of H-subunit rich ferritins to this receptor resulted in entry into endosomes and lysosomes (Li *et al.*, 2010). The third receptor involves the CXCL12 chemokines and their receprtors. It has been shown that H-subunit rich ferritins can repress chemokine receptor-mediated signal transduction and migration of lymphocytes by binding to the CXCL12 chemokine's receptor (Li *et al.*, 2006). The CXCL12 chemokines have chemotactic and various activating effects that play important roles in T-helper cell responses. H-subunit rich ferritins have been found to bind to the CXCL12's cell surface receptors (CXCR4) in the presence of CXCL12. This complex, consisting of CXCL12 and the H-subunit rich ferritin together with the receptor, are then internalized by the cell. On the inside of the cell the H-subunit rich ferritins are phosphorylated followed by nuclear translocation. Furthermore, intracellular H-subunit rich ferritins can repress CXCR4 activation followed by inhibition of lymphocyte migration (Li *et al.*, 2006).

Most of the immunomodulatory studies involving H-subunit rich ferritins seem to be of an anti-inflammatory nature. However, it was recently shown that H-subunit rich ferritins could also activate a pro-inflammatory pathway by an iron-independent mechanism (Ruddell *et al.*, 2009). Ruddell *et al.* observed that hepatic stellate cells, treated with ferritin, set in motion a pathway involving phosphatidylinositol 3-kinase (PI3-kinase) phosphorylation, protein kinase C zeta and mitogen-activated protein kinase (MAP-kinase) activation, resulting in NFκB activation and eventually in increased pro-inflammatory activity. Activation of this pro-inflammatory pathway results in the enhanced production of various pro-inflammatory mediators including Il-1β, inducible nitric oxide synthase (iNOS), the chemokine - regulated on activation normal T-cell expressed and secreted (RANTES), inhibitor of κBα and intercellular adhesion molecule 1 (iCAM1) (Ruddell *et al.*, 2009). Based on these findings ferritin has been proposed as a pro-inflammatory signal molecule.

A number of other immune-related effects have been attributed to these H-subunit rich plasma ferritins, including the down-regulation of myelopoiesis and regulation of angiogenesis (Broxmeyer *et al.*, 1984; De Domenico *et al.*, 2009b). It has specifically been shown that H-subunit rich ferritins, but not L-subunit rich ferritins, down-regulate myelopoiesis (Broxmeyer *et al.*, 1986), i.e., the growth and development of granulocytes, macrophages, erythrocytes, and platelets (Broxmeyer, 1992; Joshi & Clauberg, 1988), both *in vitro* and *in vivo*. It has been suggested that H-subunit rich ferritins constitute part of a normal inhibitory feedback mechanism for the proliferation of granulocyte-macrophage colony forming units (CFU-GM), multipotential colony forming units (CFU-GEMM), and erythroid burst forming units (BFU-E) (Broxmeyer, 1992; Jacobs *et al.*, 1984). H-subunit rich ferritin decreases the proliferation of cells during myelopoiesis by directly affecting these progenitor cells (Broxmeyer, 1992). Surface receptors specific for H-subunit rich ferritins have been shown on these progenitor cells (Fargion *et al.*, 1988). These effects of H-subunit rich ferritins are mediated *via* the ferroxidase activity of the H-subunits - most probably by inducing intracellular iron starvation (Cozzi *et al.*, 2000; Morikawa *et al.*, 1995), since addition of iron completely counteracts the inhibitory effects of the H-subunit rich ferritins (Broxmeyer *et al.*, 1991).

10. Pro-apoptotic and anti-apoptotic activity of H-subunit rich ferritins during inflammation

During inflammation the proliferation and apoptosis of specific immune cells determine the course of the inflammatory response. H-subunit rich ferritins play a role in both pro-apoptotic and anti-apoptotic pathways, not only due to its ability to donate or sequester iron, but also by mechanisms not involving iron. During inflammation, an increase in reactive oxygen species (ROS) generation by cytokines is shown to be one of the mechanisms whereby cytokines induce apoptosis in cells. Tumour necrosis factor-α (TNF-α), a pro-inflammatory cytokine, is known to induce apoptosis in many cell types during inflammation (Sharma & Anker, 2002). The mechanism by which TNF-α brings about an accumulation of ROS and apoptosis involves up-regulation of the labile iron pool (Pham *et al.*, 2004). This ROS formation induced by TNF-α is mediated by c-Jun N-terminal kinase 1-dependent (JNK1) ferritin degradation and subsequent elevation in the labile iron pool (Antosiewicz *et al.*, 2007). As H-subunit rich ferritins take-up iron faster and release iron faster than L-subunit rich ferritins it can donate or sequester iron resulting in an increase or decrease in ROS generation. In cells devoid of H-subunit rich ferritins (reduction of intracellular iron storage caused by less H-subunit rich ferritins) TNF-α can not bring about an increase in the labile iron pool, the accumulation of ROS and apoptosis. However, when TNF-α activation is accompanied by an increase in the expression of H-subunit rich ferritins, apoptosis is prevented by the sequestration of iron and the subsequent decrease in ROS production (Xie *et al.*, 2005). Thus H-subunit rich ferritins can antagonize this cytokine-induced apoptosis by sequestration of iron, preventing reactive oxygen species accumulation (Vardhan *et al*, 2010). It has been found that H-subunit rich ferritin expression is induced by NF-κB transcription factors. H-subunit rich ferritins prevent sustained c-Jun N-terminal kinase cascade activation by TNF-α by reducing the production of ROS achieved through iron sequestration (Pham *et al.*, 2004). Not only can H-subunit rich ferritins prevent apoptosis by the sequestration of iron, but H-subunit rich ferritins can also cause apoptosis by the donation of iron. H-subunit rich ferritins secreted from hepatocytes induce apoptosis by the donation of iron to the target cell. H-subunit rich ferritins are released from the hepatocyte followed by endocytosis into the target cell. The internalized H–subunit rich ferritins increase the level of intracellular iron and support the production of ROS (Bresgen *et al.*, 2010). Endocytosis of extracellular H-subunit rich ferritins increases the level of iron, promotes Fenton chemistry-based oxidative stress, induces damage to DNA, results in p53 activation, increases mitochondrial membrane permeability and activates pro-apoptotic Fas signalling (Bresgen *et al.*, 2010).

H-subunit rich ferritins have also been found to take part in the apoptotic events not involving iron or its ferroxidase activity. Upon oxidative stress, H-subuint rich ferritins increase p53 protein levels and p53 transcriptional activity in a ferroxidase activity-independent manner (Lee *et al.*, 2009). The gene coding for the H-subunit of ferritin belongs to the family of p53-regulated genes. Therefore, p53 activation can bring about an increase in H-subunit rich ferritins to support p53 in its apoptotic role (Faniello *et al.*, 2008).

11. H-subunit rich ferritins and cancer

High plasma ferritin levels have been reported for various types of cancers, irrespective of the amount of total body iron (Aulbert & Scmidt, 1985). It has even been suggested that plasma ferritin levels can be used as tumour markers for prognostic purposes and for monitoring the activity of certain types of cancer (Aulbert & Steffens, 1990; Silber *et al.*, 1991). In patients with solid tumours, such as pancreatic carcinoma, lung cancer and hepatoma, there is a particularly high incidence of elevated plasma ferritin, and in patients with breast cancer, with metastasis, ferritin plasma concentrations are commonly elevated (Worwood, 1982). It is of interest that ferritin levels in breast cancer are not only raised in the plasma, but also in breast tissue (Ionescu *et al.*, 2006; Weinstein *et al.*, 1982). Squamous cell carcinoma of the head and neck is marked by increased plasma ferritin concentrations, which remains high in patients with a poor prognosis in contrast to patients with a favourable prognosis (Maxim & Veltri, 1986). The plasma ferritin concentrations of patients with haematologic malignancies are well documented. Extremely high plasma ferritin levels were seen in acute myeloblastic leukemia whereas in complete remission ferritin plasma concentrations returned back to normal (Aulbert & Schmidt, 1985). In Hodgkin's disease, plasma ferritin concentrations are said to be related to the stage of the disease, increasing from stage 1 to stage 4 (Worwood, 1982). In non-Hodgkin's lymphoma a remarkable correlation was found between plasma ferritin concentrations and tumour histology. The highest plasma ferritin concentrations are said to be found in patients with active histiocytic lymphoma and the lowest plasma ferritin concentrations in patients with lymphocytic lymphoma whereas intermediate plasma ferritin concentrations are found in patients with mixed histology (Worwood, 1982).

Many factors are suggested to contribute to the hyperferritinaemia associated with cancer, including inflammation, hepatic necrosis due to metastasis and chemotherapy, blood transfusions and a decrease in hepatic clearance of ferritin (Vernet *et al.*, 1995). In addition, a modified and increased synthesis and secretion of ferritin by tumour cells occur (Aulbert & Steffens, 1990; Kirkali *et al.*, 1999; Vernet *et al.*, 1995; Yang *et al.*, 2001). In many instances the increased ferritin is shown to be H-subunit rich (Bevilacqua *et al.*, 1988; Higgy *et al.*, 1997; Jones *et al.*, 1980; Tripathi & Chatterjee, 1996; Vernet *et al.*, 1995; Whittaker *et al.*, 1984), and it has been suggested that the measurement of H-subunit rich ferritin may be of value in the diagnosis of malignancy (Jones *et al.*, 1980). In a study involving breast cancer patients it has been shown that H-subunit mRNA was directly related to axillary lymph node status, the presence of metastatic disease and to the clinical stage (Yang *et al.*, 2001).

The secretion of H-subunit rich ferritins in patients with cancer could be involved in the immunosupression seen in these patients. In *in vitro* studies, melanoma cells have, for instance, been found to release H-subunit rich ferritins. These H-subunit rich ferritins were able to suppress the response of peripheral blood lymphocytes stimulated by anti-CD3. These effects were mediated by the activation of regulatory T-cells to produce Il-10 (Gray *et al.*, 2003). Similar indications were seen in patients with melanoma. H-subunit rich, but not L-subunit rich ferritins, were found to be elevated in melanoma patients, with the H-subunit to L-subunit ratio correlating with the levels of regulatory T-cells (Gray *et al.*, 2003).

The most common feature of cancer is the abnormal proliferation of cells, either contained in a specific location, or following metastasis at different sites involving various organs. Iron is a necessary element for cellular proliferation and it is generally accepted that rapidly dividing cells require more iron for their growth and metabolism than resting cells, and that cells normally display an increase in cellular proliferation upon an increase in the labile iron pool (Kakhlon *et al.*, 2001). Malignant cells, because of their higher requirement for iron, are very sensitive to iron depletion (Kalinowski *et al.*, 2007). In addition, the cellular labile iron pool can modulate the magnitude of cellular proliferation by the oncogene H-ras (Kakhlon *et al.*, 2002). It is already known that iron homeostasis is dysregulated in cancerous cells. For instance, human breast cancer cells are characterised by substantial alterations in the levels

of proteins that are responsible for the maintenance of intracellular iron homeostasis, including transferrin, IRP1, IRP2, H-subunit and L-subunit of ferritin (Shpyleva *et al.*, 2011).
In view of their high need for iron, malignant cells would have mechanisms able to increase the labile iron pool. One way in which to bring about an increase in the cellular labile iron pool would be by suppression of ferritin synthesis. The transcription factor encoded by the proto-oncogene c-MYC, which is responsible for proliferation of normal cells, can during uncontrolled expression result in cellular transformation and excessive cellular proliferation. c-MYC can, where appropriate, activate or repress target genes in order to bring about cellular proliferation (Wu *et al.*, 1999). The expression of the H-subunit gene is shown to be down-regulated by c-MYC and to be essential for the control of cellular proliferation and transformation by c-MYC (Wu *et al.*, 1999). This is in agreement with the fact that H-subunit rich ferritins are responsible for controlling the labile iron pool and that down-regulation of H-subunit expression would result in an increase in the labile iron pool. The down-regulation of intracellular H-subunit rich ferritins has also been shown to be required for the pathogenesis of cancer. Epithelial-mesenchymal transition (EMT) contributes to tumour-invasive phenotypes and metastasis. The down-regulation of H-subunit rich ferritins was shown to occur between the early and highly invasive advanced stages in esophageal adenocarcinoma (Zhang *et al.*, 2009). It is suggested that an increase in the labile iron pool plays a role, since depletion of the labile iron pool and a decrease in ROS suppress the migration of tumour cells (Zhang *et al.*, 2009).
In contrast, up-regulation of intracellular H-subunit rich ferritins has been shown in several studies (Elliot *et al.*, 1993; Shpeleva *et al.*, 2011; Weinstein *et al.*, 1982). In the study by Shpeleva *et al.*, involving human breast cancer, an increase in the expression of the H-subunit and L-subunit intracellular levels of ferritin was associated with a decrease in the labile iron pool (Shpeleva *et al.*, 2011). This increase in the production of intracellular ferritin, together with an increase in the H-subunit rich ferritin in the chromatin-bound nuclear fraction, is postulated to be one of the defense mechanisms in cancer cells against iron-induced toxicity. Furthermore, the increase in intracellular ferritin production has been associated with the acquisition of a metastatic and multi-drug resistant phenotype (Shpeleva *et al.*, 2011). It was also shown that down-regulation of the H-subunit of ferritin increased the cancer cell's sensitivity to the chemotherapeutic agent Doxorubicin (Shpeleva *et al.*, 2011).
At present, many research studies support the concept that an increase in intracellular bio-available iron can augment the development and progression of cancer. Although low intracellular ferritin concentrations, and by implication high intracellular iron levels, could favour the proliferation of malignant cells, plasma ferritin levels are generally high in patients with cancer. As plasma ferritin is generally a secretory product of cells it is unlikely that intracellular ferritin levels would be low in conjunction with excessively high extracellular levels. In fact, measurements of tissue ferritin levels showed, in general, increased levels of ferritin in malignant breast tissues, at least in advanced more aggressive stages (Elliot *et al.*, 1993; Shpeleva *et al.*, 2011; Weinstein *et al.*, 1982). As a rule, one would expect these high intracellular ferritin levels to decrease bio-available iron - which is contrary to the requirement of cancer cells. The answer to this conundrum is largely still at the conjectural stage. Research is necessary to distinguish between observations that reflect attempts of malignant cells to create conditions favourable for proliferation and those of the body to protect against such proliferation. What we do know is that iron metabolism is dysregulated in cancer, and that changes occur in both intracellular and extracellular ferritin

pools. Although some work exists on the redistribution of ferritin and iron, the type of ferritin, as well as the cancer phenotype and stage of malignancy (Cade *et al.*, 1998; Kabat & Rohan, 2007; Rossiello *et al.*, 1984; Shpeleva *et al.*, 2011; Wu *et al.*, 2004), more studies are urgently needed.

12. Conclusion

Up-regulation of ferritin during the acute phase response protects against microbial growth, oxidative damage, and is involved in the regulation of immunological activity, apoptotic processes and cellular proliferation. During most of these activities the H-subunit of ferritin is differentially up-regulated, and appears to play a more important role than the L-subunit in establishing ferritin's functional properties during the acute phase response.

13. Acknowledgement

The authors would like to acknowledge the Publisher of "Archives of Physiology and Biochemistry" for permission to use adapted exerpts from the authors' own publications, Koorts, A.M. & Viljoen, M. (2007). Ferritin and ferritin isoforms I: Structure-function relationships, synthesis, degradation and secretion. *Arch Physiol Biochem*, 113(1) (2007), pp. (30-54) and Koorts, A.M. & Viljoen, M. (2007). Ferritin and ferritin isoforms II: Protection against uncontrolled cellular proliferation, oxidative damage and inflammatory processes. *Arch Physiol Biochem*, 113(2) (2007), pp. (55-64).

14. References

Agrawal, R.; Sharma, P.K. & Rao, G.S. (2001). Release of iron from ferritin by metabolites of benzene and superoxide radical generating agents. *Toxicol*, 168 (2001), pp. (223-230).

Aisen, P. (1991). Ferritin receptors and the role of ferritin in iron transport. *Targeted Diag Ther*, 4 (1991), pp. (339-354).

Ali, M.H.; Schlidt, S.A.; Chandel, N.S.; Hynes, K.L.; Schumacker, P.T. & Gewertz, B.L. (1999). Endothelial permeability and IL-6 production during hypoxia: role of ROS in signal transduction. *Am J Physiol*, 277(5) (1999), pp. (L1057-L1065).

Alvarez-Hernández, X.; Felstein, M.V. & Brock, J.H. (1986). The relationship between iron release, ferritin synthesis and intracellular iron distribution in mouse peritoneal macrophages. Evidence for a reduced level of metabolically available iron in elicited macrophages. *Biochim Biophys Acta*, 886 (1986), pp. (214-222).

Alvarez-Hernández, X.; Licéaga, J.; McKay, I.C. & Brock, J.H. (1989). Induction of hypoferremia and modulation of macrophage iron metabolism by tumor necrosis factor. *Lab Invest*, 61(3) (1989), pp. (319-322).

Antosiewicz, J.; Ziolkowski, W.; Kaczor, J.J. & Herman-Antosiewicz, A. (2007). Tumor necrosis factor-alpha-induced reactive oxygen species formation is mediated by JNK1-dependent ferritin degradation and elevation of labile iron pool. *Free Radic Biol Med*, 43(2) (2007), pp. (265-270).

Arosio, P.; Yokota, M. & Drysdale, J.W. (1976). Structural and immunological relationships of isoferritins in normal and malignant cells. *Cancer Res*, 36 (1976), pp. (1735-1739).

Arosio, P.; Levi, S.; Santambrogio, P.; Cozzi, A.; Luzzago, A.; Cesareni, G. & Albertini, A. (1991). Structural and functional studies of human ferritin H and L chains. *Curr Stud Hematol Blood Transf*, 58 (1991), pp. (127-131).

Arosio, P. & Levi, S. (2002). Ferritin, iron homeostasis, and oxidative damage. *Free Radic Biol Med*, 33(4) (2002), pp. (457-463).

Aulbert, E. & Schmidt, C.G. (1985). Ferritin - a tumor marker in myeloid leukaemia. *Cancer Detect Prev*, 8(1-2) (1985), pp. (297-302).

Aulbert, E. & Steffens, O. (1990). Serum ferritin - a tumor marker in malignant lymphomas? *Onkologie*, 13(2) (1990), pp. (102-108).

Bellotti, V.; Arosio, P.; Cazzola, M.; Cozzi, A.; Levi, S.; Meloni, F. & Zoppone, E. (1987). Characteristics of a ferritin-binding protein present in human serum. *Br J Haematol*, 65(4) (1987), pp. (489-493).

Bevilacqua, M.A.; Costanzo, F.; Buonaguro, L. & Cimino, F. (1988). Ferritin H and L mRNAs in human neoplastic tissues. *Ital J Biochem*, 37(1) (1988), pp. (1-7).

Blackwell, T.S.; Blackwell, T.R.; Holden, E.P.; Christman, B.W. & Christman, J.W. (1996). *In vivo* antioxidant treatment suppresses nuclear factor-kappa B activation and neutrophilic lung inflammation. *J Immunol*, 157(40) (1996), pp. (1630-1637).

Blake, D.R.; Lunec, J.; Ahern, M.; Ring, E.F.; Bradfield, J. & Gutteridge, J.M. (1985). Effect of intravenous iron dextran on rheumatoid synovitis. *Ann Rheum Dis*, 44(3) (1985), pp. (183-188).

Boelaert, J.R.; Vandecasteele, S.J.; Appelberg, R. & Gordeuk, V.R. (2007). The effect of the host's iron status on tuberculosis. *J Infect Dis*, 195 (2007), pp. (1745-1753).

Bomford, A.; Conlon-Hollingshead, C. & Munro, H.N. (1981). Adaptive responses of rat tissue isoferritins to iron administration. *J Biol Chem*, 256(2) (1981), pp. (948-955).

Boyd, D.; Vecoli, C.; Belcher, D.M.; Jain, S.K. & Drysdale, J.W. (1985). Structural and functional relationships of human ferritin H and L chains deduced from cDNA clones. *J Biol Chem*, 260(21) (1985), pp. (11755-11761).

Bresgen, N.; Jaksch, H.; Lacher, H.; Ohlenschlager I.; Uchida, K. & Eckl, P.M. (2010). Iron-mediated oxidative stress plays an essential role in ferritin-induced cell death. *Free Radic Biol Med*, 48(10) (2010), pp. (1347-1357).

Broxmeyer, H.E.; Gentile, P.; Listowsky, I.; Cavanna, E.; Feickert, H.J.; Dorner, M.H.; Ruggeri, G.; Cazzola, M. & Cooper, S. (1984). Acidic isoferritins in the regulation of hematopoiesis *in vitro* and *in vivo*, In: *Ferritins and isoferritins as biochemical markers*, Albertini, A.; Arosio, P.; Chiancone, E. & Drysdale, J., pp. (97-111), Elsevier Science Publishers, Amsterdam.

Broxmeyer, H.E.; Lu, L.; Bicknell, D.C.; Williams, D.E.; Cooper, S.; Levi, S.; Salfeld, J. & Arosio, P. (1986). The influence of purified recombinant human heavy-subunit and light-subunit ferritins on colony formation *in vitro* by granulocyte-macrophage and erythroid progenitor cells. *Blood*, 68(6) (1986), pp. (1257-1263).

Broxmeyer, H.E.; Cooper, S.; Levi, S. & Arosio, P. (1991). Mutated recombinant human heavy-chain ferritins and myelosuppression *in vitro* and *in vivo*: a link between ferritin ferroxidase activity and biological function. *Proc Natl Acad Sci USA*, 88 (1991), pp. (770-774).

Broxmeyer, H.E. (1992). H-ferritin: a regulatory cytokine that down-modulates cell proliferation. *J Lab Clin Med*, 120(3) (1992), pp. (367-370).

Cade, J.; Thomas, E. & Vail, A. (1998). Case-control study of breast cancer in south east England: nutritional factors. *Epidemiol Community Health*, 52 (1998), pp. (105–110).

Cairo, G.; Tacchini, L.; Pogliaghi, G.; Anzon, E.; Tomasini, A. & Bernelli-Zazzera, A. (1995). Induction of ferritin synthesis by oxidative stress: transcriptional and post-transcriptional regulation by expansion of the free iron pool. *J Biol Chem*, 270 (1995), pp. (700-703).

Cairo, G.; Castrosini, E.; Minotti, G. & Bernelli-Zazzera, A. (1996). Superoxide and hydrogen peroxide-dependent inhibition of iron regulatory protein activity: a protective strategem against oxidative injury. *FASEB J*, 10 (1996), pp. (1326-1335).

Cazzola, M.; Dezza, L.; Bergamaschi, G.; Barosi, G.; Bellotti, V.; Caldera, D.; Ciriello, M.M.; Quaglini, S.; Arosio, P. & Ascari, E. (1983). Biologic and clinical significance of red cell ferritin. *Blood*, 62(5) (1983), pp. (1078-1087).

Cazzola, M. & Ascari, A. (1986). Red cell ferritin as a diagnostic tool. *Br J Haematol*, 62(2) (1986), pp. (209-213).

Chasteen, N.D. (1998). Ferritin. Uptake, storage, and release of iron. *Met Ions Biol Syst*, 35 (1998), pp. (479-514).

Chiancone, E. & Stefanini, S. (1984). Heterogeneity of ferritin. I. Structural and functional aspects, In: *Ferritins and isoferritins as biochemical markers*, Albertini, A.; Arosio, P.; Chiancone, E. & Drysdale, J, pp. (23-32), Elsevier Science Publishers, Amsterdam.

Ciriello, M.M.; Cazzola, M.; Dezza, L.; Levi, S. & Arosio, P. (1987). Measurement of ferritin-bearing lymphocytes in man. Preliminary studies on the use of monoclonal antibodies specific for the L and H subunits of ferritin. *Tumori*, 73 (1987), pp. (37-41).

Closa, D. & Folch-Puy, E. (2004). Oxygen free radicals and the systemic inflammatory response. *IUBMB Life*, 56(4) (2004), pp. (185-191).

Coccia, E.M.; Profita, V.; Fiorucci, G.; Romeo, G.; Affabris, E.; Testa, U.; Hentze, M.W. & Battistini, A. (1992). Modulation of ferritin H-chain expression in Friend erythroleukemia cells: transcriptional and translational regulation by hemin. *Mol Cell Biol*, 12(7) (1992), pp. (3015-3022).

Cohen, L.A.; Gutierrez, L.; Weiss, A.; Leichtmann-Bardoogo, Y.; Zhang, D-L.; Crooks, D.R.; Sougrat, R.; Morgenstern, A.; Galy, B.; Hentze, M.W.; Lazaro, F.J.; Rouault, T.A. & Meyron-Holtz, E.G. (2010). Serum ferritin is derived primarily from macrophages through a nonclassical secretory pathway. *Blood*, 116(9) (2010), pp. (1574-1584).

Covell, A.M. & Worwood, M. (1984). Isoferritins in plasma, In: *Ferritins and isoferritins as biochemical markers*, Albertini, A.; Arosio, P.; Chiancone, E. & Drysdale, J., pp. (49-65), Elsevier Science Publishers, Amsterdam.

Cozzi, A.; Corsi, B.; Levi, S.; Santambrogio, P.; Albertini, A. & Arosio, P. (2000). Overexpression of wild type and mutated human ferritin H-chain in HeLa cells: *in vivo* role of ferroxidase activity. *J Biol Chem*, 275(3) (2000), pp. (25122-25129).

Cragg, S.J.; Wagstaff, M. & Worwood, M. (1981). Detection of a glycosylated subunit in human serum ferritin. *Biochem J*, 199 (1981), pp. (565-571).

Cray, C.; Zalas, J. & Altman, N.H. (2009). Acute phase response in animals: a review. *Comparative Med*, 59(6) (2009), pp. (517-526).

De Domenico, I.; Ward, D.M. & Kaplan, J. (2009a). Specific iron chelators determine the route of ferritin degradation. *Blood*, 114(20) (2009), pp. (4546-4551).

De Domenico, I.; Ward, D.M. & Kaplan, J. (2009b). Serum ferritin regulates blood vessel formation: a role beyond iron storage. *PNAS*, 106(6) (2009), pp. (1683-1684).

De Godoy, M.F.; Takakura, I.T.; Machado, R.D.; Grassi, L.V. & Nogueira, P.R. (2007). Serum ferritin and obstructive coronary artery disease: angiographic correlation. *Arq Bras Cardiol*, 88(4) (2007), pp. (430-433).

Deicher, R. & Hörl, W.H. (2006). New insights into the regulation of iron homeostasis. *Eur J Clin Invest*, 36 (2006), pp. (301-309).

Deiss, A. (1983). Iron metabolism in reticuloendothelial cells. *Semin Hematol*, 20(2) (1983), pp. (81-90).

Desiderio, S. & Yoo, J.Y. (2003). A genome-wide analysis of the acute-phase response and its regulation by Stat3β. *Ann NY Acad Sci*, 987 (2003), pp. (280-284).

Di Virgilio, F. (2004). New pathways for reactive oxygen species generation in inflammation and potential novel pharmacological targets. *Curr Pharm Design*, 10(14) (2004), pp. (1647-1652).

Dröge, W. (2002). Free radicals in the physiological control of cell function. *Physiol Rev*, 82(1) (2002), pp. (47-95).

El Kasmi, K.C.; Holst, J.; Coffre, M.; Mielke, L.; de Pauw, A.; Lhocine, N.; Smith, A.M.; Rutschman, R.; Kaushal, D.; Shen, Y.; Suda, T.; Donnelly, R.P.; Myers Jr., M.G.; Alexander, W.; Vignali, D.A.A.; Watowich, S.S.; Ernst, M.; Hilton, D.J. & Murray, P.J. (2006). General nature of STAT3-activated anti-inflammatory response. *J Immunol*, 177(11) (2006), pp. (7880-7888).

Elliot, R.L.; Elliot, M.C.; Wang, F. & Head J.F. (1993). Breast carcinoma and the role of iron metabolism. A cytochemical, tissue culture, and ultrastructural study. *Ann N Y Acad Sci*, 698 (1993), pp. (159-166).

Evenson, K.J.; Swaak, T.J. & Nossent, J.C. (2007). Increased ferritin response in adult Still's disease: specificity and relationship to outcome. *Scand J Rheumatol*, 36(2) (2007), pp. (107-110).

Fahmy, M. & Young, S.P. (1993). Modulation of iron metabolism in monocyte cell line U937 by inflammatory cytokines: changes in transferrin uptake, iron handling and ferritin mRNA. *Biochem J*, 296 (1993), pp. (175-181).

Faniello, M.C.; Di Sanzo, M.; Quaresima, B.; Baudi, F.; Di Caro, V.; Cuda, G.; Morrone, G.; Del Sal, G.; Spinelli, G.; Venuta, S. & Costanzo, F. (2008). p53-mediated downregulation of H ferritin promoter transcriptional efficiency via NF-Y. *Int J Biochem Cell Biol*, 40(10) (2008), pp. (2110-2119).

Fargion, S.; Arosio, P.; Fracanzani, A.L.; Cislaghi, V.; Levi, S.; Cozzi, A.; Piperno, A. & Fiorelli, G. (1988). Characteristics and expression of binding sites specific for ferritin H-chain on human cell lines. *Blood*, 71 (1988), pp. (753-757).

Feelders, R.A.; Vreugdenhil, G.; Eggermont, A.M.; Kuiper-Kramer, P.A.; van Eijk, H.G. & Swaak, A.J. (1998). Regulation of iron metabolism in the acute-phase response: interferon gamma and tumour necrosis factor alpha induce hypoferraemia, ferritin production and a decrease in circulating transferrin receptors in cancer patients. *Eur J Clin Invest*, 28(7) (1998), pp. (520-527).

Fillet, G.; Cook, J.D. & Finch, C.A. (1974). Storage iron kinetics. VII. A biologic model for reticuloendothelial iron transport. *J Clin Invest*, 53 (1974), pp. (1527-1533).

Fillet, G.; Beguin, Y. & Baldelli, L. (1989). Model of reticuloendothelial iron metabolism in humans: abnormal behavior in idiopathic hemochromatosis and in inflammation. *Blood*, 74(2) (1989), pp. (844-851).

Finch, C.A.; Huebers, H.A.; Cazzola, M.; Bergamaschi, G. & Bellotti, V. (1984). Storage iron, In: *Ferritins and isoferritins as biochemical markers*, Albertini, A.; Arosio, P.; Chiancone, E. & Drysdale, J., pp. (3-21), Elsevier Science Publishers, Amsterdam.

Fischbach, F.A; Gregory, D.W.; Harrison, P.M.; Hoy, T.J. & Williams, J.M. (1971). On the structure of hemosiderin and its relationship to ferritin. *J Ultrastr Res*, 37 (1971), pp. (495-503).

Ford, G.C.; Harrison, P.M.; Rice D.W.; Smith, J.M.; Treffry, A.; White, J.L. & Yariv, J. (1984). Ferritin: design and formation of an iron-storage molecule. *Phil Trans R Soc Lond*, 304 (1984), pp. (551-565).

Fuchs, D.; Zangerle, R.; Artner-Dworzak, E.; Weiss, G.; Fritsch, P.; Tilz, G.P.; Dierich, M.P. & Wachter, H. (1993). Association between immune activation, changes of iron metabolism and anaemia in patients with HIV infection. *Eur J Haematol*, 50 (1993), pp. (90-94).

Gálvez, N.; Ruiz, B.; Cuesta, R.; Colacio, E. & Dominguez-Vera, J.M. (2005). Release of iron from ferritin by aceto- and benzohydroxamic acids. *Inorg Chem*, 44(8) (2005), pp. (2706-2709).

Ganz, T. (2004). Hepcidin in iron metabolism. *Curr Opin Hematol*, 11 (2004), pp. (251-254).

Ganz, T. (2009). Iron in innate immunity: starve the invaders. *Curr Opin Immunol*, 21(1) (2009), pp. (63-67).

Gelvan, D.; Fibach, E.; Meyron-Holtz, E.G. & Konijn, A.M. (1996). Ferritin uptake by human erythroid precursors is a regulated iron uptake pathway. *Blood*, 88(8) (1996), pp. (3200-3207).

Giordano, N.; Vaccai, D.; Cintorino, M.; Minacci, C.; Magaro, L.; Battisti, E.; Marcuccil, P.; Cecconami, L. & Marcolongo, R. (1991). Histopathological study of iron deposit distribution in the rheumatoid synovium. *Clin Exp Rheumatol*, 9(5) (1991), pp. (463-467).

Goralska, M.; Holley, B.L. & McGahan, M.C. (2003). Identification of a mechanism by which lens epithelial cells limit accumulation of overexpressed ferritin H-chain. *J Biol Chem*, 278(44) (2003), pp. (42920-42926).

Goswami, B.; Tayal, D. & Mallika, V. (2009). Ferritin: A multidimensional biomarker. *Internet J Lab Med*, 3(2) (2009).

Gougerot-Pocidalo, M.A.; El Benna, J.; Elbim, C.; Chollet-Martin, S. & Dang, M.C. (2002). Regulation of human neutrophil oxidative burst by pro- and anti-inflammatory cytokines. *J Soc Biol*, 196(1) (2002), pp. (37-46).

Gray, C.P.; Arosio, P. & Hersey, P. (2003). Association of increased levels of heavy-chain ferritin with increased $CD4^+$ $CD25^+$ regulatory T-cell levels in patients with melanoma. *Clin Cancer Res*, 9 (2003), pp. (2551-2559).

Guyatt, G.; Patterson, C.; Ali, M.; Singer, J.; Levine, M.; Turpie, I. & Meyer, R. (1990). Diagnosis of iron-deficiency anemia in the elderly. *Am J Med*, 88(3) (1990), pp. (205-209).

Halliday, J.W.; Mack, U. & Powell, L.W. (1979). The kinetics of serum and tissue ferritins: relation to carbohydrate content. *Br J Haematol*, 42 (1979), pp. (535-546).

Halliday, J.W. & Powell, L.W. (1979). Serum ferritin and isoferritins in clinical medicine. *Progr Hematol*, 11 (1979), pp. (229-266).

Halliday, J.W.; Ramm, G.A.; Moss, D. & Powell, L.W. (1994). A new look at ferritin metabolism. *Adv Exp Med Biol*, 365 (1994), pp. (149-156).

Harford, J.B.; Rouault, T.A. & Klausner, R.D. (1994). The control of cellular iron homeostasis, In: *Iron metabolism in health and disease*, Brock, J.H.; Halliday, J.W.; Pippard, M.J. & Powell L.W., pp. (123-149), W.B. Saunders Company Ltd, London.

Harrison, P.M. & Arosio, P. (1996). The ferritins: molecular properties, iron storage function and cellular regulation. *Biochim Biophys Acta*, 1275 (1996), pp. (161-203).

Hershko, C. & Konijn, A.M. (1984). Serum ferritin in hematologic disorders, In: *Ferritins and isoferritins as biochemical markers*, Albertini, A.; Arosio, P.; Chiancone, E. & Drysdale, J., pp. (143-158), Elsevier Science Publishers, Amsterdam.

Hie-won, L.; Stahlhut, M.W. & Evans, A.E. (1984). Isoferritins and prognosis of neuroblastoma: the immunological role of acidic isoferritins, In: *Ferritins and isoferritins as biochemical markers*, Albertini, A.; Arosio, P.; Chiancone, E. & Drysdale, J., pp. (171-180), Elsevier Science Publishers, Amsterdam.

Higgy, N.A.; Salicioni, A.M.; Russo, I.H.; Zhang, P.L. & Russo, J. (1997). Differential expression of human ferritin H chain gene in immortal human breast epithelial MCF-10F cells. *Mol Carcinogen*, 20(4) (1997), pp. (332-339).

Hintze, K.J. & Theil, E.C. (2005). DNA and mRNA elements with complementary responses to hemin, antioxidant inducers, and iron control ferritin-L expression. *Proc Natl Acad Sci USA*, 102 (2005), pp. (15048-15052).

Hou, J.; Cliver, S.P.; Tamura, T.; Johnston, K.E. & Goldenberg, R. (2000). Maternal serum ferritin and fetal growth. *Obstet Gynecol*, 95(3) (2000), pp. (447-452).

Hynes, M.J. & Coinceanainn, M.O. (2002). Investigation of the release of iron from ferritin by naturally occurring antioxidants. *J Inorg Biochem*, 90 (2002), pp. (18-21).

Iancu, T.C. (1982). Iron overload. *Mol Aspects Med*, 6 (1982), pp. (1-100).

Iancu, T.C. (1992). Ferritin and hemosiderin in pathological tissues. *Electron Microsc Rev*, 5 (1992), pp. (209-229).

Invernizzi, R.; Caccola, M.; De Fazio, P.; Rosti, V.; Ruggeri, G. & Arosio, P. (1990). Immunocytochemical detection of ferritin in human bone marrow and peripheral blood cells using monoclonal antibodies specific for the H and L subunit. *Br J Haematol*, 76 (1990), pp. (427-432).

Ionescu, J.G.; Novotny, J.; Stejskal, V.; Latsch, A.; Blaurock-Bush, E. & Eisenmann-Klein, M. (2006). Increased levels of transition metals in breast cancer tissue. *Neuro Endocrinol Lett*, 27(Suppl1) (2006), pp. (36-39).

Iwasaki, K. & Mackenzie, E.L. (2006). Hemin-mediated regulation of an anti-oxidant-responsive element of the human ferritin H gene and role of Ref-1 during erythroid differentiation of K562 cells. *Mol Cell Biol*, 26 (2006), pp. (2845-2856).

Jacobs, A. & Worwood, M. (1975). Ferritin in serum; clinical and biochemical implications. *New Engl J Med*, 292(18) (1975), pp. (951-956).

Jacobs, A.; Hodgetts, J. & Hoy, T.G. (1984). Functional aspects of isoferritins, In: *Ferritins and isoferritins as biochemical markers*, Albertini, A.; Arosio, P.; Chiancone, E. & Drysdale, J., pp. (113-127), Elsevier Science Publishers, Amsterdam.

Jarjour, I.T. & Jarjour, L.K. (2008). Low iron storage in children and adolescents with neurally mediated syncopy. *J Pediatr*, 153 (2008), pp. (40-44).

Jones, B.M.; Worwood, M. & Jacobs, A. (1980). Serum ferritin in patients with cancer: determination with antibodies to HeLa cell and spleen ferritin. *Clin Chim Acta*, 106 (1980), pp. (203-214).

Jones, B.M.; Worwood, M. & Jacobs, A. (1983). Isoferritins in normal leucocytes. *Br J Haematol*, 55(1) (1983), pp. (73-81).

Joshi, J.G. & Clauberg, M. (1988). Ferritin: an iron storage protein with diverse functions. *Biofactors*, 1(3) (1997), pp. (207-212).

Jurado, R.L. (1997). Iron, infections, and anemia of inflammation. *Clin Infect Dis*, 25 (1997), pp. (888-895).

Kabat, C.C. & Rohan, T.F. (2007). Does excess iron play a role in breast carcinogenesis? An unresolved hypothesis. *Cancer Cause Control*, 18 (2007), pp. (1047-1053).

Kakhlon, O.; Gruenbaum, Y. & Cabantchik, Z.I. (2001). Repression of ferritin expression increase the labile iron pool, oxidative stress, and short-term growth of human erythroleukemia cells. *Blood*, 97(9) (2001), pp. (2853-2871).

Kakhlon, O.; Gruenbaum, Y. & Cabantchik, Z.I. (2002). Repression of ferritin expression modulates cell responsiveness to H-ras-induced growth. *Biochem Soc Trans*, 30(4) (2002), pp. (777-780).

Kalgaonkar, S. & Lonnerdal, B. (2009). Receptor-mediated uptake of ferritin-bound iron by human intestinal caco-2 cells. *J Nutr Biochem*, 20 (2009), pp. (304-311).

Kalinowski, D.S.; Sharpe, P.C.; Bernhardt, P.V. & Richardson, D.R. (2007). Design, synthesis, and characterization of new iron chelators with anti-proliferative activity: structure-activity relationships of novel thiohydrazone analogues. *J Med Chem*, 50(24) (2007), pp. (6212-6225).

Kato, J. & Niitsu, Y. (2002). Recent advances in molecular iron metabolism: translational disorders of ferritin. *Int J Hematol*, 76(3) (2002), pp. (208-212).

Kennedy, A.; Kohn, M.; Lammi, A. & Clarke, S. (2004). Iron status and haematological changes in adolescent female inpatients with anorexia nervosa. *J Paediatr Child Health*, 40(8) (2004), pp. (430-432).

Kew, M.C.; Torrance, J.D.; Derman, D.; Simon, M.; Macnab, G.M.; Charlton, R.W. & Bothwell, T.H. (1978). Serum and tumour ferritins in primary liver cancer. *Gut*, 19(4) (1978), pp. (294-299).

Kidane, T.Z.; Sauble, E. & Linder, M.C. (2006). Release of iron from ferritin requires lysosomal activity. *Am J Physiol Cell Physiol*, 291(3) (2006), pp. (C445-C455).

Kim, S-W.; Kim, Y-H. & Lee, J. (2001). Thermal stability of human ferritin: concentration dependence and enhanced stability of an N-terminal fusion mutant. *Biochem Biophys Res Commun*, 289 (2001), pp. (125-129).

Kirkali, Z.; Guzelsoy, M.; Mungan, M.U.; Kirkali, G. & Yorokoglu, K. (1999). Serum ferritin as a clinical marker for renal cell carcinoma: influence of tumor size and volume. *Urol Int*, 62(1) (1999), pp. (21-25).

Knickelbein, J.E.; de Souza, A.J.; Tosti, R.; Narayan, P. & Kane, L.P. (2006). Cutting edge: inhibition of T cell activation by TIM-2. *J Immunol*, 177 (2006), pp. (4966-4970).

Konijn, A.M. & Hershko, C. (1977). Ferritin synthesis in inflammation. I. Pathogenesis of impaired iron release. *Br J Haematol*, 37(1) (1977), pp. (7-16).

Konijn, A.M.; Meyron-Holtz, E.G.; Fibach, E. & Gelvan, D. (1994). Cellular ferritin uptake: a highly regulated pathway for iron assimilation in human erythroid precursor cells. *Adv Exp Med Biol*, 356 (1994), pp. (189-197).

Kosmidou, I.; Vassilakopoulos, T.; Xagorari, A.; Zakynthinos, S; Papapetropoulos, A. & Roussos, C. (2002). Production of interleukin-6 by skeletal myotubes: role of reactive oxygen species. *Am J Resp Cell Mol Biol*, 26(5) (2002), pp. (587-593).

Kotagal, S. & Silber, M.H. (2004). Childhood-onset restless legs syndrome. *Ann Neurol*, 56(6) (2004), pp. (803-807).

Lee, J.H.; Jang, H.; Cho, E.J. & Youn, H.D. (2009). Ferritin binds and activates p53 under oxidative stress. *Biochem Biophys Res Commun*, 389(3) (2009), pp. (399-404).

Leimberg, M.J.; Prus, E.; Konijn, A.M. & Fibach, E. (2008). Macrophages function as a ferritin iron source for cultured human erythroid precursors. *J Cell Biochem*, 103(4) (2008), pp. (1211-1218).

Levi, S.; Santambrogio, P.; Cozzi, A.; Rovida, E.; Corsi, B.; Tamborini, E.; Spada S.; Albertini, A. & Arosio P. (1994). The role of the L-chain in ferritin iron incorporation; studies of homo and heteropolymers. *J Mol Biol*, 238 (1994), pp. (649-654).

Levi, S.; Cozzi, A. & Arosio, P. (2005). Neuroferritinopathy: a neurodegenerative disorder associated with L-ferritin mutation. *Best Pract Res Clin Hamatol*, 18(2) (2005), pp. (265-276).

Li, J.Y.; Paragas, N.; Ned, R.M.; Qiu, A.; Viltard, M.; Leete, T. Drexler, I.R.; Chen, X.; Sanna-Cherchi, S.; Mohammed, F.; Williams, D.; Lin, C.S.; Schmidt-Ott, K.M.; Andrews, N.C. & Barasch, J. (2009). Scara5 is a ferritin receptor mediating non-transferrin iron delivery. *Dev Cell*, 16(1) (2009), pp. (35-46).

Li, L.; Fang, C.J.; Ryan, J.C.; Niemi, E.C.; Lebron, J.A.; Bjorkman, P.J.; Arase, H.; Torti, F.M.; Torti, S.V.; Nakamura, M.C. & Seaman, W.E. (2010). Binding and uptake of H-ferritin are mediated by human transferrin receptor-1. *Proc Natl Acad Sci USA*, 107(8) (2010), pp. (3505-3510).

Li, R.; Luo, C.; Mines, M.; Zhang, J. & Fan, G.H. (2006). Chemokine CXCL12 induces binding of ferritin heavy chain to the chemokine receptor CXCR4, alters CXCR4 signaling, and induces phosphorylation and nuclear translocation of ferritin heavy chain. *J Biol Chem*, 281(49) (2006), pp. (37616-37627).

Lipschitz, D.A.; Simon, M.O.; Lynch, S.R.; Dugard, J.; Bothwell, T.H. & Charlton, R.W. (1971). Some factors affecting the release of iron from reticuloendothelial cells. *Br J Haematol*, 21 (1971), pp. (289-303).

Liu, H. & Pope, R.M. (2004). Phagocytes: mechanisms of inflammation and tissue destruction. *Rheum Dis Clin North Am*, 30(1) (2004), pp. (19-39).

Liu, X.; Jin, W. & Theil, E.C. (2003). Opening protein pores with chaotropes enhances Fe reduction and chelation of Fe from the ferritin biomineral. *PNAS*, 100(7) (2003), pp. (3653-3658).

Ludwiczek, S.; Aigner, E.; Theurl, I. & Weiss, G. (2003). Cytokine-mediated regulation of iron transport in human monocytic cells. *Blood*, 101(10) (2003), pp. (4148-4154).

MacKenzie, E.L.; Ray, P.D. & Tsuji, Y. (2008). Role and regulation of ferritin H in rotenone-mediated mitochondrial oxidative stress. *Free Radic Biol Med*, 44(9) (2008), pp. (1762-1771).

Massover, W.H. (1994). Alpha-2-macroglobulin: a ferritin binding protein. *Ann N Y Acad Sci*, 737 (1994), pp. (468-471).

Maxim, P.E. & Veltri, R.W. (1986). Serum ferritin as a tumor marker in patients with squamous cell carcinoma of the head and neck. *Cancer*, 57(2) (1986), pp. (305-311).

Mehlhase, J.; Sandig, G.; Pantopoulos, K. & Grune, T. (2005). Oxidation-induced ferritin turnover in microglial cells: role of proteasome. *Free Radic Biol Med*, 38 (2005), pp. (276-285).

Meyron-Holtz, E.G.; Fibach, E.; Gelvan, D. & Konijn, A.M. (1994). Binding and uptake of exogenous isoferritins by cultured human erythroid precursor cells. *Br J Haematol*, 86 (1994), pp. (635-641).

Meyron-Holtz, E.G.; Vaisman, B.; Cabantchik, Z.I.; Fibach, E.; Rouault, T.A.; Hershko, C. & Konijn, A.M. (1999). Regulation of intracellular iron metabolism in human erythroid precursors by internalized extracellular ferritin. *Blood*, 94(9) (1999), pp. (3205-3211).

Miller, L.L.; Miller, S.C.; Torti, S.V.; Tsuji, Y. & Torti, F.M. (1991). Iron-independent induction of ferritin H chain by tumor necrosis factor. *Proc Natl Acad Sci USA*, 88(11) (1991), pp. (4946-4950).

Miyazaki, E.; Kato, J.; Kobune, M.; Okumura, K.; Sasaki, K.; Shintani, N.; Arosio, P. & Niitsu, Y. (2002). Denatured H-ferritin subunit is a major constituent of haemosiderin in the liver of patients with iron overload. *Gut*, 50 (2002), pp. (413-419).

Morikawa, K.; Oseko, F. & Morikawa, S. (1995). A role for ferritin in hematopoiesis and the immune system. *Leuk Lymphoma*, 18 (2005), pp. (429-433).

Niitsu, Y.; Onodera, Y.; Kohgo, Y.; Goto, Y.; Watanabe, N. & Urushizaki, I. (1984). Isoferritins in malignant diseases, In: *Ferritins and isoferritins as biochemical markers*, Albertini, A.; Arosio, P.; Chiancone, E. & Drysdale, J., pp. (113-127), Elsevier Science Publishers, Amsterdam.

Noyes, W.D.; Bothwell, T.H. & Finch, C.A. (1960). The role of the reticulo-endothelial cell in iron metabolism. *Br J Haematol*, 6 (1960), pp. (43-55).

Orino, K.; Lehman, L.; Tsuji, Y.; Ayaki, H.; Torti, S.V. & Torti, F.M. (2001). Ferrritin and the response to oxidative stress. *Biochem J*, 357 (2001), pp. (241-247).

Pang, J-H.S.; Jiang, M-J.; Chen, Y-L.; Wang, F-W.; Wang, D.L.; Chu, S-H. & Chau, L-Y. (1996). Increased ferritin gene expression in atherosclerotic lesions. *J Clin Invest*, 97(10) (1996), pp. (2204-2212).

Parthasara, N.; Torti, S.V. & Torti, F.M. (2002). Ferritin binds to light chain of human H-kininogen and inhibits kallikrein-mediated bradykinin release. *Biochem J*, 365 (2002), pp. (279-286).

Pham, C.G.; Bubici, C.; Zazzeroni, F.; Papa, S.; Jones, J.; Alvarez, K.; Jayawardena, S.; De Smaele, E.; Cong, R.; Beaumont, C.; Torti, F.M.; Torti, S.V. & Franzoso, G. (2004). Ferritin heavy chain upregulation by NF-κB inhibits TNFα-induced apoptosis by suppressing reactive oxygen species. *Cell*, 119 (2004), pp. (529-542).

Piñero, D.J.; Hu, J.; Cook, B.M.; Scaduto Jr., R.C. & Connor, J.R. (2000). Interleukin-1β increases binding of the iron regulatory protein and the synthesis of ferritin by increasing the labile iron pool. *Biochim Biophys Acta*, 1497 (2000), pp. (279-288).

Ponka, P.; Beaumont, C. & Richardson, D.R. (1998). Function and regulation of transferrin and ferritin. *Semin Hematol*, 35(1) (1998), pp. (35-54).

Powell, L.W.; Alpert, E.; Isselbacher, K.J. & Drysdale, J.W. (1975). Human isoferritins: organ specific iron and apoferritin distribution. *Br J Haematol*, 30 (1975), pp. (47-132).

Prentice, A.M. (2008). Iron metabolism, malaria, and other infections. What is all the fuss about? *J Nutr*, 138 (2008), pp. (2537-2541).

Radisky, D.C. & Kaplan, J. (1998). Iron in cytosolic ferritin can be recycled through lysosomal degradation in human fibroblasts. *Biochem J*, 336 (1998), pp. (201-205).
Ramadori, G. & Christ, B. (1999). Cytokines and the hepatic acute-phase response. *Semin Liver Dis*, 19(2) (1999), pp. (141-155).
Richter, G.W. (1978). The iron-loaded cell - the cytopathology of iron storage. *Am J Pathol*, 91(2) (1978), pp. (363-404).
Richter, G.W. (1984). Studies of iron overload; rat liver siderosome ferritin. *Lab Invest*, 50(1) (1984), pp. (26-35).
Ringeling, P.L.; Cleton, M.I.; Kroos, M.J.; Sorber, L.W.; de Bruyn, W.C.; Harrison, P.M. & van Eijk, H.G. (1989). Lysosomal and cytosolic ferritins. A biochemical and electron-spectroscopic study. *Biol Metals*, 2 (1989), pp. (114-121).
Rogers, J.T.; Bridges, K.R.; Durmowicz, G.P.; Glass, J.; Auron, P.E. & Munro, H.N. (1990). Translational control during the acute phase response; ferritin synthesis in response to interleukin-1. *J Biol Chem*, 265(24) (1990), pp. (14572-14578).
Rogers, J.; Lacroix, L.; Durmowitz, G.; Kasschau, K.; Andriotakis, J. & Bridges, K.R. (1994). The role of cytokines in the regulation of ferritin expression. *Adv Exp Med Biol*, 356 (1994), pp. (127-132).
Rogers, J.T. (1996). Ferritin translation by interleukin-1 and interleukin-6: the role of sequences upstream of the start codons of the heavy and light subunit genes. *Blood*, 87(6) (1996), pp. (2525-2537).
Rossiello, R.; Carriero, M.V. & Giordano, G.G. (1984). Distribution of ferritin, transferrin and lactoferrin in breast carcinoma tissue. *J Clin Pathol*, 37 (1984), pp. (51-55).
Rousseau, I. & Puntarulo, S. (2009). Ferritin-dependent radical generation in rat liver homogenates. *Toxicol*, 264(3) (2009), pp. (155-161).
Rowley, D.; Gutteridge, J.M.; Blake, D.; Farr, M. & Halliwell, B. (1984). Lipid peroxidation in rheumatoid arthritis: thiobarbituric acid-reactive material and catalytic iron salts in synovial fluid from rheumatoid patients. *Clin Sci*, 66(6) (1984), pp. (691-695).
Rubin, C.; Wood, P.J.; Archer, T. & Rowe, D.J. (1984). Changes in serum ferritin and other acute phase proteins following major surgery. *Ann Clin Biochem*, 21(Pt 4) (1984), pp. (290-294).
Ruddell, R.G.; Hoang-Le, D.; Barwood, J.M.; Rutherford, P.S.; Piva, T.J.; Watters, D.J.; Santambrogio, P.; Arosio, P. & Ramm, G.A. (2009). Ferritin functions as a proinflammatory cytokine via iron-independent protein kinase C zeta/nuclear factor kappaB-regulated signaling in rat hepatic stellate cells. *Hepatol*, 49(3) (2009), pp. (887-900).
Ruggeri, G.; Iacobello, C.; Albertini, A.; Brocchi, E.; Levi, S.; Gabri, E. & Arosio, P. (1984). Studies of human isoferritins in tissues and body fluids, In: *Ferritins and isoferritins as biochemical markers*, Albertini, A.; Arosio, P.; Chiancone, E. & Drysdale, J., pp. (67-78), Elsevier Science Publishers, Amsterdam.
Ruggeri, G.; Santambrogio, P.; Bonfiglio, F.; Levi, S.; Bugari, G.; Verardi, R.; Cazzola, M.; Invernizzi, R.; Zambelli, L.M.; Albertini, A. & Arosio, P. (1992). Antibodies for denatured human H-ferritin stain only reticuloendothelial cells within the bone marrow. *Br J Haematol*, 81 (1992), pp. (118-124).
Sammarco, M.C.; Ditch, S.; Banerjee, A. & Grabczyk, E. (2008). Ferritin H and L subunits are differentially regulated on a post-transcriptional level. *J Biol Chem*, 283(8) (2008), pp. (4578-4587).

Sánchez, P.; Gálvez, N.; Colacio, E.; Miñones, E. & Domínguez-Vera, J.M. (2005). Catechol releases iron(III) from ferritin by direct chelation without iron(II) production. *Dalton Trans*, (2005), pp. (811-813).

Savarino, A.; Pescarmona, G.P. & Boelaert, J.R. (1999). Iron metabolism and HIV infection: reciprocal interactions with potentially harmful consequences. *Cell Biochem Funct*, 17 (1999), pp. (279-287).

Sekigwa, I.; Suzuki, J.; Nawata, M.; Ikeda, K.; Koike, M.; Lida, N.; Hashimoto, H. & Oshimi, K. (2001). Hemophagocytosis in autoimmune disease. *Clin Exp Rheumatol*, 19(3) (2001), pp. (333-338).

Sharma, R. & Anker, S.D. (2002). Cytokines, apoptosis and cachexia: the potential for TNF antagonism. *Int J Cardiol*, 85 (2002), pp. (161-171).

Shpyleva, S.I.; Tryndyak, V.P.; Kovalchuk, O.; Starlard-Davenport, A.; Chekhun, V.F.; Beland, F.A. & Pogribny, I.P. (2011). Role of ferritin alterations in human breast cancer cells. *Breast Cancer Res Treat*, 126 (2011), pp. (63-71).

Sibile, J.C.; Kondo, H. & Aisen, P. (1988). Interaction between isolated hepatocytes and Kupffer cells in iron metabolism: a possible role for ferritin as an iron carrier protein. *Hepatol*, 8 (1988), pp. (296-301).

Silber, J.H.; Evans, A.E. & Fridman, M. (1991). Models to predict outcome from childhood neuroblastoma: the role of serum ferritin and tumor histology. *Cancer Res*, 51(5) (1991), pp. (1426-1433).

Speyer, B.E. & Fielding, J. (1979). Ferritin as a cytosol iron transport intermediate in human reticulocytes. *Br J Haematol*, 42 (1979), pp. (255-267).

Stijlemans, B.; Vankrunkelsven, A.; Brys, L.; Magez, S. & De Baetselier, P. (2008). Role of iron homeostasis in trypanosomiasis-associated anemia. *Immunobiol*, 213(9-10) (2008), pp. (823-835).

Stites, S.W.; Plautz, M.W.; Bailey, K.; O'Brien-Ladner, A.R. & Wesselius, L.J. (1999). Increased concentrations of iron and isoferritins in the lower respiratory tract of patients with stable cystic fibrosis. *Am J Resp Crit Care Med*, 160(3) (1999), pp. (796-801).

Tapia, G.; Fernández, V.; Varela, P.; Cornejo, P.; Guerrero, J. & Videla, L.A. (2003). Thyroid hormone-induced oxidative stress triggers nuclear factor-κB activation and cytokine gene expression in rat liver. *Free Radic Biol Med*, 35(3) (2003), pp. (257-265).

Theil, E.C. (1990). The ferritin family of iron storage proteins. *Adv Enzymol Relat Areas Mol Biol*, 63 (1990), pp. (421-449).

Thurnham, D.I.; McCabe, L.D.; Haldar, S.; Wieringa, F.T.; Northrop-Clewes, C.A. & McCabe, G.P. (2010). Adjusting plasma ferritin concentrations to remove the effects of subclinical inflammation in the assessment of iron deficiency: a meta-analysis. *Am J Clin Nutr*, 92(3) (2010), pp. (546-555).

Tilg, H.; Dinarello, C.A. & Mier, J.W. (1997). Il-6 and APPs: Anti-inflammatory and immunosuppressive mediators. *Immunol Today*, 18 (1997), pp. (428-432).

Torrance, J.D.; Charlton, R.W.; Simon, M.O.; Lynch, S.R. & Bothwell, T.H. (1978). The mechanism of endotoxin-induced hypoferremia. *Scand J Haematol*, 21 (1978), pp. (403-410).

Torti, S.V. & Torti, F.M. (1994). Iron and ferritin in inflammation and cancer. *Adv Inorg Biochem*, 10 (1994), pp. (119-137).

Torti, F.M. & Torti, S.V. (2002). Regulation of ferritin genes and protein. *Blood*, 99(10) (2002), pp. (3505-3516).

Tripathi, P.K. & Chatterjee, S.K. (1996). Elevated expression of ferritin H-chain mRNA in metastatic ovarian tumor. *Can Invest*, 14(6) (1996), pp. (518-526).

Truty, J.; Malpe, R. & Linder, M.C. (2001). Iron prevents ferritin turnover in hepatic cells. *J Biol Chem*, 276(52) (2001), pp. (48775-48780).

Tsuji, Y.; Ayaki, H.; Whitman, S.P.; Morrow, C.S.; Torti, S.V. & Torti, F.M. (2000). Coordinate transcriptional and translational regulation of ferritin in response to oxidative stress. *Mol Cell Biol*, 20(16) (2000), pp. (5818-5827).

Turkson, J. & Jove, R. (2000). STAT proteins: novel molecular targets for cancer drug discovery. *Oncogene*, 19(56) (2000), pp. (6613-6626).

Vardhan, H.; Bhengraj, A.R.; Jha, R.; Srivastava, P.; Jha, H.C. & Mittal, A. (2010). Higher expression of ferritin protects Chlamydia trachomatis infected HeLa 229 cells from reactive oxygen species mediated cell death. *Biochem Cell Biol*, 88(5) (2010), pp. (835-842).

Vernet, M.; Renversez, J.C.; Lasne, Y.; Revenant, M.C.; Charlier de Bressing, C.; Guillemin, C.; Pressac, M. & Rymer, J.C. (1995). Comparison of six serum ferritin immunoassays and isoferritin spectrotypes in malignancies. *Ann Biol Clin*, 53 (1995), pp. (419-427).

Wagstaff, M.; Worwood, M. & Jacobs, A. (1982). Iron and isoferritins in iron overload. *Clin Sci*, 62(5) (1982), pp. (529-540).

Wang, W.; Knovich, M.A.; Coffman, L.G.; Torti, F.M. & Torti, S.V. (2010). Serum ferritin: past, present and future. *Biochim Biophys Acta*, 1800 (2010), pp. (760-769).

Watt, G.D.; Frankel, R.B. & Papaefthymiou, G.C. (1985). Reduction of mammalian ferritin. *Proc Natl Acad Sci USA*, 82 (1985), pp. (3640-3643).

Weinstein, R.E.; Bond, B.H. & Silberberg, B.K. (1982). Tissue ferritin concentrations in cancinoma of the breast. *Cancer*, 50(11) (1982), pp. (2406-2409).

Weir, M.P.; Sharp, G.A. & Peters, T.J. (1985). Electron microscopic studies of human haemosiderin and ferritin. *J Clin Pathol*, 38 (1985), pp. (915-918).

Weiss, G. & Goodnough, L.T. (2005). Anemia of chronic disease. *New Engl J Med*, 352(10) (2005), pp. (1011-1023).

White, K. & Munro, H.N. (1988). Induction of ferritin subunit synthesis by iron is regulated at both the transcriptional and translational levels. *J Biol Chem*, 263(18) (1988), pp. (8938-8942).

Whittaker, D.; Torrance, J.D. & Kew, M.C. (1984). Isolation of ferritin from human hepatocellular carcinoma. *Scand J Haematol*, 33(5) (1984), pp. (432-439).

Wilkinson IV, J.; Di, X., Schönig, K.; Buss, J.L.; Kock, N.D.; Cline, J.M.; Saunders, T.L.; Bujard, H.; Torti, S.V. & Torti, F.M. (2006). Tissue-specific expression of ferritin H regulates cellular iron homeostasis *in vivo*. *Biochem J*, 395 (2006), pp. (501-507).

Wixom, R.L.; Prutkin, L. & Munro, H.N. (1980). Hemosiderin: nature, formation, and significance. *Int Rev Exp Pathol*, 22 (1980), pp. (193-225).

World Health Organization, Centers for Disease Control and Prevention. Assessing the iron status of populations. Geneva, Switzerland, WHO Press, 2004.

World Health Organization, Centers for Disease Control and Prevention. Assessing the iron status of populations. Geneva, Switzerland, WHO Press, 2007.

Worwood, M.; Dawkins, S.; Wagstaff, M. & Jacobs, A. (1976). The purification and properties of ferritin from human serum. *Biochem J*, 157 (1976), pp. (97-103).

Worwood, M. (1982). Ferritin in human tissues and serum. *Clin Haematol*, 11(2) (1982), pp. (275-307).

Worwood, M. (1990). Ferritin. *Blood Rev*, 4 (1990), pp. (259-269).

Wu, K.J.; Polack, A. & Dalla-Favera, R. (1999). Coordinated regulation of iron-controlling genes, H-ferritin and IRP-2, by c-MYC. *Sci*, 283(5402) (1999), pp. (676-679).

Wu, T.; Sempos, C.T.; Freudenheim, J.L.; Muti, P. & Smit, E. (2004). Serum iron, copper and zinc concentrations and risk of cancer mortality in US adults. *Ann Epidemiol*, 14 (2004), pp. (195-201).

Xie, C.; Zhang, N.; Zhou, H.; Li, J.; Li, Q.; Zarubin, T.; Lin, S.C. & Han, J. (2005). Distinct roles of basal steady-state and induced H-ferritin in tumor necrosis factor-induced death in L929 cells. *Mol Cell Biol*, 25(15) (2005), pp. (6673-6681).

Yang, D.; Elner, S.G.; Bian, Z.M.; Till, G.O.; Petty, H.R. & Elner, V.M. (2007). Pro-inflammatory cytokines increase reactive oxygen species through mitochondria and NADPH oxidase in cultured RPE cells. *Exp Eye Res*, 85(4) (2007), pp. (462-472).

Yang, D.C.; Wang, F.; Elliott, R.L. & Head, J.F. (2001). Expression of transferrin receptor and ferritin H-chain mRNA are associated with clinical and histopathological prognostic indicators in breast cancer. *Anticancer Res*, 21(1B) (2001), pp. (541-549).

Zhang, K-H.; Tian, H-Y.; Gao, X.; Lei, W-W.; Hu, Y.; Wang, D-M.; Pan, X-C.; Yu, M-L. Xu, G-J.; Zhao, F-K. & Song, J-G. (2009). Ferritin heavy chain-mediated iron homeostasis and subsequent increase in reactive oxygen species production are essential for epithelial-mesenchymal transition. *Cancer Res*, 69(13) (2009), pp. (5340-5348).

Zhang, Y.; Mikhael, M.; Xu, D.; Li, Y.; Soe-Lin, S.; Ning, B.; Li, W.; Nie, G.; Zhao, Y. & Ponka, P. (2010). Lysosomal proteolysis is the primary degradation pathway for cytosolic ferritin and cytosolic ferritin degradation is necessary for iron exit. *Antioxid Redox Sign*, 13(7) (2010), pp. (999-1009).

Zhao, G.; Arosio, P. & Chasteen, N.D. (2006). Iron(II) and hydrogen peroxide detoxification by human H-chain ferritin. An EPR spin-trapping study. *Biochem*, 45(10) (2006), pp. (3429-3436).

8

The Hepatic Acute Phase Response to Thermal Injury

Marc G. Jeschke
Ross Tilley Burn Centre,
Sunnybrook Health Sciences Centre,
Department of Surgery, Division of Plastic Surgery University of Toronto
Canada

1. Introduction

A thermal injury represents one of the most severe forms of trauma and occurs in over two million people in the United States of America per year (1). According to the World Health Organization (WHO), an estimated 330,000 deaths per year worldwide are related to thermal injury (2). Over 440,000 children receive medical attention for burn injuries each year in the United States (3). With approximately 1,100 children dying of burn-related injuries in the United States every year (4), severe burns represent the third most common cause of death in the pediatric patient population (5) and account for a significant number of hospital admissions in the United States (6, 7). A severe burn, therefore, represents a devastating injury affecting nearly every body organ system and leads to significant patient morbidity and mortality (8). Burn produces a profound hypermetabolic stress response characterized by increased glucose production via glycogenolysis and gluconeogenesis, lipolysis, and protein catabolism (7-9). The hypermetabolic stress response is driven by the inflammatory response, which encompasses hormones, cytokines, and acute phase proteins (10-12). Clinical studies have shown that sustained or increased hypermetabolic, inflammatory, and acute phase responses can be life threatening with the uncontrolled and prolonged action of counterregulatory stress hormones (cortisol, catecholamines, glucagon), cytokines and acute phase proteins contributing to multi-organ failure, hypermetabolism, hypercatabolism, morbidity, and mortality (11-13).

Over the last two decades, burn research focused on areas such as hypermetabolism, resuscitation, wound healing, pulmonary support, and infection (7). Advances in these areas improved post-burn outcomes, but severe burn is still associated with significant morbidity and mortality. We are (14-17) proposing that an integral part of the post-burn response has not been determined and, therefore, focused our research on the role of the liver. The liver, with its metabolic, inflammatory, immune, and acute phase functions, plays a pivotal role in patient survival and recovery by modulating multiple pathways (13). The role of the liver during the post-burn response is essentially unknown and we, therefore, initiated a variety of studies to determine the function and role of the liver during the post-burn response. This review aims to discuss the liver and its role during the post-burn response.

2. Liver anatomy, function and physiology

2.1 Anatomy

The liver constitutes approximately one-fiftieth of total body weight (2%) and weighs approximately 1,500 g in the adult. Its size reflects its complexity of its functions. The American system (lobar anatomy) divides the liver anatomically, based on the distribution of the intrahepatic branches of the hepatic artery, portal vein and bile ducts; the right lobe is divided into an anterior section and a posterior section, and the left lobe into a medial section and lateral section. The French system divides the liver into VIII segments (Soupault and Couinaud's segmental system). The afferent blood supply to the liver arises from two sources: (a) *The hepatic artery* which carries oxygenated blood and accounts for approximately 25% of the hepatic blood flow, and (b) *The portal vein* drains the splanchnic circulation and accounts for 75% of the hepatic blood flow (18).

2.2 Physiology

The liver has a unique spectrum of functions. The liver regulates the amount of energy, stores, distributes, and disposes various nutrients and synthesizes, transforms and metabolizes many endogenous substrates and pollutants. The liver consists of 5 physiologic–anatomic units that are interrelated (18, 19).

1. The circulatory system. A dual blood supply nourishes the liver and acts as a vehicle for material absorbed from the intestinal tract to be utilized in the metabolic pool. Blood vessels are accompanied by lymphatics and nerve fibers that contribute to the regulation of blood flow and intrasinusoidal pressure. The liver expends approximately 20% of the body's energy and consumes 20% to 25% of the total utilized oxygen, which is due to the remarkable hepatic architecture and the blood supply. The hepatocellular organelles in plasma membranes permit specific functions and at the same time, interrelate with an extracellular matrix, which facilitates metabolic exchange between blood and hepatocytes (18, 19). The liver receives blood from the arterial and portal circulation; processes nutrients and metabolizes toxins and wastes, stores and transforms, and distributes them to the vascular, biliary or lymphatic circulations. Mean total hepatic blood flow has been estimated to be 100 to 130 ml/kg/min. Seventy to 75% of total hepatic blood flow comes from the portal vein, while the remainder comes from the hepatic artery. There is a reciprocal increase in hepatic arterial blood flow in response to a reduction in the portal flow, but the reverse does not occur (13, 18). To a large extent, portal venous flow into the liver is regulated by extrahepatic factors such as the rate of flow from the intestines and spleen. Food, bile salts, secretin, cholecystokinin, pentagastrin, epinephrine, vasoactive intestinal peptide and glucagon all increase portal blood flow. The liver serves as a physiologic reservoir of blood with 25% to 30% of its volume composed of blood. During acute blood loss, 300 ml or more can be released into the systemic circulation without adverse effects on liver function. Conversely, in the state of right-sided heart failure, up to 1000 ml of blood can be stored in the liver without affecting its function (18-20).
2. Biliary system. These serve as channels of exit for material secreted by the liver cells, including bilirubin, cholesterol and detoxified drugs. This system originates with the Golgi apparatus adjacent to the microvilli of the bile canaliculi and eventually terminates in the common bile duct. Bile secretion is an active process, relatively independent of total liver blood flow, except in conditions of shock. Bile is formed at

two sites: a) the canalicular membrane of the hepatocyte and b) the bile ductules or ducts. Total unstimulated bile flow in a 70-kg man has been estimated to be 0.41 to 0.43 ml/min. Eighty percent of the total daily production of bile (approximately 1500 ml) is secreted by hepatocytes and 20% is secreted by the bile duct epithelial cells. The principal organic compounds in bile are the conjugated bile acids, cholesterol, phospholipid and protein. As bile passes through the biliary ductules or ducts, it is modified by secretion or absorption of epithelial cells. The best characterized hormone to stimulate bile secretion is secretin. The bile is then being secreted into the gallbladder, which only functions to concentrate and store bile during fasting. Approximately 90% of the water in gallbladder bile is absorbed in 4 h. Most of the bile salt is absorbed into the enterohepatic circulation. The liver extracts the bile acids and transports them back to the canalicular membrane where they are re-secreted back into the biliary system. Total bile pool size in humans is 2 to 5 g and undergoes this circulation 2 to 3 times per meal and 6 to 10 times a day, depending on the dietary habit. In addition, 0.2 to 0.6 g are lost in the stool per day, and this quantity is replaced by newly synthesized bile acids (20). Bilirubin is a breakdown product of heme and is almost completely excreted in the bile. With hepatocellular disease or extrahepatic biliary obstruction, free bilirubin may accumulate in blood and tissues. Approximately 75% of bilirubin is derived from senescent red blood cells. Bilirubin circulates bound to albumin, which protects tissue from its toxicity. It is rapidly removed from the plasma by the liver through a carrier transport system. In the hepatocyte, bilirubin is conjugated with glucuronide and secreted in bile. Conjugated bilirubin may form a covalent bound with albumin, so called delta bilirubin. In the intestine, bilirubin is reduced by bacteria to mesobilirubin and stercobilirubin, collectively termed urobilinogen. These are both excreted in the stool. A part of urobilinogen is oxidized to urobilin, which is a brown pigment and gives stool its normal color (18-21).

3. The reticuloendothelial system (RES). This system has 60% of its cellular elements in the liver and includes the phagocytic, Kupffer cells, and endothelial cells. The Kupffer cells of the liver are part of the RES. The RES is part of the immune system and consists of the phagocytic cells located in reticular connective tissue, primarily monocytes and macrophages. The RES is divided into primary and secondary lymphoid organs. The liver is a secondary lymphoid organ. The function of the secondary lymphoid structures is to survey all entering or circulating antigen and to mobilize an immune response against foreign antigen upon its discovery.
4. The functioning liver cells (hepatocytes), which are capable of a wide variation of activity. The metabolic pool in the liver serves the needs of the entire body. The cells perform both anabolic and catabolic activities, secrete, and stores metabolites. The large amount of energy required for these transformations result from the conversion of adenosine triphosphate to adenosine diphosphate.
5. Liver as a hormone producing and secreting unit. Various hormones are synthesized and secreted by the liver, such as insulin-like growth factor-I (IGF-I), insulin-like growth factor binding proteins (IGFBPs), hepatocyte growth factor (HGF). Further, the liver interacts with various other hormonal systems thus playing a central role in the hormonal axes.

2.3 Metabolic system

2.3.1 Acute phase response

The acute phase response is a cascade of events initiated to prevent tissue damage and to activate repair processes (13, 22). Initiated is the acute phase response by activated phagocytic cells, fibroblasts, and endothelial cells, which release proinflammatory cytokines leading to the systemic phase of the acute phase response (13, 22). The systemic reaction affects the hypothalamus which leads to fever, the pituitary-adrenal axis to release steroid hormones, the liver which causes the synthesis and secretion of acute phase proteins, the bone marrow which promulgates further hemopoietic responses, and the immune system which allows the activation of the RES and the stimulation of lymphocytes (13, 22). However, a crucial step in this cascade of reactions involves the interaction between the site of injury and the liver, which is the principle organ responsible for producing acute phase proteins and modulating the systemic inflammatory response. The acute phase response usually encompasses positive acute phase proteins, whose expression is increased, e.g. C-reactive protein, α2-macroglobulin, haptoglobin, etc. and negative acute phase proteins, whose expression is decreased, e.g. albumin and pre-albumin, transferrin, retinol-binding protein, etc.

2.3.2 Carbohydrate metabolism

The liver has a central role in energy metabolism: it provides glucose as a readily available source of energy to the central nervous system, red blood cells and adrenal medulla. During fed state, results of intestinal carbohydrates digestion (glucose: 80%; galactose and fructose: 20%) are delivered to the liver, with galactose and fructose rapidly converted into glucose. Glucose absorbed by the hepatocyte is converted directly into glycogen for storage up to a maximum of 65 g of glycogen per kg of liver mass. Excess glucose is converted to fat. Glycogen is also produced by skeletal muscles, but this is not available for use by any other tissues. During the fasting state, glycogen is the primary source of glucose. However, after 48 h of fasting, liver glycogen is reduced, and the body uses fat and proteins which are mobilized to meet the metabolic need. In the muscle, mainly alanine is mobilized which then is converted by the liver to glucose (23, 24).

Glycogenesis, glycogenolysis, and the conversion of galactose into glucose all represent hepatic functions, which ensures adequate glucose synthesis and, therefore, hypoglycemia is rare and only when associated with extensive hepatic disease. Hyperglycemia, however, is common with severe liver disease due to deficient glycogenesis. Lactate by anaerobic metabolism is metabolized only in the liver. Ordinarily, it is converted to pyruvate and subsequently back into glucose. This shuttling of glucose and lactate between liver and peripheral tissue is carried out in the Cori cycle. The brain does not participate in the cycle and a continuous source of glucose for the brain must come at the expense of muscle proteins. In liver disease, the metabolism of glucose is often deranged. Frequently, in patients with cirrhosis the portal-systemic shunting causes decreased exposure of portal blood to the hepatocytes, producing an abnormal result of the oral glucose tolerance test. In fulminate hepatic failure, however, there is extensive loss of hepatocyte mass and function, and hypoglycemia supervenes as gluconeogenesis fails (21).

2.3.3 Lipid metabolism

There are three sources of free fatty acids (FFA) available to the liver: fat absorbed from the gut, fat liberated from adipocytes in response lipolysis, and fatty acids synthesized from carbohydrates and amino acids. These fatty acids are etherified with glycerol to form triglyceride. The export of triglycerides (TG) is dependent on the synthesis of very low density lipoproteins. In cases of excess supply of fatty acid, there is lipid accumulation in the liver because there is an imbalance of triglyceride relative to very low density lipoproteins. This is seen in obesity, corticosteroid use, pregnancy, diabetes, and total parenteral nutrition. Simple protein malnutrition or protein-calories imbalance may also result in fatty change of liver, based on decreased export of TG, because of limited supply of precursors for hepatic synthesis of lipoproteins (21, 25).

Synthesis of both the phospholipid and cholesterol takes place in the liver, and the latter serves as a standard for the determination of lipid metabolism. The liver is the major organ involved in the synthesis, esterification, and excretion of cholesterol. In the presence of parenchymal damage, both the total cholesterol and the percentage of esterified fraction decreased. The biliary obstruction results in the rise in cholesterol, and the most pronounced elevations are noted in the primary biliary cirrhosis and the cholangiolitis accompanying toxic reactions to the phenothiazine derivatives (20, 21).

2.3.4 Protein metabolism

At least 17 of the major plasma proteins are synthesized and secreted by the liver. The liver is the only organ that produces serum albumin and α-globulin, and it synthesizes most the urea in the body. Production of various serum proteins is an important index of liver function. Albumin is the most abundant serum protein, its synthesis accounting for 11% to 15% of total hepatic synthesis. Synthesis of albumin is influenced by nutrition, thyroxin, insulin, glucagons, cortisol, and cytokines produced during the systemic inflammatory response (16, 26). Hepatic cells are responsible for the synthesis of albumin, fibrinogen, prothrombin, and other factors involved in blood clotting. A reduction of serum albumin is one of the most accurate reflections of liver disease and the effects of medical therapy. Because the half-life of albumin is 21 days, impairment of hepatic synthesis must be present for at least 3 weeks before liver synthetic abnormalities can be reflected in relative decrease in serum albumin concentrations. The correlation between total protein and disease of the liver is not as close as that between the serum albumin level and liver disease, since albumin is produced only by hepatic cells and a reduction is frequently compensated for by the increase in the level of globulin (21).

2.3.5 Vitamin metabolism

The liver has many important roles of uptake, storage, and mobilization of vitamins. Most important are the fat-soluble vitamins A, E, D, and K. The absorption of these vitamins is dependent on bile salts. The vitamins appear in the thoracic duct 2 to 6 h after oral administration. Vitamin A is exclusively stored in the liver, and excess ingestion of Vitamin A may be associated with significant liver injury. A role for storage of Vitamin A in the Ito cells (fat-storing cells) has been suggested. Initial step in Vitamin D activation occurs in the liver where Vitamin D_3 is converted 25-hydroxycholecalciferol. Vitamin K is essential for the γ-carboxylation of the Vitamin K-dependent coagulation factors II, VII, IX and X. These factors are inactive without γ-carboxylation (see paragraph below) (20, 21). A vitamin that has gained attention is Vitamin E, because Vitamin E has been shown to be a very potent anti-oxidant, which could reduce oxidative stress post-trauma or thermal injury.

2.3.6 Coagulation

The liver produces multiple coagulation factors, which can be altered or being defect in the state of liver disease. In the state of jaundice, Vitamin K resorption is decreased resulting in a decreased synthesis of prothrombin, or when the liver is severely damaged, in the state of hepatocellular dysfunction prothrombin is not synthesized at all. The diagnosis of pathological prothrombin synthesis is made by the prothrombin time. Decreases in factors V, VII, IX and fibrinogen also have been noted in hepatic disease (20, 21).

2.4 Hormonal system

Multiple hormones are either synthesized, secreted, or interact with the liver. Angiotensinogen is made and secreted into the bloodstream by the liver. The liver also is actively involved in Vitamin D synthesis by hydroxylation of *cholecalciferol to 25-hydroxycholecaciferol by the enzyme 25-hydroxylase.* IGF-I and IGFBPs are important hormones that play a role in the growth and development that are synthesized and secreted in the liver. The main stimulus for IGF-I production is growth hormone (GH). Lastly, HGF, a major hepatic regenerative growth factor, is synthesized in the liver (27).

3. Hepatic changes in response to a burn and the hepatic acute phase response

3.1 Liver damage and morphological changes

After a thermal injury, a variable degree of liver injury is present and it is usually related to the severity of the thermal injury. By which mechanisms a thermal injury induces, fatty changes is not entirely defined by and we suggest that fatty changes are associated with hepatic apoptosis (described in detail below). Fatty changes and hepatomegaly (Figure 1), a very common finding are, per se, reversible and their significance depends on the cause and severity of accumulation (28). However, autopsies of burned children who died have shown that fatty liver infiltration was associated with increased bacterial translocation, liver failure, and endotoxemia (29).

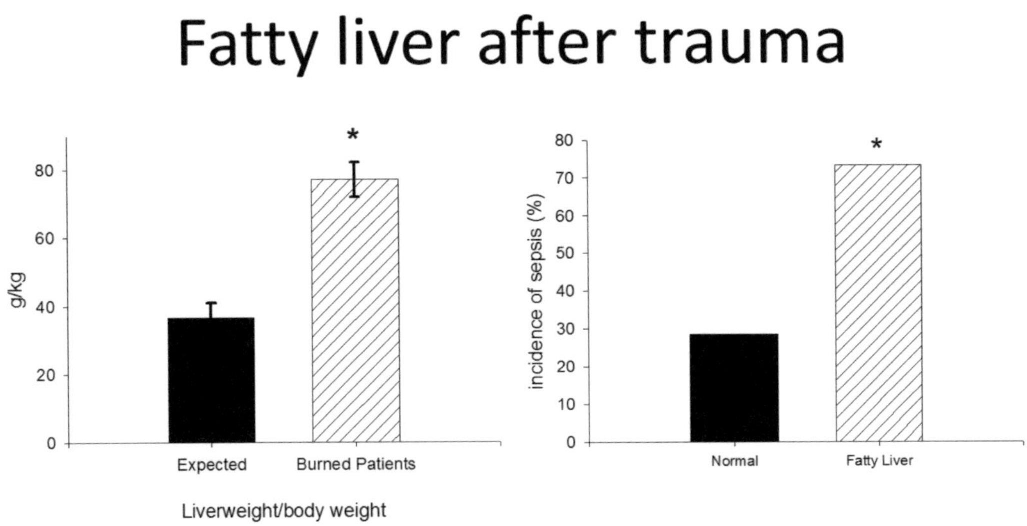

(*) significant difference burn patients with fatty liver vs. no fatty liver, p<0.001

Fig. 1. Fatty liver is associated with increased hepatomegaly and incidence of sepsis.

Immediately after burn, the damage of the liver may be associated with an increased hepatic edema formation. Jeschke *et al.* (15) have shown that the liver weight and liver/body-weight significantly increased 2 to 7 days after burn when compared to controls. As hepatic protein concentration was significantly decreased in burned rats, we suggest that the liver weight gain is due to increased edema formation rather than increases in the number of hepatocytes or protein levels. An increase in edema formation may lead to cell damage, with the release of the hepatic enzymes. Liver enzymes, such as aspartate aminotransferase (AST) and alanine aminotransferase (ALT) are the most sensitive indicators of hepatocyte injury. Both ALKP can be elevated in patients with mass bone resorption and children growing. Therefore, alterations in hepatic enzymes need to be carefully evaluated.

AST and ALT are normally present in low concentrations. However, with cellular injury or changes in cell membrane permeability, these enzymes leak into circulation. Of the two, the ALT is the more sensitive and specific test for hepatocyte injury as AST can be also elevated in the state of cardiac arrest or muscle injury. Serum glutamate dehydrogenase is also a marker and is elevated in the state of severe hepatic damage. Serum alkaline phosphatase (ALKP) provides an elevation of the patency of the bile channels at all levels, intrahepatic and extrahepatic. Elevation is demonstrated in patients with obstruction of the extrahepatic biliary tract or caliculi. In general, serum levels are elevated in hepatobiliary disease. Thermal injury causes liver damage by edema formation, hypoperfusion, pro-inflammatory cytokines or other cell death signals with the release of the hepatic enzymes. Serum AST, ALT and ALKP are elevated between 50 to 200% from baseline when compared with normal levels (Figure 2). Jeschke *et al.* (16, 26) observed that serum AST and ALT peaked during the first day post-burn and ALKP during the second day post-burn. During hepatic regeneration all enzymes returned to baseline during acute hospitalization. A limitation of the use of hepatic enzymes is that they could be elevated due other reasons. For example, ALKP can be elevated in patients with mass bone resorption and children growing. Therefore, alterations in hepatic enzymes need to be carefully evaluated.

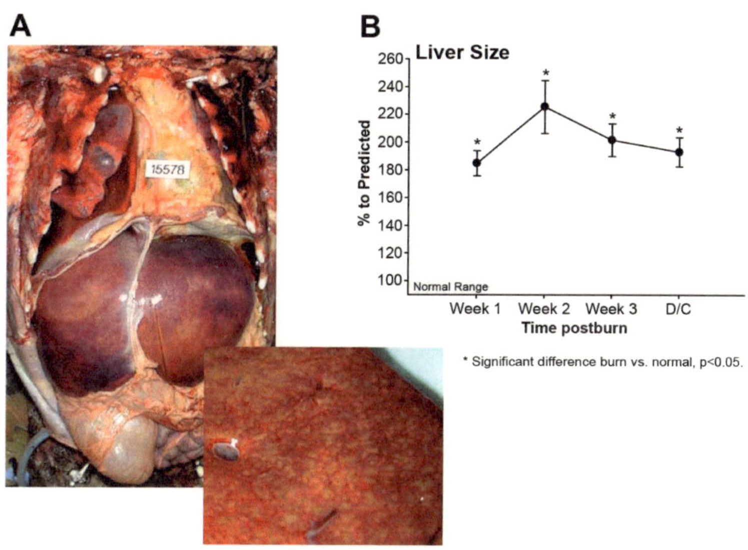

Fig. 2. (A) Massive hepatomegaly (upper Figure 2A) and hepatic fatty infiltration (lower Figure 2A) of a burn victim at autopsy. (B) Liver size increases throughout acute hospitalization by over 200% in 242 surviving burn patients.

Liver damage has been associated with increased hepatocyte cell death (15). In general, cell death occurs by two distinctly different mechanisms-programmed cell death (apoptosis) or necrosis (30). Apoptosis is characterized by cell shrinkage, DNA fragmentation, membrane blebbing, and phagocytosis of the apoptotic cell fragments by neighboring cells or extrusion into the lumen of the bowel without inflammation. This is in contrast to necrosis, which involves cellular swelling, random DNA fragmentation, lysosomal activation, membrane breakdown, and extrusion of cellular contents into the interstitium. Membrane breakdown and cellular content release induced inflammation with the migration of inflammatory cells and release of pro-inflammatory cytokines and free radicals, which leads to further tissue breakdown. Pathological studies found that 10% to 15% of thermally injured patients show signs of liver necrosis at autopsy (28). The necrosis is generally focal or zonal, central or paracentral, sometimes microfocal, and related to burn shock and sepsis. The morphological differences between apoptosis and necrosis are used to differentiate the two processes.

A cutaneous thermal injury induces liver cell apoptosis associated with caspase activation (15). This increase in hepatic programmed cell death is compensated for by an increase in hepatic cell proliferation, suggesting that the liver attempts to maintain homeostasis. Despite the attempt to compensate increased apoptosis by increased hepatocyte proliferation, the liver cannot regain hepatic mass and protein concentration, as we found a significant decrease in hepatic protein concentration in burned rats. It has been shown that a cutaneous burn induces small bowel epithelial cell apoptosis (31, 32). In the same study, the authors showed that small bowel epithelial cell proliferation was not increased, leading to a loss of mucosal cells and hence mucosal mass (31, 32). Similar findings were demonstrated in the heart (33, 34). Burn-induced cardiocyte apoptosis; however, cardiocyte proliferation remained unchanged causing cardiac impairment and dysfunction (33, 34).

The mechanisms whereby a cutaneous burn induces programmed cell death in hepatocytes are not defined. Studies suggested that in general hypoperfusion and ischemia-reperfusion are associated to promote apoptosis (35-38). After a thermal injury, it has been shown that the blood flow to the bowel decreases by nearly 60% of baseline and stays decreased for approximately 4 h (31). It can be surmised that the hepatic blood flow also decreases, thus causing programmed cell death. In addition, proinflammatory cytokines such as IL-1 and tumor necrosis factor (TNF)-α have been described to be an apoptotic signal (30, 39-42). After a thermal injury serum and hepatic concentration of proinflammatory cytokines such as IL-1α/β, IL-6 and TNF-α are increased (14, 43-45) and we, therefore, suggest that two possible mechanisms are involved in increased hepatocyte apoptosis, decreased splanchnic blood-flow, and elevation of pro-inflammatory cytokines, initiating intracellular signaling mechanisms. Signals that may be involved encompass many signals that play an important role during the acute phase response.

Studies now focus on the identification by which molecular mechanisms a thermal injury leads to hepatocyte apoptosis and dysfunction (Figure 3) (46) and found that burn injury leads to ER stress and gross alterations in ER calcium with increased cytosolic calcium concentrations. Increased cytosolic calcium induces mitochondrial damage which releases cytochrome c. Cytochrome c binds to the IP3R augmenting the depletion of ER calcium stores. ER stress/UPR leads to cell apoptosis and activation of JNK which phosphorylates the serine IRS-1, blocking phosphorylation of tyrosine IRS-1. ER stress/UPR also impairs the pro-survival PI3K/Akt signaling, resulting in an increased activation of the IP3R increasing

ER stress/UPR. This finding is of therapeutic significance because limiting the unfolded protein burden with "chemical chaperones" may promote hepatocyte survival (47). Furthermore, the ongoing development of pharmacologic agents which limit pro-apoptotic ER stress signaling pathways may have a therapeutic benefit to improve organ function and patient survival (48).

3.2 Effects on biliary system

In trauma and sepsis, intrahepatic cholestasis occurs frequently and appears to be an important pathophysiologic factor and occurs without demonstrable extrahepatic obstruction. This phenomenon has been described in association with a number of processes, such as hypoxia, drug toxicity, or total parenteral nutrition (49). The mechanisms of intrahepatic cholestasis seem to be associated with an impairment of basolateral and cunicular hepatocyte transport of bile acids and organic anions (50, 51). This is most likely due to decreased transporter protein and RNA expression thus leading to increased bile. Intrahepatic cholestasis, which is one of the prime manifestations of hepatocellular injury, was present in 26% in a clinical study (28).

3.3 Reticuloendothelial system (RES)

Severe burn is associated with a compromised immune system that can lead to infections and sepsis (52-54). Burn has furthermore been shown to depress RES phagocytic activity (55, 56). The exact mechanism by which a burn causes RES dysfunction is not known. Trop *et al.* (55, 56) investigated some possible mechanisms by which a burn causes RES dysfunction and found that hemolysis may play a role in the alterations in RES phagocytic activity. Others and we (15, 16, 22, 43, 57) have shown that the liver also contributes to the inflammatory and acute phase response by expressing proinflammatory cytokines and acute phase proteins indicating the central role of the liver in the inflammatory, acute phase, and immune response.

4. Metabolic system

4.1 Glucose, protein, and lipid metabolism

Severe burns covering more than 40% total body surface area (TBSA) are typically followed by a period of stress, inflammation and hypermetabolism, characterized by a hyperdynamic circulatory response with increased body temperature, glycolysis, proteolysis, glycogenolysis and gluconeogenesis lipolysis and futile substrate cycling (58-60). These responses are present in all trauma, surgical, or critically ill patients, but the severity, length, and magnitude is unique for burn patients (7). Marked and sustained increases in catecholamine, glucocorticoid, glucagon, and dopamine secretion are thought to initiate the cascade of events leading to the acute hypermetabolic response with its ensuing catabolic state (7, 8, 26, 61-63). The cause of this complex response is not well understood. However, interleukin (IL)-1 and IL-6, platelet-activating factor, TNF, endotoxin, neutrophil-adherence complexes, reactive oxygen species, nitric oxide and coagulation as well as complement cascades have also been implicated in regulating this response to thermal injury (64). Once these cascades are initiated, their mediators and by-products appear to stimulate the persistent and increased metabolic rate associated with altered glucose metabolism seen after severe thermal injury (65).

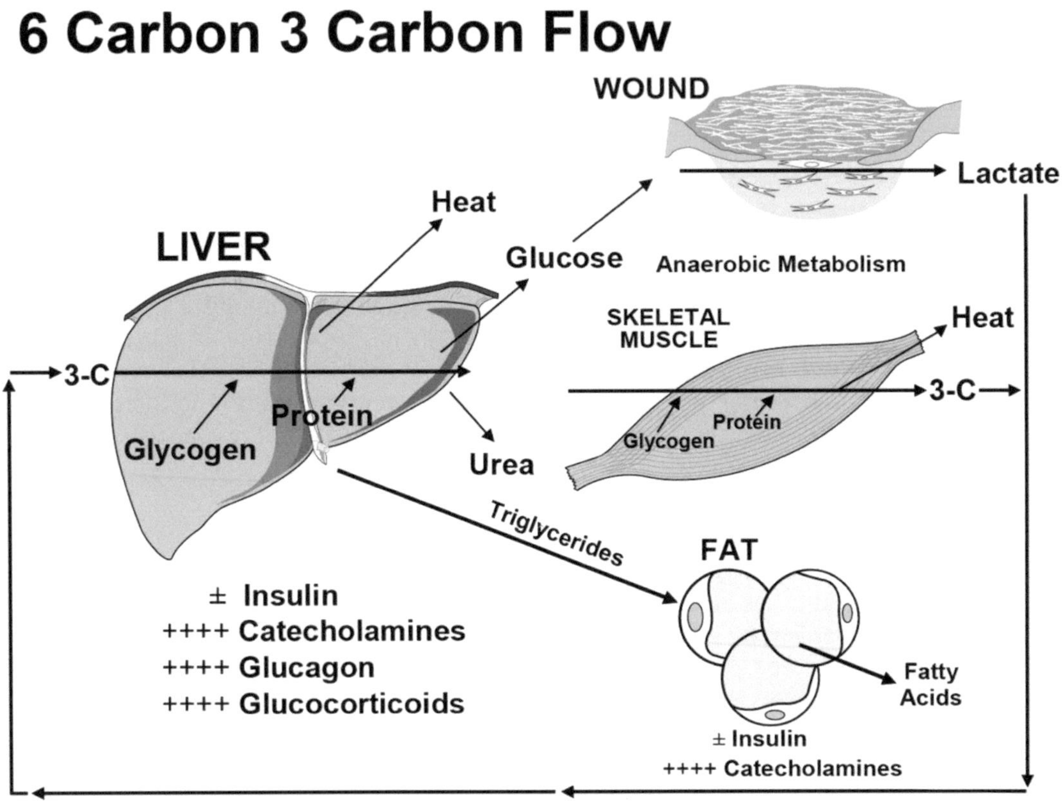

Fig. 3. Metabolic changes post-burn with the liver playing an essential role.

Several studies have indicated that these metabolic phenomena post-burn occur in a timely manner, suggesting two distinct pattern of metabolic regulation following injury (26, 66). The first phase occurs immediately post severe thermal injury and lasts for about 12 to 14 h and has classically been called the "ebb phase" (66-68), and is characterized by decreases in cardiac output, oxygen consumption, and metabolic rate as well as impaired glucose tolerance associated with its hyperglycemic state. These metabolic variables gradually increase within the first five days post-injury to a plateau phase (called the "flow" phase), characteristically associated with hyperdynamic circulation and the above mentioned hypermetabolic state (66). Insulin release, during this time period, was found to be twice that of controls in response to glucose load (26, 69) and plasma glucose levels are markedly elevated, indicating the development of an insulin-resistance (26, 69). Current understanding has been that these metabolic alterations resolve soon after complete wound closure. However, recent studies found that the hypermetabolic response to thermal injury may last for at least 12 months after the initial event (16, 58, 70, 71).

Glucose metabolism in healthy subjects is tightly regulated: under normal circumstances, a postprandial increase in blood glucose concentration stimulates release of insulin from pancreatic β-cells. Insulin mediates peripheral glucose uptake into skeletal muscle and adipose tissue and suppresses hepatic gluconeogenesis, thereby maintaining blood glucose homeostasis (72, 73). In critical illness, however, metabolic alterations can cause significant changes in energy substrate metabolism. In order to provide glucose, a major fuel source to vital organs, release of the above mentioned stress mediators oppose the anabolic actions of insulin (74). By enhancing adipose tissue lipolysis (75) and skeletal muscle proteolysis (76), they increase gluconeogenic substrates, including glycerol, alanine and lactate, thus augmenting hepatic glucose production in burned patients (72, 73, 77). Hyperglycemia fails to suppress hepatic glucose release during this time (23) and the suppressive effect of insulin on hepatic glucose release is attenuated, significantly contributing to post-trauma hyperglycemia (78). Catecholamine-mediated enhancement of hepatic glycogenolysis, as well as direct sympathetic stimulation of glycogen breakdown, can further aggravate the hyperglycemia in response to stress (73). Catecholamines have also been shown to impair glucose disposal via alterations of the insulin signaling pathway and GLUT-4 translocation muscle and adipose tissue, resulting in peripheral insulin resistance (72, 79). Cree *et al.* (69) showed an impaired activation of Insulin Receptor Substrate-1 at its tyrosine binding site and an inhibition of Akt in muscle biopsies of children at seven days post-burn. Work of Wolfe *et al.* (23, 75, 78, 80) indicates links between impaired liver and muscle mitochondrial oxidative function, altered rates of lipolysis, and impaired insulin signaling post-burn attenuating both the suppressive actions of insulin on hepatic glucose production and on the stimulation of muscle glucose uptake. Another counter-regulatory hormone of interest during stress of the critically ill is glucagon. Glucagon, like epinephrine, leads to increased glucose production through both gluconeogenesis and glycogenolysis (81). The action of glucagons alone is not maintained over time; however, its action on gluconeogenesis is sustained in an additive manner with the presence of epinephrine, cortisol, and GH (74, 81). Likewise, epinephrine and glucagon have an additive effect on glycogenolysis (81). Recent studies found that proinflammatory cytokines contribute indirectly to post-burn hyperglycemia via enhancing the release of the above mentioned stress hormones (82-85). Other groups showed that inflammatory cytokines, including TNF, IL-6 and Monocyte Chemotactic Protein-1 also act via direct effects on the insulin signal transduction pathway through modification of signaling properties of insulin receptor substrates, contributing to post-burn hyperglycemia via liver and skeletal muscle insulin resistance (86-88). Alterations in metabolic pathways as well as proinflammatory cytokines, such as TNF, have also been implicated in significantly contributing to lean muscle protein breakdown, both during the acute and convalescent phases in response to thermal injury (11, 12, 89, 90). In contrast to starvation, in which lipolysis and ketosis provide energy and protect muscle reserves, thermal injury considerably reduces the ability of the body to utilize fat as an energy source. Counter regulatory hormones such as glucagons, cortisone, and etc. post severe thermal injury vary in their concentration. While glucagons appears to be decreased Norbury *et al.* (63) and Gauglitz *et al.* (91) have recently shown that cortisone levels are markedly increased up to three years post severe thermal injury. The major mechanisms by which thermal injury causes hyperglycemia is probably not due to the hormonal system but rather on a molecular level associated with impaired insulin receptor signaling (92).

Skeletal muscle is thus the major source of fuel in the burned patient, which leads to marked wasting of lean body mass (LBM) within days after injury (7, 93). This muscle breakdown has been demonstrated with whole body and cross leg nitrogen balance studies in which pronounced negative nitrogen balances persisted for 6 and 9 months after injury (58). Since skeletal muscle has been shown to be responsible for 70–80% of whole-body insulin-stimulated glucose uptake, decreases in muscle mass may significantly contribute to this persistent insulin resistance post-burn (94). The correlation between hyperglycemia and muscle protein catabolism has been also supported by Flakoll *et al.* (95) in which an isotopic tracer of leucine was utilized to index whole-body protein flux in normal volunteers. The group showed a significant increase in proteolysis rates occurring without any alteration in either leucine oxidation or non-oxidative disposal (an estimate of protein synthesis), suggesting a hyperglycemia-induced increase in protein breakdown (95). Flakoll *et al.* (95) further demonstrated that elevations of plasma glucose levels resulted in a marked stimulation of whole body proteolysis during hyperinsulinemia. A 10-15% loss in LBM has been shown to be associated with significant increases in infection rate and marked delays in wound healing (96). The resultant muscle weakness was further shown to prolong mechanical ventilatory requirements, inhibit sufficient cough reflexes and delay mobilization in protein-malnourished patients, thus markedly contributing to the incidence of mortality in these patients. Persistent protein catabolism may also account for delay in growth frequently observed in our pediatric patient population for up to 2 years post-burn (61, 96-99).

Of great interest is the change in fat metabolism, serum triglycerides and FFA, all of which are significantly altered throughout almost the entire acute hospital stay. Fat transporter proteins are decreased post-burn while triglycerides and FFA are increased which could explain the fatty infiltration of the liver and other organs post-burn. Barret *et al.* (29) have shown that hepatomegaly with fatty infiltration is associated with increased incidence of sepsis and mortality implying the importance of organ integrity and function. The occurrence of triglycerides accumulation in the liver has been documented by direct liver biopsy in critically ill patients (100) and in autopsies of patients who died from severe thermal injury (29, 101, 102). Several investigators (29, 101-103) have shown in a clinical study that the size of the liver may be increased by 4-fold or more in burn patients. The rate of gain of liver triglycerides in severely burned patients far exceeds the rate of gain in any other pathological circumstance in which hepatic steatosis develops. The mechanisms leading to hepatic triglycerides accumulation after thermal injury are an excessive delivery of fatty acids to the liver as a consequence of β-adrenergic mediated stimulation of lipolysis (104, 105) and a diminished effectiveness of insulin (from carbohydrate intake) in suppressing lipolysis (101). Uptake of fatty acids across the liver was found to be proportionate to delivery in both pigs (106) and human patients (25) so that accelerated delivery of fatty acids due to lipolysis resulted in hepatic uptake at a rate well in excess of the requirement for oxidation. Thus, fatty acids taken up by the liver were channeled to triglycerides synthesis at a markedly accelerated rate in both pigs and humans (105, 106). The process of hepatic triglycerides deposition is accelerated when a high proportion of the diet is fat (107). However, substitution of dietary fat with carbohydrate results in the stimulation of de novo fatty acid synthesis, which also contributes to hepatic triglycerides (25). Thus, it appears production of liver triglycerides is a result of the metabolic response to thermal injury, rather than a simple consequence of nutritional support. Nonetheless, accelerated hepatic triglycerides synthesis does not necessarily translate to increased liver triglycerides. In normal individuals, accelerated hepatic triglycerides synthesis is accompanied by increased VLDL- triglycerides secretion, thereby minimizing hepatic accumulation of triglycerides. In contrast, VLDL- triglycerides secretion is low in burn patients and unresponsive to increased hepatic triglycerides synthesis (105). Consequently, it can be predicted that reduction of delivery of FFA to the liver would be the most effective approach to minimizing hepatic triglycerides accumulation. Interestingly, excessive glucose intake and uncontrolled hyperglycemia may also lead to fat deposition in the liver augmenting fatty infiltration of the liver post severe thermal injury (108).

In summary, the liver clearly plays a central role in orchestrating and modulating metabolic processes post-burn. The liver is responsible for glucose, fat, and protein metabolism post-burn and alterations in glucose, fat, and protein metabolism have been detrimental outcomes. We, therefore, propose that the liver, with its metabolic function, is one of the essential organs and can determine outcomes of severely burned patients.

4.2 Acute phase response

After major trauma, such as a severe burn, hepatic protein synthesis shifts from hepatic constitutive proteins, such as albumin, pre-albumin, transferrin, and retinol-binding protein to acute phase proteins (13, 16, 22, 26) (Fig. 4). Previously, acute phase proteins were divided into type I acute phase proteins, such as haptoglobin and α1-acidglycoprotein, mediated by IL-1-like cytokines (IL-1 and TNF) and type II acute phase proteins, such as α2-macroglobulin and fibrinogen, which are mediated by IL-6-like cytokines (IL-6, IL-11) (13). It is unclear whether this division holds true with the discovery of new cytokines and signal transcription factors. Furthermore, it appears that there is a lot of cross-communication between the two responses indicating that that this strict division is not functional and reflecting the ongoing responses. However, the upregulation of acute phase proteins represents a redirection of the liver in order to fulfill immune functions, metabolic responses, coagulation, and wound healing processes (13, 16, 22, 26).

In contrast to acute phase proteins, constitutive hepatic proteins are downregulated (109-112). After a thermal injury, albumin and transferrin decrease by 50-70% below normal levels (109-112) (Fig. 5). Studies have shown that two mechanisms are responsible for the decrease of constitutive hepatic proteins: one is that the liver re-prioritizes its protein synthesis from constitutive hepatic proteins to acute phase proteins. This could be shown in many studies in which the mRNA synthesis for constitutive hepatic proteins is decreased. The other mechanism for decreased constitutive hepatic protein concentration is the capillary leakage and the loss of constitutive hepatic proteins into the massive extravascular space and burn wound. Albumin and transferrin, however, have important physiologic functions as they serve as transporter proteins and contribute to osmotic pressure and plasma pH (109-112). Their downregulation after trauma has been described as potentially harmful and the synthesis of these proteins has been used as a predictor of mortality and indicators of recovery (11, 12, 112-115).

Mediators of the acute phase response are cytokines. In several studies, the biphasic time course of proinflammatory cytokines has been demonstrated. Immediately after burn, IL-1, IL-6, IL-8, and TNF increase 2- to 10-fold above normal levels, decrease slightly after approximately 12 h, increase again and then start to decrease. Animal and human studies demonstrated that cytokines can either approach normal levels within 2 days after trauma or can be elevated up to 2 weeks after thermal injury (10, 16, 26, 44, 70, 116). The signal transcription cascade includes various pro- and anti-inflammatory signal transcription factors such as c-jun/c-fos, nuclear factor-kappa B (NF-κB), CCAAT/enhancer-binding-

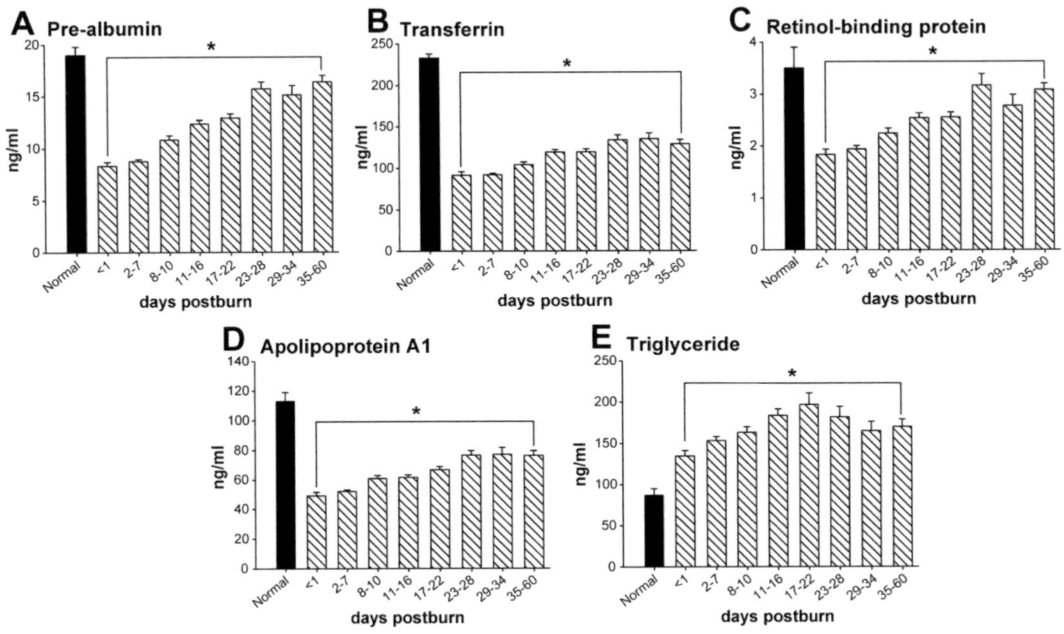

Fig. 4. Changes in constitutive hepatic proteins in severely burned patients over time. Burn caused profound decrease in constitutive hepatic protein such as pre-albumnin, transferrin,retinol-binding protein. There are furthermore alterations in the lipid associated proteins, apolipoprotein a1 was significantly decreased while triglycerides were increased indicating that a severe injury affects constitutive hepatic protein synthesis.

proteins (C/EBPs), tyrosine phosphorylation and activation of intracellular tyrosine kinases (JAKs), latent cytoplasmic transcription factors, STAT1, STAT3, and STAT5 (signal transducer and activator of transcription), or mitogen-activated protein (57, 109, 110, 117-121). These signals activate transcription, translation and expression of acute phase proteins. Particularly IL-6 has been speculated to be the main mediating cytokine. IL-6 activates glycoprotein 130 (gp 130) and the JAK-kinases (JAK-1) leading to activation of STAT 1 and 3 translocating to the nucleus. Intranuclear, the genes for acute phase proteins are turned on. The aim of the acute phase response is to protect the body from further damage, and the aim will be achieved when all elements of the acute phase response coalesce in a balanced fashion. However, a prolonged increase in proinflammatory cytokines and acute phase proteins has been shown to be indicative of a hypercatabolic state, associated with an increased risk of sepsis, multi-organ failure, morbidity and mortality (11, 12, 112-114).

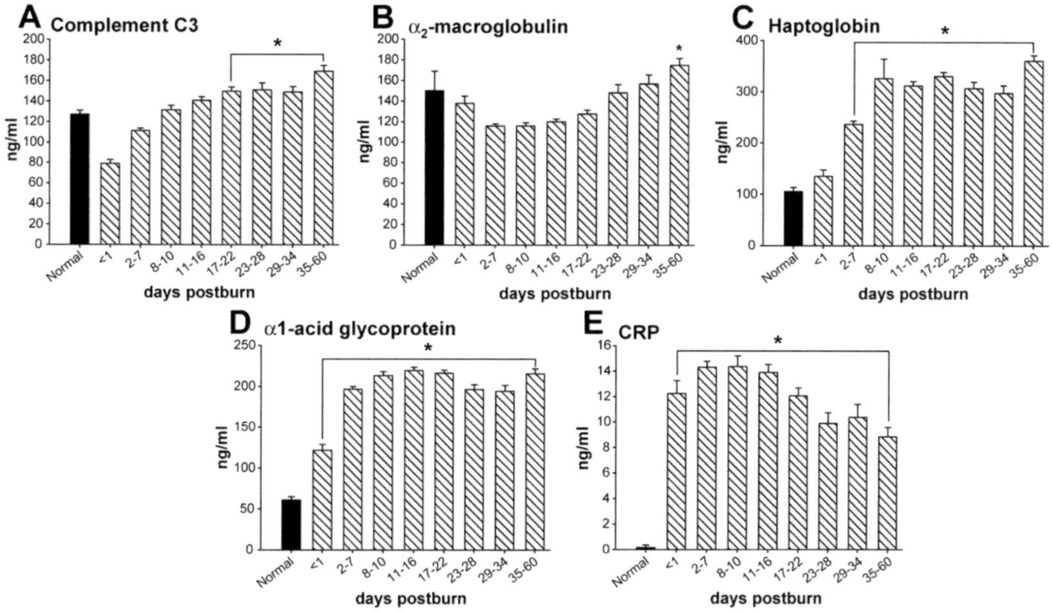

Fig. 5. Changes in acute phase hepatic proteins in severely burned patients over time. Burn caused profound increases in acute phase protein such as complement c3, alpha2 macroglobulin, haptoglobin, alpha1 acid glycoprotein and c-reactive protein. Indicating that a severe injury affects hepatic acute phase protein synthesis.

4.3 Vitamin metabolism

Vitamins play an important role in wound healing, energy, metabolism, inflammation, and antioxidants. Post-burn hypermetabolism causes a vitamin deficiency requiring substitution (122-124). There are decreased Vitamin A levels in burn patients. This is perhaps due to a reduction of retinol binding protein, which is a Vitamin A transporter. Vitamin A has been shown to enhance wound healing, thus its substitution is important for dermal wound repair. Vitamin E encompasses anti-oxidant properties, and in animal experiments, its administration has been shown to reduce lung injury. After a thermal injury its concentration is decreased, thus its substitution is suggested. Vitamin D, with its crucial function in the ossear cascade, is also decreased after thermal injury; however, its substitution has not been proven. Thiamin and Riboflavin are vitamins that affect energy and protein metabolism and wound healing. Both factors are decreased after trauma. Thiamin serves as a cofactor in the Krebs cycle and for the oxidation of glucose, thus its needs is related to the energy intake. Thiamin is further necessary for the lysyl oxidase function to form collagen. Riboflavin is involved as a coenzyme in oxidation-reduction reactions. Riboflavin is decreased after burn and an increased need for burn victims has been shown (122-124). Folic acid is depleted after a burn and can lead to impaired synthesis of DNA and RNA. Inadequate supplies of Vitamin B_{12} and the indispensable amino acid, methionine, impair folate utilization. Thus, a deficiency of either of these nutrients can produce signs of folate deficiency. Vitamin B complex with B_6 and B_{12} serve as coenzymes in the energy and protein metabolic process. Vitamin B_6 is involved of amino acid metabolism, Vitamin B_{12} in the catabolism of odd-chain-long fatty acids. Both should be substituted in form of a multi-vitamin complex, as both are decreased in the post-burn hypermetabolic response. Vitamin C plays an important role during the post-burn hypermetabolic response. During that period, oxygen-free radicals such as superoxide, peroxide, and hydroxyl may cause increased post-burn vascular permeability. Vitamin C administration, a free radical scavenger, has thus been suggested to be beneficial in terms of reducing microvascular permeability and thus required fluid volume (125).

4.4 Coagulation and clotting factors

Homeostasis of clotting is complex and has been recently investigated in thermally injured patients (126). Thrombotic and fibrinolytic mechanisms are activated after burn and the extent of activation increased with the severity of the thermal injury. Most homeostatic markers fell during the early shock phase of burns due to dilutional effects, loss and degradation of plasma proteins. Clotting factors return to normal levels after the aggressive resuscitation period. Later in the post-burn, course thrombogenicity has been suggested to be increased due to a decrease in antithrombin III, protein C, and protein S levels while fibrinolysis activation occurs via increases in tissue plasminogen activation factor, thus leading to an increased risk of thrombosis. The hypercoagulable state places many thermally injured patients at risk for disseminated intravascular coagulation (DIC). DIC has been described post mortem in 30% of the examined cases. Alterations in clotting factors indicate liver damage and should raise concern in terms of poor outcomes.

4.5 Hormones

Several hormones are produced or interact with the liver. HGF has been shown to accelerate hepatic regeneration, improve hepatic function and modulate the acute phase response in vivo and in vitro (127-129). Within 30 to 60 min of injury, plasma HGF is elevated presumably sending a strong mitogenic signal to the hepatocytes (127-129). The cause of the increase in plasma HGF is currently unknown, however, has been postulated to be due either to increased production of HGF in extrahepatic organs such as lung, spleen, kidney, or gut, or to a decrease in hepatic HGF excretion (127-129). The rapid increase in HGF stimulates hepatocyte mitogenesis, motogenesis, and DNA synthesis (27). HGF administered to normal rats only stimulates a small number of hepatocytes to enter the DNA synthesis cycle, indicating that hepatocytes in normal livers are not ready to respond to mitogenic signals without the priming events that switch them into a responsive mode (27).

Our group has shown that rhHGF administration restores homeostasis of the acute phase response post-burn (128) by increasing constitutive hepatic proteins and decreasing acute phase proteins. The exact mechanisms by which HGF stimulates constitutive hepatic proteins are unknown; however, HGF is capable of regulating the synthesis of several transcription factors, one of which is C/EBPs (130). Activation of C/EBPα during the acute phase response leads to stimulation of constitutive hepatic proteins (130) while blockade of the C/EBPβ leads to decreased synthesis of acute phase proteins (130). HGF, furthermore, exerted beneficial effects after thermal injury by increasing liver weight, liver weight per 100-g body weight and higher total hepatic protein content compared to rats receiving saline. HGF, furthermore, demonstrated no increase in liver triglyceride content, a phenomenon associated with thermal injury (15, 16).

Another hormone that is synthesized in the liver is IGF-I. IGF-I is a 7.7-kDa single-chain polypeptide of 70 amino acids with sequence homology to proinsulin (131). In the system, 95-99% of IGF-I is bound and transported with one of its six binding proteins IGFBP 1-6 (131, 132). The IGF-I system is synthesized in the liver and its production is stimulated by

GH (131-133). IGF-I has been shown to improve cell recovery, muscle protein synthesis, gut and immune function, and exert pro-mitogenic functions not only after burn, but also in various other pathological states (7, 134-137). Recent evidence suggests that IGF-I is instrumental in the early phases of liver regeneration after trauma and modulates the hepatic acute phase response in burned rats restoring hepatic homeostasis and improving hepatic morphology (136, 137). Hormones, therefore, play an important function in hepatic recovery and regeneration.

5. Importance of the liver for post-burn outcomes

In the sections above, we have described that the liver has multiple essential functions, but the question remains, is liver function and integrity essential for burn outcomes? The significance of the liver post-burn is essentially unknown. There is evidence based on the retrospective study from Price *et al.* (138) that liver function and integrity and function affect outcomes of burn victims, but no prospective evidence exists. We, therefore, conducted several studies to examine whether hepatic function can affect burn outcomes. In our first study, Barret *et al.* (29) reviewed autopsies of pediatric burn patients and determined the incidence of hepatomegaly, fatty liver, and sepsis. All patients had hepatomegaly at autopsy, while 80% had fatty infiltration of the liver. Barret *et al.* (29) further found that patients with severe hepatic fatty infiltration had a higher incidence of sepsis indicating that fatty infiltration of the liver is associated with an increased incidence of sepsis. We then asked whether hepatomegaly is specific for non-survivors or does it occur in burn patients that recover. In a large prospective study, Jeschke *et al.* (16) found that post-burn liver size significantly increased starting the first week post-burn (+185±5%), peaked at 2 weeks post-burn (+226±19%) and was increased by +189±10% at discharge. At 6, 9 and 12 months post-burn, liver weight was increased by 140%-150% compared to predicted liver weight indicating prolonged alterations in liver structure. Hepatic protein synthesis was affected up to 12 months after burn (16). We, therefore, concluded that the liver demonstrates a significant enlargement accompanied by impairment in hepatic protein synthesis.

In order to determine whether hepatomegaly and hepatic steatosis play a role in burn outcomes, Mittendorfer *et al.* (107) designed an experiment in rodents. Fatty liver was induced by nutritional manipulation and mortality after a 60% TBSA burn was determined. Our data showed that a high-fat diet caused hepatomegaly and induced fatty liver. In rats with hepatomegaly and hepatic steatosis, mortality was 40% while there were no deaths in the control group. We concluded that hepatomegaly and hepatic steatosis and dysfunction in severely burned rats are associated with increased mortality after thermal injury. Data indicated that liver integrity and function are crucial for survival post-burn (107). That the liver is important for survival was also demonstrated in other diseases (139). Deutschman *et al.* (139) demonstrated in a mouse sepsis model that IL-6 knockout mice demonstrated a tremendously increased mortality when compared to normal littermates (IL-6 competent). When the authors evaluated hepatic changes, they found that CLP induced cholestasis, steatosis, and hepatocellular injury in IL-6 -/-, but not IL-6 +/+, mice. Regeneration was absent following CLP in IL-6 -/- animals but occurred in IL-6 +/+ mice. The authors concluded that the absence of IL-6 is an important determinant of hepatic dysfunction and mortality in sepsis, but more interestingly is the fact that hepatic damage and dysfunction was associated with a 3- to 4-fold increase in mortality (139). Others and we (140, 141) hypothesize that Fas/Fas Ligand is involved in hepatic failure and hepatic apoptosis. Song *et al.* (141) elegantly demonstrated that RNA interference targeting Fas protected mice from fulminant hepatitis. The authors further showed that Fas silencing prevents death from fulminant hepatitis and concluded that hepatic dysfunction contributes to mortality and restoring hepatic function will improve mortality (141). The function of Fas/FasL in burns is not fully investigated but there is strong evidence that burn induces Fas/FasL (142) representing one possible pathay by which burn induces hepatic apoptosis and dysfunction.

As the association between organ impairment and mortality is difficult to make in animal experiments, we conducted prospective clinical studies to determine whether liver function affects post-burn outcomes. In the first study, we conducted in collaboration with the Inflammation and the Host Response to Injury group (Glue grant) (Finnerty, submitted to Nature Medicine). From a cohort of 75 patients with burns over ≥20% of the TBSA requiring surgical treatment, 16 non-survivors were identified and matched to 16 survivors. We analyzed plasma proteins by high throughput proteomic analysis in order to screen for specific protein expression and to identify a proteomic signature that can predict survival or non-survival in severely burned patients (Finnerty, submitted to Nature Medicine). The profiling of the 32 samples led to a total of 4,163 different peptides corresponding to 602 different plasma proteins. Our analysis identified 39 proteins that were statistically different between the two groups. We found that 23 of these proteins are produced in the liver and are either part of the coagulation cascade, the complement response, hepatic acute phase response signaling, and hepatic fibrosis and stellate cell activation. These data indicate that the proteomic signature associated with outcomes predicts outcomes. Furthermore, data indicate that the majority of the 39 proteins differentially expressed in non-survivors after burn are produced in the liver. This strongly supports the hypothesis in a randomized multicenter trial, that the liver function and integrity play orchestrates and determines post-burn outcomes and survival. As mortality represents a very strong outcome, we then asked whether liver protein could further predict the incidence of multi-organ failure. Twenty-two patients with similar burn size and injury severity were divided into burn with multi-organ failure (MOF) (DENVER >4) and no MOF. We determined the proteomic signature at admit and at peak DENVER. We found that 20 proteins were differently expressed in burn patients with MOF and burn patients without MOF. Of these 20 proteins, 15 proteins are produced in the liver and can be categorized into acute phase proteins, coagulation, inflammation, and liver metabolism (unpublished data). This finding indicates that liver function and protein production not only determines survival, but also the incidence of MOF, delineating the importance of the liver post-burn.

Lastly, we conducted a large follow-up study and divided 100 control patients (receiving no anabolic or experimental drug) into survivors and non-survivors. In order to screen for possible serum biomarkers predictors, we studied data sets comprising hormones, proteins, cytokines, and electrolytes. Different supervised and unsupervised feature extraction techniques and quadratic discriminant analysis (QDA) were applied to classify data using all the features. We used the plot for the empirical cumulative distribution (CDF) of the p-values to decide the number of features needed for our study for the purpose of data reduction. Patient demographic and injury severity was similar between the two groups. We found using 38 serum biomarkers that eight "features" have strong discrimination. Biomarkers free fatty acid, retinol binding protein, pre-albumin/albumin, α1-acid glycoprotein, alanine amino transferase, apolipoprotein A1, and haptoglobin are the most significant and important proteins indicating if the patient is in a higher risk to die in the early-stage post-burn. We calculated the probability to survive based on the fitted model and the performance was >0.97. These data from severely burned pediatric patients confirm the data from burned adults and again emphasize the importance of hepatic proteins on survival and post-burn outcomes.

6. Conclusion

In summary, a severe burn represents a devastating injury affecting nearly every organ system and leading to significant morbidity and mortality (7). In this review, we delineated the central role of the liver during the post-burn response. The liver has not only one myriad functions that are each essential for survival. All of these hepatic functions are affected by a thermal injury, and we have strong evidence that hepatic biomarkers predict and determine morbidity and mortality in severely burned patients. We, therefore, believe that the liver is central for post-burn outcome and we propose that attenuation of liver damage and restoration of liver function will improve morbidity and mortality of severely burned patients. Our hypothesis is being supported by a recent book on the liver in which Will Self writes, "Our livers are more valuable than we are, more able, more alive" (143).

7. Acknowledgments

This review paper was supported by the Shriners Hospitals for Children 8660, 8760, and 9145, NIH RO1 GM087285-01A2. CFI Leader's Opportunity Fund application (Project # 25407) and Physicians' Services Incorporated Foundation - Health Research Grant Program - Author has no disclosures to declare.

8. References

[1] Bringham PA, McLoughlin E. (1996) Burn incidence and medical care use in the United States: estimates, trends and data sources. *J Burn Care Rehabil* 17: 95-107.

[2] (2002) World Health Organization (WHO). A graphical overview of the global burden of injuries. The Injury Chart Book, Geneva.

[3] Palmieri TL, Greenhalgh DG. (2002) Topical treatment of pediatric patients with burns: a practical guide. *Am J Clin Dermatol* 3: 529-534.

[4] Nelson KJ, Beierle EA. (2005) Exhaust system burn injuries in children. *J Pediatr Surg* 40: E43-46.

[5] Foglia RP, Moushey R, Meadows L, Seigel J, Smith M. (2004) Evolving treatment in a decade of pediatric burn care. *J Pediatr Surg* 39: 957-960.

[6] Miller SF, *et al.* (2006) National Burn Repository 2005: a ten-year review. *J Burn Care Res* 27: 411-436.

[7] Herndon DN, Tompkins RG. (2004) Support of the metabolic response to burn injury. *Lancet* 363: 1895-1902.

[8] Herndon DN, Hart DW, Wolf SE, Chinkes DL, Wolfe RR. (2001) Reversal of catabolism by beta-blockade after severe burns. *N Engl J Med* 345: 1223-1229.

[9] Van den Berge G, *et al.* (2001) Intensive insulin therapy in critically ill patients. *New Engl J Med* 345: 1359-1367.

[10] Finnerty CC, *et al.* (2006) Cytokine expression profile over time in severely burned pediatric patients. *Shock* 26: 13-19.

[11] Tracey KJ, *et al.* (1987) Anti-cachectin/TNF monoclonal antibodies prevent septic shock during lethal bacteraemia. *Nature* 330: 662-664.
[12] Tracey KJ, *et al.* (1987) Cachectin/tumor necrosis factor induces lethal shock and stress hormone responses in the dog. *Surg Gynecol Obstet* 164: 415-422.
[13] Moshage H. (1997) Cytokines and the hepatic acute phase response. *J Pathol* 181: 257-266.
[14] Jeschke MG, Klein D, Herndon DN. (2004) Insulin treatment improves the systemic inflammatory reaction to severe trauma. *Ann Surg* 239: 553-560.
[15] Jeschke MG, *et al.* (2001) Cell proliferation, apoptosis, NF-kappaB expression, enzyme, protein, and weight changes in livers of burned rats. *Am J Physiol Gastrointest Liver Physiol* 280: G1314-1320.
[16] Jeschke MG, Micak RP, Finnerty CC, Herndon DN. (2007) Changes in liver function and size after a severe thermal injury. *Shock* 28: 172-177.
[17] Jeschke MG, *et al.* (2005) Insulin prevents liver damage and preserves liver function in lipopolysaccharide-induced endotoxemic rats. *J Hepatol* 42: 870-879.
[18] Moll KJ. (2008) Anatomie. Leber. Jungjohann Verlag, München.
[19] Winkeltau G, Kraas E. (2006) Leber. In: *Chirurgie*. Schumpelick V, Bleese NM, Mommsen U (eds.) Enke Verlag, Stuttgart, pp. 658-675.
[20] Schwartz SI. (1999) Liver. In: *Principles of Surgery*. Schwartz SI, Shires GT, Spencer FC, Daly JM, Fischer JE, Galloway AC (eds.) McGraw-Hill, New York, pp. 1395-1436.
[21] Küttler T. (2004) Biochemie. In: *Biochemie*. Küttler T (ed.) Jungjohann Verlag, München, pp. 240-265.
[22] Jeschke MG, Barrow RE, Herndon DN. (2004) Extended hypermetabolic response of the liver in severely burned pediatric patients. *Arch Surg* 139: 641-647.
[23] Wolfe RR, Durkot MJ, Allsop JR, Burke JF. (1979) Glucose metabolism in severely burned patients. *Metabolism* 28: 1031-1039.
[24] Wolfe RR, Herndon DN, Jahoor F, Miyoshi H, Wolfe M. (1987) Effect of severe burn injury on substrate cycling by glucose and fatty acids. *N Engl J Med* 317: 403-408.
[25] Aarsland A, Chinkes D, Wolfe RR. (1996) Contributions of de novo synthesis of fatty acids to total VLDL-triglyceride secretion during prolonged hyperglycemia/hyperinsulinemia in normal man. *J Clin Invest* 98: 2008-2017.
[26] Jeschke MG, *et al.* (2008) Pathophysiologic response to severe burn injury. *Ann Surg* 248: 387-401.
[27] Gomez-Lechon MJ, *et al.* (1995) Effects of hepatocyte growth factor on the growth and metabolism of human hepatocytes in primary culture. *Hepatology* 21: 1248-1254.
[28] Linares H. (1991) Autopsy finding in burned children. In: *Burns in Children*. Carvajal H, Parks D (eds.) Year Book Medical, Chicago, pp. 1-25.
[29] Barret JP, Jeschke MG, Herndon DN. (2001) Fatty infiltration of the liver in severely burned pediatric patients: autopsy findings and clinical implications. *J Trauma* 51: 736-739.
[30] Steller H. (1995) Mechanisms and genes of cellular suicide. *Science* 267: 1445-1449.
[31] Ramzy PI, *et al.* (2000) Gut epithelial apoptosis after severe burn: effects of gut hypoperfusion. *J Am Coll Surg* 190: 281-287.
[32] Wolf SE, *et al.* (1999) Cutaneous burn increases apoptosis in the gut epithelium of mice. *J Am Coll Surg* 188: 10-16.

[33] Horton JW. (2004) Left ventricular contractile dysfunction as a complication of thermal injury. *Shock* 22: 495-507.
[34] Horton JW, *et al.* (1999) Calcium antagonists improve cardiac mechanical performance after thermal trauma. *J Surg Res* 87: 39-50.
[35] Baron P, *et al.* (1994) Gut failure and translocation following burn and sepsis. *J Surg Res* 57: 197-204.
[36] Baron PW, Barrow RE, Pierre EJ, Herndon DN. (1997) Prolonged use of propranolol safely decreases cardiac work in burned children. *J Burn Care Rehabil* 18: 223-227.
[37] Ikeda H, *et al.* (1998) Apoptosis is a major mode of cell death caused by ischaemia and ischaemia/reperfusion injury to the rat intestinal epithelium. *Gut* 42: 530-537.
[38] Noda T, Iwakiri R, Fujimoto K, Matsuo S, Aw TY. (1998) Programmed cell death induced by ischemia-reperfusion in rat intestinal mucosa. *Am J Physiol* 274: G270-276.
[39] Bellas RE, FitzGerald MJ, Fausto N, Sonenshein GE. (1997) Inhibition of NF-kappa B activity induces apoptosis in murine hepatocytes. *Am J Pathol* 151: 891-896.
[40] Boehning D, *et al.* (2003) Cytochrome c binds to inositol (1,4,5) trisphosphate receptors, amplifying calcium-dependent apoptosis. *Nat Cell Biol* 5: 1051-1061.
[41] Strasser A, O'Connor L, Dixit VM. (2000) Apoptosis signaling. *Annu Rev Biochem* 69: 217-245.
[42] Yoneda T, *et al.* (2001) Activation of caspase-12, an endoplastic reticulum (ER) resident caspase, through tumor necrosis factor receptor-associated factor 2-dependent mechanism in response to the ER stress. *J Biol Chem* 276: 13935-13940.
[43] Klein D, Schubert T, Horch RE, Jauch KW, Jeschke MG. (2004) Insulin treatment improves hepatic morphology and function through modulation of hepatic signals after severe trauma. *Ann Surg* 240: 340-349.
[44] Gauglitz GG, *et al.* (2008) Characterization of the inflammatory response during acute and post-acute phases after severe burn. *Shock* 30: 503-507.
[45] Jeschke MG, Boehning DF, Finnerty CC, Herndon DN. (2007) Effect of insulin on the inflammatory and acute phase response after burn injury. *Crit Care Med* 35: S519-523.
[46] Jeschke MG, *et al.* (2009) Calcium and ER stress mediate hepatic apoptosis after burn injury. *J Cell Mol Med*: [Epub ahead of print].
[47] Ozcan U, *et al.* (2006) Chemical chaperones reduce ER stress and restore glucose homeostasis in a mouse model of type 2 diabetes. *Science* 313: 1137-1140.
[48] Wiseman RL, Balch WE. (2005) A new pharmacology--drugging stressed folding pathways. *Trends Mol Med* 11: 347-350.
[49] Cano N, Gerolami A. (1983) Intrahepatic cholestasis during total parenteral nutrition. *Lancet* 1: 985.
[50] Bolder U, *et al.* (2006) Heat stress enhances recovery of hepatocyte bile acid and organic anion transporters in endotoxemic rats by multiple mechanisms. *Cell Stress Chaperones* 11: 89-100.
[51] Bolder U, Ton-Nu HT, Schteingart CD, Frick E, Hofmann AF. (1997) Hepatocyte transport of bile acids and organic anions in endotoxemic rats: impaired uptake and secretion. *Gastroenterology* 112: 214-225.

[52] Knox J, Demling R, Wilmore D, Sarraf P, Santos A. (1995) Increased survival after major thermal injury: the effect of growth hormone therapy in adults. *J Trauma* 39: 526-532.

[53] Kobayashi M, *et al.* (2002) An increase in the susceptibility of burned patients to infectious complications due to impaired production of macrophage inflammatory protein 1 alpha. *J Immunol* 169: 4460-4466.

[54] Kobayashi M, *et al.* (2006) Bacterial sepsis and chemokines. *Curr Drug Targets* 7: 119-134.

[55] Trop M, Schiffrin EJ, Callahan RJ, Strauss HW, Carter EA. (1990) Effect of acute burn trauma on reticuloendothelial system phagocytic activity in rats. II: Comparison of uptake of radiolabelled colloid and bacteria. *Burns* 16: 278-280.

[56] Trop M, Schiffrin EJ, Carter EA. (1990) Role of skin in the burn-induced reduction of reticuloendothelial phagocytic activity in rats. *Burns* 16: 57-59.

[57] Klein D, Einspanier R, Bolder U, Jeschke MG. (2003) Differences in the hepatic signal transcription pathway and cytokine expression between thermal injury and sepsis. *Shock* 20: 536-543.

[58] Hart DW, *et al.* (2000) Determinants of skeletal muscle catabolism after severe burn. *Ann Surg* 232: 455-465.

[59] Reiss E, Pearson E, Artz CP. (1956) The metabolic response to burns. *J Clin Invest* 35: 62-77.

[60] Haze K, Yoshida H, Yanagi H, Yura T, Mori K. (1999) Mammalian transcription factor ATF6 is synthesized as a transmembrane protein and activated by proteolysis in response to endoplasmic reticulum stress. *Mol Biol Cell* 10: 3787-3799.

[61] Hart DW, *et al.* (2000) Persistence of muscle catabolism after severe burn. *Surgery* 128: 312-319.

[62] Norbury WB, Herndon DN. (2007) Modulation of the hypermetabolic response after burn injury. In: *Total Burn Care.* Herndon DN (ed.) Saunders Elsevier, New York, pp. 420-433.

[63] Norbury WB, Herndon DN, Branski LK, Chinkes DL, Jeschke MG. (2008) Urinary cortisol and catecholamine excretion following burn injury in children. *J Clin Endocrinol Metab* 93: 1270-1275.

[64] Sherwood ER, Toliver-Kinsky T. (2004) Mechanisms of the inflammatory response. *Best Pract Res Clin Anaesthesiol* 18: 385-405.

[65] Pereira CT, Herndon DN. (2005) The pharmacologic modulation of the hypermetabolic response to burns. *Adv Surg* 39: 245-261.

[66] Wolfe RR. (1981) Review: acute versus chronic response to burn injury. *Circ Shock* 8: 105-115.

[67] Cuthbertson DP, Angeles Valero Zanuy MA, Leon Sanz ML. (2001) Post-shock metabolic response. 1942. *Nutr Hosp* 16: 176-182.

[68] Tredget EE, Yu YM. (1992) The metabolic effects of thermal injury. *World J Surg* 16: 68-79.

[69] Cree MG, *et al.* (2007) Insulin sensitivity and mitochondrial function are improved in children with burn injury during a randomized controlled trial of fenofibrate. *Ann Surg* 245: 214-221.

[70] Jeschke MG, *et al.* (2007) Burn size determines the inflammatory and hypermetabolic response. *Crit Care* 11: R90.

[71] Mlcak RP, Jeschke MG, Barrow RE, Herndon DN. (2006) The influence of age and gender on resting energy expenditure in severely burned children. *Ann Surg* 244: 121-130.
[72] Gearhart MM, Parbhoo SK. (2006) Hyperglycemia in the critically ill patient. *AACN Clin Issues* 17: 50-55.
[73] Robinson LE, van Soeren MH. (2004) Insulin resistance and hyperglycemia in critical illness: role of insulin in glycemic control. *AACN Clin Issues* 15: 45-62.
[74] Khani S, Tayek JA. (2001) Cortisol increases gluconeogenesis in humans: its role in the metabolic syndrome. *Clin Sci (Lond)* 101: 739-747.
[75] Wolfe RR, *et al.* (1987) Regulation of lipolysis in severely burned children. *Ann Surg* 206: 214-221.
[76] Gore DC, Jahoor F, Wolfe RR, Herndon DN. (1993) Acute response of human muscle protein to catabolic hormones. *Ann Surg* 218: 679-684.
[77] Carlson GL. (2001) Insulin resistance and glucose-induced thermogenesis in critical illness. *Proc Nutr Soc* 60: 381-388.
[78] Cree MG, *et al.* (2008) Human mitochondrial oxidative capacity is acutely impaired after burn trauma. *Am J Surg* 196: 234-239.
[79] Hunt DG, Ivy JL. (2002) Epinephrine inhibits insulin-stimulated muscle glucose transport. *J Appl Physiol* 93: 1638-1643.
[80] Cree MG, *et al.* (2007) PPAR-alpha agonism improves whole body and muscle mitochondrial fat oxidation, but does not alter intracellular fat concentrations in burn trauma children in a randomized controlled trial. *Nutr Metab (Lond)* 4: 9.
[81] Gustavson SM, *et al.* (2003) Glucagon's actions are modified by the combination of epinephrine and gluconeogenic precursor infusion. *Am J Physiol Endocrinol Metab* 285: E534-544.
[82] Akita S, *et al.* (2006) Elevated circulating leukemia inhibitory factor in patients with extensive burns. *J Burn Care Res* 27: 221-225.
[83] Lang CH. (1992) Sepsis-induced insulin resistance in rats is mediated by a beta-adrenergic mechanism. *Am J Physiol* 263: E703-711.
[84] Lang CH, Dobrescu C, Bagby GJ. (1992) Tumor necrosis factor impairs insulin action on peripheral glucose disposal and hepatic glucose output. *Endocrinology* 130: 43-52.
[85] Lang CH, Frost RA, Vary TC. (2007) Regulation of muscle protein synthesis during sepsis and inflammation. *Am J Physiol Endocrinol Metab* 293: E453-459.
[86] Fan J, Li YH, Wojnar MM, Lang CH. (1996) Endotoxin-induced alterations in insulin-stimulated phosphorylation of insulin receptor, IRS-1, and MAP kinase in skeletal muscle. *Shock* 6: 164-170.
[87] del Aguila LF, Claffey KP, Kirwan JP. (1999) TNF-alpha impairs insulin signaling and insulin stimulation of glucose uptake in C2C12 muscle cells. *Am J Physiol* 276: E849-855.
[88] Sell H, Dietze-Schroeder D, Kaiser U, Eckel J. (2006) Monocyte chemotactic protein-1 is a potential player in the negative cross-talk between adipose tissue and skeletal muscle. *Endocrinology* 147: 2458-2467.
[89] Jahoor F, Desai M, Herndon DN, Wolfe RR. (1988) Dynamics of the protein metabolic response to burn injury. *Metabolism* 37: 330-337.
[90] Jahoor F, Herndon DN, Wolfe RR. (1986) Role of insulin and glucagon in the response of glucose and alanine kinetics in burn-injured patients. *J Clin Invest* 78: 807-814.

[91] Gauglitz GG, Herndon DN, Kulp GA, Meyer WJ, 3rd, Jeschke MG. (2009) Abnormal insulin sensitivity persists up to three years in pediatric patients post-burn. *J Clin Endocrinol Metab*: [Epub ahead of print].

[92] Ikezu T, Okamoto T, Yonezawa K, Tompkins RG, Martyn JA. (1997) Analysis of thermal injury-induced insulin resistance in rodents. Implication of postreceptor mechanisms. *J Biol Chem* 272: 25289-25295.

[93] Saffle JR, Graves C. (2007) Nutritional support of the burned patient. In: *Total Burn Care*. Herndon DN (ed.) Saunders Elsevier, London, pp. 398-419.

[94] DeFronzo RA, *et al.* (1981) The effect of insulin on the disposal of intravenous glucose. Results from indirect calorimetry and hepatic and femoral venous catheterization. *Diabetes* 30: 1000-1007.

[95] Flakoll PJ, Hill JO, Abumrad NN. (1993) Acute hyperglycemia enhances proteolysis in normal man. *Am J Physiol* 265: E715-721.

[96] Chang DW, DeSanti L, Demling RH. (1998) Anticatabolic and anabolic strategies in critical illness: a review of current treatment modalities. *Shock* 10: 155-160.

[97] Hart DW, *et al.* (2000) Determinants of skeletal muscle catabolism after severe burn. *Ann Surg* 232: 455-465.

[98] Przkora R, *et al.* (2006) Body composition changes with time in pediatric burn patients. *J Trauma* 60: 968-971.

[99] Przkora R, *et al.* (2005) Metabolic and hormonal changes of severely burned children receiving long-term oxandrolone treatment. *Ann Surg* 242: 384-391.

[100] Wolfe BM, Walker BK, Shaul DB, Wong L, Ruebner BH. (1988) Effect of total parenteral nutrition on hepatic histology. *Arch Surg* 123: 1084-1090.

[101] Aarsland A, *et al.* (1998) Insulin therapy in burn patients does not contribute to hepatic triglyceride production. *J Clin Invest* 101: 2233-2239.

[102] Barrow RE, Mlcak R, Barrow LN, Hawkins HK. (2004) Increased liver weights in severely burned children: comparison of ultrasound and autopsy measurements. *Burns* 30: 565-568.

[103] Barrow RE, Wolfe RR, Dasu MR, Barrow LN, Herndon DN. (2006) The use of beta-adrenergic blockade in preventing trauma-induced hepatomegaly. *Ann Surg* 243: 115-120.

[104] Aarsland A, *et al.* (1996) Beta-blockade lowers peripheral lipolysis in burn patients receiving growth hormone. Rate of hepatic very low density lipoprotein triglyceride secretion remains unchanged. *Ann Surg* 223: 777-789.

[105] Morio B, Irtun O, Herndon DN, Wolfe RR. (2002) Propranolol decreases splanchnic triacylglycerol storage in burn patients receiving a high-carbohydrate diet. *Ann Surg* 236: 218-225.

[106] Martini WZ, *et al.* (2001) Alteration of hepatic fatty acid metabolism after burn injury in pigs. *JPEN J Parenter Enteral Nutr* 25: 310-316.

[107] Mittendorfer B, Jeschke MG, Wolf SE, Sidossis LS. (1998) Nutritional hepatic steatosis and mortality after burn injury in rats. *Clin Nutr* 17: 293-299.

[108] Deng QG, *et al.* (2005) Steatohepatitis induced by intragastric overfeeding in mice. *Hepatology* 42: 905-914.

[109] Gilpin DA, Hsieh CC, Kuninger DT, Herndon DN, Papaconstantinou J. (1996) Effect of thermal injury on the expression of transcription factors that regulate acute phase

response genes: the response of C/EBP alpha, C/EBP beta, and C/EBP delta to thermal injury. *Surgery* 119: 674-683.

[110] Gilpin DA, Hsieh CC, Kuninger DT, Herndon DN, Papaconstantinou J. (1996) Regulation of the acute phase response genes alpha 1-acid glycoprotein and alpha 1-antitrypsin correlates with sensitivity to thermal injury. *Surgery* 119: 664-673.

[111] Hiyama DT, *et al.* (1991) Synthesis of albumin and acute-phase proteins in perfused liver after burn injury in rats. *J Burn Care Rehabil* 12: 1-6.

[112] Livingston DH, Mosenthal AC, Deitch EA. (1995) Sepsis and multiple organ dysfunction syndrome: a clinical-mechanistic overview. *New Horiz* 3: 257-266.

[113] De Maio A, Mooney ML, Matesic LE, Paidas CN, Reeves RH. (1998) Genetic component in the inflammatory response induced by bacterial lipopolysaccharide. *Shock* 10: 319-323.

[114] De Maio A, Torres MB, Reeves RH. (2005) Genetic determinants influencing the response to injury, inflammation, and sepsis. *Shock* 23: 11-17.

[115] Selzman CH, *et al.* (1998) Therapeutic implications of interleukin-10 in surgical disease. *Shock* 10: 309-318.

[116] Finnerty CC, Herndon DN, Chinkes DL, Jeschke MG. (2007) Serum cytokine differences in severely burned children with and without sepsis. *Shock* 27: 4-9.

[117] Siebenlist U, Franzoso G, Brown K. (1994) Structure, regulation and function of NF-kappa B. *Annu Rev Cell Biol* 10: 405-455.

[118] Kishimoto T, Taga T, Akira S. (1994) Cytokine signal transduction. *Cell* 76: 253-262.

[119] Niehof M, *et al.* (2001) Interleukin-6-induced tethering of STAT3 to the LAP/C/EBPbeta promoter suggests a new mechanism of transcriptional regulation by STAT3. *J Biol Chem* 276: 9016-9027.

[120] Janes KA, *et al.* (2005) A systems model of signaling identifies a molecular basis set for cytokine-induced apoptosis. *Science* 310: 1646-1653.

[121] Mori K, Ma W, Gething MJ, Sambrook J. (1993) A transmembrane protein with a cdc2+/CDC28-related kinase activity is required for signaling from the ER to the nucleus. *Cell* 74: 743-756.

[122] Chan MM, Chan GM. (2009) Nutritional therapy for burns in children and adults. *Nutrition* 25: 261-269.

[123] Nguyen TT, *et al.* (1993) Free radical activity and loss of plasma antioxidants, vitamin E, and sulfhydryl groups in patients with burns: the 1993 Moyer Award. *J Burn Care Rehabil* 14: 602-609.

[124] Manning AJ, Meyer N, Klein GL. (2007) Vitamin and trace element homeostasis following burn injury. In: *Total Burn Care.* Herndon DN (ed.) WB Saunders, Philadelphia, pp. 251-255.

[125] Matsuda T, *et al.* (1991) Reduced fluid volume requirement for resuscitation of third-degree burns with high-dose vitamin C. *J Burn Care Rehabil* 12: 525-532.

[126] Sherwood ER, Traber DL. (2007) The systemic inflammatory response syndrome. In: *Total Burn Care.* Herndon DN (ed.) WB Saunders, Philadelphia, pp. 292-309.

[127] Guillen MI, Gomez-Lechon MJ, Nakamura T, Castell JV. (1996) The hepatocyte growth factor regulates the synthesis of acute-phase proteins in human hepatocytes: divergent effect on interleukin-6-stimulated genes. *Hepatology* 23: 1345-1352.

[128] Jeschke MG, *et al.* (2000) Hepatocyte growth factor modulates the hepatic acute-phase response in thermally injured rats. *Crit Care Med* 28: 504-510.

[129] Yamashita Y, Jeschke MG, Wolf SE. (2000) Differential expression of hepatocyte growth factor in liver, kidney, lung, and spleen following burn in rats. *Cytokine* 12: 1293-1298.

[130] Cho MK, Kim SG. (2003) Hepatocyte growth factor activates CCAAT enhancer binding protein and cell replication via PI3-kinase pathway. *Hepatology* 37: 686-695.

[131] Humbel RE. (1990) Insulin-like growth factors I and II. *Eur J Biochem* 190: 445-462.

[132] Baxter RC. (1990) Circulating levels and molecular distribution of the acid-labile (alpha) subunit of the high molecular weight insulin-like growth factor-binding protein complex. *J Clin Endocrinol Metab* 70: 1347-1353.

[133] Jeschke MG, Chrysopoulo MT, Herndon DN, Wolf SE. (1999) Increased expression of insulin-like growth factor-I in serum and liver after recombinant human growth hormone administration in thermally injured rats. *J Surg Res* 85: 171-177.

[134] Herndon DN, *et al.* (1999) Muscle protein catabolism after severe burn, effects of IGF-1/IGFBP3 treatment. *Ann Surg* 229: 713-720.

[135] Jeschke MG, *et al.* (2008) Combination of recombinant human growth hormone and propranolol decreases hypermetabolism and inflammation in severely burned children. *Pediatr Crit Care Med* 9: 209-216.

[136] Jeschke MG, Herndon DN, Barrow RE. (2000) Insulin-like growth factor I in combination with insulin-like growth factor binding protein 3 affects the hepatic acute phase response and hepatic morphology in thermally injured rats. *Ann Surg* 231: 408-416.

[137] Jeschke MG, *et al.* (2001) IGF-I/BP-3 administration preserves hepatic homeostasis after thermal injury which is associated with increases in no and hepatic NF-kappa B. *Shock* 16: 373-379.

[138] Price LA, Thombs B, Chen CL, Milner SM. (2007) Liver disease in burn injury: evidence from a national sample of 31,338 adult patients. *J Burns Wounds* 7: e1.

[139] Deutschman CS, Cereda M, Ochroch EA, Raj NR. (2006) Sepsis-induced cholestasis, steatosis, hepatocellular injury, and impaired hepatocellular regeneration are enhanced in interleukin-6 -/- mice. *Crit Care Med* 34: 2613-2620.

[140] Cheng J, *et al.* (1994) Protection from Fas-mediated apoptosis by a soluble form of the Fas molecule. *Science* 263: 1759-1762.

[141] Song E, *et al.* (2003) RNA interference targeting Fas protects mice from fulminant hepatitis. *Nat Med* 9: 347-351.

[142] Jeschke MG, *et al.* (2007) Gut mucosal homeostasis and cellular mediators after severe thermal trauma and the effect of insulin-like growth factor-I in combination with insulin-like growth factor binding protein-3. *Endocrinology* 148: 354-362.

[143] Self W. (2008) Liver: A Fictional Organ with a Surface Anatomy of Four Lobes. In: Self W (ed.). Viking Books, New York.

9

Adipocytokines in Severe Sepsis and Septic Shock

Hanna Dückers, Frank Tacke,
Christian Trautwein and Alexander Koch
Department of Medicine III, RWTH-University Hospital Aachen, Germany

1. Introduction

Among the different conditions of critical illness leading to admission to an Intensive Care Unit (ICU), sepsis remains the leading cause of death at the non-coronary medical ICU [1]. Even with optimal therapy, mortality rates of severe sepsis and septic shock are about 40 to 50% [2, 3]. Although there are numerous studies with varying methods from different countries, the incidence of severe sepsis is constantly approximately one out of ten admissions to all ICUs worldwide [4]. With millions of individuals concerned every year, worldwide sepsis is one of the major healthcare problems today. The proportion of severe sepsis, and case fatal outcomes increased during the last years [2]. It is crucial to establish the diagnosis sepsis as early as possible and to identify its origin, in order to initiate an appropriate therapy permitting to achieve the best possible outcome [5].

Sepsis is defined as a systemic inflammatory response syndrome (SIRS) caused by an infection. The association with organ dysfunction or sepsis-induced hypotension is termed severe sepsis. Septic shock, as a subset of severe sepsis, is characterized by sepsis-induced hypotension, persisting despite adequate fluid resuscitation [6]. Early differentiation between sepsis and SIRS is a considerable problem in the treatment of patients on ICU. Due to the early systemic release of inflammatory cytokines as compared with synthesis of acute-phase-proteins, cytokines have been widely investigated for their diagnostic potential in predicting sepsis [7]. Nevertheless, until now the perfect biomarker for differentiation of sepsis and SIRS has not been found yet and ongoing research focuses on identification of appropriate diagnostic biomarkers for sepsis [8].

Despite a growing number of studies, the physiopathology of sepsis is not satisfyingly understood. Data show that physiopathology is characterized by a large number of pro- and anti-inflammatory cytokines and mediators of inflammation with complex interactions [9]. For instance, the application of a single bolus i.v. infusion of endotoxin to a healthy individual leads to the expression of 3147 genes, (> 10% of the human genome) [10]. These mediators and cytokines lead to endothelial dysfunction and activation of inflammatory and coagulation pathways as reaction to the invasion of a pathogen [11]. In order to reduce the sepsis-related high mortality, a better understanding of common pathogenic mechanisms of sepsis and other critical diseases is needed, potentially resulting in more effective treatment options.

2. Obesity in critical disease

At present, obesity is regarded as a low-grade proinflammatory state with oxidative stress caused by glucose and macronutrient intake. In this setting various proinflammatory cytokines and acute phase reactants are induced, e.g. TNF-α and IL-6, which are mainly derived from the macrophages as part of the white adipose tissue [11, 12]. Oxidative stress leads to the production of reactive oxygen species (ROS) with NADPH oxidase as major vascular source of ROS [13]. ROS are particularly important for endothelial dysfunction and can cause cellular injury [14]. For these reasons the reaction to sepsis in obese individuals is different than those in individuals without chronic inflammatory state [11].

Obesity has been suggested as a prominent risk factor for mortality in critically ill patients, especially in sepsis [15, 16]. Singer et al. hypothesized that continuous low-grade chronic inflammation primes blood and endothelial cells to reply more rapidly to any additional inflammatory stimulus, such as sepsis [17]. However, recent publications on critical disease, only reported an influence of obesity on morbidity, but not on mortality [18, 19]. This means that obese and very obese patients acquired more frequently ICU-associated infections and had a longer length-of-stay, but there was no evidence for a higher 60-day in-hospital mortality compared with normal weighted patients in the study of Sakr et al. [19] .

3. Hyperglycemia and insulin resistance in critical disease

As in obesity, hyperglycemia, impaired glucose tolerance and insulin resistance are common findings in critically ill patients after surgery or with sepsis [20]. This feature has also been termed "diabetes of injury" [21, 22]. Hyperglycemia in hospitalized patients is known to lead to various adverse effects (e.g. fluid imbalance, alterations of immune function and inflammation), which are commonly improved by glucose control [23] (Table).

Adverse effects of Acute Hyperglycemia
Blood-flow abnormalities
Increase of vascular permeability
Electrolyte disturbances
Fluid shifts
Acid-base disturbances
Proinflammatory gene expression
Immune dysfunction
Impairment of complement activity
Inhibition of opsonization
Catabolism

Table 1. Adverse effects of Acute Hyperglycemia in critical illness (modified from [23])

In case of critical disease or trauma hepatic gluconeogenesis is increasing despite hyperglycemia and high insulin levels, whereas insulin-dependent glucose uptake in skeletal muscle and heart is impaired. In critically ill patients the overall glucose-uptake is elevated but mainly in tissues which do not depend on insulin for glucose uptake [24]. Hyperglycemia in critically ill patients has been related to mediators of stress, but there is growing evidence for causative defects in glucose metabolism [25] (Fig.1). Moreover, proinflammatory cytokines can affect glucose metabolism by changing insulin receptor signaling and by boosting counterregulatory hormone secretion [21, 26]. Likely, adipocytokines link hyperglycemia and insulin resistance to inflammation in sepsis.

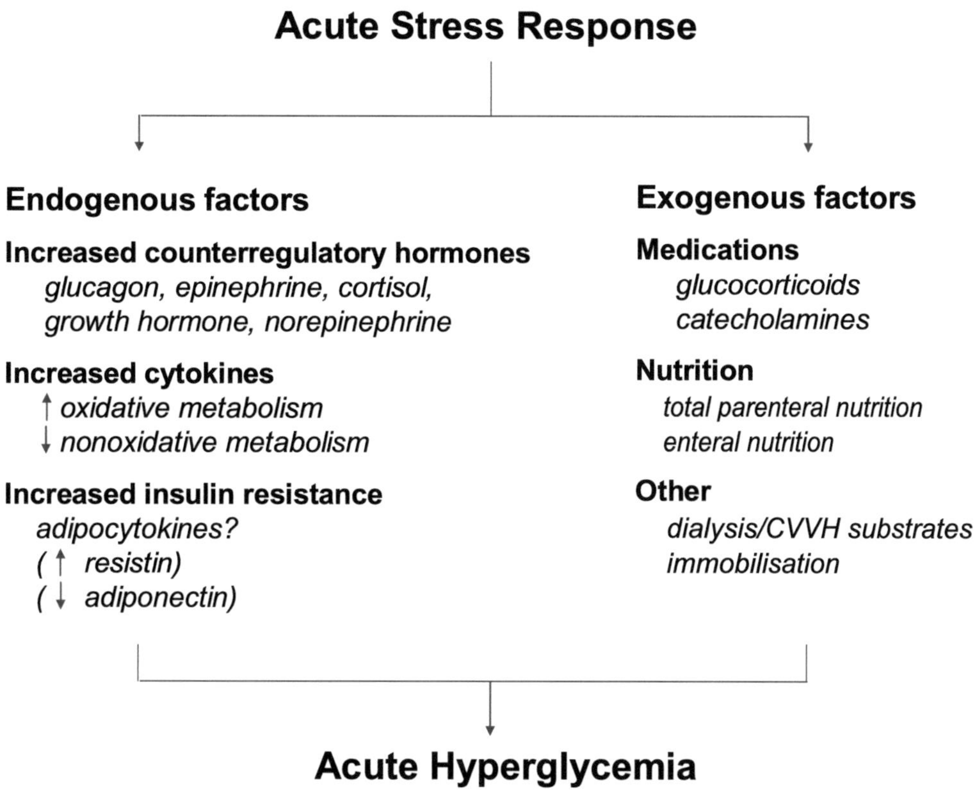

Fig. 1. Etiology of acute hyperglycemia. Acute stress response is characterized by complex interactions of counter-regulatory hormones, cytokines and insulin sensitivity (modified from [23]).

In 2001 a milestone study from van den Berghe et al. showed that tight control of hyperglycemia during critical illness in a cohort of cardiac surgery patients significantly improved outcome in terms of morbidity and mortality. Adjustment of hyperglycemia resulted in less severe nosocomial infections, renal and hepatic dysfunction, critical illness polyneuropathy, muscle weakness, and anemia [27, 28]. Increasing hyperglycemia paralleled increase in rates of mortality in critical illness [27]. Nevertheless, consecutive studies in medical ICU patients demonstrated higher mortality for intensive insulin therapy, potentially due to severe hypoglycemia [29]. Therefore, control of hyperglycemia by insulin therapy in a moderate range of blood glucose levels of 140-180 mg/dL is at present part of standard therapy in critically ill patients.

4. Adipose tissue as a hormonally active organ

Historically, adipose tissue was solely considered to store excess energy. Most recent data emphasize the role of adipose tissue as a hormonally active system, influencing inflammation, metabolism, body weight, and lipid and glucose metabolism [30]. Proteins mainly secreted by adipocytes are called adipokines [11]. Matsuzawa and colleagues reported that approximately 30% of all genes expressed in visceral fat encode secretory proteins [31]. An increasing number of soluble mediators ("adipocytokines") mainly derived from adipocytes itself or other cell types from adipose tissue (e.g. stromavascular fraction, adipose precursor cells and macrophages in the adipose tissue) have been identified. Adipocytokines are important mediators linking chronic inflammatory conditions to systemic insulin resistance in obesity and diabetes mellitus type 2 [18, 32] (Fig.2).

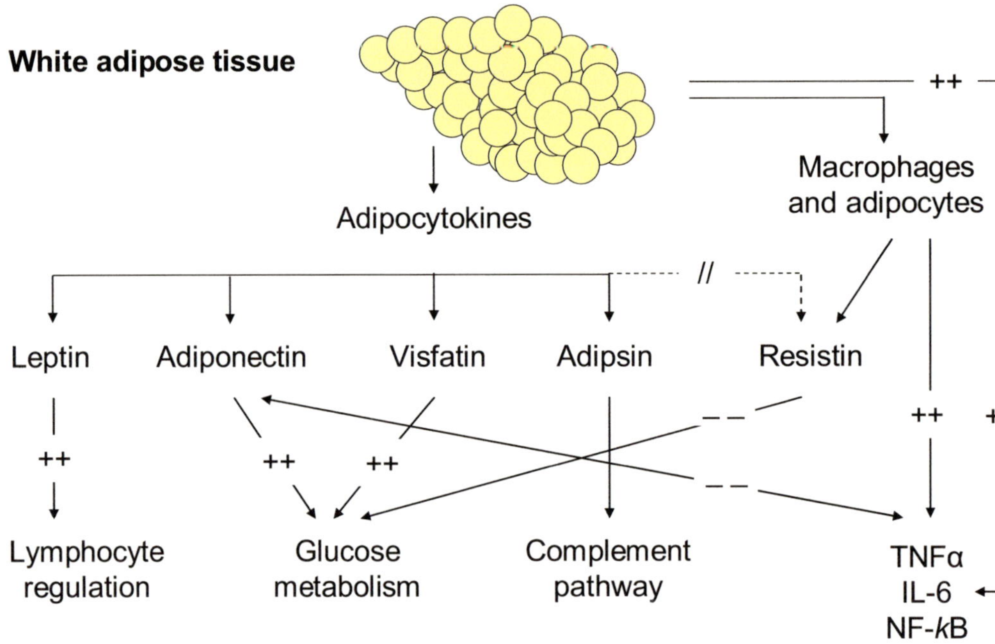

Fig. 2. Secretion of adipocytokines and 'classic' inflammatory cytokines by white adipose tissue. Although regarded as an adipokine resistin is in humans mainly derived from macrophages. TNF, tumor necrosis factor; IL, interleukin; NF, nuclear factor (modified from [11]).

Potentially relevant factors released from fat tissue include hormones, adipocytokines, chemokines, growth factors, transcription factors, enzymes and participants of the coagulation cascade [33]. Many of these factors signal to organs of metabolic importance and the immune system and thus contribute to the phenomenon of insulin resistance [30] as proved for TNF-α and IL-6 [34, 35]. A recent study demonstrated similar high adipocytokine profiles in septic patients as well as in morbidly obese [36]. Most validated data are available for Interleukins-1,-6,-8 and -10, TNF-α, Resistin, Adiponectin, Leptin, Leptin-Rezeptor, RBP4, Osteopontin, Visfatin, Omentin, Adipsin, Sfrp5, Adipophilin and VASPIN (visceral adipose-tissue-derived serine protease inhibitor).

In critically ill patients adipocytokines seem to be involved in the regulation of inflammation and metabolism and by this directly influence the clinical outcome of ICU patients. For critical illness, especially severe sepsis and septic shock, most valid data are available for resistin, leptin, leptin-receptor, and adiponectin.

5. Resistin

Up to now, resistin is the most widely studied adipocytokine in critical illness. Human resistin is mainly derived from macrophages and neutrophils as recently reported [37] and not from adipocytes (like in mice [38]) and has been implicated in glucose metabolism and insulin sensitivity. It is named for mediating resistance to insulin through the exacerbation of the adipose tissue inflammation in humans [39]. In a knock-out mouse model it has been demonstrated that the lack of resistin protects against diet-induced insulin resistance and type 2 diabetes mellitus [40].

Elevated resistin serum levels have been found in critically ill patients with significantly higher concentrations in sepsis than in non-sepsis patients and peak values in septic shock [37, 41]. Likely, resistin seems to act as an acute-phase protein and might be part of the systemic inflammatory response, as it has been correlated to IL-6, IL-10, TNF-α, C-reactive protein and procalcitonin [42].

Data concerning the correlation between resistin, obesity, insulin resistance, hyperglycemia and diabetes mellitus are controversially discussed at present. Several studies found a positive correlation between resistin serum levels and hyperinsulinemia, hyperglycemia and insulin resistance in patients who suffer from obesity and type 2 diabetes [43, 44], but these findings could not be confirmed in other studies [45, 46]. Interestingly, resistin levels have been recently found to be independent of pre-existing diabetes mellitus or body-mass index (BMI) in critically ill, especially in septic patients [41, 42].

Resistin serum levels have been correlated to renal and liver functions [47, 48], implicating renal and hepatic elimination or degradation of resistin. Resistin is considered as a part of the systemic inflammatory response from adipocytes, but in the critical illness response, resistin seems to be mainly derived from macrophages and not from adipocytes [42].

For critically ill, non-septic patients, high resistin serum concentrations have been identified as an adverse prognostic indicator for the ICU- as well as overall survival. Potentially, high resistin levels could indicate an excess of inflammatory reaction that might be of considerable harm, even in the absence of infection [42].

6. Leptin and leptin-receptor

Since its identification in 1994 leptin has been known for its role in controlling body weight and food intake through hypothalamic pathways [49, 50]. The name leptin derived from the Greek language, as the word leptos means thin [51]. In mouse models, deficiency of leptin or leptin-receptor resulted in a hyperphagic, morbidly obese, and lethargic phenotype with significantly reduced macrophage phagocytic activity [52-54]. Circulating leptin levels directly reflect adipose tissue mass in non-critically ill subjects [55]. The same result applies in critical disease, in which leptin has also been found to closely correlate with adipose tissue mass; moreover, an inverse association between circulating leptin-receptor and the BMI in critically ill patients has been reported [56].

Little is known about the mechanisms of leptin expression. It is secreted not only from white adipocytes, but also from placenta and stomach [57]. In not critically ill individuals leptin serum concentrations correlate with impaired insulin sensitivity, increased inflammatory markers, and coronary artery disease [58]. Various central and peripheral effects of leptin via leptin-receptors in brain and leptin-receptors in pancreas, liver, adipose tissue, and in the immune system, especially in human peripheral blood mononuclear cells, have been described [59]. Therefore, leptin is not only involved in control of body weight and energy expenditure, but also in glucose homeostasis and immunoregulation. Leptin is able to modulate the immune response by proliferation and activation of the mononuclear cells. Moreover, it activates the production of proinflammatory cytokines in cultured monocytes, protects monocytes against apoptosis and influences RNA metabolism. The leptin-receptor itself is similar to members of the class I cytokine family and exists in six isoforms [60]. Leptin is regarded as a proinflammatory cytokine itself [61], whose action in the central nervous system is necessary for an adequate systemic immune response [62].

In animal and human studies administration of endotoxin and TNF-α as inducers of severe systemic inflammation resulted in significant elevation of serum leptin levels [63]. Yousef and colleagues also reported increased values for IL-6, CRP, TNF-α and leptin at admission to ICU, with leptin threshold values of 38 μg/l for distinguishing between SIRS and sepsis [7]. Controversially, among other studies, a study from Denmark revealed low leptin levels - and also low adiponectin and RBP4 levels - at admission to the ICU, possibly due to an acute stress response [64]. The absence of increasing leptin levels in these studies may be due to the short duration of the experiments, given that a delay is needed to observe an increase of leptin following a LPS-stimulation [65]. Another study in critically ill patients, including septic and non-septic groups didn't report differences in leptin and leptin-receptor serum concentrations as compared with healthy controls [56].

Besides the suggested potential role as a diagnostic parameter leptin and leptin-receptor seem to have a prognostic impact, as high leptin-receptor serum concentrations at admission to ICU have been identified as an adverse prognostic indicator for survival [56]. Bornstein and colleagues noticed earlier that low levels of leptin might indicate a poor prognosis in septic patients [66]. Other studies had similar findings with exogenous leptin administration as a protective factor in leptin-deficient mice [67, 68]. These results are in conflict with observations from other investigators. Shapiro et al. reported a decrease in survival rates after application of exogenous leptin in murine sepsis models, whereas leptin-receptor deficient mice showed a better outcome with higher survival rates [60].

Despite the strong evidence that leptin takes part in the cell-mediated immunity response and in cytokine crosstalk [69] additional studies for clearing the role of leptin and its receptors in sepsis and SIRS are warranted.

7. Adiponectin

Adiponectin is the most abundant adipocytokine in humans with high serum concentrations, normally accounting for about 0.01% of total plasma protein [70]. There are three different molecular forms of circulating adiponectin [30]. It is exclusively secreted by adipocytes with higher serum concentration in females [71]. Interestingly, despite sole adipocytic origin, adiponectin has been found to be inversely correlated to the BMI in healthy individuals and in critically ill patients as well [72]. Until now, this so called "adiponectin paradox" - exclusive synthesis in adipocytes but low adiponectin levels in obesity - has not been solved yet [73]. Secretion of adiponectin is boosted several folds by insulin [70], but interestingly in type 2 diabetes - as in obesity - adiponectin serum concentrations are reduced [74]. Reduced adiponectin levels and an association with pre-existing diabetes mellitus have been reported in critically ill patients as well [72].

Adiponectin has been found as an anti-atherogenic agent with positive correlation to high-density lipoprotein cholesterol and inverse correlations to low-density lipoprotein cholesterol, triglycerides, insulin resistance, and diastolic blood pressure. Moreover, adiponectin seems to exert direct anti-atherogenic effects on the endothelial cells [75]. Studies in rodents also demonstrated protective functions of adiponectin in obesity and insulin resistance [76]. In a study with nondiabetic, but obese patients with varying degrees of insulin resistance, the presence of adiponectin resulted in an increase of insulin-sensitivity. Concomitantly to higher adiponectin serum concentrations in lean individuals, serum levels of TNF-α are decreased [74]. As TNF-α is presently known for its implication in insulin resistance, reduced serum concentrations might affect higher insulin sensitivity as well [77].

Additionally, adiponectin seems to have anti-inflammatory functions in animal models of sepsis. It has been reported as a potent inhibitor of cytokine production in porcine macrophages [78]. Furthermore, adiponectin-knockout mice had significantly higher mortality rates and serum levels of inflammatory markers in polymicrobial sepsis [79]. In a study of Teoh and colleagues the administration of adiponectin to adiponectin-knockout mice led to an improved outcome in experimentally generated sepsis. As concluded by the authors, low adiponectin levels potentially link obesity and the (discussed) worse outcome of obese patients in sepsis [80]. Glucocorticoids, inflammation, and oxidative stress - commonly associated with critical disease - are known for reducing adiponectin synthesis [81]. Matching these facts, some studies reported low adiponectin levels in patients with critical disease of pulmonary origin and also in rats with sepsis (without analyzing the impact of the measured low values on mortality or outcome) [64, 82]. Nevertheless, there are conflicting data concerning the role of adiponectin in critical illness. In a large monocenter clinical study there was no difference in adiponectin serum levels in critically ill patients compared to healthy controls and furthermore no difference between septic and non septic patients. In the same study low adiponectin serum concentrations at admission to ICU have been found as a positive prognostic indicator for ICU and overall survival in contrast to the above mentioned theory of low adiponectin levels worsening the outcome of critically ill patients [72].

Interestingly, no correlation of adiponectin with cytokines or mediators of inflammation have been reported in critically ill patients [64, 72]. The mechanisms of adiponectin excretion and biodegradation in critical disease are presently unclear. Due to a reported correlation between adiponectin levels and markers of cholestasis and cystatin C as a marker of renal function, hepatic and renal elimination have been discussed in critically ill patients [72]. Other studies in non-ICU patients with liver cirrhosis, animal models and uremic patients confirm the theory of partially biliary and renal excretion of adiponectin [83, 84]. Yuan et al. reported a direct suppression of adiponectin gene expression by C-reactive protein in a concentration- and time-dependent manner [85], which might be an important finding for understanding adiponectin in critical disease, especially in sepsis, in which extremely high CRP levels are frequently found.

As a result of the entirety of conflicting data, up to now it remains unclear whether circulating adiponectin is pathogenetically involved in mechanisms of critical disease leading to higher mortality rates. Maybe it is an epiphenomenon of variables such as adiposity, yet unknown functions of adipose tissue or metabolic alterations in critical illness [72].

8. Retinol binding protein 4 (RBP4)

Retinol binding protein 4 is secreted by adipose tissue and liver. Although it is named an adipocytokine for its derivation of adipocytes, the main source of RBP4 in humans is the liver [86]. Besides serving as a transport protein for vitamin A (retinol), RBP4 has been implicated in the development of insulin resistance in rodent models and in humans [87, 88]. Von Eynatten et al. found elevated gene expression for RBP4 in the adipose tissue, but not in the liver of insulin-resistant mice, whereas the application of RBP4 to other mice led to insulin resistance [87]. Another study demonstrated down-regulation of the insulin-responsive glucose-transporter GLUT4 in adipocytes in obesity, resulting in increased secretion of RBP4 by a yet unknown regulatory mechanism [88]. RBP4 has been identified as a marker of insulin resistance in individuals with various clinical presentations, but not yet manifested diabetes mellitus. The strong correlation to insulin resistance in case of obesity, impaired glucose tolerance, type 2 diabetes and even in lean subjects seems to be more specific than the correlation of other adipocytokines like leptin and adiponectin to insulin resistance [89].

As a consequence of its main derivation from the liver, RBP4 serum levels are reduced in case of chronic and acute liver diseases or dysfunction [86, 90]. But also renal function seems to be important for the RBP4 metabolism with increasing levels in case of impaired renal function [91].

In critical disease RBP4 serum levels have been found decreased compared to healthy controls, independent of the origin of critical illness [64, 92]. During the course of disease, serum levels normalized with resolving critical illness [64]. Langouche and colleagues hypothesized that reduced synthesis or increased removal might be the reason for the decreased serum levels. In sepsis, capillary leakage has been considered as a possible mechanism for reducing the levels of adipocytokines in general [64]. As shown in another study the decrease in serum concentrations of RBP4 is independent of the origin of critical illness. There was no difference between concentrations in septic and non-septic patients requiring intensive care medicine, so capillary leakage as a well-known problem in sepsis seems not to be the main reason [92]. Instead, a strong correlation between liver and kidney function and serum RBP4 concentrations was found, reflecting the above mentioned relation of RBP4 to liver and kidney function observed in not critically ill patients [92]. As RBP4 levels were inversely correlated with markers of inflammation, RBP4 seems potentially to be a member of the negative acute-phase reactants described by Richie et al. [93], what might be another explanation for decreased levels in critical disease [92]. At present, no association between RBP4 and other adipokines like adiponectin and resistin has been reported, suggesting that the adipose tissue does not contribute to a great extent to serum RBP4 concentrations in critical disease [92].

Recently, despite a missing association of RBP4 with preexisting diabetes mellitus or obesity, a study reported a correlation with C-peptide levels, reflecting endogenous insulin production, and with insulin resistance (HOMA index) [92]. The hypothesis of RBP4 interaction in glucose metabolism is supported by a recent finding, that during intensive insulin therapy the raise of RBP4 levels in the course of critical illness is blunted [64].

Importantly, high serum concentrations of RBP4 at admission to the ICU have been identified as a positive predictor of ICU-survival [92]. Maybe this is due to the fact that higher RBP4 levels just represent preserved liver function and are not pathogenetically involved in the course of critical disease, as liver function itself is clearly linked to survival rates in critical disease [94]. Further studies are needed to definitely clarify the regulatory pathways of RBP4, its role in the pathogenesis of critical illness, and its significance as a potential novel biomarker for ICU patients.

9. Visfatin

Initially known as Pre-B-cell colony-enhancing factor (PBEF) this recently described adipocytokine was found in high concentrations in visceral fat, therefore renamed visfatin [95]. The third name for this eclectic protein is Nampt (nicotinamide phosphoribosyltransferase) [96]. Interestingly, visfatin has a unique structure without homology to other known proteins [96]. The number of names already indicates the divers properties exerted by this protein.
As Nampt, this protein acts intracellular as the rate-limiting part of the NAD (nicotinamide adenine dinucleotide) production in mice [97]. NAD is an essential cofactor in numerous fundamental intracellular processes [98]. Moreover Kitani et al. proposed a role for PBEF in cell cycle regulation because of its varying intracellular distribution due to the growth phase of the cell [99].
As characteristic for adipocytokines visfatin is involved in the glucose metabolism. By binding to the insulin-receptor it shows insulin-mimetic effects in mice and cultured cells [100]. In question of reproducibility of these effects of visfatin, this publication had to be retracted recently [101], but Xie et al. demonstrated an insulin-like effect of visfatin on cultured osteoblasts [102]. Furthermore, other authors reported a correlation between visfatin serum levels and obesity, diabetes mellitus, and visceral fat mass [103-105]. Therefore, visfatin seems to be involved in a number of metabolic processes, but the definite role remains to be clarified.
Initially PBEF was discovered by Samal et al. (1994) as a mediator of maturation of B-cells precursors, secreted by activated lymphocytes in bone marrow stromal cells. Its gene was found mainly transcribed in human bone marrow, liver tissue, and muscle [106]. Even though the characteristic signal peptide required for extracellular secretion of mature protein is missing, PBEF shows other properties which allow allocation of it to the class of cytokines [106]. PBEF has been found as an inhibitor of apoptosis of neutrophils in experimental inflammation and clinical sepsis by Jia et al. [107]. The excess of neutrophils in sepsis accounts for inflammatory tissue damage, e.g. for respiratory distress syndromes as often observed in sepsis [108]. The prolonged survival of neutrophils in sepsis due to inhibition of apoptosis mediated by PBEF even amplifies these destructive effects [107]. Furthermore increased PBEF was found in swollen or infected human fetal membranes indicating cytokine functions [109]. It exerts chemotactic activity and up-regulates the serum levels of other pro-inflammatory cytokines [110]. Garcia and Vinasco demonstrated a crucial role for PBEF in acute lung injury (ALI), which is usually caused by sepsis [111]. In these critical ill patients they found elevated concentrations of PBEF in bronchoalveolar lavage and serum. They identified two single nucleotide polymorphisms in the PBEF promoter, which seems to enhance the susceptibility for the development of ALI in septic patients.
Although the role of PBEF as a cytokine is incompletely understood today, this protein seems to have a magnitude of properties contributing to the complex mechanisms accounting for the course of critical disease. Not at least this is underlined by the fact that PBEF is highly conserved through evolution as it could be identified in bacteria [112], invertebrate sponges [113], fishes [114], chickens and mammals [115].

10. Adipsin

When adipsin was initially identified in 1983, this was the first evidence for the potential role of adipose tissue in regulation of immune system biology [116]. Spiegelman and colleagues discovered adipsin mRNA in cultured mouse adipocyte cell lines [117]. Just a short time after its identification the similarity between the novel serin protease adipsin in mice and human complement factor D was shown [118]. Factor D is a serin protease accounting for the activation of the alternative pathway of complement activation. It constitutes the initial obligatory, rate-limiting catalytic activity of this activation by cleaving complement factor B when B is complexed with an activated form of complement component C3 [119]. The complement system is the key in innate immunity with important properties in enhancing adaptive immunity and in the clearance of bacteria and apoptotic cells [120]. In dissimilarity to mouse adipsin, which is only expressed by adipose tissue, human complement factor D it mainly derived from macrophages and monocytes [121]. So the potential involvement of this adipocytokine in critical disease seems obvious. Adipsin-deficiency abolishes alternative-pathway dependent complement activation, in case of infection with *Neisseria meningitidis* leading to an increased susceptibility for invasive meningococcal disease [122, 123].

Adipsin also seems to play an important role in energy balance as it has been found to be decreased in fat from genetically obese and diabetic mice in comparison to normal lean mice and also in serum levels of varying animal models in obesity [124, 125]. Its serum concentrations decline during infusion of glucose which results in a hyperglycemic and hyperinsulinemic state [124]. Interestingly, the serum adipsin concentrations are reduced in case of genetically and chemical induced obesity, whereas in the state of adiposity resulting from pure overfeeding there is no change leading to the conclusion that adipsin could be a marker for distinguishing between obesity caused by metabolic disorders or caused just by overfeeding [124].

11. Conclusion

Overall, adipocytokines in critical illness seem to fulfill various functions which are at present not satisfyingly understood. The interaction of metabolic and inflammatory mediators has been found of prognostic impact in these patients. More and more functions of adipocytokines and their interaction in insulin resistance, obesity and immune reactions have been unraveled by an increasing number of clinical and animal studies. Nevertheless, further future research is crucial to understand the complex effects of adipocytokines and their role as a link between inflammation and metabolism in critical disease.

12. References

[1] Angus DC, Linde-Zwirble WT, Lidicker J, Clermont G, Carcillo J, Pinsky MR: Epidemiology of severe sepsis in the United States: analysis of incidence, outcome, and associated costs of care. *Crit Care Med* 2001, 29(7):1303-1310.

[2] Dombrovskiy VY, Martin AA, Sunderram J, Paz HL: Rapid increase in hospitalization and mortality rates for severe sepsis in the United States: a trend analysis from 1993 to 2003. *Crit Care Med* 2007, 35(5):1244-1250.

[3] Vincent JL, Sakr Y, Sprung CL, Ranieri VM, Reinhart K, Gerlach H, Moreno R, Carlet J, Le Gall JR, Payen D: Sepsis in European intensive care units: results of the SOAP study. *Crit Care Med* 2006, 34(2):344-353.

[4] Linde-Zwirble WT, Angus DC: Severe sepsis epidemiology: sampling, selection, and society. *Crit Care* 2004, 8(4):222-226.

[5] Claus RA, Otto GP, Deigner HP, Bauer M: Approaching clinical reality: markers for monitoring systemic inflammation and sepsis. *Curr Mol Med* 2010, 10(2):227-235.
[6] Bone RC, Balk RA, Cerra FB, Dellinger RP, Fein AM, Knaus WA, Schein RM, Sibbald WJ: Definitions for sepsis and organ failure and guidelines for the use of innovative therapies in sepsis. The ACCP/SCCM Consensus Conference Committee. American College of Chest Physicians/Society of Critical Care Medicine. 1992. *Chest* 2009, 136(5 Suppl):e28.
[7] Yousef AA, Amr YM, Suliman GA: The diagnostic value of serum leptin monitoring and its correlation with tumor necrosis factor-alpha in critically ill patients: a prospective observational study. *Crit Care* 2010, 14(2):R33.
[8] Pierrakos C, Vincent JL: Sepsis biomarkers: a review. *Crit Care* 2010, 14(1):R15.
[9] Cavaillon JM, Adib-Conquy M, Fitting C, Adrie C, Payen D: Cytokine cascade in sepsis. *Scand J Infect Dis* 2003, 35(9):535-544.
[10] Calvano SE, Xiao W, Richards DR, Felciano RM, Baker HV, Cho RJ, Chen RO, Brownstein BH, Cobb JP, Tschoeke SK *et al*: A network-based analysis of systemic inflammation in humans. *Nature* 2005, 437(7061):1032-1037.
[11] Vachharajani V, Vital S: Obesity and sepsis. *J Intensive Care Med* 2006, 21(5):287-295.
[12] Dandona P, Aljada A, Bandyopadhyay A: Inflammation: the link between insulin resistance, obesity and diabetes. *Trends Immunol* 2004, 25(1):4-7.
[13] Furukawa S, Fujita T, Shimabukuro M, Iwaki M, Yamada Y, Nakajima Y, Nakayama O, Makishima M, Matsuda M, Shimomura I: Increased oxidative stress in obesity and its impact on metabolic syndrome. *J Clin Invest* 2004, 114(12):1752-1761.
[14] Cooper D, Stokes KY, Tailor A, Granger DN: Oxidative stress promotes blood cell-endothelial cell interactions in the microcirculation. *Cardiovasc Toxicol* 2002, 2(3):165-180.
[15] El-Solh A, Sikka P, Bozkanat E, Jaafar W, Davies J: Morbid obesity in the medical ICU. *Chest* 2001, 120(6):1989-1997.
[16] Bercault N, Boulain T, Kuteifan K, Wolf M, Runge I, Fleury JC: Obesity-related excess mortality rate in an adult intensive care unit: A risk-adjusted matched cohort study. *Crit Care Med* 2004, 32(4):998-1003.
[17] Singer G, Granger DN: Inflammatory responses underlying the microvascular dysfunction associated with obesity and insulin resistance. *Microcirculation* 2007, 14(4-5):375-387.
[18] Akinnusi ME, Pineda LA, El Solh AA: Effect of obesity on intensive care morbidity and mortality: a meta-analysis. *Crit Care Med* 2008, 36(1):151-158.
[19] Sakr Y, Madl C, Filipescu D, Moreno R, Groeneveld J, Artigas A, Reinhart K, Vincent JL: Obesity is associated with increased morbidity but not mortality in critically ill patients. *Intensive Care Med* 2008, 34(11):1999-2009.
[20] Van Cromphaut SJ, Vanhorebeek I, Van den Berghe G: Glucose metabolism and insulin resistance in sepsis. *Curr Pharm Des* 2008, 14(19):1887-1899.
[21] McCowen KC, Malhotra A, Bistrian BR: Stress-induced hyperglycemia. *Crit Care Clin* 2001, 17(1):107-124.
[22] Thorell A, Nygren J, Ljungqvist O: Insulin resistance: a marker of surgical stress. *Curr Opin Clin Nutr Metab Care* 1999, 2(1):69-78.
[23] Kovalaske MA, Gandhi GY: Glycemic control in the medical intensive care unit. *J Diabetes Sci Technol* 2009, 3(6):1330-1341.

[24] Van den Berghe G: How does blood glucose control with insulin save lives in intensive care? *J Clin Invest* 2004, 114(9):1187-1195.
[25] Falciglia M: Causes and consequences of hyperglycemia in critical illness. *Curr Opin Clin Nutr Metab Care* 2007, 10(4):498-503.
[26] Marette A: Mediators of cytokine-induced insulin resistance in obesity and other inflammatory settings. *Curr Opin Clin Nutr Metab Care* 2002, 5(4):377-383.
[27] Krinsley JS: Association between hyperglycemia and increased hospital mortality in a heterogeneous population of critically ill patients. *Mayo Clin Proc* 2003, 78(12):1471-1478.
[28] van den Berghe G, Wouters P, Weekers F, Verwaest C, Bruyninckx F, Schetz M, Vlasselaers D, Ferdinande P, Lauwers P, Bouillon R: Intensive insulin therapy in the critically ill patients. *N Engl J Med* 2001, 345(19):1359-1367.
[29] Finfer S, Chittock DR, Su SY, Blair D, Foster D, Dhingra V, Bellomo R, Cook D, Dodek P, Henderson WR *et al*: Intensive versus conventional glucose control in critically ill patients. *N Engl J Med* 2009, 360(13):1283-1297.
[30] Badman MK, Flier JS: The adipocyte as an active participant in energy balance and metabolism. *Gastroenterology* 2007, 132(6):2103-2115.
[31] Matsuzawa Y, Shimomura I, Kihara S, Funahashi T: Importance of adipocytokines in obesity-related diseases. *Horm Res* 2003, 60 Suppl 3:56-59.
[32] Shoelson SE, Herrero L, Naaz A: Obesity, inflammation, and insulin resistance. *Gastroenterology* 2007, 132(6):2169-2180.
[33] Fantuzzi G, Mazzone T: Adipose tissue and adipokines in health and disease. Totowa, NJ: Humana Press Inc.; 2007.
[34] Hotamisligil GS, Murray DL, Choy LN, Spiegelman BM: Tumor necrosis factor alpha inhibits signaling from the insulin receptor. *Proc Natl Acad Sci U S A* 1994, 91(11):4854-4858.
[35] Klover PJ, Clementi AH, Mooney RA: Interleukin-6 depletion selectively improves hepatic insulin action in obesity. *Endocrinology* 2005, 146(8):3417-3427.
[36] Hillenbrand A, Knippschild U, Weiss M, Schrezenmeier H, Henne-Bruns D, Huber-Lang M, Wolf AM: Sepsis induced changes of adipokines and cytokines - septic patients compared to morbidly obese patients. *BMC Surg* 2010, 10:26.
[37] Johansson L, Linner A, Sunden-Cullberg J, Haggar A, Herwald H, Lore K, Treutiger CJ, Norrby-Teglund A: Neutrophil-derived hyperresistinemia in severe acute streptococcal infections. *J Immunol* 2009, 183(6):4047-4054.
[38] Savage DB, Sewter CP, Klenk ES, Segal DG, Vidal-Puig A, Considine RV, O'Rahilly S: Resistin / Fizz3 expression in relation to obesity and peroxisome proliferator-activated receptor-gamma action in humans. *Diabetes* 2001, 50(10):2199-2202.
[39] Qatanani M, Szwergold NR, Greaves DR, Ahima RS, Lazar MA: Macrophage-derived human resistin exacerbates adipose tissue inflammation and insulin resistance in mice. *J Clin Invest* 2009.
[40] Banerjee RR, Rangwala SM, Shapiro JS, Rich AS, Rhoades B, Qi Y, Wang J, Rajala MW, Pocai A, Scherer PE *et al*: Regulation of fasted blood glucose by resistin. *Science* 2004, 303(5661):1195-1198.
[41] Sunden-Cullberg J, Nystrom T, Lee ML, Mullins GE, Tokics L, Andersson J, Norrby-Teglund A, Treutiger CJ: Pronounced elevation of resistin correlates with severity of disease in severe sepsis and septic shock. *Crit Care Med* 2007, 35(6):1536-1542.

[42] Koch A, Gressner OA, Sanson E, Tacke F, Trautwein C: Serum resistin levels in critically ill patients are associated with inflammation, organ dysfunction and metabolism and may predict survival of non-septic patients. *Crit Care* 2009, 13(3):R95.

[43] McTernan PG, Fisher FM, Valsamakis G, Chetty R, Harte A, McTernan CL, Clark PM, Smith SA, Barnett AH, Kumar S: Resistin and type 2 diabetes: regulation of resistin expression by insulin and rosiglitazone and the effects of recombinant resistin on lipid and glucose metabolism in human differentiated adipocytes. *J Clin Endocrinol Metab* 2003, 88(12):6098-6106.

[44] Fujinami A, Obayashi H, Ohta K, Ichimura T, Nishimura M, Matsui H, Kawahara Y, Yamazaki M, Ogata M, Hasegawa G *et al*: Enzyme-linked immunosorbent assay for circulating human resistin: resistin concentrations in normal subjects and patients with type 2 diabetes. *Clin Chim Acta* 2004, 339(1-2):57-63.

[45] Pfutzner A, Langenfeld M, Kunt T, Lobig M, Forst T: Evaluation of human resistin assays with serum from patients with type 2 diabetes and different degrees of insulin resistance. *Clin Lab* 2003, 49(11-12):571-576.

[46] Stejskal D, Adamovska S, Bartek J, Jurakova R, Proskova J: Resistin - concentrations in persons with type 2 diabetes mellitus and in individuals with acute inflammatory disease. *Biomed Pap Med Fac Univ Palacky Olomouc Czech Repub* 2003, 147(1):63-69.

[47] Axelsson J, Bergsten A, Qureshi AR, Heimburger O, Barany P, Lonnqvist F, Lindholm B, Nordfors L, Alvestrand A, Stenvinkel P: Elevated resistin levels in chronic kidney disease are associated with decreased glomerular filtration rate and inflammation, but not with insulin resistance. *Kidney Int* 2006, 69(3):596-604.

[48] Yagmur E, Trautwein C, Gressner AM, Tacke F: Resistin serum levels are associated with insulin resistance, disease severity, clinical complications, and prognosis in patients with chronic liver diseases. *Am J Gastroenterol* 2006, 101(6):1244-1252.

[49] Friedman JM, Halaas JL: Leptin and the regulation of body weight in mammals. *Nature* 1998, 395(6704):763-770.

[50] Zhang Y, Proenca R, Maffei M, Barone M, Leopold L, Friedman JM: Positional cloning of the mouse obese gene and its human homologue. *Nature* 1994, 372(6505):425-432.

[51] Sone M, Osamura RY: Leptin and the pituitary. *Pituitary* 2001, 4(1-2):15-23.

[52] Considine RV, Caro JF: Leptin and the regulation of body weight. *Int J Biochem Cell Biol* 1997, 29(11):1255-1272.

[53] Houseknecht KL, Baile CA, Matteri RL, Spurlock ME: The biology of leptin: a review. *J Anim Sci* 1998, 76(5):1405-1420.

[54] Loffreda S, Yang SQ, Lin HZ, Karp CL, Brengman ML, Wang DJ, Klein AS, Bulkley GB, Bao C, Noble PW *et al*: Leptin regulates proinflammatory immune responses. *FASEB J* 1998, 12(1):57-65.

[55] Havel PJ, Kasim-Karakas S, Mueller W, Johnson PR, Gingerich RL, Stern JS: Relationship of plasma leptin to plasma insulin and adiposity in normal weight and overweight women: effects of dietary fat content and sustained weight loss. *J Clin Endocrinol Metab* 1996, 81(12):4406-4413.

[56] Koch A, Weiskirchen R, Zimmermann HW, Sanson E, Trautwein C, Tacke F: Relevance of serum leptin and leptin-receptor concentrations in critically ill patients. *Mediators Inflamm* 2010, pii: 473540

[57] Leininger MT, Portocarrero CP, Bidwell CA, Spurlock ME, Houseknecht KL: Leptin expression is reduced with acute endotoxemia in the pig: correlation with glucose,

insulin, and insulin-like growth factor-1 (IGF-1). *J Interferon Cytokine Res* 2000, 20(1):99-106.

[58] Wallace AM, McMahon AD, Packard CJ, Kelly A, Shepherd J, Gaw A, Sattar N: Plasma leptin and the risk of cardiovascular disease in the west of Scotland coronary prevention study (WOSCOPS). *Circulation* 2001, 104(25):3052-3056.

[59] Bjorbaek C, Kahn BB: Leptin signaling in the central nervous system and the periphery. *Recent Prog Horm Res* 2004, 59:305-331.

[60] Shapiro NI, Khankin EV, Van Meurs M, Shih SC, Lu S, Yano M, Castro PR, Maratos-Flier E, Parikh SM, Karumanchi SA *et al*: Leptin exacerbates sepsis-mediated morbidity and mortality. *J Immunol* 2010, 185(1):517-524.

[61] Sanchez-Margalet V, Martin-Romero C, Santos-Alvarez J, Goberna R, Najib S, Gonzalez-Yanes C: Role of leptin as an immunomodulator of blood mononuclear cells: mechanisms of action. *Clin Exp Immunol* 2003, 133(1):11-19.

[62] Tschop J, Nogueiras R, Haas-Lockie S, Kasten KR, Castaneda TR, Huber N, Guanciale K, Perez-Tilve D, Habegger K, Ottaway N *et al*: CNS leptin action modulates immune response and survival in sepsis. *J Neurosci* 2010, 30(17):6036-6047.

[63] Finck BN, Kelley KW, Dantzer R, Johnson RW: In vivo and in vitro evidence for the involvement of tumor necrosis factor-alpha in the induction of leptin by lipopolysaccharide. *Endocrinology* 1998, 139(5):2278-2283.

[64] Langouche L, Vander Perre S, Frystyk J, Flyvbjerg A, Hansen TK, Van den Berghe G: Adiponectin, retinol-binding protein 4, and leptin in protracted critical illness of pulmonary origin. *Crit Care* 2009, 13(4):R112.

[65] Anderson PD, Mehta NN, Wolfe ML, Hinkle CC, Pruscino L, Comiskey LL, Tabita-Martinez J, Sellers KF, Rickels MR, Ahima RS *et al*: Innate immunity modulates adipokines in humans. *J Clin Endocrinol Metab* 2007, 92(6):2272-2279.

[66] Bornstein SR, Licinio J, Tauchnitz R, Engelmann L, Negrao AB, Gold P, Chrousos GP: Plasma leptin levels are increased in survivors of acute sepsis: associated loss of diurnal rhythm, in cortisol and leptin secretion. *J Clin Endocrinol Metab* 1998, 83(1):280-283.

[67] Faggioni R, Fantuzzi G, Gabay C, Moser A, Dinarello CA, Feingold KR, Grunfeld C: Leptin deficiency enhances sensitivity to endotoxin-induced lethality. *Am J Physiol* 1999, 276(1 Pt 2):R136-142.

[68] Wang W, Poole B, Mitra A, Falk S, Fantuzzi G, Lucia S, Schrier R: Role of leptin deficiency in early acute renal failure during endotoxemia in ob/ob mice. *J Am Soc Nephrol* 2004, 15(3):645-649.

[69] Haas P, Straub RH, Bedoui S, Nave H: Peripheral but not central leptin treatment increases numbers of circulating NK cells, granulocytes and specific monocyte subpopulations in non-endotoxaemic lean and obese LEW-rats. *Regul Pept* 2008, 151(1-3):26-34.

[70] Scherer PE, Williams S, Fogliano M, Baldini G, Lodish HF: A novel serum protein similar to C1q, produced exclusively in adipocytes. *J Biol Chem* 1995, 270(45):26746-26749.

[71] Wajchenberg BL: Subcutaneous and visceral adipose tissue: their relation to the metabolic syndrome. *Endocr Rev* 2000, 21(6):697-738.

[72] Koch A, Sanson E, Voigt S, Helm A, Trautwein C, Tacke F: Serum adiponectin upon admission to the intensive care unit may predict mortality in critically ill patients. *J Crit Care* 2011, 26(2):166-174
[73] Owecki M: Fat tissue and adiponectin: new players in critical care? *Crit Care* 2009, 13(4):174.
[74] Kern PA, Di Gregorio GB, Lu T, Rassouli N, Ranganathan G: Adiponectin expression from human adipose tissue: relation to obesity, insulin resistance, and tumor necrosis factor-alpha expression. *Diabetes* 2003, 52(7):1779-1785.
[75] Yamamoto Y, Hirose H, Saito I, Tomita M, Taniyama M, Matsubara K, Okazaki Y, Ishii T, Nishikai K, Saruta T: Correlation of the adipocyte-derived protein adiponectin with insulin resistance index and serum high-density lipoprotein-cholesterol, independent of body mass index, in the Japanese population. *Clin Sci (Lond)* 2002, 103(2):137-142.
[76] Berg AH, Combs TP, Du X, Brownlee M, Scherer PE: The adipocyte-secreted protein Acrp30 enhances hepatic insulin action. *Nat Med* 2001, 7(8):947-953.
[77] Cawthorn WP, Sethi JK: TNF-alpha and adipocyte biology. *FEBS Lett* 2008, 582(1):117-131.
[78] Wulster-Radcliffe MC, Ajuwon KM, Wang J, Christian JA, Spurlock ME: Adiponectin differentially regulates cytokines in porcine macrophages. *Biochem Biophys Res Commun* 2004, 316(3):924-929.
[79] Uji Y, Yamamoto H, Tsuchihashi H, Maeda K, Funahashi T, Shimomura I, Shimizu T, Endo Y, Tani T: Adiponectin deficiency is associated with severe polymicrobial sepsis, high inflammatory cytokine levels, and high mortality. *Surgery* 2009, 145(5):550-557.
[80] Teoh H, Quan A, Bang KW, Wang G, Lovren F, Vu V, Haitsma JJ, Szmitko PE, Al-Omran M, Wang CH *et al*: Adiponectin deficiency promotes endothelial activation and profoundly exacerbates sepsis-related mortality. *Am J Physiol Endocrinol Metab* 2008, 295(3):E658-664.
[81] Swarbrick MM, Havel PJ: Physiological, pharmacological, and nutritional regulation of circulating adiponectin concentrations in humans. *Metab Syndr Relat Disord* 2008, 6(2):87-102.
[82] Tsuchihashi H, Yamamoto H, Maeda K, Ugi S, Mori T, Shimizu T, Endo Y, Hanasawa K, Tani T: Circulating concentrations of adiponectin, an endogenous lipopolysaccharide neutralizing protein, decrease in rats with polymicrobial sepsis. *J Surg Res* 2006, 134(2):348-353.
[83] Tacke F, Wustefeld T, Horn R, Luedde T, Srinivas Rao A, Manns MP, Trautwein C, Brabant G: High adiponectin in chronic liver disease and cholestasis suggests biliary route of adiponectin excretion in vivo. *J Hepatol* 2005, 42(5):666-673.
[84] Chudek J, Adamczak M, Karkoszka H, Budzinski G, Ignacy W, Funahashi T, Matsuzawa Y, Cierpka L, Kokot F, Wiecek A: Plasma adiponectin concentration before and after successful kidney transplantation. *Transplant Proc* 2003, 35(6):2186-2189.
[85] Yuan G, Chen X, Ma Q, Qiao J, Li R, Li X, Li S, Tang J, Zhou L, Song H *et al*: C-reactive protein inhibits adiponectin gene expression and secretion in 3T3-L1 adipocytes. *J Endocrinol* 2007, 194(2):275-281.

[86] Smith FR, Goodman DS: The effects of diseases of the liver, thyroid, and kidneys on the transport of vitamin A in human plasma. *J Clin Invest* 1971, 50(11):2426-2436.

[87] von Eynatten M, Humpert PM: Retinol-binding protein-4 in experimental and clinical metabolic disease. *Expert Rev Mol Diagn* 2008, 8(3):289-299.

[88] Wolf G: Serum retinol-binding protein: a link between obesity, insulin resistance, and type 2 diabetes. *Nutr Rev* 2007, 65(5):251-256.

[89] Graham TE, Yang Q, Bluher M, Hammarstedt A, Ciaraldi TP, Henry RR, Wason CJ, Oberbach A, Jansson PA, Smith U *et al*: Retinol-binding protein 4 and insulin resistance in lean, obese, and diabetic subjects. *N Engl J Med* 2006, 354(24):2552-2563.

[90] Tacke F, Weiskirchen R, Trautwein C: Liver function critically determines serum retinol-binding protein 4 (RBP4) levels in patients with chronic liver disease and cirrhosis. *Hepatology* 2008, 48(5):1724-1725; author reply 1725-1726.

[91] Henze A, Frey SK, Raila J, Tepel M, Scholze A, Pfeiffer AF, Weickert MO, Spranger J, Schweigert FJ: Evidence that kidney function but not type 2 diabetes determines retinol-binding protein 4 serum levels. *Diabetes* 2008, 57(12):3323-3326.

[92] Koch A, Weiskirchen R, Sanson E, Zimmermann HW, Voigt S, Duckers H, Trautwein C, Tacke F: Circulating retinol binding protein 4 in critically ill patients before specific treatment: prognostic impact and correlation with organ function, metabolism and inflammation. *Crit Care* 2010, 14(5):R179.

[93] Ritchie RF, Palomaki GE, Neveux LM, Navolotskaia O, Ledue TB, Craig WY: Reference distributions for the negative acute-phase serum proteins, albumin, transferrin and transthyretin: a practical, simple and clinically relevant approach in a large cohort. *J Clin Lab Anal* 1999, 13(6):273-279.

[94] Vincent JL, Moreno R: Clinical review: scoring systems in the critically ill. *Crit Care* 2010, 14(2):207.

[95] Pilz S, Mangge H, Obermayer-Pietsch B, Marz W: Visfatin/pre-B-cell colony-enhancing factor: a protein with various suggested functions. *J Endocrinol Invest* 2007, 30(2):138-144.

[96] Luk T, Malam Z, Marshall JC: Pre-B cell colony-enhancing factor (PBEF)/visfatin: a novel mediator of innate immunity. *J Leukoc Biol* 2008, 83(4):804-816.

[97] Rongvaux A, Shea RJ, Mulks MH, Gigot D, Urbain J, Leo O, Andris F: Pre-B-cell colony-enhancing factor, whose expression is up-regulated in activated lymphocytes, is a nicotinamide phosphoribosyltransferase, a cytosolic enzyme involved in NAD biosynthesis. *Eur J Immunol* 2002, 32(11):3225-3234.

[98] Ziegler M: New functions of a long-known molecule. Emerging roles of NAD in cellular signaling. *Eur J Biochem* 2000, 267(6):1550-1564.

[99] Kitani T, Okuno S, Fujisawa H: Growth phase-dependent changes in the subcellular localization of pre-B-cell colony-enhancing factor. *FEBS Lett* 2003, 544(1-3):74-78.

[100] Fukuhara A, Matsuda M, Nishizawa M, Segawa K, Tanaka M, Kishimoto K, Matsuki Y, Murakami M, Ichisaka T, Murakami H *et al*: Visfatin: a protein secreted by visceral fat that mimics the effects of insulin. *Science* 2005, 307(5708):426-430.

[101] Fukuhara A, Matsuda M, Nishizawa M, Segawa K, Tanaka M, Kishimoto K, Matsuki Y, Murakami M, Ichisaka T, Murakami H *et al*: Retraction. *Science* 2007, 318(5850):565.

[102] Xie H, Tang SY, Luo XH, Huang J, Cui RR, Yuan LQ, Zhou HD, Wu XP, Liao EY: Insulin-like effects of visfatin on human osteoblasts. *Calcif Tissue Int* 2007, 80(3):201-210.

[103] Chen MP, Chung FM, Chang DM, Tsai JC, Huang HF, Shin SJ, Lee YJ: Elevated plasma level of visfatin/pre-B cell colony-enhancing factor in patients with type 2 diabetes mellitus. *J Clin Endocrinol Metab* 2006, 91(1):295-299.

[104] Haider DG, Schindler K, Schaller G, Prager G, Wolzt M, Ludvik B: Increased plasma visfatin concentrations in morbidly obese subjects are reduced after gastric banding. *J Clin Endocrinol Metab* 2006, 91(4):1578-1581.

[105] Sandeep S, Velmurugan K, Deepa R, Mohan V: Serum visfatin in relation to visceral fat, obesity, and type 2 diabetes mellitus in Asian Indians. *Metabolism* 2007, 56(4):565-570.

[106] Samal B, Sun Y, Stearns G, Xie C, Suggs S, McNiece I: Cloning and characterization of the cDNA encoding a novel human pre-B-cell colony-enhancing factor. *Mol Cell Biol* 1994, 14(2):1431-1437.

[107] Jia SH, Li Y, Parodo J, Kapus A, Fan L, Rotstein OD, Marshall JC: Pre-B cell colony-enhancing factor inhibits neutrophil apoptosis in experimental inflammation and clinical sepsis. *J Clin Invest* 2004, 113(9):1318-1327.

[108] Weiss SJ: Tissue destruction by neutrophils. *N Engl J Med* 1989, 320(6):365-376.

[109] Ognjanovic S, Bao S, Yamamoto SY, Garibay-Tupas J, Samal B, Bryant-Greenwood GD: Genomic organization of the gene coding for human pre-B-cell colony enhancing factor and expression in human fetal membranes. *J Mol Endocrinol* 2001, 26(2):107-117.

[110] Moschen AR, Kaser A, Enrich B, Mosheimer B, Theurl M, Niederegger H, Tilg H: Visfatin, an adipocytokine with proinflammatory and immunomodulating properties. *J Immunol* 2007, 178(3):1748-1758.

[111] Garcia JG, Moreno Vinasco L: Genomic insights into acute inflammatory lung injury. *Am J Physiol Lung Cell Mol Physiol* 2006, 291(6):L1113-1117.

[112] Martin PR, Shea RJ, Mulks MH: Identification of a plasmid-encoded gene from Haemophilus ducreyi which confers NAD independence. *J Bacteriol* 2001, 183(4):1168-1174.

[113] Muller WE, Perovic S, Wilkesman J, Kruse M, Muller IM, Batel R: Increased gene expression of a cytokine-related molecule and profilin after activation of Suberites domuncula cells with xenogeneic sponge molecule(s). *DNA Cell Biol* 1999, 18(12):885-893.

[114] Fujiki K, Shin DH, Nakao M, Yano T: Molecular cloning and expression analysis of the putative carp (Cyprinus carpio) pre-B cell enhancing factor. *Fish Shellfish Immunol* 2000, 10(4):383-385.

[115] McGlothlin JR, Gao L, Lavoie T, Simon BA, Easley RB, Ma SF, Rumala BB, Garcia JG, Ye SQ: Molecular cloning and characterization of canine pre-B-cell colony-enhancing factor. *Biochem Genet* 2005, 43(3-4):127-141.

[116] Costa JV, Duarte JS: [Adipose tissue and adipokines]. *Acta Med Port* 2006, 19(3):251-256.

[117] Spiegelman BM, Frank M, Green H: Molecular cloning of mRNA from 3T3 adipocytes. Regulation of mRNA content for glycerophosphate dehydrogenase and other differentiation-dependent proteins during adipocyte development. *J Biol Chem* 1983, 258(16):10083-10089.

[118] Niemann MA, Bhown AS, Bennett JC, Volanakis JE: Amino acid sequence of human D of the alternative complement pathway. *Biochemistry* 1984, 23(11):2482-2486.

[119] Lesavre PH, Hugli TE, Esser AF, Muller-Eberhard HJ: The alternative pathway C3/C5 convertase: chemical basis of factor B activation. *J Immunol* 1979, 123(2):529-534.

[120] Liu B, Zhang J, Tan PY, Hsu D, Blom AM, Leong B, Sethi S, Ho B, Ding JL, Thiagarajan PS: A computational and experimental study of the regulatory mechanisms of the complement system. *PLoS Comput Biol* 2011, 7(1):e1001059.

[121] Whaley K: Biosynthesis of the complement components and the regulatory proteins of the alternative complement pathway by human peripheral blood monocytes. *J Exp Med* 1980, 151(3):501-516.

[122] Sprong T, Roos D, Weemaes C, Neeleman C, Geesing CL, Mollnes TE, van Deuren M: Deficient alternative complement pathway activation due to factor D deficiency by 2 novel mutations in the complement factor D gene in a family with meningococcal infections. *Blood* 2006, 107(12):4865-4870.

[123] Hiemstra PS, Langeler E, Compier B, Keepers Y, Leijh PC, van den Barselaar MT, Overbosch D, Daha MR: Complete and partial deficiencies of complement factor D in a Dutch family. *J Clin Invest* 1989, 84(6):1957-1961.

[124] Flier JS, Cook KS, Usher P, Spiegelman BM: Severely impaired adipsin expression in genetic and acquired obesity. *Science* 1987, 237(4813):405-408.

[125] Rosen BS, Cook KS, Yaglom J, Groves DL, Volanakis JE, Damm D, White T, Spiegelman BM: Adipsin and complement factor D activity: an immune-related defect in obesity. *Science* 1989, 244(4911):1483-1487.

10

Haptoglobin Function and Regulation in Autoimmune Diseases

Georgina Galicia and Jan L. Ceuppens
Catholic University of Leuven
Clinical Immunology Department, Leuven
Belgium

1. Introduction

Haptoglobin (Hp) is an acute phase protein, primarily synthesized in the liver and secreted into the plasma. Hp is also produced in other tissues including lung, skin, spleen, brain, intestine, arterial vessels and kidney, but to a lesser extent (D'Armiento et al., 1997; Pelletier et al., 1998; Yang et al., 2000). The normal concentration in human plasma ranges from 0.3- 3 mg/ml and increases several fold in the occurrence of local or systemic inflammation. Increased production of Hp is the result of transcriptional activation of the Hp gene (Baumann & Jahreis, 1983; Oliviero et al., 1987) by pro-inflammatory cytokines such as interleukin(IL)-1β, IL-6, and Tumor Necrosis factor (TNF) (Baumann et al., 1989). The result of pro-inflammatory cytokine signalling is the activation of essential transcription factors that are needed for the expression of Hp (STAT, C/EBP, PEA3). Among vertebrate species, the promoter of the Hp gene is conserved and contains three key regulatory elements that include two C/EBPβ recognition sequences that flank a STAT binding site (Wang et al., 2001).

2. Haptoglobin structure and polymorphism

Hp is composed of four chains: 2 α-chains (~9kDa each) and 2 β-chains (~33kDa each). Alpha and beta chains are encoded by a single gene and are synthesized as a single polypeptide chain that is proteolytically cleaved into a short α-chain and a long β-chain that remain connected through a disulfide bond. In addition an α-β unit is linked to another α-β unit also by a disulphide bond (Wejman et al., 1984).

In humans, Hp is characterized by a genetic polymorphism which arises from differences in α-chains while β–chains are identical in all Hp types. The Hp locus is located on chromosome 16 (16q22.1). Two common alleles exist for Hp, Hp1 and Hp2 that give rise to three major phenotypes. Individuals that are homozygous for allele Hp1 express the phenotype 1-1, those homozygous for allele Hp2, express phenotype Hp2-2, and heterozygous individuals express phenotype Hp1-2. The Hp1 allele is organized in 5 exons. The first 4 exons encode for the α-subunit while exon 5 encodes for the β-subunit. The Hp2 allele consists of 7 exons, the first 6 exons encode for a larger form of α–subunit and exon 7 encodes for the β-subunit. The larger form of the Hp α-subunit seems to originate from an intragenic duplication of exons 3 and 4. As a consequence, the Hp1-1 phenotype consists of homodimers of two α-β units, but Hp1-2 and Hp2-2 consist of polymers, as the cysteine that forms the disulfide bond between α-subunits is duplicated in Hp2. The resultant stoichiometry is for Hp1-1 homodimers of (α1-β)2; for Hp2-1 linear polymers of (α1-β)2 + (α2+β)n (n=0,1,2, etc); and for Hp2-2 cyclic polymers (α2+β)n (n=3,4 etc) (Van et al., 2004). The distribution of Hp1 and Hp2 alleles in the world population differs according to the racial origin. Native populations in South America have the highest frequency of the Hp1 allele (0.7), while Asian populations have the lowest frequency of the Hp1 allele (0.2). The European population has a Hp1 allele frequency of 0.4 with a phenotypic distribution of approximately 15% Hp1-1, 50% Hp 1-2, and 35% Hp2-2 (Carter & Worwood, 2007). Importantly, the three different Hp phenotypes exhibit functional differences that can have clinical and biological consequences.

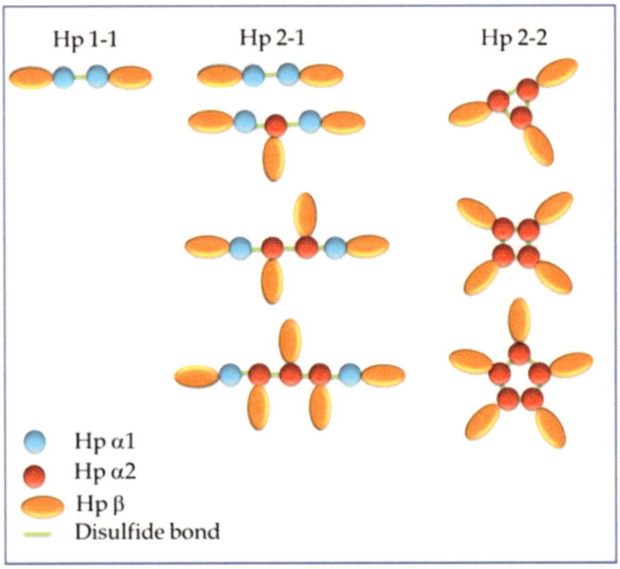

Fig. 1. Schematic representation of the structure of the different haptoglobin polymers determined by phenotype.

3. Haptoglobin: Biological functions

3.1 Haptoglobin prevents oxidative stress

Hp scavenges free hemoglobin (Hb) in the event of intravascular and/or extravascular hemolysis or during normal red blood cell turnover. In plasma, free Hb instantly binds Hp with extremely high affinity (KD ~10^{-15} M) but low dissociation speed, in a ratio of 1Hp:1Hb, to form the Hp-Hb complexes. These complexes are rapidly cleared and degraded by macrophages via the CD163 cell-surface receptor. CD163 receptor is expressed in monocytes and mature tissue macrophages. Hb-Hp complexes once internalized by tissue macrophages are degraded in lysosomes. The heme fraction is converted by heme oxygenase into bilirubin, carbon monoxide, and iron (Buehler et al., 2009). By doing so, Hp prevents the oxidative damage caused by free Hb. Free Hb is highly toxic due to its content of iron-heme that in the presence of H_2O_2 can generate reactive hydroxyl radicals (Fenton reaction) that in turn cause damage to lipids, proteins and DNA (Lim et al., 2001). Additionally, free Hb acts as a potent scavenger of nitric oxide (NO), an endogenous antioxidant and a regulator of vascular homeostasis, via deoxygenation. NO depletion by Hb has severe consequences such as blood vessel constriction and pulmonary and systemic hypertension, thrombosis, platelet activation, and smooth muscle responses (Alayash, 2011). NO is also important as a toxic defence molecule against infectious organisms and regulates the functional activity, growth and death of many immune and inflammatory cell types that results in an anti-inflammatory effect. The consumption of nitric oxide by Hb reduces the anti-inflammatory properties of NO (Tripathi, 2007).

Independently of its binding capacity to Hb, Hp is an effective antioxidant molecule of Cu2+ and AAPH-induced LDL oxidation. Hp also plays a role in cellular resistance to oxidative stress since its expression renders cells more resistant to damage by oxidative stress induced by hydrogen peroxide (Tseng et al., 2004).

Its capacity of Hp to prevent oxidative stress is directly related to its phenotype. Hp1-1 has been demonstrated to provide superior protection against Hb-iron driven peroxidation than Hp2-2. The superior antioxidant capacity of Hp1-1 seems not to be related with a dissimilar affinity with Hb but the functional differences may be explained by the restricted distribution of Hp2-2 in extravascular fluids as a consequence of its high molecular mass (Melamed-Frank et al., 2001).

The lessened antioxidant function of Hp2-2 is translated into clinical consequences. For instance, low levels of Hp (hypo-haptoglobinemia) and the Hp2-2 phenotype are associated with idiopathic familial and posttraumatic epilepsy. The mechanism behind this association can be the defective inhibition of Hb-driven brain-lipid peroxidation after micro-haemorrhage events within the central nervous system (CNS) caused by the null or low concentration of Hp in this tissue as a result of the low diffusion of Hp2-2 high molecular mass-polymers into the interstitial compartment of the CNS (Panter et al., 1985; Sadrzadeh et al., 2004). In subarachnoid haemorrhage (SAH) and intracerebral haemorrhage (ICH), Hp is important for protecting brain from damage caused by free Hb. In experimental SAH Hp1-1 showed higher protection of the brain tissue from vasospasm, inflammation and improved survival compared to Hp2-2 (Levy et al., 2007). In the ICH model, lack of Hp promoted axonal and oligodendroglia damage (Zhao et al., 2009).

3.2 Haptoglobin beyond its antioxidative role

Besides its anti-oxidative capacity, Hp has been demonstrated to exert direct angiogenic properties and to be involved in arterial restructuring. Hp has been shown to stimulate angiogenesis in both *in vitro* and *in vivo* models. Hp is implicated in arterial restructuring through the formation of a temporary gelatin-based matrix that enhances cell migration (De Kleijn et al., 2002). Additionally, Hp has been reported to function as an extracellular chaperone as it inhibits the heat and stress-induced precipitation of a wide variety of purified proteins by forming soluble high molecular weight complexes with missfolded proteins. All three phenotypes of Hp have efficient chaperone function, however Hp1-1 has the highest efficacy (Yerbury et al., 2005). Moreover, Hp can inhibit formation of amyloid fibrils from diverse proteins by interacting with prefibrillar species to maintain the solubility of amylodogenic proteins, avoiding the incorrect accumulation of proteins in extracellular spaces (Yerbury et al., 2009).

Haptoglobin forms part of the innate unspecific defence against pathogenic bacteria. Hp has a bacteriostatic role by binding Hb and preventing the utilization of iron by pathogenic bacteria that require iron for their growth (Eaton et al., 1982). Hp2-2 can bind the T4 antigen on the surface of streptoccocus bacterium and agglutinates this pathogen, thus inhibiting its growth (Delanghe, J. et al., 1998). However, Hp can also have a detrimental function in parasite infection. Hp-Hb complexes bind a receptor expressed on *Trypanosoma brucei* surface. Parasites seem to acquire heme from Hp-Hb complexes in order to increase their growth rate and resistance to the oxidative response of the host to eliminate parasites. On the other hand, a highly similar protein to Hp called "haptoglobin related protein" (Hpr) binds Hb and also associates with trypanosome lytic factor (TLF). TLF is a deadly toxic molecule for parasites. The penetration of TLF into the parasite is mediated by Hpr-Hb complexes. Hpr-Hb complexes are recognized by the same trypanosomal receptor that binds Hp-Hb complexes (Pays & Vanhollebeke, 2009).

The secretion of Hp is enhanced in inflammatory states, and at the same time, Hp has important anti-inflammatory properties. As a consequence of macrophage activation, a variety of inflammatory mediators are released, including prostaglandins, leukotrienes, and platelet-activating factor, which are products of the metabolism of the membrane polyunsaturated fatty acid arachidonic acid (AA) by 5-lipoxygenase (5-LO), cyclooxygenase (COX) or cytochrome P450 epoxygenase activity. Leukotrienes have chemotactic, chemokinetic, vasoactive and immunomodulatory properties. Hp possesses significant inhibitory activity on the biosynthesis of prostaglandins via COX and on 12-hydroxyeicosatetrenoate (12-HETE) via lipoxygenase (Saeed et al., 2007). Consequently, during the initial events of inflammation, Hp participates actively in reducing tissue damage.

During the inflammatory process and tissue injury, proteases such as cathepsin B are released. Cathepsin B is an abundantly expressed cysteine peptidase involved in many physiological processes, such as remodelling of the extracellular matrix (wound healing), apoptosis, and activation of thyroxin and rennin. Cathepsin B importantly participates in many pathological processes, such as inflammation, parasite infection and cancer, where it is highly up-regulated. Hp specifically inhibits cathepsin B activity (Kalsheker et al., 1981; Pagano et al., 1980; Snellman & Sylven, 1967). Therefore, Hp might have a regulatory role in tissue proteolysis associated with the inflammatory reaction.

Neutrophils are recruited at sites of inflammation within minutes after injury or infection. In this context Hp suppresses neutrophil function. Hp is synthesized in myelocytes/metamyelocytes during granulocyte differentiation, stored in specific granules of fully differentiated neutrophils and exocytosed immediately in response to activation. Hp binding to activated neutrophils inhibits not only the activity of both 5-LO and COX but also calcium influx and subsequent generation of reactive oxygen species. Hp inhibits respiratory burst activity in neutrophils stimulated with fMLP, arachidonic acid, and opsonized zymosan (Oh et al., 1990). Hp also inhibits the chemotactic response of human granulocytes and differentiated HL-60 cells to fMLP, but does not affect chemotaxis by IL-8. Hp inhibits phagocytosis and reduces intracellular bactericidal activities of granulocytes (Rossbacher et al., 1999; Theilgaard-Monch et al., 2006). Thus, Hp secreted at sites of injury or inflammation mitigates potential tissue damage locally.

4. Haptoglobin expression, polymorphism and disease

Expression of Hp has been associated with diverse inflammatory autoimmune diseases and as a marker of disease activity. Also, genetic polymorphism of Hp has been shown to influence the course of several inflammatory pathologies.

Infection

Patients infected with HIV-1 and with Hp2-2 phenotype have a worse prognosis, related to a more rapid rate of viral replication, than HIV-1 infected patients with the Hp1-1 phenotype. Hp2-2 patients also show higher iron levels and oxidize more vitamin C. It is possible that the less efficient protection against heme-driven oxidative stress by Hp2-2 may stimulate the viral replication (Delanghe, J. R. et al., 1998).

Cancer

High amounts of Hp in plasma and locally in tumoral tissue have been observed in diverse types of malignancies including, lung, bladder, breast cancer, leukemia, glioblastoma, malignant lymphoma, and ovarian cancer (Abdullah et al., 2009; Carter & Worwood, 2007; Kumar et al., 2010; Smeets et al., 2003). The suggested functions of Hp in cancer are as a biomarker of malignancy, as a regulator of the immune response against tumor cells, and as a facilitator of metastasis, since Hp seems to participate in cell migration and angiogenesis (Cid et al., 1993; De Kleijn et al., 2002).

Atherosclerosis

In cross sectional studies, the Hp2-2 phenotype is also associated with an increased risk of atherosclerotic vascular disease and acute myocardial infarction. The lower antioxidant capacity of Hp2-2 together with a lower capacity of Hp2-2 in stimulating macrophages to secrete anti-inflammatory cytokines after binding CD163, might be the reason why individuals with Hp2-2 phenotype are more susceptible for cardiovascular diseases (Levy et al., 2007).

Myasthenia gravis

High serum levels of Hp have been found in patients with myasthenia gravis. Hp serum level is directly correlated with the severity of the disease. This correlation could be explained by the presence of high levels of pro-inflammatory cytokines during active disease. To determine the Hp serum levels in patients with myasthenia can be useful to monitor the severity of the disease (Oliveira et al., 2008).

Arthritis

In patients with active rheumatoid arthritis, high serum levels of Hp have been found. Levels of Hp correlate with clinical disease activity (Cylwik et al., 2010). In juvenile idiopathic arthritis (JIA), a heterogeneous group of inflammatory diseases, Hp was found in inflamed joints. Hp was locally produced in synovial fluid of patients with JIA. Moreover, Hp was expressed differentially between JIA subtypes. Hp expression was increased in systemic JIA. The presence of Hp in the inflamed tissue suggests that Hp plays a role in the progression and pathology of the disease and can also be used as a biomarker of disease activity (Rosenkranz et al., 2010).

Psoriasis

In psoriasis, a structure modification of Hp was described that might impair the Hb binding function and also the activity of the lecithin-cholesterol acyltransferase (LCTA) enzyme (Cigliano et al., 2008). The structural modification of Hp in psoriasis patients is an abundance or structure change of specific glycans that differ or do not exist in Hp from healthy donors. These changes are associated with altered function of that might have an impact on the disease activity (Maresca et al., 2010). Interestingly, it was found that there is no higher prevalence of any of the three phenotypes of Hp in psoriasis.

Lupus

It has been shown that in systemic lupus erythematosus (SLE) patients, Hp plasma levels correlate with severity of the disease and that the Hp2-2 phenotype is over-represented in SLE patients (Pavon et al., 2006; Rantapaa et al., 1988). The association of the Hp2-2 phenotype with SLE can have several implications. SLE is an autoimmune disease mediated by B cells that secrete self-reactive pathogenic antibodies. Individuals with the Hp2-2 phenotype seem to have a higher number of CD22 binding sites compared to other Hp phenotypes. Additionally, it is known that cardiovascular disease is a common complication of SLE. The finding that Hp2-2 has lower anti-oxidant capacity (Van et al., 2004) might be an explication for this.

Celiac disease

The frequency of the Hp1-2 phenotype in celiac disease patients has been reported to be higher than in the general population. However, Hp2-2 phenotype was associated with a more severe clinical course of the disease (Papp et al., 2008). The structural differences and the functional differences between Hp phenotypes may account for phenotype association of Hp to the more severe form of celiac disease. Hp2-2-Hb complexes upon binding CD163 induce lower expression of IL-10 compared to Hp1-1-Hb complexes. Hp2-2 is as well associated to a stronger immune response (Guetta et al., 2007).

Diabetes type I

In patients with a long duration of type I diabetes, an increased risk of cardiovascular disease was observed in patients with the Hp2-2 phenotype. Again, as Hp2-2 has low anti-oxidant capacity and a low efficiency in preventing heme release, this can contribute to the higher cardiovascular risk in type I diabetes (Costacou et al., 2008). Also, it was shown that the Hp phenotype may be an independent determinant of early renal function decline and progression to end-stage renal disease (Costacou et al., 2009).

Inflammatory bowel diseases (IBD)

Inflammatory bowel disease (IBD) is a chronic, relapsing intestinal inflammatory condition that is classified into two major forms, Crohn's disease (CD) and ulcerative colitis (UC). The etiology is unknown, but the pathogenesis is likely dependent on the interaction between local immune reaction and environmental factors in susceptible individuals. To explore a possible role of Hp in IBD patients we recently studied polymorphisms in the Hp locus in a cohort of CD and UC patients. It was found that the Hp2 locus was overrepresented in CD and UC patients compared to healthy individuals (Marquez, et al. in press). These results indicate that Hp phenotype can be a risk factor for IBD. Since Hp phenotypes differ in their function, further research is necessary to understand how Hp genotype modulates IBD pathogenesis.

5. Haptoglobin and the immune response

Disease associations mentioned above are strongly suggestive for a modulatory effect of Hp on immune responses. Several experimental data support this concept.

5.1 Receptors for Hp on immune cells

The Hb-Hp complex is removed from the circulation by binding to CD163 expressed on the monocyte-macrophage system. CD163 is a member of the SRCR family class B and is expressed on most subpopulations of mature tissue macrophages. Triggering CD163 by ligand binding (Hb-Hp) results in a protein tyrosine kinase-dependent signal and secretion of IL-6 and IL-10. Moreover, IL-6 and IL-10 are known to up-regulate CD163 and this might function as a positive feedback mechanism for CD163 induction. In fact, CD163 has an important immunomodulatory function. The Hp genotype modulates the balance of Th1 and Th2 cytokines produced by macrophages exposed to free Hb via a CD163 dependent mechanism. The Hp1-1–Hb complex stimulated the secretion of significantly more IL-6 and IL-10 than the Hp2-2–Hb complex (Guetta et al., 2007). Moreover, CD163 also exerts an immunomodulatory role by degradation of heme which results in the production of metabolites with suggested anti-inflammatory effects (Moestrup & Moller, 2004; Nielsen et al., 2007).

Hp also binds to the integrin adhesion receptor, Mac-1 (Macrophage-1 antigen, integrin alphaMbeta2, CD11b/CD18) (El Ghmati et al., 1996) which is expressed on dendritic cells, neutrophils, monocytes, macrophages, NK cells, and a small subset of T cells. Mac-1 is involved in maturation, phagocytosis and adhesion of monocytes and is required for adhesion and transmigration of monocytes into tissues. Engagement of Mac-1 by its ligands initiates an intracellular signalling cascade that results in activation and cytokine secretion (Shi et al., 2004; Shi & Simon, 2006).

Hp is a ligand of CD22 on B cells and CD22 is implicated in B cell activation and survival (Langlois et al., 1997). By binding CD22, Hp can inhibit the interaction with other CD22 ligands and as a consequence may negatively modulate the B cell function (Hanasaki et al., 1995).

Hp has also been demonstrated to bind a not-yet-identified receptor on mast cells interfering with their spontaneous proliferation (El-Ghmati et al., 2002), and perhaps with other functions that have not been explored.

5.2 Immunomodulatory effects of Hp

Hp participates actively in several processes of the immune response, from activation of the innate and adaptive immune response to tissue repair and regeneration. Hp released locally and systemically modulates numerous cellular activities, including prostaglandin synthesis, leukocyte activation, recruitment and migration, modulation of cytokine patterns, and tissue repair (Wang et al., 2001). Hp rises during inflammatory process, including those caused by autoimmunity, and the general picture is that Hp has an anti-inflammatory effect (Arredouani et al., 2005; Quaye, 2008; Wang et al., 2001).

An anti-proliferative capacity of Hp on lymphocytes has been demonstrated in a variety of conditions. Purified Hp or Hp present in sera and ascites fluid of cancer patients has been shown to inhibit the polyclonal proliferation of mitogen-stimulated T cells (Arredouani et al., 2003; Oh, S. K. et al., 1987b). Hp modifies the T helper Th1/Th2 balance (Arredouani et al., 2003; Oh, S. K. et al., 1987a; Oh, S. K. et al., 1987b). Furthermore, Hp inhibits or enhances proliferation of B-cells in response to bacterial endotoxins, depending on its concentration (Quaye, 2008; Wang et al., 2001).

Dendritic cells (DC) are central regulators of immune responses and the bridge between innate and adaptive immune response. It has been demonstrated that Hp prevents epidermal Langerhans cells (LC) from spontaneous functional maturation in the skin. Hp is stored in the epidermal LC cytoplasm, but LC do not produce Hp. Though, Hp is produced in keratinocytes (KC). KC play an important role in regulating the function of LC and T cells in the skin by producing cytokines and possibly by expressing Hp (Li et al., 2005; Wang et al., 2005; Xie et al., 2000).

5.3 Haptoglobin has a negative regulatory role in a CNS-autoimmune response

Experimental autoimmune encephalomyelitis (EAE) is a model for organ specific autoimmunity. The immunopathological events of EAE encompass the initial T-cell priming in the secondary lymphoid organs, followed by the recruitment of primed T-cells in the CNS and the subsequent effector phase. Systemic immunisation with myelin antigens in CFA is sufficient to prime myelin-reactive T cells. Neuroantigen-reactive T cells recognize their cognate antigen presented by professional antigen-presenting cells (APCs) within secondary lymphoid organs where those cells are activated and expanded (Becher et al., 2006). Once myelin-reactive T cells are activated in the periphery, they migrate to the CNS traversing the blood brain barrier (BBB). Activated T cells in the CNS recruit other lymphocytes, monocytes, and granulocytes by secreting inflammatory mediators. All inflammatory immune cells orchestrate damage to myelin that covers axons, a process called demyelination. In turn, demyelination leads to a variety of neurological symptoms including paralysis as a final result.

Until recently there were no studies yet that specifically analyzed the effect of Hp on development and course of CNS autoimmune inflammatory disease. We aimed to characterize the role of Hp in EAE induced by immunisation with MOG35-55 peptide in C57BL/6 mice. We immunised wild-type (WT) and Hp-/- C57BL/6 mice with MOG35-55 in complete Freunds adjuvans (CFA) and showed that Hp influences the severity of EAE, as the lack of Hp results in clinically and in pathologically exacerbated EAE (Galicia et al., 2009). Our further results indicated that Hp has an important modulatory effect on the infiltration of mononuclear cells into the CNS and on the production of Th1 cytokines and IL-17A by auto-reactive T cells. Exacerbated disease in Hp-/- mice was related to an increased expression of IFN–γ, IL-6 and IL-17A in the CNS of these animals. Furthermore, the number of IL-17+ cells in the CNS was increased (Galicia et al., 2009). Neutralization of IL-17A with anti-IL-17A monoclonal antibodies (mAbs) in Hp-/- mice significantly reduced the severity of the disease but did not completely block it as it did in WT animals (Fig2) (unpublished data).

These results strongly suggest that Hp has a protective role in reducing the severity of an autoimmune inflammatory process, and this protection is related with the suppression of auto-aggressive cells that produce inflammatory cytokines.

5.4 Haptoglobin has a regulatory role in experimental colitis

Several animal models of inflammatory bowel disease have been developed, in which colitis can be induced using chemical compounds such as dextran sulphate sodium (DSS) or oxazolone in susceptible strains of mice. The resulting inflammation is mediated by polymorphonuclear cells, macrophages, and lymphocytes. Interestingly, Hp is expressed by intestinal epithelial cells (Pelletier et al., 1998).

To study whether Hp has an effect on the course of inflammatory colitis, we induced colitis with DSS and oxazolone in wild-type and in Hp deficient mice. We found that in both forms of colitis, the severity of the disease was exacerbated in Hp-/- mice compared to WT. The more severe inflammation in Hp-/- mice was related to high mRNA expression of IL-17, IFN-γ, TNF and IL-6 in colonic tissue in Hp-/- DSS colitis mice, while there was a slight increase in IL-13 mRNA in Hp-/- mice with oxazolone-induced colitis. In order to determine the immunological mechanisms for the protective role of Hp in these models, draining lymph nodes from DSS or oxazolone colitis mice were cultured in the presence of IL-23, a cytokine that contributes to the survival and effector functions of IL-17-producing cells (Th17). Cells obtained from DSS and oxazolone colitis Hp-/- mice produced high amounts of IL-17 compared with WT mice, suggesting the presence of increased numbers of Th17 cells in Hp-/- mice. However, we found that *in vitro* Hp does not interfere with Th17 differentiation but that it rather suppresses IL-17 production (Marquez, et al. in press). Thus again, Hp exerts n immunomodulatory function by reducing the activity of pro-inflammatory lymphocytes.

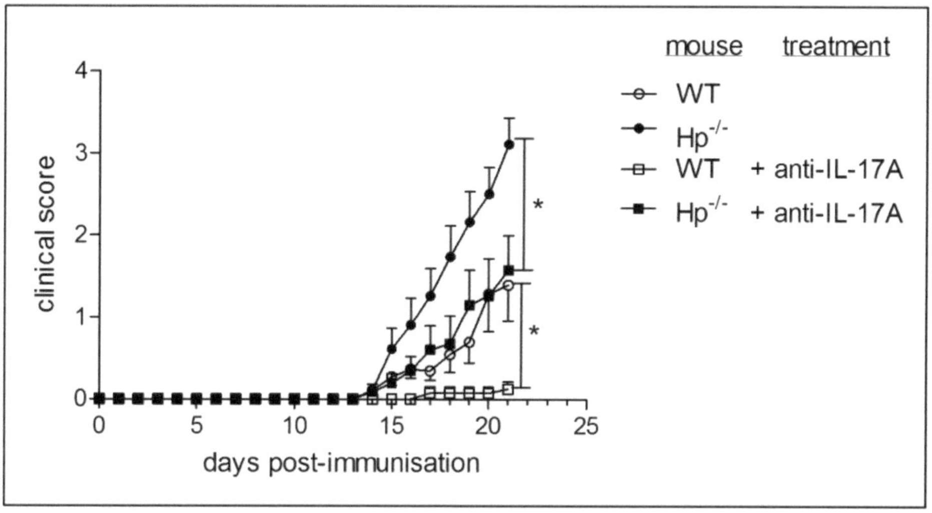

Fig. 2. Blockade of IL-17A reduces the severity of EAE in WT and Hp-/- mice. Clinical scores of WT and Hp-/- mice immunised with MOG35-55/CFA untreated or treated with murine anti-mouse IL-17A mAbs. Anti-IL-17A mAb was administered intra peritoneally two times per week (0.2 mg/mouse) from day 7 until day 21 after immunisation. Data shown are from two different experiments (n=10). *p≤ 0.05. (Galicia, et al. unpublished data)

5.5 Hp is required to induce mucosal tolerance

The immune response serves primarily to protect the organism from foreign invading pathogens and tumor cells. Reduced or absent responsiveness of the immune system against self-antigens is necessary to allow the immune system to mount an effective response to eliminate infectious invaders while leaving host tissues intact. This condition is known as immune tolerance. Self-tolerance is maintained by central (thymus-dependent) and by peripheral mechanisms. The mechanism of central tolerance is the deletion of self-reactive T cells in the thymus during T cell maturation. During ontogeny auto-reactive cells encounter self-antigens in the medullary-cortical junction in the thymus, and those cells that react with high affinity to the antigen are eliminated in a process called negative selection (Kyewski & Klein, 2006). Nevertheless, some self-reactive T cells can escape from deletion in the thymus. These auto-reactive cells must be kept in a state of reduced or absent responsiveness to avoid pathogenic immune reactivity. Peripheral tolerance provides a second line of protection against autoimmune responses by regulating potentially pathogenic autoreactive lymphocytes, a process in which regulatory T cells have a major role (Li & Boussiotis, 2006). When self-tolerance is broken, the immune reaction against self-antigens can lead to autoimmune disease.

Mucosal tolerance induction is a naturally occurring immunological phenomenon that originates from mucosal contact with inhaled or ingested proteins. The largest areas of the body exposed to the external environment are the mucosal surfaces. Regular contact of antigens with mucosal surfaces prevents harmful inflammatory responses to non-dangerous proteins, such as food components, harmless environmental inhaled antigens and symbiotic microorganisms. The lymphoid tissue associated to the mucosa of the gastrointestinal tract and to the airway system mucosa therefore plays an important role in tolerance maintenance (Dubois et al., 2005). Administration of antigens by either oral or nasal route, in the absence of costimulatory signals, leads to specific suppression of systemic immune responses against these antigens in mice. The induction of oral or nasal tolerance to antigens is an active process that results in anergy, generation of antigen-specific suppressive T lymphocytes, production of anti-inflammatory cytokines such as IL-4, IL-10 and TGF-β, and deletion of antigen reactive T cells (Dubois et al., 2005; Faria & Weiner, 2006). On the contrary, mucosal tolerance induction is abrogated by applying the antigen in the presence of an adjuvant, such as LPS or cholera toxin (Kraal et al., 2006).

Oral and nasal tolerance has been used successfully to prevent a number of experimental autoimmune diseases including, arthritis, diabetes, uveitis, and EAE (Faria & Weiner, 2006). Particularly, administration of MOG35-55 peptide by the nasal route is highly efficient in suppressing EAE (Shi et al., 1998; Xu et al., 2000). Shortly after intranasal antigen instillation of a soluble, harmless antigen, it can be detected in the nose-draining lymph nodes. The majority of inhaled antigen detected in lymph nodes is associated with a variety of dendritic cells (DC), such as CD8αlow CD205+, plasmacytoid DCs and CD8αhigh DC (Wikstrom & Stumbles, 2007). These DC play a pivotal role in induction of tolerance through the differential expression of surface molecules and cytokines that make them able of inducing T-regulatory cells (Coombes et al., 2007). After antigen presentation under non-inflammatory conditions to antigen-specific naïve CD4+ T cells, those T cells proliferate transiently and become tolerant. The CD4+ T cell population that arises after harmless antigen administration in the nose is able to transfer tolerance and to suppress specific immune responses in naïve animals (Unger et al., 2003). The draining lymph nodes of the nose which are the internal jugular (IJLN) and superficial cervical lymph (CLN) nodes are essential for tolerance induction towards inhaled antigens. Removing these lymph nodes abrogates the capacity of nasal tolerance induction and their function cannot be restored by peripheral lymph nodes when transplanted to this site (Kraal et al., 2006; Wolvers et al., 1999). Importantly, Hp expression is increased in cervical lymph nodes shortly after nasal protein antigen instillation without adjuvant (Boots et al., 2004). Thus, Hp might have an important function in nasal tolerance induction.

Several murine models of autoimmune diseases can be prevented by nasally administering the self-antigens prior to disease induction with the same antigen, including EAE (Li et al., 1998; Shi et al., 1998). To study the participation of Hp in nasal tolerance induction, we administrated 100μg of MOG35-55 to Hp-/- and WT sex-age matched mice by nasal instillation at day 7, 5, and 3 before EAE induction by immuniszation with MOG in CFA. The control group was given PBS as vehicle control. We found that Hp-/- mice were partly resistant to the development of nasal tolerance induction, as Hp-/- mice that received nasally MOG peptide in the nose still developed severe EAE, while the WT mice were protected. These data suggest that Hp is a critical modulator of mucosal tolerance induction (Fig3) (Galicia, et al. unpublished data). Lack of immune tolerance in Hp-/- mice was associated with deficient suppression of antigen-dependent IL-17A production by T cells (unpublished data).

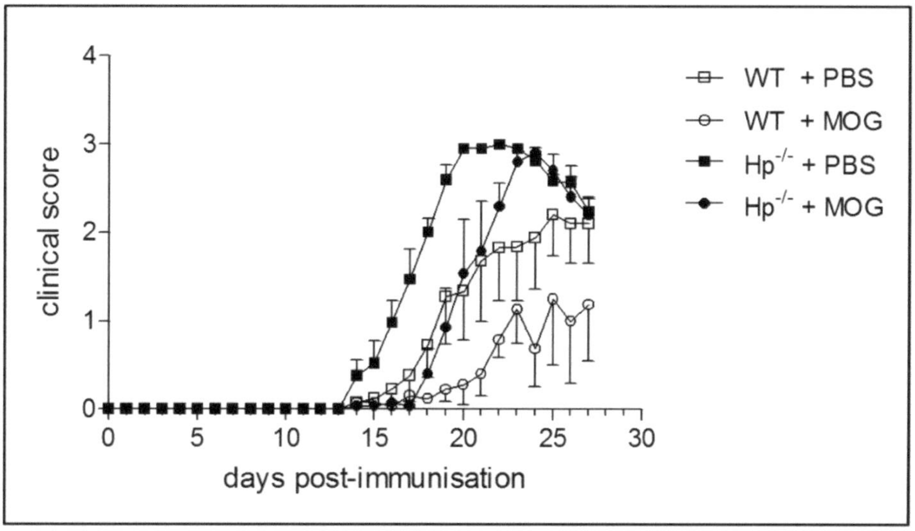

Fig. 3. Lack of Hp hampers induction of nasal tolerance. Mice received 100µg MOG35-55 or PBS by nasal instillation, on day 7, 5 and 3 before MOG-immunisation. EAE was induced by injection of MOG35-55 in CFA in the footpads. Clinical score was assessed daily. A representative experiment out of three independent experiments with similar results is shown. Each experimental group consisted of 5 mice. WT+PBS vs WT+MOG: p=0.0066; WT+PBS vs Hp-/- +PBS: p=0.048. Hp-/-+PBS vs Hp-/-+MOG: p=0.06.

6. Conclusion

Apart from the Hb scavenger function of Hp, several recent studies have revealed new functions of Hp on immune responses and in autoimmunity. Furthermore, Hp polymorphism seems to be related with the outcome of various autoimmune diseases. The differential capacity to prevent oxidative stress, modulation of immune responses, and control of inflammation by the three major Hp phenotypes (Van et al., 2004) can account for differences in susceptibility to, or severity of the autoimmune inflammation. Previously, our laboratory demonstrated that Hp was able to modulate not only the function of T cells, by regulating *in vivo* and *in vitro* the Th1/Th2 response, but also macrophage cytokine secretion. Whereas in some cells the Hp binding receptor is known (Mac-1 on macrophages, dendritic cells; CD22 on B cells), additional receptors might exist. However, the evidence that Hp acts directly on immune cells points out that Hp plays an important negative regulatory role in immune response and likely in autoimmunity. To explore this hypothesis we used models of organ-specific autoimmunity mediated by T cells. We showed in two different models of autoimmune inflammation that Hp has a crucial role in controlling inflammation mediated by Th1 and Th17 cells. Though the mechanism behind exacerbated

Th1/Th17 responses is still not clear, we propose that Hp may regulate differentiation and/or activity of T cells indirectly through the negative regulation of dendritic cell and macrophage functions.

Dendritic cells are the most efficient cells in driving the activation and differentiation of naïve T cells (Ueno et al., 2007). Hp has been described as an alternative low affinity ligand for the CD11b/CD18 (Mac-1) integrin (El Ghmati et al., 1996). Moreover, Mac-1 has been demonstrated to play an important role in the function of Mac-1 expressing cells and in migration and phagocytosis. Thus, it is likely that Hp, by binding Mac-1, may negatively regulate the function of dendritic cells, macrophages, and any cell that express Mac-1. Consequently, we propose that the lack of Hp allows for a stronger activation of DC, and therefore more potent activation and differentiation of auto-aggressive T cells with a pro-inflammatory cytokine profile (Fig4).

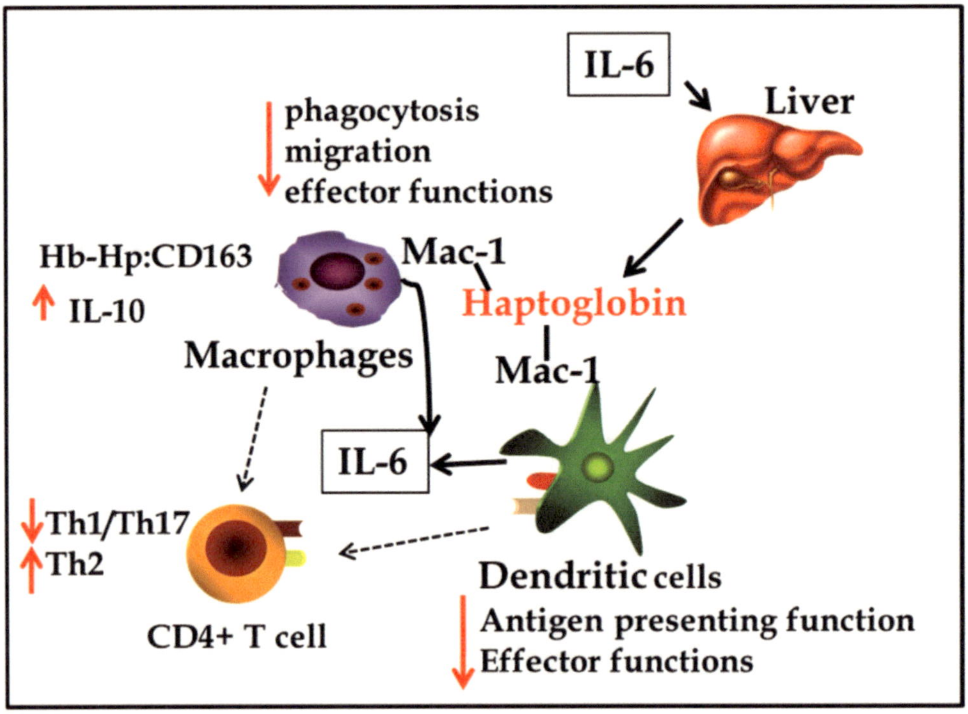

Fig. 4. Diagrammatic scheme of the potential mechanism of Hp regulation of immune cell functions. Hp is proposed to act through binding Mac-1 on dendritic cells and macrophages, thus reducing their activity and IL-6 secretion. Dotted arrows indicate an indirect effect of Hp on T cells through function modulation of macrophages and dendritic cells, resulting in decreased Th1 and Th17 activity.

Our results imply that Hp can be considered as a highly relevant player in controlling immunity and inflammation. Additionally, we showed that Hp polymorphism is associated with inflammatory bowel disease. Finally, we also demonstrated that Hp is an essential component for the mucosal tolerance induction. Further studies are needed to obtain more insight into the mechanism through which Hp restrain the Th1/Th17 response and how Hp is relevant in creating a proper environment in the lymph nodes to induce tolerance.

7. Acknowledgments

This work was supported by the Fund for scientific research Vlaanderen and by the SCAP foundation for allergy research.

8. References

Abdullah, M., Schultz, H., Kahler, D., Branscheid, D., Dalhoff, K., Zabel, P., Vollmer, E., & Goldmann, T. (2009). Expression of the acute phase protein haptoglobin in human lung cancer and tumor-free lung tissues. *Pathololog*y *research and practice*. 205:639-647

Alayash, A.I. (2011). Haptoglobin: Old protein with new functions. *Clinica Chimica Acta*. 412:493-498

Arredouani, M., Matthijs, P., Van, H.E., Kasran, A., Baumann, H., Ceuppens, J.L., & Stevens, E. (2003). Haptoglobin directly affects T cells and suppresses T helper cell type 2 cytokine release. *Immunology*. 108:144-151

Arredouani, M.S., Kasran, A., Vanoirbeek, J.A., Berger, F.G., Baumann, H., & Ceuppens, J.L. (2005). Haptoglobin dampens endotoxin-induced inflammatory effects both in vitro and in vivo. *Immunology*. 114:263-271

Baumann, H. and Jahreis, G.P. (1983). Regulation of mouse haptoglobin synthesis. *The Journal of Cell Biology*. 97:728-736

Baumann, H., Prowse, K.R., Marinkovic, S., Won, K.A., & Jahreis, G.P. (1989). Stimulation of hepatic acute phase response by cytokines and glucocorticoids. *Ann.N.Y.Acad.Sci.* 557:280-95, discussion

Becher, B., Bechmann, I., & Greter, M. (2006). Antigen presentation in autoimmunity and CNS inflammation: how T lymphocytes recognize the brain. *J Mol.Med*. 84:532-543

Boots, A.M., Verhaert, P.D., tePoele, R.J., Evers, S., Coenen-deRoo, C.J., Cleven, J., & Bos, E.S. (2004). Antigens up the nose: identification of putative biomarkers for nasal tolerance induction functional studies combined with proteomics. *J.Proteome Res.* 3:1056-1062.1535-3893

Buehler, P.W., Abraham, B., Vallelian, F., Linnemayr, C., Pereira, C.P., Cipollo, J.F., Jia, Y., Mikolajczyk, M., Boretti, F.S., Schoedon, G., Alayash, A.I., & Schaer, D.J. (2009). Haptoglobin preserves the CD163 hemoglobin scavenger pathway by shielding hemoglobin from peroxidative modification. *Blood*. 113:2578-2586

Carter, K. and Worwood, M. (2007). Haptoglobin: a review of the major allele frequencies worldwide and their association with diseases. *Int.J.Lab Hematol*. 29:92-110

Cid, M.C., Grant, D.S., Hoffman, G.S., Auerbach, R., Fauci, A.S., & Kleinman, H.K. (1993). Identification of haptoglobin as an angiogenic factor in sera from patients with systemic vasculitis. *The Journal of Clinical Investigation*. 91:977-985

Cigliano, L., Maresca, B., Salvatore, A., Nino, M., Monfrecola, G., Ayala, F., Carlucci, A., Pugliese, R.C., Pedone, C., & Abrescia, P. (2008). Haptoglobin from psoriatic patients exhibits decreased activity in binding haemoglobin and inhibiting lecithin-cholesterol acyltransferase activity. *J.Eur.Acad.Dermatol.Venereol*. 22:417-425

Coombes, J.L., Siddiqui, K.R., rancibia-Carcamo, C.V., Hall, J., Sun, C.M., Belkaid, Y., & Powrie, F. (2007). A functionally specialized population of mucosal CD103+ DCs induces Foxp3+ regulatory T cells via a TGF-beta and retinoic acid-dependent mechanism. *J Exp.Med*. 204:1757-1764

Costacou, T., Ferrell, R.E., Ellis, D., & Orchard, T.J. (2009). Haptoglobin genotype and renal function decline in type 1 diabetes. *Diabetes*. 58:2904-2909

Costacou, T., Ferrell, R.E., & Orchard, T.J. (2008). Haptoglobin genotype: a determinant of cardiovascular complication risk in type 1 diabetes. *Diabetes*. 57:1702-1706

Cylwik, B., Chrostek, L., Gindzienska-Sieskiewicz, E., Sierakowski, S., & Szmitkowski, M. (2010). Relationship between serum acute-phase proteins and high disease activity in patients with rheumatoid arthritis. *Adv.Med.Sci.* 55:80-85

D'Armiento, J., Dalal, S.S., & Chada, K. (1997). Tissue, temporal and inducible expression pattern of haptoglobin in mice. *Gene*. 195:19-27

De Kleijn, D.P., Smeets, M.B., Kemmeren, P.P., Lim, S.K., Van Middelaar , B.J., Velema, E., Schoneveld, A., Pasterkamp, G., & Borst, C. (2002). Acute-phase protein haptoglobin is a cell migration factor involved in arterial restructuring. *FASEB J.* 16:1123-1125

Delanghe, J., Langlois, M., Ouyang, J., Claeys, G., De, Buyzere M., & Wuyts, B. (1998). Effect of haptoglobin phenotypes on growth of Streptococcus pyogenes. *Clin.Chem.Lab Med.* 36:691-696

Delanghe, J. R., Langlois, M. R., Boelaert, J. R., Van, Acker J., Van, Wanzeele F., van der Groen, G., Hemmer, R., Verhofstede, C., De, Buyzere M., De, Bacquer D., Arendt, V., & Plum, J. (1998). Haptoglobin polymorphism, iron metabolism and mortality in HIV infection. *AIDS*. 12:1027-1032

Dubois, B., Goubier, A., Joubert, G., & Kaiserlian, D. (2005). Oral tolerance and regulation of mucosal immunity. *Cell Mol.Life Sci.* 62:1322-1332

Eaton, J.W., Brandt, P., Mahoney, J.R., & Lee, J.T., Jr. (1982). Haptoglobin: a natural bacteriostat. *Science*. 215:691-693

El Ghmati, S.M., Van Hoeyveld, E.M., Van Strijp, J.G., Ceuppens, J.L., & Stevens, E.A. (1996). Identification of haptoglobin as an alternative ligand for CD11b/CD18. *J Immunol.* 156:2542-2552

El-Ghmati, S.M., Arredouani, M., Van Hoeyveld, E.M., Ceuppens, J.L., & Stevens, E.A. (2002). Haptoglobin interacts with the human mast cell line HMC-1 and inhibits its spontaneous proliferation. *Scand.J.Immunol.* 55:352-358

Faria, A.M. and Weiner, H.L. (2006). Oral tolerance: therapeutic implications for autoimmune diseases. *Clin.Dev.Immunol.* 13:143-157

Galicia, G., Maes, W., Verbinnen, B., Kasran, A., Bullens, D., Arredouani, M., & Ceuppens, J.L. (2009). Haptoglobin deficiency facilitates the development of autoimmune inflammation. *Eur.J.Immunol.* 39:3404-3412

Guetta, J., Strauss, M., Levy, N.S., Fahoum, L., & Levy, A.P. (2007). Haptoglobin genotype modulates the balance of Th1/Th2 cytokines produced by macrophages exposed to free hemoglobin. *Atherosclerosis*. 191:48-53

Hanasaki, K., Powell, L.D., & Varki, A. (1995). Binding of human plasma sialoglycoproteins by the B cell-specific lectin CD22. Selective recognition of immunoglobulin M and haptoglobin. *J.Biol.Chem.* 270:7543-7550

Kalsheker, N.A., Bradwell, A.R., & Burnett, D. (1981). The inhibition of cathepsin B by plasma haptoglobin biochemistry (enzymes, metabolism). *Experientia*. 37:447-448

Kraal, G., Samsom, J.N., & Mebius, R.E. (2006). The importance of regional lymph nodes for mucosal tolerance. *Immunol.Rev.* 213:119-130

Kumar, D.M., Thota, B., Shinde, S.V., Prasanna, K.V., Hegde, A.S., Arivazhagan, A., Chandramouli, B.A., Santosh, V., & Somasundaram, K. (2010). Proteomic identification of haptoglobin alpha2 as a glioblastoma serum biomarker: implications in cancer cell migration and tumor growth. *J. Proteome. Res.* 9:5557-5567

Kyewski, B. and Klein, L. (2006). A central role for central tolerance. *Annu. Rev. Immunol.* 24:571-606

Langlois, M., Delanghe, J., Philippe, J., Ouyang, J., Bernard, D., De, B.M., Van, N.G., & Leroux-Roels, G. (1997). Distribution of lymphocyte subsets in bone marrow and peripheral blood is associated with haptoglobin type. Binding of haptoglobin to the B-cell lectin CD22. *Eur.J.Clin. Chem. Clin. Biochem.* 35:199-205

Levy, A.P., Levy, J.E., Kalet-Litman, S., Miller-Lotan, R., Levy, N.S., Asaf, R., Guetta, J., Yang, C., Purushothaman, K.R., Fuster, V., & Moreno, P.R. (2007). Haptoglobin genotype is a determinant of iron, lipid peroxidation, and macrophage accumulation in the atherosclerotic plaque. *Arterioscler. Thromb. Vasc. Biol.* 27:134-140

Li, H.L., Liu, J.Q., Bai, X.F., vn der Meide, P.H., & Link, H. (1998). Dose-dependent mechanisms relate to nasal tolerance induction and protection against experimental autoimmune encephalomyelitis in Lewis rats. *Immunology.* 94:431-437

Li, L. and Boussiotis, V.A. (2006). Physiologic regulation of central and peripheral T cell tolerance: lessons for therapeutic applications. *J Mol. Med.* 84:887-899

Li, P., Gao, X.H., Chen, H.D., Zhang, Y., Wang, Y., Wang, H., Wang, Y., & Xie, Y. (2005). Localization of haptoglobin in normal human skin and some skin diseases. *Int. J Dermatol.* 44:280-284

Lim, S.K., Ferraro, B., Moore, K., & Halliwell, B. (2001). Role of haptoglobin in free hemoglobin metabolism. *Redox.Rep.* 6:219-227

Maresca, B., Cigliano, L., Corsaro, M.M., Pieretti, G., Natale, M., Bucci, E.M., Dal, P.F., Balato, N., Nino, M., Ayala, F., & Abrescia, P. (2010). Quantitative determination of haptoglobin glycoform variants in psoriasis. *Biol. Chem.* 391:1429-1439

Melamed-Frank, M., Lache, O., Enav, B.I., Szafranek, T., Levy, N.S., Ricklis, R.M., & Levy, A.P. (2001). Structure-function analysis of the antioxidant properties of haptoglobin. *Blood.* 98:3693-3698

Moestrup, S.K. and Moller, H.J. (2004). CD163: a regulated hemoglobin scavenger receptor with a role in the anti-inflammatory response. *Ann. Med.* 36:347-354

Nielsen, M.J., Petersen, S.V., Jacobsen, C., Thirup, S., Enghild, J.J., Graversen, J.H., & Moestrup, S.K. (2007). A unique loop extension in the serine protease domain of haptoglobin is essential for CD163 recognition of the haptoglobin-hemoglobin complex. *J Biol. Chem.* 282:1072-1079

Oh, S. K., Leung, M. F., Knee, T., & Williams, J. M. (1987a). Biological properties of suppressive E-receptor factor on lymphokine function. *Eur.J Immunol.* 17:1403-1409

Oh, S.K., Pavlotsky, N., & Tauber, A.I. (1990). Specific binding of haptoglobin to human neutrophils and its functional consequences. *J Leukoc. Biol.* 47:142-148

Oh, S. K., Very, D. L., Walker, J., Raam, S., & Ju, S. T. (1987b). An analogy between fetal haptoglobin and a potent immunosuppressant in cancer. *Cancer Res.* 47:5120-5126

Oliveira, L.H., Franca Jr, M.C., Nucci, A., Oliveira, D.M., Kimura, E.M., & Sonati, M.F. (2008). Haptoglobin study in myasthenia gravis. *Arq Neuropsiquiatr.* 66:229-233

Oliviero, S., Morrone, G., & Cortese, R. (1987). The human haptoglobin gene: transcriptional regulation during development and acute phase induction. *EMBO J.* 6:1905-1912

Pagano, M., Engler, R., Gelin, M., & Jayle, M.F. (1980). Kinetic study of the interaction between rat haptoglobin and rat liver cathepsin B. *Can.J Biochem.* 58:410-417

Panter, S.S., Sadrzadeh, S.M., Hallaway, P.E., Haines, J.L., Anderson, V.E., & Eaton, J.W. (1985). Hypohaptoglobinemia associated with familial epilepsy. *J.Exp.Med.* 161:748-754

Papp, M., Foldi, I., Nemes, E., Udvardy, M., Harsfalvi, J., Altorjay, I., Mate, I., Dinya, T., Varvolgyi, C., Barta, Z., Veres, G., Lakatos, P.L., Tumpek, J., Toth, L., Szathmari, E., Kapitany, A., Gyetvai, A., & Korponay-Szabo, I.R. (2008). Haptoglobin polymorphism: a novel genetic risk factor for celiac disease development and its clinical manifestations. *Clin. Chem.* 54:697-704

Pavon, E.J., Munoz, P., Lario, A., Longobardo, V., Carrascal, M., Abian, J., Martin, A.B., Arias, S.A., Callejas-Rubio, J.L., Sola, R., Navarro-Pelayo, F., Raya-Alvarez, E., Ortego-Centeno, N., Zubiaur, M., & Sancho, J. (2006). Proteomic analysis of plasma from patients with systemic lupus erythematosus: increased presence of haptoglobin alpha2 polypeptide chains over the alpha1 isoforms. *Proteomics.* 6 Suppl 1:S282-S292

Pays, E. and Vanhollebeke, B. (2009). Human innate immunity against African trypanosomes. *Curr.Opin.Immunol.* 21:493-498

Pelletier, N., Boudreau, F., Yu, S.J., Zannoni, S., Boulanger, V., & Asselin, C. (1998). Activation of haptoglobin gene expression by cAMP involves CCAAT/enhancer-binding protein isoforms in intestinal epithelial cells. *FEBS Lett.* 439:275-280

Quaye, I.K. (2008). Haptoglobin, inflammation and disease. *Trans.R.Soc.Trop.Med.Hyg.* 102:735-742

Rantapaa, D.S., Beckman, G., & Beckman, L. (1988). Serum protein markers in systemic lupus erythematosus. *Hum.Hered.* 38:44-47

Rosenkranz, M.E., Wilson, D.C., Marinov, A.D., Decewicz, A., Grof-Tisza, P., Kirchner, D., Giles, B., Reynolds, P.R., Liebman, M.N., Kolli, V.S., Thompson, S.D., & Hirsch, R. (2010). Synovial fluid proteins differentiate between the subtypes of juvenile idiopathic arthritis. *Arthritis Rheum.* 62:1813-1823

Rossbacher, J., Wagner, L., & Pasternack, M.S. (1999). Inhibitory effect of haptoglobin on granulocyte chemotaxis, phagocytosis and bactericidal activity. *Scand.J Immunol.* 50:399-404

Sadrzadeh, S.M., Saffari, Y., & Bozorgmehr, J. (2004). Haptoglobin phenotypes in epilepsy. *Clin.Chem.* 50:1095-1097

Saeed, S.A., Ahmad, N., & Ahmed, S. (2007). Dual inhibition of cyclooxygenase and lipoxygenase by human haptoglobin: its polymorphism and relation to hemoglobin binding. *Biochem.Biophys.Res.Commun.* 353:915-920

Shi, C. and Simon, D.I. (2006). Integrin signals, transcription factors, and monocyte differentiation. *Trends Cardiovasc.Med.* 16:146-152

Shi, C., Zhang, X., Chen, Z., Sulaiman, K., Feinberg, M.W., Ballantyne, C.M., Jain, M.K., & Simon, D.I. (2004). Integrin engagement regulates monocyte differentiation through the forkhead transcription factor Foxp1. *J Clin.Invest.* 114:408-418

Shi, F.D., Bai, X.F., Xiao, B.G., van der Meide, P.H., & Link, H. (1998). Nasal administration of multiple antigens suppresses experimental autoimmune myasthenia gravis, encephalomyelitis and neuritis. *J Neurol.Sci.* 155:1-12

Smeets, M.B., Fontijn, J., Kavelaars, A., Pasterkamp, G., & De Kleijn, D.P. (2003). The acute phase protein haptoglobin is locally expressed in arthritic and oncological tissues. *Int.J.Exp.Pathol.* 84:69-74

Snellman, O. and Sylven, B. (1967). Haptoglobin acting as a natural inhibitor of cathepsin B activity. *Nature.* 216:1033

Theilgaard-Monch, K., Jacobsen, L.C., Nielsen, M.J., Rasmussen, T., Udby, L., Gharib, M., Arkwright, P.D., Gombart, A.F., Calafat, J., Moestrup, S.K., Porse, B.T., & Borregaard, N. (2006). Haptoglobin is synthesized during granulocyte differentiation, stored in specific granules, and released by neutrophils in response to activation. *Blood.* 108:353-361

Tripathi, P. (2007). Nitric oxide and immune response. *Indian J Biochem.Biophys.* 44:310-319

Tseng, C.F., Lin, C.C., Huang, H.Y., Liu, H.C., & Mao, S.J. (2004). Antioxidant role of human haptoglobin. *Proteomics.* 4:2221-2228

Ueno, H., Klechevsky , E., Morita, R., Aspord, C., Cao, T., Matsui, T., Di, P.T., Connolly, J., Fay, J.W., Pascual, V., Palucka, A.K., & Banchereau, J. (2007). Dendritic cell subsets in health and disease. *Immunol.Rev.* 219:118-142

Unger, W.W., Hauet-Broere, F., Jansen, W., van Berkel, L.A., Kraal, G., & Samsom, J.N. (2003). Early events in peripheral regulatory T cell induction via the nasal mucosa. *J.Immunol.* 171:4592-4603

Van, V.H., Langlois, M., & Delanghe, J. (2004). Haptoglobin polymorphisms and iron homeostasis in health and in disease. *Clin.Chim.Acta.* 345:35-42

Wang, H., Gao, X.H., Wang, Y.K., Li, P., He, C.D., Xie, Y., & Chen, H.D. (2005). Expression of haptoglobin in human keratinocytes and Langerhans cells. *Br.J Dermatol.* 153:894-899

Wang, Y., Kinzie, E., Berger, F.G., Lim, S.K., & Baumann, H. (2001). Haptoglobin, an inflammation-inducible plasma protein. *Redox.Rep.* 6:379-385

Wejman, J.C., Hovsepian, D., Wall, J.S., Hainfeld, J.F., & Greer, J. (1984). Structure of haptoglobin and the haptoglobin-hemoglobin complex by electron microscopy. *J.Mol.Biol.* 174:319-341

Wikstrom, M.E. and Stumbles, P.A. (2007). Mouse respiratory tract dendritic cell subsets and the immunological fate of inhaled antigens. *Immunol.Cell Biol.* 85:182-188

Wolvers, D.A., Coenen-de Roo, C.J., Mebius, R.E., van der Cammen, M.J., Tirion, F., Miltenburg, A.M., & Kraal, G. (1999). Intranasally induced immunological tolerance is determined by characteristics of the draining lymph nodes: studies with OVA and human cartilage gp-39. *J.Immunol.* 162:1994-1998

Xie, Y., Li, Y., Zhang, Q., Stiller, M.J., Wang, C.L., & Streilein, J.W. (2000). Haptoglobin is a natural regulator of Langerhans cell function in the skin. *J Dermatol.Sci.* 24:25-37

Xu, L.Y., Yang, J.S., Huang, Y.M., Levi, M., Link, H., & Xiao, B.G. (2000). Combined nasal administration of encephalitogenic myelin basic protein peptide 68-86 and IL-10 suppressed incipient experimental allergic encephalomyelitis in Lewis rats. *Clin.Immunol.* 96:205-211

Yang, F., Ghio, A.J., Herbert, D.C., Weaker, F.J., Walter, C.A., & Coalson, J.J. (2000). Pulmonary expression of the human haptoglobin gene. *Am.J.Respir.Cell Mol.Biol.* 23:277-282

Yerbury, J.J., Kumita, J.R., Meehan, S., Dobson, C.M., & Wilson, M.R. (2009). alpha2-Macroglobulin and haptoglobin suppress amyloid formation by interacting with prefibrillar protein species. *J.Biol.Chem.* 284:4246-4254

Yerbury, J.J., Rybchyn, M.S., Easterbrook-Smith, S.B., Henriques, C., & Wilson, M.R. (2005). The acute phase protein haptoglobin is a mammalian extracellular chaperone with an action similar to clusterin. *Biochemistry*. 44:10914-10925

Zhao, X., Song, S., Sun, G., Strong, R., Zhang, J., Grotta, J.C., & Aronowski, J. (2009). Neuroprotective role of haptoglobin after intracerebral hemorrhage. *J.Neurosci.* 29:15819-15827

11

Acute-Phase Proteins: Alpha -1- Acid Glycoprotein

C. Tesseromatis[1], A. Alevizou[2], E. Tigka[1] and A. Kotsiou[3]
[1]*Department of Pharmacology, Medical School, University of Athens*
[2]*Attiko University Hospital, Athens*
[3]*Pharmacy Dpt, Aretaieion Univ. Hospital, Athens*
Greece

1. Introduction

Acute-phase proteins are proteins whose plasma concentrations increase in response to inflammation. The variability in protein plasma levels, and following impact on drug binding extent, cause modifications in the mode of drug action, distribution, disposition and elimination. One of the most important acute phase proteins is a1-acid glycoprotein (AAG or AGP), principal binding protein for basic drugs.

Although plasma concentration of AAG is much lower than that of albumin, AAG can become the major drug binding macromolecule in plasma with significant clinical implications. Moreover AAG is involved in drug-drug interactions, especially in the displacement of drugs and endogenous substances from their binding sites, with important pharmacokinetic and clinical consequences.

AAG is an acidic glycoprotein of about 41 kDa , a single chain of 183 amino acids, the tertiary structure of which partially resembles those of cellular beta 2-agonist receptors. The carbohydrate content (glycans) represents 45% of its molecular weight. The biological function of AGP remains unknown; however, a number of activities of possible physiological significance, such as various immunomodulating effects, have been described. The immunomodulatory as well as the binding activities of AGP have been shown to be mostly dependent on its carbohydrate composition. AAG is one of the plasma acute phase proteins synthesized by the liver and is mainly secreted by hepatocytes and its serum concentration increases in response to systemic tissue injury, inflammation, infection or cancer.

Human alpha1-acid glycoprotein displays genetic polymorphism. AGP of most individuals exists as a mixture of two or three main genetic variants (i.e. A variant and F1 and/or S variants). Concerning native human AGP composition, the relative occurrence of the three main phenotypes in the population was found to be about 50% for F1+S+A, 35% for F1+A and 15% for S+A. Different drug binding properties of the two main genetic products (F1-S and A variants) have been demonstrated.

Various drug molecules have different selectivity in binding affinities for the genetic variants, ranging from the lack of selectivity to the total preference of one of the variants. In binding competition experiments performed by dialysis, radioactive imipramine and warfarin were chosen as high-affinity selective marker ligands for the A variant and the F1-S variant mixture, respectively. Since the majority of the published AGP drug binding results relate to the mixture of the variants, structure–binding relationships at the molecular level are not well understood.

Expression of the AGP gene is controlled by a combination of the major regulatory mediators, i.e. glucocorticoids and a cytokine network involving mainly interleukin-1 beta (IL-1 beta), tumor necrosis factor-alpha (TNF alpha), interleukin-6 and IL-6 related cytokines.

A-1-acid glycoprotein (AAG) is of particular interest as a major binding protein for several basic drugs, including lidocaine, verapamil, imipramine, propranolol and others. AGP binds numerous neutral lipophilic drugs from endogenous (steroid hormones) and exogenous origin. In contrast, findings suggest that regarding fentanyl, although a basic drug with a pKa value of 8.43, its binding to alpha 1-acid glycoprotein is of minor importance. Seven binding sites of AAG have been described. In addition AAG can also bind acidic drugs such as phenobarbital.

The pharmacokinetic-pharmacodynamic relationship of the model drug S(-)-propranolol with structural similarities to AAG's molecule was evaluated, using mechanism-based estimations of in vivo receptor affinity under conditions of altered plasma protein binding resulting from different levels of alpha-1-acid glycoprotein.

If plasma AAG concentration increases or changes rapidly, plasma drug concentration and drug effect may be unpredictable. Under these circumstances an estimate of free drug fraction may be clinically helpful.

In myocardial infarction elevated AAG concentration may result in clinical toxicity of lidocaine. It has been shown that the rise in alpha-1-acid glycoprotein after myocardial infarction is associated with lidocaine accumulation, but increased plasma binding attenuates the rise in free drug. The co-administration of lidocaine with propranalol or clonidine has been documented to induce rise in lidocaine levels. This suggests that the toxicologic implications of lidocaine accumulation may have been exaggerated and therapeutic monitoring of total plasma levels may be misleading and must be interpreted appropriately. This provides the strongest rationale for monitoring free rather than total drug concentration as an aid in lidocaine therapy.

Studies in normal subjects and patients with myocardial infarction, renal disease, hepatic failure and receiving antiepileptic drug therapy have all shown a remarkably good relationship between AAG concentration and the binding ratio for lidocaine.

Possible elevation of serum concentrations of the acute-phase reactant a1-acid glycoprotein may be experienced, between many other physiologic derangements, by cigarette smokers. The results of the relevant studies are controversial, some reported elevated AAG concentrations in cigarette smokers, whereas others found no effect of smoking.

Basic drugs competing for the same binding site on AGP molecule may enhance the pharmacological active free fraction of the less affinity drug, with critical consequences for the therapeutic management of the patients.

The large variations observed in the binding ratios of basic drugs in plasma in several physiological and pathological states are correlated with the large variations in the plasma level of AGP with implications for the monitoring of their free fractions of basic drugs during clinical therapy.

AAG serum concentration, which is stable in physiological conditions, increases several-fold during acute-phase reactions and its plasma levels can be used as a diagnostic and prognostic parameter, during clinical therapy (e.g. free or relapse intervals in cancer

treatment). Furthermore AGP levels estimation may interfere in the proper dosage adjustment, in order to obtain the optimum therapeutic target.
The binding of drugs to plasma proteins has been recognized as one of the major determinants of drug action, distribution, and disposition. Initially albumin was considered as the main binding protein, but alpha 1-acid glycoprotein (AAG) has increasingly become important although its plasma concentration is much lower than that of albumin. Serum albumin is the principal binding protein for acidic compounds and a1-acid glycoprotein (AAG) or (AGP) or orosomucoid (ORM) is the principal binding protein for basic drugs. [1]
AAG was first described in 1950 by Karl Schmid and Richard J. Winzler and colleagues [2,3]

2. AAG properties and activities

AAG is an acidic glycoprotein of about 41 kDa in molecular weight, has a normal plasma concentration between 0.6-1.2 mg/mL (1-3% of plasma proteins) and its tertiary structure partially resembles those of cellular beta2-agonist receptors. Fig 1 Human AAG is a single polypeptide chain of 183 amino acids and consists approximately of 45% carbohydrate attached in the form of five complex-type *N*-linked glycans. A notable characteristic of AAG is its unusually high solubility in water and in many polar organic solvents. The biological function of AAG is not only the ability to bind basic drugs and many other molecules like steroid hormones (leading to the suggestion that AAG might be a member of the lipocalin family) but it also exert various immunomodulating effects. [4]
The binding as well as the immunomodulatory activities of AGP have been shown to be mostly dependent on its carbohydrate composition. Different forms of AGP can be distinguished in serum depending on the type of glycosylation and multiple amino acid substitutions. [5,6]
AAG serum concentration which is stable in physiological conditions (about 1 g/l in humans and 0.2 g/l in rats) increases several-fold during acute-phase reactions and AGP is considered as a major member of the positive acute phase protein family and its plasma levels can be used as a diagnostic and prognostic parameter, during clinical therapy. [5,7]

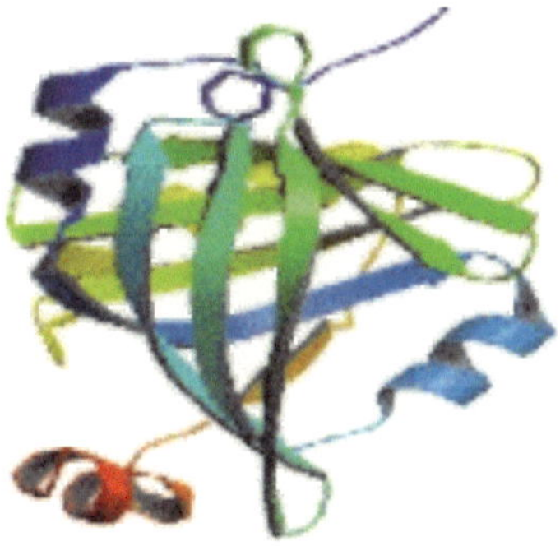

Fig. 1. Alpha-1-acid glycoprotein (AAG) a simplified name for orosomucoid (ORM) consisting of 183 amino acid and 5 sugar chains.

3. AGP production

Alpha-1 acid glycoprotein is one of the plasma proteins synthesized by the liver and is mainly secreted by hepatocytes, although extra-hepatic AGP gene expression has also been reported. Hepatic production of AAG and other acute phase proteins is increased following the response to various stressful stimuli: physical trauma, such as surgery or wounding, bacterial infection, or various other unspecific inflammatory stimuli. Extra-hepatic production of AGP and of other acute phase proteins has been described but the hepatic expression remains the most abundant. [8,9]

The first evidence of the presence of AAG as well as other serum glycoproteins in extra-hepatic tissues was probably done by investigators examining qualitative and quantitative alterations of normal serum glycoproteins in cancer.[10]

AGP gene expression is modulated quantitatively (protein levels) as well as qualitatively (microheterogeneity of the glycan chains) in various physiological and pathological disorders. Studies in transgenic mice by Dente et al. [11,12]showed that both *cis*-acting regulatory elements and cellular environment (diffusible factors, cell–cell interaction) are responsible for the liver specificity of AGP gene expression. Finally, AGP gene expression appears to be highly conserved since it is expressed in all the species studied including *Euglena gracilis*, an ancestral eucaryote unicellular alga. [13]

Among the AAG of animals the rat AGP is a protein of 187 amino acids (mature form) sharing 59% amino acid sequence homology with human AGP and its molecular weight is 40–44 kDa [14]

4. AAG genetic polymorphism and mediators

Native AGP isolated from plasma is not homogeneous; beside the high heterogeneity of glycans, the protein part shows genetic polymorphism and the different forms of AGP in serum depend on the type of glycosylation and multiple amino acid substitutions. In human population two variants of AGP (ORM1 and ORM2) were detected reflecting a gene polymorphism. A 22 amino acid difference was detected between these two variants of AAG encoded by two different genes . In addition, at position 32 and 47, other amino acids can be present. [15]

AGP of most individuals exists as a mixture of two or three main genetic variants (i.e. A variant and F1 and/or S variants). Concerning native human AGP composition the relative occurrence of the three main phenotypes in the population was found to be about 50% for F1+S+A, 35% for F1+A and 15% for S+A. [16]

12–20 glycoforms of AGP has been detected in normal human serum and this micro-heterogeneity is strongly dependent on the pathophysiological conditions. For example, substantial increases in glycoforms expressing di-antennary glycans are apparent in the early phase of an acute-phase reaction as well as an increase in the degree of 3-fucosylation, since fucose is a terminating sugar. These changes in glycosylation could of course affect the biological properties of AGP. [17]

Changes in glycosylation of AGP occur in a wide variety of various pathophysiological conditions like pregnancy, severe rheumatoid arthritis, alcoholic liver cirrhosis and hepatitis. [18,19]

Expression of the AGP gene is controlled by a combination of the major regulatory mediators, i.e. glucocorticoids and a cytokine network involving mainly interleukin-1 beta (IL-1 beta), tumour necrosis factor-alpha (TNF alpha), interleukin-6 and IL-6 related cytokines. It is now well established that the acute phase response may take place in extra-hepatic cell types, and may be regulated by inflammatory mediators as observed in hepatocytes. [4]

5. Drug binding to AGP

Due to its physical-chemical properties, AGP mainly binds basic drugs like tamoxifen [20] and propanolol [21]but also acidic drugs, such as phenobarbital [22] and endogenous steroids (cortisol). [23] AGP as a drug carrier for steroids has been demonstrated since the end of the sixties [24]. AGP was found to also bind synthetic steroids (RU486) [23]. Up to seven binding sites have been described for estradiol - depending on the isolation method used [25]- while in vitro studies provided evidence that two classes of binding sites for basic and neutral drugs are present on AGP. From the literature, it appeared that there is only one binding site on AGP for acidic drugs [26]except for phenobarbital for which two sites have been described. [22]

The presence of two binding sites on AGP for propranolol may reflect differences in the binding characteristics of the stereoisomers. [27]

The nature of drug binding to AGP has been the subject of several studies and has mainly pointed to hydrophobic bindings due to hydrophobic residues near the AGP binding site. However, the binding capacity of AGP depends upon the conformational change of the protein, the polarity of the ligand (interaction is weakest for the steroid with the highest polarity), the temperature, and several other amino acid residues lying at the periphery of the hydrophobic domains of AGP. Although the binding of drugs to AGP has been shown to be mostly hydrophobic in nature, several data also point to an electrostatic interaction and a lot of studies have reported that in plasma, drug bindings are stereoselective, especially in the case of basic drugs. Among factors influencing the characteristics of drug bindings to AGP, pH is one of the important parameters, i.e. drug binding in plasma increases with increasing pH [28]. Desialylation can also affect binding [29]; it reduced the propanolol binding, whereas the progesterone binding did not change.

Much of the inter-individual variability in the extent of plasma protein binding of basic drugs is due to variability in plasma levels of AAG. [27]

5.1 Drug binding of the two main genetic AGP variants

Different drug binding properties of the two main genetic products, F1-S and A variants, have been demonstrated. Various drug molecules have different selectivities in binding affinities for the genetic variants, ranging from the lack of selectivity to the total preference of one of the variants. Since the majority of the published AGP drug binding competition experiments results relate to the A variant and the F1-S variant mixture, structure–binding relationships at the molecular level are not well understood. [30,31]

Concerning the binding of various basic drugs to the F(1)S and A genetic variants of alpha(1)-acid glycoprotein, it was found that , the higher the affinity of basic drugs for AGP, the more they inhibit the binding of other basic drugs, and further, the inhibitory potency depends on the selectivity of binding to the AGP variants. [32]

During specific circular dichroism (CD) probes, dicumarol and acridine orange were found to specifically bind to the F1-S and A variants, respectively. Dicumarol binding to the F1-S variant produced induced Cotton effects originating from the favored chiral conformation of the bound label. Acridine orange gave induced biphasic Cotton effects due to chiral intermolecular exciton interaction between label molecules bound to the A variant. Displacement of the CD probes by specific marker ligands was demonstrated. The induced CD spectrum of dicumarol was found to change sign in the presence of imipramine, as a manifestation of high-affinity ternary complex formation on the F1-S variant. Warfarin was found to bind selectively to the F1-S variant of AGP. The structurally related compound dicumarol could be expected to prefer this variant, and it was confirmed by the results obtained here. While the binding of dicumarol to the A variant is weak and non-specific, the binding of dicumarol to the F1-S genetic variant is highly specific. The induced characteristic polyphasic Cotton effects reported for native AGP can be attributed to this fraction, amounting to about 70% of the native AGP. This is in agreement with the binding site number of 0.6 found previously in CD binding studies performed with native AGP. This induced CD of dicumarol can be used for selective binding interaction studies, provided that the intrinsic or extrinsic Cotton effects of the other ligands are negligible. It was shown that in the presence of imipramine the induced CD of dicumarol bound to the F1-S variant is inverted and it is accompanied with mutually enhanced binding of both ligands. This phenomenon detected previously with native AGP was explained by ternary complex formation on a wide and flexible drug binding area, where the binding sites of acidic and basic drugs are partially overlapping. It was proved that this interaction takes place on the F1-S variant, which is known to be the low-affinity isoprotein in the AGP binding of imipramine. It also means that in the presence of dicumarol the preference of A variant in the binding of imipramine to native AGP is less pronounced. [33]

The pharmacokinetic-pharmacodynamic relationship of the model drug S(-)-propranolol was evaluated using mechanism-based estimations of in vivo receptor affinity, under conditions of altered plasma protein binding resulting from different levels of alpha-1-acid glycoprotein (AGP). Male Wistar Kyoto rats with isoprenaline-induced tachycardia received an intravenous infusion of S(-)-propranolol, on postsurgery day 2 ($n = 7$) and day 7 ($n = 8$) with elevated and normal plasma protein binding, respectively. Serial blood samples were taken in parallel to heart rate measurements. AGP concentration was a covariate for intercompartmental clearance for the third compartment of the pharmacokinetic model of S(-)-propranolol. It was confirmed that, plasma protein binding restricts the pharmacodynamics of S(-)-propranolol. [34]

5.2 AGP drug binding in disease states

The large variations observed in the binding ratios of basic drugs in plasma during several physiological and pathological states are correlated with the large variations in the plasma level of AGP, defining the pharmacokinetics and ultimately the pharmacodynamic effect of the drugs used. The binding of several drugs has been shown to increase following surgical interventions, inflammation and stress, and this increased binding is due to an increase in the plasma concentration of AGP. [35, 36]

Piafsky at al have already since 1978 demonstrated the importance of disease-induced increases in plasma concentrations of α_1 acid glycoprotein. The propranolol binding in plasma was increased in patients with Crohn's disease , inflammatory arthritis and with chronic renal failure, compared with healthy controls. Chlorpromazine binding yielded similar results. Percentage of free drug and α_1 acid glycoprotein concentration were inversely correlated ($r = -0.77$ with propranolol, $P<0.001$, and $r = -0.69$ with chlorpromazine, $P<0.001$). Increases in plasma protein binding in patients with inflammatory disease appear mediated by increases in α_1 acid glycoprotein concentration, which may influence drug kinetics. [37]

The AAG levels' variations have implications for the monitoring of the free fractions of basic drugs during clinical therapy. The consequences of elevated serum AGP levels, often seen in

several disease states, on the pharmacokinetic of drugs have been investigated using transgenic animals. Holladay et al. studied steady-state kinetics of imipramine in transgenic mice expressing serum AGP levels about 9-fold elevated over normal. [38,39]
It was found that of the many physiologic derangements experienced by cigarette smokers, possible elevation of serum concentrations of the acute-phase reactant a, alpha-1-acid glycoprotein (AAG) is of particular interest because AAG is a major binding protein for several basic drugs, including lidocaine, amitriptyline, verapamil, and perhaps others. [40]
It is generally assumed that in plasma, acidic drugs are mainly bound to human serum albumin. However, binding to AGP will contribute significantly to the total plasma binding of these drugs, especially in diseases in which the concentration of AGP increases and/or of human serum albumin decreases.Cited By in Scopus[6,41] It should be mentioned that warfarin binding affinity to AAG increases with decreasing Ph indicating that one of the intermolecular forces by which AAG binds its ligands (be they basic or acidic) is the donation of a hydrogen bond. [42]

5.3 AAG binding experimental studies

The binding of drugs at therapeutic concentrations to alpha-1 acid glycoprotein in vitro at physiological and non physiological concentrations, consistent with those that might be seen in a variety of clinical conditions was investigated.
In a study with the antiarrythmic verapamil there was a good correlation (r = 0.83) between the binding ratio and AAG concentration, suggesting that AAG could bind verapamil. While the data indicate that AAG is responsible for most of the variability in plasma verapamil binding, which in turn contributes somewhat to variation in effectiveness of a given total plasma concentration, neither of these causes of individual variations is likely to have a major clinical impact in patients who, apart from arrhythmia, are otherwise healthy. [43]
The same was observed in studies with the antiarrythmic quinidine. [44]
Concerning the opiate meperidine binding to AAG did not have any important impact upon fetal and maternal concentrations.[45]
The binding of prednisolone to alpha 1-acid glycoprotein (AGP) was determined in vitro by equilibrium dialysis and indicated the both low affinity and low capacity of AGP for prednisolone. Overall, contribution of AGP to the total plasma binding of prednisolone is less than 3% when considered in the competitive protein binding system with transcortin and albumin. Disease induced alterations of AGP concentrations are relatively unimportant regarding plasma protein binding of prednisolone. [46]
Acetaminophen, phenobarbital, theophylline, and valproic acid showed negligible binding to alpha-1 acid glycoprotein whereas lidocaine and phenytoin demonstrated binding to this protein, and increases in the alpha-1 acid glycoprotein concentration produced decreases in the unbound (free) or "active" concentration of these two drugs. These findings are significant when lidocaine, phenytoin, phenobarbital, theophylline, or valproic acid are used in patients with clinical conditions that may affect the concentration of the binding proteins. [47]
The relationship between binding ratio of imipramine and plasma alpha 1-acidglycoprotein (AAG) was determined in normal subjects, patients with chest pain syndrome, and patients after myocardial infarction. Binding ratio of imipramine significantly correlated with plasma AAG concentration, but not with plasma albumin. In addition, binding ratio of imipramine and pure AAG was significantly related, indicating AAG is an important determinant for

imipramine binding. If plasma AAG concentration increases or changes rapidly, plasma drug concentration and drug effect may be unpredictable. Under these circumstances an estimate of free drug fraction may be clinically helpful and can be estimated from the formula. y = 7.95 + 0.03 X AAG. [48]

The binding of taxol to plasma proteins was studied by equilibrium dialysis. Human serum albumin and alpha 1-acid glycoprotein were found to contribute about equally to the binding, with a minor contribution from lipoproteins. The binding was found to be extensive (about 95%), concentration independent, indicating nonspecific hydrophobic binding, without a significant difference between healthy volunteers and cancer patients. None of the drugs commonly co administered with (dexamethasone, diphenhydramine, ranitidine, doxorubicin, 5-fluorouracil and cisplatin) altered the binding of taxol significantly. The protein binding of taxol was found to dramatically decrease the red blood cell uptake of taxol. Fig 2.[49]

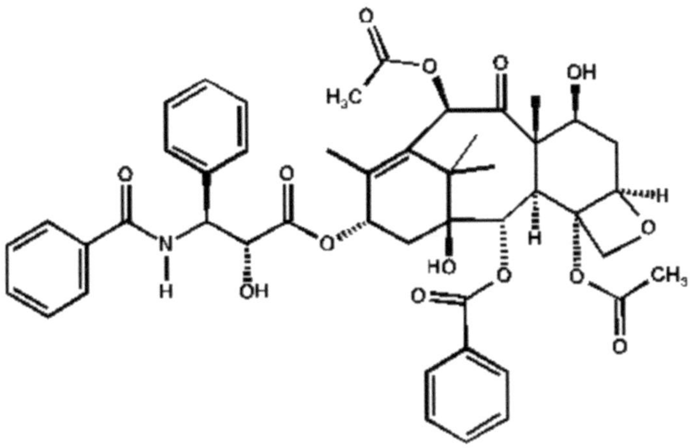

Fig. 2. Taxol, a potent anticancer natural product with activity against a number of leukeamias and solid tumors.

Disopyramide, a drug with narrow therapeutic range, used for cardiac arrhythmias, is more than 90% bound to AAG and less than 10 % to albumin. Changing the AAG level therefore has clinical significance for this drug and similars bound to AAG (danger for toxic effects). [50]

In contrast to other basic drugs, fentanyl binding to alpha 1-acid glycoprotein is of minor importance. Due to unspecific binding of fentanyl by hydrophobic interactions, a major role of albumin, which amounts to about 60% of total protein, seems to be evident. [51]

Gimatecan, a camptothecin with a lipophilic substitution in position 7, is orally absorbed and its variable plasma levels seem to be related to AAG plasma concentrations. Data obtained in mice, together with the fact that AAG levels largely exceeded gimatecan plasma concentrations, suggest that the increased gimatecan levels in patients with high AAG levels are not related to the binding of the drug to AAG with consequent reduced tissue drug distribution, but possibly to other mechanism associated with inflammation being AAG simply a marker of the inflammation process. [52]

Ropivacaine is a long-acting local anesthetic used frequently for peripheral nerve blocks (continuous peripheral nerve block catheters). In a study, the free ropivacaine drug levels

over time were evaluated in trauma patients, by measuring the serum concentration of bound and unbound local anesthetic.There was no correlation between free ropivacaine concentration and alpha-1-acid glycoprotein concentration except in patients who had already been receiving ropivacaine infusions before entering the study. Despite this lack of correlation, the total duration of local anesthetic infusion did not seem to influence the free concentration of the drug. [53]
High-performance affinity chromatography was used to study binding by the drug lidocaine to human serum albumin (HSA) and alpha(1)-acid glycoprotein (AGP). AGP had strong binding to lidocaine. Fig 3 Lidocaine had weak to moderate binding to HSA. Competitive experiments with site selective probes showed that lidocaine was interacting with Sudlow site II of HSA and the propranolol site of AGP and provided a better quantitative understanding of how lidocaine binds to these serum proteins and is transported in the circulation. Fig. 4 [54]

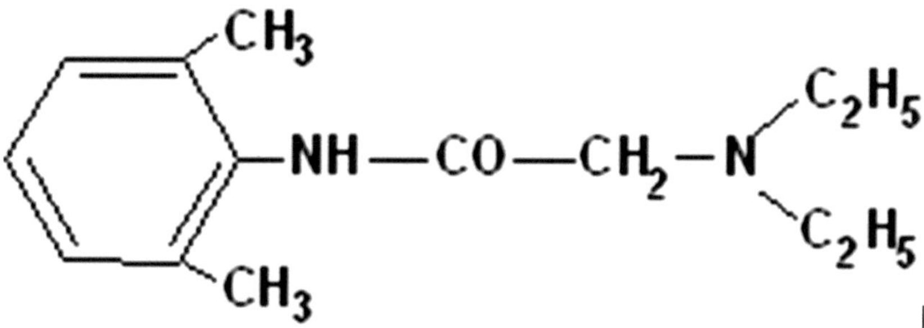

Fig. 3. Lidocaine a local anesthetic chemically designated as 2-(diethylamino)-N-(2,6-dimethyl-phenyl)-acetamide with the above structural formula.

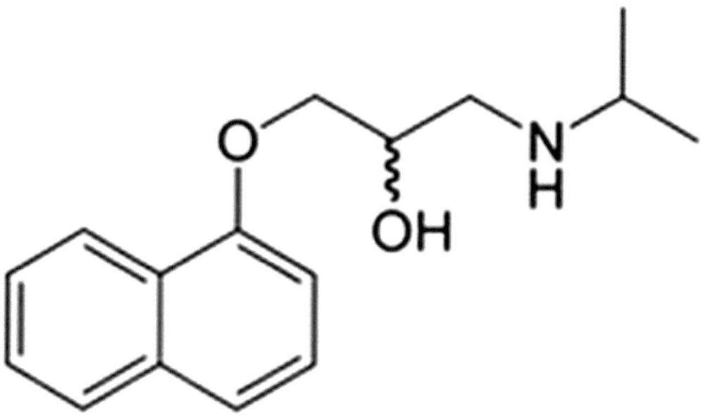

Fig. 4. Propranolol a "beta-adrenergic antagonist

Studies in normal subjects and patients with myocardial infarction, renal disease, hepatic failure and receiving antiepileptic drug therapy have all shown a remarkably good relationship between AAG concentration and the degree of plasma binding of lidocaine. In situations where AAG is altered, particularly myocardial infarction, the usual therapeutic range for total plasma lidocaine concentrations may not apply and must be interpreted appropriately. This provides the strongest rationale for monitoring free rather than total drug concentration as an aid in lidocaine therapy. [55]

In patients with confirmed myocardial infarction, alpha-1-acid glycoprotein rose significantly from 117 mg/dL at admission to 140 mg/dL at 36 hours (p less than 0.01)The patients were given prolonged infusions of lidocaine (2 mg/min).In patients with myocardial infarction, the rise in plasma alpha 1-acid glycoprotein concentration was associated with increased lidocaine binding and a rise in total lidocaine concentrations between 12 and 48 hours (p less than 0.05). Because of the binding changes, however, the rise in free drug concentration (31.2%) was significantly less than the 56.3% rise in total drug level (p less than 0.05). No changes in alpha 1-acid glycoprotein or lidocaine disposition were seen between12 and 48 hours in the control subjects. The results show that the rise in alpha 1-acid glycoprotein after myocardial infarction is associated with lidocaine accumulation, but increased plasma binding attenuates the rise in free drug. This suggests that the toxicologic implications of lidocaine accumulation may have been exaggerated and therapeutic monitoring of total plasma levels may be misleading. [56]
Three models of stressor stimuli (experimental mandible osteotomy , forced cold swimming stress and Freund's adjuvant induced arthritis) were performed in order to investigate the discrepancy of lidocaine plasma concentration in comparison to the control. Lidocaine was administered at 5 doses of 3 mg/kg intramuscularly every 2 hours. Lidocaine levels and its binding to proteins were estimated in plasma and mandible. In groups under stress, lidocaine concentrations in serum showed a marked elevation. In addition, these animals demonstrated a significant decrease in the percent of lidocaine binding in the mandible. [57]

Drug	Drug Characteristics	elevated AAG dependent activity
lidocaine	antiarrythmic	total plasma lidocaine cumulation [55-58]
propranolol	beta blocker	reduced unbound propranolol fraction [37]
imipramine	antidepressant	reduced free drug fraction [48]
disopyramide	antiarrhythmic	reduced free drug fraction [50]
phenytoin	antiepileptic	reduced free drug fraction [47]
paclitaxel	cancer medication	reduced free drug fraction [49]

Table 1. Drugs' documented AAG dependent activity

Moreover role of stress (trauma, cold swimming, and adjuvant rheumatoid arthritis) on lidocaine concentrations as well as lidocaine's protein binding in heart and liver tissues in male Wistar rats was investigated. Since lidocaine is a cationic molecule it is bound to AGP. The levels of AGP are increased mainly in inflammatory conditions and the protein binding of lidocaine was increased and consequently its free plasma concentration was reduced. [58]
In co-administration of lidocaine and clonidine, a significant increase of lidocaine free fraction is documented. Both drugs are cationic (clonidine pKa =8.25 and lidocaine pKa=7.9) and have higher binding affinity to alpha- acid glycoprotein than to albumin. Probably a displacement process takes place and lidocaine is displaced by clonidine from its binding sites in serum and tissue proteins thereby leading to rise in its free fraction. [59].
Drugs that are documented to be of AAP depended activity are presented in the following table (1)

6. AAG clinical aspect

Alpha-1-Acid glycoprotein is found in increased amounts in patients with a variety of cancers. The application of discriminated analysis to the comparison of plasma levels of AAG in patients with lung cancer and patients without known cancer, yielded a sensitivity of 89% and specificity of 84% in the detection of active lung cancer via AAG measurement. In addition it was demonstrated that normalization of alpha-1-acid glycoprotein levels during antineoplastic therapy correlates with a significantly prolonged relapse-free survival in lung cancer patients. [60]

Alpha-1-acid glycoprotein is suggested to provide prognostic information in patients with glioblastoma multiform since it was higher in patients with glioblastoma multiform who died within one year after admission than in those with a longer survival time. [61]

Unlike other cancers, patients with breast cancer were found to have normal glycoprotein levels with early disease and elevated levels when the disease was advanced (positive bone scans), suggesting that such investigations may be useful in selecting patients with truly localized disease. Most reported estimates of serum glycoprotein levels in disease have been based on biochemical estimates of protein-bound sugars in serum fractions and estimates of serum protein-bound fucose have been advocated as a means of differentiating between benign and malignant breast disease(AAG is a specific glycoprotein containing fucose in its molecule). [62]

The effect of altered concentrations of serum proteins in malignant disease was studied on drug binding with lidocaine, a basic drug and tolbutamide, an acidic drug. Patients with cancer had increased serum concentrations of AAG and lowered serum concentration of albumin. Lidocaine binding was increased at all concentrations studied and that of tolbutamide was decreased at the highest concentration. Not all of the increase in lidocaine binding was explicable on the basis of increased serum AAG concentration. Estimation of binding parameters with a model with two independent sites showed increased affinity at the high affinity site in cancer patients with no change in the calculated number of binding sites. Therefore, in cancer there is increased lidocaine binding in association with increased AAG concentrations. [63]

AGP as a pool of cationic drugs may play an important role with clinical impact in various medication regiments, since its discrepancy may represent a prognostic index of the therapy procedure and furthermore may interfere in the proper dosage adjustment in order to obtain the optimum therapeutic target.

7. References

[1] Israili ZH, Dayton PG. Human alpha-1-glycoprotein and its interactions with drugs. Drug Metab Rev. 2001 May;33(2):161-235. (1)

[2] Schmid K.J. Am. Chem. Soc. 72 (1950), p. 2816.

[3] Weimer H.E., Mehl J.W. and Winzler R.J. J. Biol. Chem. 185 (1950), pp. 561–568.

[4] Fournier T, Medjoubi-N N, Porquet D. Alpha-1-acid glycoprotein. Biochim Biophys Acta. 2000, 18;1482(1-2):157-71.

[5] Schmid K., Nimberg R.B., Kimura A.,. Yamaguchi H and. Binette J.P. Biochim. Biophys. Acta 492 (1977), pp. 291–302.

[6] Yoshima H., Matsumoto A., Mizuochi T., Kawasaki T. and Kobata A.. J. Biol. Chem. 256 (1981), pp. 8476–8484.

[7] Schwick H.G., Haupt H., in: F.W. Putnam (Ed.), The Plasma Proteins, Vol. IV, 2nd edn., Academic Press, New York, 1984, pp. 167–200.
[8] Kushner I. Ann. New York Acad. Sci. 389 (1982), pp. 39–49.
[9] Fey G.H and Füller G.M. Mol. Biol. Med. 4 (1987), pp. 323–338.
[10] P.O. Alminquist and E. Lausing. *Scand. J. Clin. Lab. Invest.* 9 (1957), pp. 179–183.
[11] L. Dente, U. Ruther, M. Tripodi, E.F. Wagner and R. Cortese. Genes Dev. 2 (1988), pp. 259–266. and by Dewey et al. (12)
[12] M.J. Dewey, C. Rheaume, F.G. Berger and H. Baumann. J. Immunol. 144 (1990), pp. 4392–4398.
[13] G. Durand, C. Delranc, J. Bonaly, H. Chacun, D. Porquet and J.P. Barque. Biochem. Biophys. Res. Commun. 234 (1997), pp. 544–548.
[14] G.A. Ricca, R.W. Hamilton, J.W. McLean, A. Conn, J.E. Kalinyak and J.M. Taylor. J. Biol. Clin. 256 (1981), pp. 10362–10368.
[15] Schmid K, in: F.W. Putman (Ed.): The Plasma Proteins, Academic Press, New York, 1975, pp. 183–288.
[16] C.B. Eap, C. Cuendet and P. Baumann, Orosomucoid (alpha-1-acid glycoprotein) phenotyping by use of immobilized pH gradients with 8 M urea and immunoblotting. A new variant encountered in a population study. Hum. Genet. 80 (1988), pp. 183–185.
[17] W. Van Dijk. Glycoconj. J. 12 (1995), pp. 227–233.
[18] M. Jezeguel, N.S. Seta, M.M. Corbic, J.M. Féger and G. Durand. Clin. Chim. Acta 176 (1988), pp. 49–57.
[19] J.M. Wieruszeski, B. Fournet, D. Konan, D. Biou and G. Durand. FEBS Lett. 238 (1988), pp. 390–394.
[20] K. Schmid, H. Kaufman, S. Isemura, F. Bauer, J. Emura, T. Motoyama, M. Ishiguro and S. Nanno. Biochemistry 12 (1973), pp. 2711–2724.
[21] F. Albani, R. Riva, R.M. Contin and A. Baruzzi. Br. J. Clin. Pharmacol. 18 (1984), pp. 244–246.
[22] J. Schley and B. Mueller-Oerlinghausen. Pharmacopsychiatry 16 (1983), pp. 82–85.
[23] B. Grimaldi, C. Hamberger and D. Tremblay. Prog. Clin. Biol. Res. 300 (1989), pp. 445–448.
[24] U. Westphal, in: F. Gross, A. Labhart, T. Mann, L.T. Samuels, J. Sander (Eds.), Monographs on Endocrinology, Vol. 4, Springer, New York, 1971, pp. 375–433.
[25] J. Kerkay and U. Westphal. Biochim. Biophys. Acta 170 (1968), pp. 324–333.
[26] J. Schley and B. Mueller-Oerlinghausen. J. Pharm. Pharmacol. 38 (1986), pp. 102–106
[27] Gillis A M., YEE Y.G ,. Kates R E. Binding of antiarrhythmic drugs to purified human a1-acid glycoprotein .*Biochemicall Pharmacology,*1985, 34, (24), 4279-4282.
[28] K.V. Ponganis and D.R. Stanski. J. Pharm. Sci. 74 (1985), pp. 57–60.
[29] A.K.L. Wong and J.C. Hsia. Can. J. Biochem. Cell Biol. 61 (1983), pp. 1114–1116
[30] C.D. Eap, C. Cuendet and P. Baumann, Selectivity in the binding of psychotropic drugs to the variants of human alpha-1-acid glycoprotein. Naunyn Schmiedebergs Arch. Pharmacol. 337 (1988), pp. 220–224.
[31] C.D. Eap, C. Cuendet and P. Baumann, Binding of amitriptyline to α1-acid glycoprotein and its variants. J. Pharm. Pharmacol. 40 (1988), pp. 767–770.
[32] Ishizaki J, Fukaishi A, Fukuwa C, Yamazaki S, Tabata M, Ishida T, Suga Y, Arai K,Yokogawa K, Miyamoto K. Evaluation of selective competitive binding of basic drugs to alpha1-acid glycoprotein variants. Biol Pharm Bull. 2010 Jan;33(1):95-9.

[33] Fitos I, Visy J, Zsila F, Bikádi Z, Mády G, Simonyi M. Specific ligand binding on genetic variants of human alpha1-acid glycoprotein studied by circular dichroism spectroscopy. Biochem Pharmacol. 2004 Feb 15;67(4):679-88.
[34] van Steeg TJ, Krekels EH, Freijer J, Danhof M, de Lange EC. Effect of altered AGP plasma binding on heart rate changes by S(-)-propranolol in rats using mechanism-based estimations of in vivo receptor affinity (K(B,vivo)). J Pharm Sci. 2010 May;99(5): 2511-20.
[35] K.M. Piafsky, Disease-induced changes in the plasma binding of basic drugs, Clin Pharmacokinetics 5 (1980), pp. 246–262
[36] Otagiri M. Study on binding of drug to serum protein Yakugaku Zasshi 2009 Apr;129(4):413-25.
[37] Piafsky K. M, Borgå O.D, Odar-Cederlöf I. Johansson, C, and Sjöqvist F. Increased Plasma Protein Binding of Propranolol and Chlorpromazine Mediated by Disease-Induced Elevations of Plasma α_1 Acid Glycoprotein N Engl J Med 1978; 299:1435-1439.
[38] J.W. Holladay, M.J. Dewey and S.D. Yoo. Pharm. Res. 13 (1996), pp. 1313–1316. and pharmacokinetics and antidepressant activity of fluoxetine .
[39] J.W. Holladay, M.J. Dewey and S.D. Yoo. Drug. Metab. Dispos. 26 (1998), pp. 20–24.
[40] Parish RC, Terrell JR, Brown WJ Jr. Clinical pharmacokinetics of theophylline and levels of alpha 1-acid glycoprotein in smokeless tobacco users. Chest. 1989 Jun;95(6): 1253-6.
[41] S. Urien, E. Albengres, J.L. Pinquier and J.P. Tillement. Clin. Pharmacol. Ther. 39 (1986), pp. 683–689.
[42] Urien S, Bree F, Testa B, and Tillement JP. pH-dependence of warfarin binding to ax-acid glycoprotein (orosomucoid). Biochem. J. (1993) 289, 767-770
[43] McGowan FX, Reiter MJ, Pritchett EL, Shand DG. Verapamil plasma binding: relationship to alpha 1-acid glycoprotein and drug efficacy. Clin Pharmacol Ther. 1983 Apr;33(4):485-90.
[44] Nilsen OG, Leren P, Aakesson I, Jacobsen S. Binding of quinidine in sera with different levels of triglycerides, cholesterol, and orosomucoid protein. Biochem Pharmacol. 1978 Mar 15;27(6):871-6.
[45] Nation RL. Meperidine binding in maternal and fetal plasma. Clin Pharmacol Ther. 1981 Apr;29(4):472-9.
[46] Milsap RL, Jusko WJ. Binding of prednisolone to alpha 1-acid glycoprotein. J Steroid Biochem. 1983 Feb;18(2):191-4.
[47] Bailey DN, Briggs JR. The binding of selected therapeutic drugs to human serum alpha-1 acid glycoprotein and to human serum albumin in vitro. Ther Drug Monit. 2004 Feb;26(1):40-3.
[48] Freilich DI, Giardina EG. Imipramine binding to alpha-1-acid glycoprotein in normal subjects and cardiac patients. Clin Pharmacol Ther. 1984;35(5):670-4
[49] Kumar GN, Walle UK, Bhalla KN, Walle T. Binding of taxol to human plasma, albumin and alpha 1-acid glycoprotein. Res Commun Chem Pathol Pharmacol. 1993 Jun;80(3):337-44.
[50] A. Nomura, H. Yasuda , T. Kobayashi I , S. Kishino , N. Kohri , K. Iseki , and K. Miyazaki. Serum alpha-l-acid glycoprotein and protein binding of disopyramide in patients with congestive heart failure. Eur J Clin Pharmacol (1992) 42:115-116
[51] Wiesner G, Taeger K, Peter K. Serum protein binding of fentanyl. The effect of postoperative acute phase reaction with elevated alpha 1-acid glycoprotein and

methodologic problems in determination by equilibrium dialysis. Anaesthesist. 1996 Apr;45(4):323-9.
[52] Frapolli R, Zucchetti M, Sessa C, Marsoni S, Viganò L, Locatelli A, Rulli E,Compagnoni A, Bello E, Pisano C, Carminati P, D'Incalci M. Clinical pharmacokinetics of the new oral camptothecin gimatecan: the inter-patient variability is related to alpha1-acid glycoprotein plasma levels. Eur J Cancer. 2010 Feb;46(3):505-16.
[53] Bleckner LL, Bina S, Kwon KH, McKnight G, Dragovich A, Buckenmaier CC 3rd.Serum ropivacaine concentrations and systemic local anesthetic toxicity in trauma patients receiving long-term continuous peripheral nerve block catheters.Anesth Analg. 2010 Feb 1;110(2):630-
[54] Soman S, Yoo MJ, Jang YJ, Hage DS. Analysis of lidocaine interactions with serum proteins using high-performance affinity chromatography. J Chromatogr B Analyt Technol Biomed Life Sci. 2010 (1);878(7-8):705-8.
[55] Shand DG. alpha 1-Acid glycoprotein and plasma lidocaine binding. Clin Pharmacokinet. 1984 Jan;9 Suppl 1:27-31.
[56] Routledge PA, Stargel WW, Wagner GS, Shand DG. Increased alpha-1-acid glycoprotein and lidocaine disposition in myocardial infarction. Ann Intern Med. 1980 Nov;93(5):701-4.
[57] Saranteas T, Mourouzis C, Dannis C, Alexopoulos C, Lolis E, Tesseromatis C. Effect of various stress models on lidocaine pharmacokinetic properties in the mandible after masseter injection.
[58] Saranteas T, Tesseromatis C, Potamianou A, Mourouzis C, Varonos D. Stress-induced lidocaine modification in serum and tissues. *Eur J Drug Metab Pharmacokinet* ; 27:229-32.
[59] Tigka E, Kotsiou A, Saranteas T, Mourouzis J, Kostopanagiotou G, Tesseromatis C. Clonidine changes lidocaine free concentrations in rat myocardium without affecting heart function measured by echocardiography. Eur J Drug Metab Pharmacokinet. 2009 Jul-Sep;34(3-4):229-32.
[60] Ganz PA, Baras M, Ma PY, Elashoff RM. Monitoring the therapy of lung cancer with alpha-1-acid glycoprotein. Cancer Res. 1984 ;44(11):5415-21.
[61] H Matsuura and S Nakazawa. Prognostic significance of serum alpha 1-acid glycoprotein in patients with glioblastoma multiforme: a preliminary communication. Neurol Neurosurg Psychiatry. 1985 August; 48(8): 835–837. Neurol Neurosurg Psychiatry. 1985 August; 48(8): 835–837.
[62] Roberts J. G, Keyser W. Baum M. Serum a-I-acid glycoprotein as an index of dissemination in- breast cancer. Br. J. Surg. Vol. 62 (1975) 816-81
[63] Jackson PR, Tucker GT, Woods HF. Altered plasma drug binding in cancer: role of alpha 1-acid glycoprotein and albumin. Clin Pharmacol Ther. 1982 ;32(3):295-302.

12

Haptoglobin and Hemopexin in Heme Detoxification and Iron Recycling

Deborah Chiabrando, Francesca Vinchi, Veronica Fiorito and Emanuela Tolosano
Molecular Biotechnology Center, University of Torino
Italy

1. Introduction

The acute phase reaction is an early response aimed at the defence of the organism and at the re-establishment of homeostasis in response to acute infection, inflammation and other pathological states (Kushner, 1982).

The putative mechanism responsible for this reaction is based on an initial signal derived from macrophages and other cells that synthesize and secrete several factors (probably cytokines) capable of inducing, in hepatocytes, a series of events. One of the most important mediators of the liver acute phase response is the monokine Interleukin (IL)-6 (Gauldie et al., 1987). The acute phase response consists in a change in the concentration of several plasma proteins, generally synthesized in the liver, including α_1-glycoprotein (AGP), complement factor C3, serum amyloid A, Haptoglobin and Hemopexin.

2. Haptoglobin

2.1 Gene structure

The Haptoglobin (Hp) locus is located on chromosome 16 in humans (chromosome 8 in mice) and shows an unusual polymorphism involving duplication, and, rarely, also triplication of parts of the coding region. Some Hp polymorphisms are linked to cardio-vascular and renal diseases.

A second gene exists, adjacent to the Hp gene and highly homologous to it, called Hpr (Haptoglobin related). Hpr arose by gene duplication and subsequent modification by a 7-kilobase retrovirus-like insertion into the first intron of the Hp gene (Marinkovic and Baumann, 1990). Both Hp and Hpr gene are transcribed in liver, but Hpr transcript level is only approximately 6% of that of Hp (Nielsen and Moestrup, 2009).

Although the primary site of Hp expression is the liver, it can also be detected in several other organs, including the nervous system, lung, spleen, thymus and heart (Nielsen and Moestrup, 2009).

2.2 Protein structure

Hp is a tetrachain ($\alpha_2\beta_2$) glycoprotein synthesized in the adult (but not fetal) liver and secreted into the plasma. The pro-Hp form is proteolytically processed into an α– and a β–chain. The two α-subunits and the two β-subunits of Hp protein are joined by inter-chain disulfide bonds. In humans, the precise structure of Hp protein is different according to the different Hp alleles, that give rise to an (αβ)-dimer or to various (αβ)-multimers (Figure 1). Hp has a high binding affinity for hemoglobin that is bound to the β-chain (Adams and Weiss, 1969; Nielsen and Moestrup, 2009).

2.3 Gene, mRNA and protein regulation

Regulation of the expression of the Hp gene occurs at least at three levels: (i) developmental control, responsible for the lack of expression in fetal liver; (ii)tissue-specific control, responsible for the selectivity of the expression of the gene in the hepatocyte; (iii)modulation of its expression during the acute phase reaction (Oliviero et al., 1987).

A short DNA segment of the 5' flanking region of Hp gene contains sufficient information for tissue-specific expression and transcriptional activation by acute phase stimuli (Oliviero et al., 1987). Among these cis-acting elements in the Hp promoter, there are two IL-6 responsive elements, accounting for dramatic increase of Hp mRNA levels in the presence of this monokine (Oliviero and Cortese, 1989). Hp production is also regulated by glucocorticoids, but no information is available about a glucocorticoid-responsive element (GRE) in the human Hp gene (Marinkovic and Baumann, 1990). Transcription factor C/EBPβ and the nuclear matrix protein p55 were identified as the major proteins that bound the hormone-responsive cis-element of Hp gene during the acute phase response, at least in rat (Poznanovic et al., 1999).

The Hp gene is transcribed quite selectively in hepatocytes about fifty times more in adult than in fetal liver nuclei, compared to about a twenty-fold increase in the case of the hemopexin gene (Oliviero et al., 1987). As a consequence, Hp is found in very low concentrations in fetal plasma, whereas its levels in the adult are about 0.45-3 mg/ml.

Regarding cell lines, the Hp mRNA is present in some human hepatoma cell lines, such as HepG2, but it is completely absent in others, such as Hep3B.

Finally, ectopic production of Hp was reported in cases of inflammation and cancer. In fact, the expression of Hp mRNA was observed in a small number of pancreatic cancer cell lines. Moreover, some pancreatic cancer cells, thanks to secretion of IL-6, are able to induce the production of fucosylated Hp in hepatoma cell lines and, according to this, high levels of fucosylated Hp can be found in sera from patients with pancreatic cancer (Narisada et al., 2008). A similar condition is also common in cases of advanced ovarian cancer, mammary carcinomas and severe inflammation diseases, such as rheumatic arthritis and inflammatory bowel disease.

2.4 Conservation of gene, protein and regulation

New World primates and rats possess only a single Hp gene, while Old World monkeys carry two to three tightly clustered Hp genes. In humans, four structural alleles have been identified: HplS, HplF, Hp2, and Hp3. Hp2 and Hp3 differ from Hp1 by having seven rather than five exons resulting in an increase of the α-subunit amino acids content.

Hp1 and Hp2 are the two major allelic forms of human Hp and they can give rise to three major Hp genotypes: Hp1-1, Hp2-1 and Hp2-2 (Nielsen and Moestrup, 2009).

An extensive study has been made on rat Hp, demonstrating that rat Hp cDNA sequence shows a high degree of similarity to the human Hp1 allele and that no Hpr gene can be found in rat genome. The rat Hp shows 75% amino acid sequence homology for the α-subunit and 86% for the β-subunit when compared with the human Hp1 gene product. Rat β-subunit contains two potential N-glycosylation sites, in contrast to the human β-subunit, which has four sites. Finally, rat Hp gene responsiveness to IL-6 is lower than in humans, and in rat cells the combination of IL-1, IL-6 and glucocorticoids (as dexamethasone) is required for maximal Hp expression (Marinkovic and Baumann, 1990).

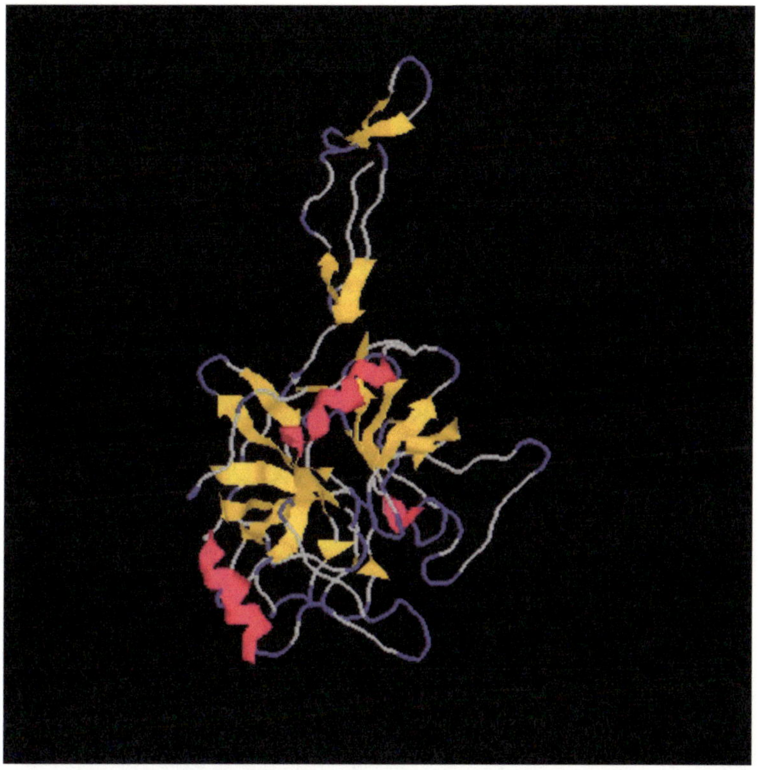

Fig. 1. Model of the human Haptoglobin isoform 1 monomer. α-Helices and β-strands are shown in pink and yellow, respectively. Loops are drawn in blue. The Hp model was generated using CPHmodels available at http://www.expasy.org/tools. The model was drawn with the Rasmol available at http://www.expasy.org/tools.

3. Hemopexin

3.1 Gene structure

The Hemopexin (Hx) gene is an 11Kb long gene located on human chromosome 11 (chromosome 7 in mice), the same location as the β-globin gene cluster (Law et al., 1988).
It is mainly expressed in the liver and, to a lesser extent, in neurons and astrocytes of the central nervous system, ganglionic and photoreceptor cells of the retina, Schwann and fibroblast-like cells of the peripheral nervous system, kidney mesangial cells and skeletal muscle (Tolosano et al., 1996).

3.2 Protein structure

Hx is a plasma 60-kD β-1B-glycoprotein composed of a single 439 amino acids long peptide chain, which forms two domains resembling two thick disks that lock together at a 90° angle and are joined by an interdomain linker peptide.

It contains about 20% carbohydrate, including sialic acid, mannose, galactose, and glucosamine and it does not present free sulfhydryl groups (Takahashi et al., 1984). Twelve cysteine residues were found in the protein sequence, probably accounting for six disulfide bridges.

The structure of human Hx is characterized by its unique clustering of histidine and tryptophan residues. The histidine residues are present in His-Gly sequences presumably exposed at the surface, while tryptophan mostly occurs in four clusters (Takahashi et al., 1984) (Figure 2).

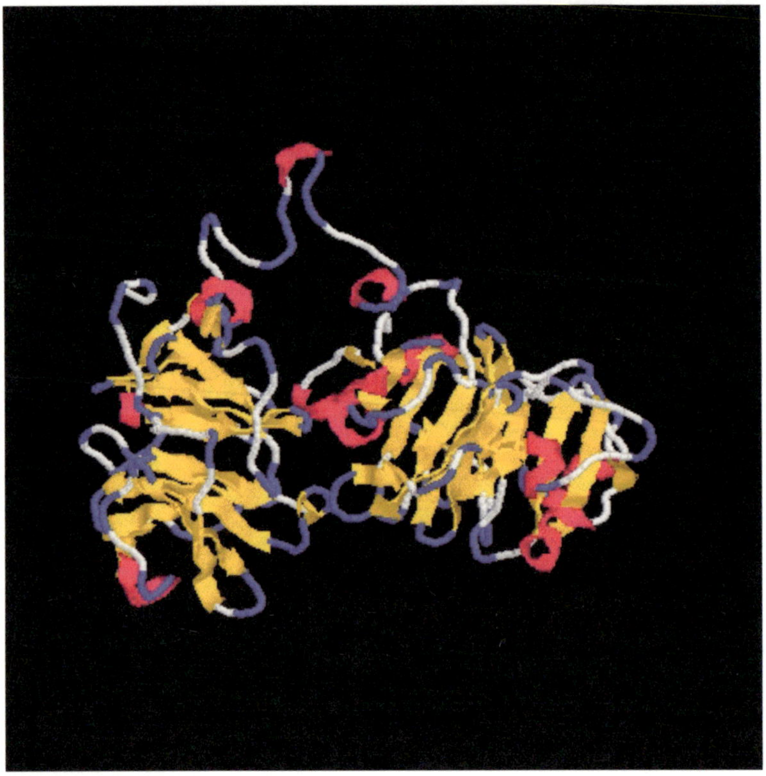

Fig. 2. Model of the human Hemopexin precursor. α-Helices and β-strands are shown in pink and yellow, respectively. Loops are drawn in blue. The Hx model was generated using CPH models available at http://www.expasy.org/tools. The model was drawn with the Rasmol available at http://www.expasy.org/tools.

Hx has the highest known heme affinity (Kd<1 pM) of any characterized heme-binding protein. It binds heme in an equimolar ratio, but there is no evidence that heme is covalently bound to the protein (Takahashi et al., 1984). The heme ligand is bound between the two domains of Hx in a pocket formed by the interdomain linker peptide. Heme binding and release results from opening and closing of the heme binding pocket, through movement of the two domains and/or interdomain linker peptide. The heme affinity decreases on lowering pH, on reduction of the heme iron atom, on nitric oxide (NO) binding to the ferrous heme iron atom, and in the presence of the chloride anion and of divalent metal ions, while the sodium cation increases the heme affinity for Hx (Tolosano et al., 2010).

Other than heme, Hx can also interact with a wide variety of natural and synthetic metalloporphyrins. As in cytochrome b5 (with which Hx shares several chemical and physical properties), two histidines in the N-terminal domain are proposed to be the ligands to heme iron, while tryptophan residues seem to reinforce the interaction of Hx with heme (Takahashi et al., 1984).
Regarding the C-terminal domain, its structure is common to that found in other proteins such as metalloproteinases which, for this reason, are indicated as "hemopexin-like domain" containing proteins (Bode, 1995).

3.3 Gene, mRNA and protein regulation

In murine development, Hx mRNA expression appears in the fetal life and the hepatic production of the protein and its serum concentration increase considerably during postnatal development, reaching the maximum level in the adult (Takahashi et al., 1984).
Similarly, Nikkilä et al. showed that hepatic Hx mRNA in rat is first detected on day 14 after gestation. Hx gene expression is not present in yolk sac, placenta, decidua, uterus or early embryonic tissues (Nikkila et al., 1991).
Apart from liver, other sites of Hx synthesis are the nervous system, skeletal muscle, retina and kidney, while Hx mRNA is not detectable in lung, heart, gastrointestinal tract and spleen (Poli et al., 1986).
Among human hepatoma cell lines, Hep3B cells have been shown to produce the highest amount of Hx mRNA (Poli et al., 1986).
After its synthesis, Hx is released in plasma where it can reach a concentration of about 0.5-1mg/ml. Its level can, however, increase during hemolyses or inflammatory events (Tolosano and Altruda, 2002; Tolosano et al., 1996).
Hx production is known to be regulated in large part at the transcriptional level. The tissue specific and the temporal expression of the Hx gene is directed by a 500bp fragment located upstream of the transcription start point in the Hx promoter. This region contains a specific cis-acting element, called Hpx A site, which, apart from being important for the cell-specific transcription of Hx, is also responsible for its regulation during the acute phase response (Poli et al., 1989).
Among inducers of Hx expression there are the cytokines IL-6, IL-11, leukaemia inhibitory factor (LIF), oncostatin M, IL-1β and Tumor Necrosis Factor (TNF)α (Immenschuh et al., 1995), while unlike most acute-phase proteins the serum amount of Hx is only slightly affected by dexamethasone. The regulation of Hx expression in response to IL-6 is mediated by a liver specific nuclear protein, IL6DBP (a member of the C/EBP family), which binds to the Hpx A site, and by the IL6RE-BP, an inducible nuclear factor which binds to another similar, but functionally distinct, IL6-responsive element in the Hx promoter (Tolosano et al., 1996).
Besides being regulated during inflammation, Hx production increases in response to extracorpuscular heme, while the levels of other acute-phase proteins remain unchanged after this kind of stimulus. Interestingly, rat Hx expression is also promoted by hyperoxia (Nikkila et al., 1991).

3.4 Conservation of gene, protein and regulation

The physiological importance of Hx is suggested by the extensive homologies in the sequence of this protein in different species and by the fact that its structure is very similar in all vertebrates.

As an example, the N-terminal domain of Hx has been identified as the heme-binding domain in human, rabbit and pig. Moreover, human and rat Hx share a high degree of homology at the amino acid level (76%) and a comparison of the interdomain disulfide bond formation reveals a similarity in their N-terminal and C-terminal domain structure.
Finally, the perfect conservation of the cysteine residues of rat and human Hx indicates that the same disulfide configuration is present in both proteins (Nikkila et al., 1991).
Beside protein structure conservation, gene expression regulation was maintained during evolution. Indeed, at least in human, rabbit, rat and chicken Hx gene expression is quite entirely confined to the liver and follows a peculiar temporal pattern during development, increasing several folds from fetal to adult life.

4. Haptoglobin and Hemopexin function into the bloodstream

4.1 Antioxidant and cytoprotective function of both Haptoglobin and Hemopexin

Hp and Hx belong to the acute-phase proteins whose expression can be induced by various cytokines in a context of inflammatory processes and act as soluble scavengers of free hemoglobin and heme, respectively.
Before starting to discuss in detail the role of Hp and Hx in heme metabolism, we want to open a short parenthesis on why heme scavenging from circulation is crucial.

4.1.1 Heme

Heme (protoporphyrin IX and iron) plays critical roles in several biological processes as it is the prosthetic group of a lot of essential proteins, such as hemoglobin, myoglobin, catalases, peroxidases and cytochromes (Tsiftsoglou et al., 2006).
On the other hand, free heme is highly toxic as it is a source of redox-active iron. In the cytoplasm, iron can participate in the Fenton reaction to produce the highly toxic reactive oxygen species (ROS) that damage lipid membranes, proteins and nucleic acids (Papanikolaou and Pantopoulos, 2005). Heme toxicity is further exacerbated by its ability to intercalate into lipid membranes. Heme-iron may initially lodge within the hydrophobic interstices of the phospholipid bilayer. Within this highly oxidizable matrix, iron catalyzes the oxidation of cell membrane constituents and assists in the formation of cytotoxic lipid peroxide, which enhances permeability and membrane disorder. Oxidation of membrane components may promote cell lysis and death.
Free heme is also a potent hemolytic agent. It affects erythrocyte membrane stability as a result of ROS formation and oxidative membrane damage thus shortening erythrocyte life span. Finally, free heme is an important source of iron for pathogenic microorganisms, predisposing to infections (Kumar and Bandyopadhyay, 2005).
Release of hemoglobin into the bloodstream is a physiologic process due to intravascular hemolysis that occurs during enucleation of erythroblasts and destruction of senescent erythrocytes. It has been calculated that, even if senescent red blood cells are mostly phagocytosed by macrophages, intravascular hemolysis accounts for at least 10% of red cell breakdown in normal individuals. However intravascular hemolysis becomes a severe pathological complication when it is accelerated in various disorders, such as hemorrhage, hemolytic anemia and hemoglobinopathies, polycitemia vera, malaria, ischemia reperfusion and muscle injury (Ascenzi et al., 2005; Stuart and Nagel, 2004). Under physiologic conditions, released hemoglobin is bound by Hp and transported to macrophages and hepatocytes. After massive hemolysis, when the buffering capacity of plasma Hp is

overwhelmed, hemoglobin is quickly oxidised to ferrihemoglobin, which releases free heme (Tolosano et al., 2010). Ferriheme then binds to albumin [Kd~10nM] and is subsequently transferred to Hx [Kd<1pM]. Heme is initially associated with albumin, presumably because the molar concentration of albumin in plasma is considerably greater than that of Hx (300 μM vs. 20 μM). After heme binding, Hx specifically delivers heme to the liver (Figure 3).

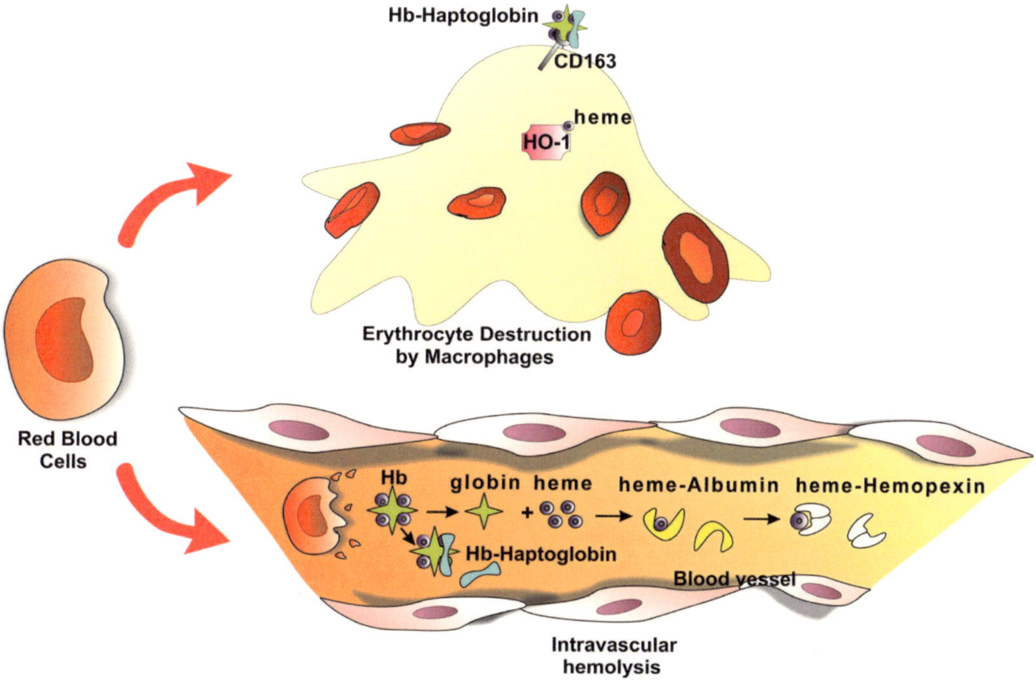

Fig. 3. Hemoglobin catabolism. Heme contained in red blood cells is mostly recycled by macrophages through erythrophagocytosis. During this process heme is degraded by HO-1 and iron recycled. A minor part of erythrocytes undergoes intravascular destruction, releasing hemoglobin which is bound by Hp and the complexes are subsequently delivered to hepatocytes and macrophages of the reticuloendothelial system, where they are internalized through CD163 receptor–mediated endocytosis. When the buffering capacity of Hp is exceeded, hemoglobin liberates heme, which binds to albumin and is subsequently transferred to Hx. (Hb: hemoglobin).

Under these conditions, the physiological mechanisms of removing free hemoglobin and heme from the circulation collapses, allowing nonspecific hemoglobin and heme uptake and heme catalyzed oxidation reactions (Kumar and Bandyopadhyay, 2005; Wagener et al., 2003b).

The vasculature is one of the most susceptible tissue to heme-mediated oxidative injury as it is continuously exposed to circulating erythrocytes, exogenous hemoglobin and heme released by damaged cells, (Balla et al., 2000; Jeney et al., 2002; Ogita and Liao, 2004; Wagener et al., 2001a). Heme can threaten vascular endothelial cell integrity directly by promoting intracellular ROS formation (Balla et al., 2000; Stocker and Keaney, 2004; Wagener et al., 2001a; Wagener et al., 2003a) and indirectly by its ability to oxidize low density lipoproteins (LDLs) (Grinshtein et al., 2003). The initial step of heme-mediated LDL oxidation involves the spontaneous insertion of heme into LDL particles. The inserted heme directly promotes extensive oxidative modification of LDL. Accordingly, when endothelial cells are exposed to LDL from plasma containing hemoglobin or free heme, oxidative endothelial damage ensures (Grinshtein et al., 2003).

Under physiological condition, the endothelial layer is non-adhesive for leukocytes. However, when exposed to free heme, activated endothelial cells increase the surface expression of adhesion molecules, as Intercellular Cell Adhesion Molecule (ICAM)-1, Vascular Cell Adhesion Molecule (VCAM)-1 and selectins (Belcher et al., 2003; Wagener et al., 2001a) which may subsequently promote the recruitment of leukocytes at the site of inflammation. By enhancing adhesion molecule expression and generating oxidative stress known to damage cells, heme also acts as a pro-inflammatory molecule and starts the inflammatory cascades (Wagener et al., 2001b). Finally free heme is considered a trigger of vasopermeabilization, which results from the partial retraction of endothelial cells of venules in the vicinity of inflammation, leaving small intercellular gaps. Vascular leakage results in slower blood flow by allowing the passage of water, salts and small proteins from the plasma into the damaged area (Mehta and Malik, 2006).

Other than for the vessels, free heme is also highly toxic for other tissues and organs causing oxidative stress and damage.

4.1.2 Haptoglobin

Following intravascular hemolysis, stable hemoglobin-Hp complexes are formed in plasma and are delivered to the reticuloendothelial system by CD163 receptor-mediated endocytosis and to liver parenchymal cells through a yet unidentified receptor. CD163 is a member of the cysteine-rich scavenger receptor family and is exclusively expressed by cells of monocyte/macrophages lineage (Kristiansen et al., 2001; Nielsen and Moestrup, 2009). The existence of another receptor for hemoglobin-Hp complexes in hepatocytes has been hypothesized as it has been demonstrated that after injection of labeled hemoglobin-Hp complexes in rats, most of labeled hemoglobin is taken up by liver parenchymal cells (Higa et al., 1981; Kino et al., 1982; Ship et al., 2005; Weinstein and Segal, 1984). In macrophages, upon endocytosis, the receptor–ligand complex enters early endosomes where hemoglobin-Hp complexes are released from CD163. The receptor then recycles to the cell surface while hemoglobin-Hp complexes continue through the endocytic pathway to end up in lysosomes where the protein moieties and the ligand are degraded (Nielsen and Moestrup, 2009).

In this manner, Hp reduces the loss of hemoglobin through the renal glomeruli hence protecting against peroxidative kidney injury and allows heme-iron recovery.

This has been extensively confirmed by studies in Hp-null mice which have shown that the loss of Hp did not affect hemoglobin clearance (Fagoonee et al., 2005; Lim et al., 1998) but influences the pattern of hemoglobin distribution. Following the injection of low doses of labeled hemoglobin, hemoglobin-Hp complexes are mainly delivered to hepatocytes and Kupffer cells in the liver and to macrophages in the spleen of wild-type animals; in the absence of Hp, hemoglobin is mainly recovered by the kidney instead of the liver and spleen suggesting that Hp is important for the delivery of hemoglobin complexes to the liver and spleen. In a similar way, when high doses of labeled hemoglobin were injected into wild-type mice, causing the saturation of Hp binding capacity, in addition to the liver and spleen, hemoglobin is also delivered to the kidney thus mimicking what occurs during pathological conditions such us chronic hemolysis.

The role of Hp in preventing hemoglobin filtration through the glomerular barrier is further supported by the observation that Hp-null mice develops kidney iron overload with ageing (Fagoonee et al., 2005). Particularly, hemoglobin derived iron accumulate mainly in the proximal tubular cells of the kidney. Similarly, HO-1 knockout mice which completely lack macrophages expressing the hemoglobin-Hp receptor CD163 also develop kidney iron loading (Kovtunovych et al., 2010).

Moreover, excessive hemolysis or transfusion of hemoglobin solution have been shown to result in Hp depletion and subsequent renal failure, particularly acute tubular necrosis (Tam and Wong, 1988).

In the absence of Hp, hemoglobin is filtered through the glomerular barrier and is reabsorbed by proximal tubular cells through the endocytic receptors megalin and cubilin. Megalin and cubilin are multiligand endocytic receptors expressed at the apical membrane of proximal tubules. Their primary function is to reabsorb small molecules that pass the glomerular filtration barrier. It has been previously demonstrated that hemoglobin is one of their ligands (Christensen and Birn, 2001; Gburek et al., 2002). Once in tubular cells, hemoglobin is degraded in the endosomal compartment and heme is catabolized by heme oxygenase (HO) (Figure 4).

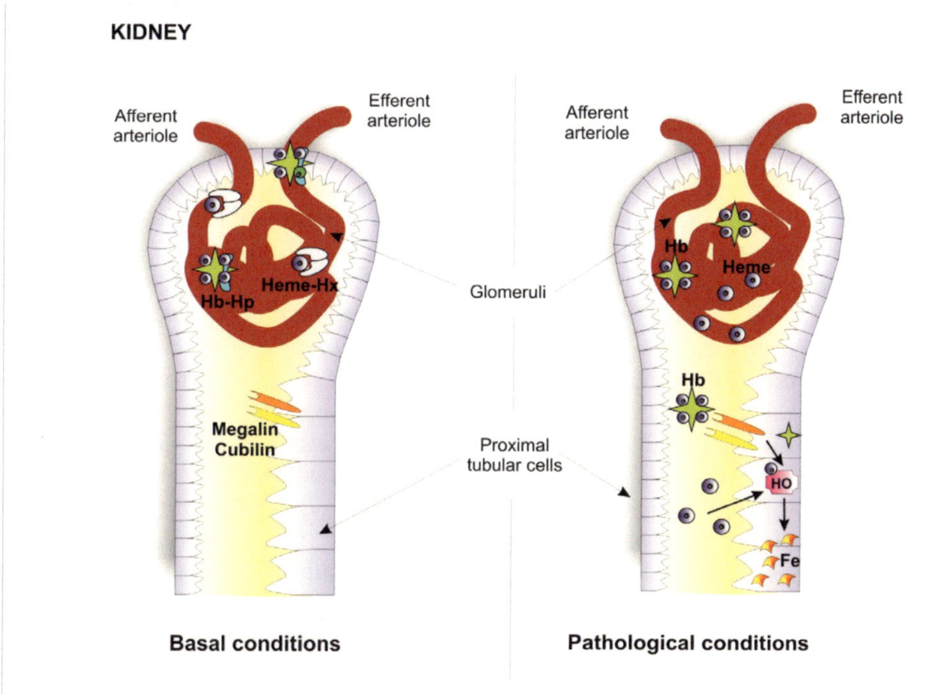

Fig. 4. Haptoglobin and Hemopexin prevent kidney iron loading. Under basal conditions hemoglobin and heme are targeted to macrophages and hepatocytes by Hp and Hx, respectively. Under pathologic conditions when Hp and Hx binding capacity is overwhelmed, hemoglobin and heme are filtered through the glomerular barrier and are re-absorbed by proximal tubular cells. Hemoglobin is recognized by the endocytic receptors megalin and cubilin while heme enters into the cells through a yet unidentified mechanism. Into the cells, heme is degraded by HO and iron stored bound to ferritin (Ft).

In agreement with renal iron loading, Hp-null mice show higher basal level of renal lipid peroxidation and suffered greater tissue damage, as evidenced by the induction of the hepatic acute phase response resulting in increased AGP levels (Lim et al., 1998). Moreover, these mice showed increased susceptibility to acute hemolysis induced by phenylhydrazine treatment and are more sensitive to kidney injury than wild-type animals. Accordingly, an increased susceptibility to hemoglobin driven lipid peroxydation has been observed in human patients with hypo- or anhaptoglobinemia.

4.1.3 Hemopexin

Hx represents the primary line of defence against heme toxicity thanks to its ability to bind heme with high affinity and to function as a heme specific carrier from the bloodstream to the liver (Tolosano et al., 2010). The formation of heme-Hx complexes has been demonstrated to promote heme delivery to the parenchymal cells of the liver (Smith and Morgan, 1978, 1979). On the contrary, the heme-albumin complex appears to act only as a heme depository, before transport to the liver as heme-Hx, and there is no experimental evidence that albumin has a transport function in vivo (Smith and Morgan, 1981). Nowadays, several lines of evidence support the fact that the liver is the main target tissue for heme-Hx complex internalization and heme-derived iron recycling. In vivo studies showed that the liver is the major site of radioactive heme uptake after intravenous injection of ^{55}Fe-heme-^{125}I-Hx: nearly 90% of the administered heme is transported to the liver within 2 hours (K_D700nM) without significant urinary excretion of either isotope (Smith and Ledford, 1988; Smith and Morgan, 1978, 1979, 1981, 1984). Hx-mediated heme uptake by the liver has been shown in vivo and in vitro to be a saturable process: saturation is indicative of an interaction with a rate-limiting step and a finite number of binding sites and is characteristic of receptor-mediated uptake. Furthermore, heme-Hx internalization has been demonstrated to be a highly tissue-specific process, time-, temperature- and energy-dependent (Smith and Morgan, 1978, 1979). Occurring within minutes, the association is on the same time scale as the receptor-mediated uptake of asialoglycoproteins (LaBadie et al., 1975) and of iron-transferrin complexes (Gardiner and Morgan, 1974). Nowadays, the only known Hx receptor on hepatocytes is represented by the LDL receptor-related protein 1 (LRP1), a multi-ligand scavenger receptor, involved in the metabolism of lipoprotein and expressed in several cell types including macrophages, hepatocytes and neurons (Boucher et al., 2003; Lillis et al., 2005). LRP1 has been shown to mediate heme-Hx internalization, resulting in cellular heme uptake (Hvidberg et al., 2005). Once entered the cell, the heme-Hx complex is dissociated by lysosomal activity: LRP1 is then recycled to the plasma membrane, whereas Hx destiny, after complex internalization, is somewhat controversial. Some studies have suggested that Hx can be recycled as an intact molecule to the extracellular milieu (Smith and Morgan, 1979). However, it has also been proposed that following hepatic uptake of heme from heme-Hx, varying proportion of the protein are either returned to the circulation or degraded in the liver (Potter et al., 1993). Recently, Hvidberg et al. have shown that most Hx is degraded in lysosomes (Hvidberg et al., 2005). Accordingly, in a model of heme overload, plasma Hx level has been found to decrease, thus indicating that Hx is actively involved in heme scavenging and subjected to degradation (Vinchi et al., 2008). Furthermore, a decrease in plasma Hx concentration reflects a recent release of heme compounds in the extracellular compartment. Invariably, high concentrations of heme are associated with low concentration of Hx (Muller-Eberhard et al., 1968). Hx is in fact found to decrease in plasma after hemolytic stress associated to pathologies like hemolytic anemias, acute intermittent porphyria and chronic neuromuscular diseases.

As a consequence of Hx-mediated heme delivery to the liver, heme deleterious effects are efficiently counteracted as demonstrated by several experimental data. First, heme binding to Hx has been demonstrated to reduce the heme-mediated free radical formation from organic peroxides (Timmins et al., 1995). Furthermore, in vitro studies demonstrated that Hx strongly decreases the peroxidative and catalatic activity of heme by forming inactive heme-protein complexes. Interestingly, these hemin activities were found to be inhibited by 80-90% with Hx but only by 50-60% with either human or bovine albumin (Grinberg et al., 1999). The marked effectiveness of Hx at inhibiting heme toxicity was most probably the result of its very high affinity to heme with a dissociation constant K_D of 10^{-13}M. Moreover, binding to Hx was shown to inhibit heme-catalyzed lipid peroxidation in artificial liposomes (Gutteridge and Smith, 1988), rat liver microsomes (Vincent et al., 1988) and plasma LDL (Miller et al., 1996). Thus, Hx has an essential role in the prevention of heme-induced oxidative damage and cell death (Eskew et al., 1999).

Many experimental evidences also support the antioxidant function of Hx in vivo. Hx-null mice have been demonstrated to be particularly sensitive to heme overload and more prone to heme-induced oxidative damage and inflammation during hemolytic processes (Tolosano et al., 1999; Vinchi et al., 2008). Furthermore, in vivo studies showed that the most damaged tissues upon heme overload conditions are the vasculature, the liver and the kidney.

It has been demonstrated that Hx has a crucial role in the protection of the endothelial wall against heme toxicity. It has been observed an increased induction of the adhesion molecules ICAM-1 and VCAM-1 in the endothelium and increased vascular permeability in Hx-null mice compared to wild-type mice, after intravenous heme injection (Vinchi et al., 2008), thus demonstrating that Hx activity is required to prevent heme-induced vasopermeabilization and endothelial activation.

Oxidative stress has already been shown to induce vascular HO-1 expression in rats, mice, and humans. Even if HO-1 induction is significantly higher in the vascular endothelium of Hx-null mice compared to controls, it cannot prevent endothelial damage (Vinchi et al., 2008). On the other hand, the induction of HO-1 before intravenous heme injection preserved endothelial integrity in Hx-null mice, thus indicating that the lack of Hx may be tolerated if the cells are already equipped to metabolize an excess of heme and suggesting that Hx and HO-1 work in sequence to counteract the toxic effect of heme, Hx being the first line of defence.

Besides the vasculature, other tissues have been described as particularly sensitive to heme-mediated damage. Studies on Hx-null mice have demonstrated that these animals are particularly sensitive to acute hemolysis. These mice recover more slowly after phenylhydrazine-induced hemolysis and suffer from more severe renal damage compared to wild-type mice. In fact, after hemolytic stimulus, Hx-null mice present prolonged hemoglobinuria, higher kidney iron loading and lipid peroxidation than wild-type mice (Tolosano et al., 1999). These findings emphasize the protective role of Hx in hemolytic processes. Moreover, Hx-null kidneys exhibit increased lipid peroxidation not only after phenylhydrazine treatment but also after intravenous injection of hemin (Vinchi et al., 2008). Therefore Hx, together with Hp, plays a fundamental role in the kidney during hemolysis: Hp has a major function in the protection of renal tubules from hemoglobin-mediated oxidative damage; then, once Hp disappears from the circulation, the delayed presence of Hx in the plasma takes on a relevant role in the protection against heme derived from hemoglobin oxidation.

Interestingly Hx and Hp compound mutant mice subjected to phenylhydrazine-induced hemolysis presented, other than kidney damage, a more severe injury in the liver characterized by inflammation, necrosis and fibrosis (Tolosano et al., 2002). The liver is also the most sensitive organ to heme overload in Hx-null mice. Indeed the liver of heme-overloaded Hx-null mice developed a marked congestion characterized by red blood cell stasis and sinusoidal dilation around the centrolobular area (Figure 5). Hepatic congestion was found to be associated with abnormal iron deposits, increased lipid peroxidation and massive leukocyte infiltrates (Vinchi et al., 2008).

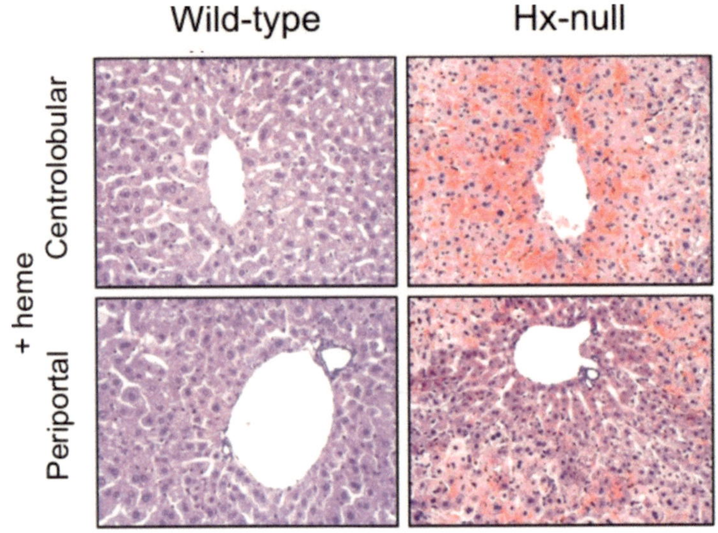

Fig. 5. Liver congestion in heme-overloaded Hemopexin-null mice. Liver sections of a wild-type and a Hx-null mouse injected with heme into the tail vein and sacrificed 6 hours later. Note the marked congestion around the centrolobular vein in Hx-null animal. Hematoxylin and eosin staining; X200.

This phenotype underlines the increased susceptibility of Hx-null mice to acute hepatic damage in condition of heme overload and highlights a role for Hx in the protection from liver injury. Liver damage in Hx-null mice may be prevented by induction of HO-1 before heme overload, thus confirming once again that Hx and HO-1 work together to ensure tissue protection against heme toxicity.

The congestion observed in the liver of heme-overloaded Hx-null mice resembles the hepatic phenotype of patients suffering from vaso-occlusive diseases like veno-occlusive disease (VOD) (Bayraktar et al., 2007; Senzolo et al., 2007) and Budd-Chiari syndrome (BCS) (Aydinli and Bayraktar, 2007; Hillmen et al., 1995) or experienced painful vaso-occlusive crises associated with hemoglobinopathies (Ahn et al., 2005; Dampier et al., 2004). Particularly, in sickle cell disease, vascular occlusions are the major causes of the pain, morbidity, and mortality (Stuart and Nagel, 2004).

Since all the disorders mentioned above are usually related to pathological conditions wherein extracellular hemoglobin and free heme are released in massive amounts, it could be speculated that heme represent a predisposing factor for vaso-occlusion and that Hx is important to counteract its pro-occlusive effects. This hypothesis is also in agreement with the mentioned role of Hx as a detoxification mechanism that prevents endothelial damage by removing free heme from circulation.

In conclusion in vivo studies highlight the critical importance of Hx in preventing firstly vascular inflammation and acute liver injury and secondly renal damage, thanks to its ability to limit heme-induced oxidative stress. Interestingly all the toxic effects of heme are exacerbated in Hx-null mice, indicating not only that Hx has an important protective role in plasma but also that none of the plasma proteins able to bind heme (ie, albumin, α1-microglobulin, high- and low-density lipoproteins) may substitute for Hx after heme overload.

4.2 Role of Haptoglobin and Hemopexin in iron recycling

4.2.1 Haptoglobin- and Hemopexin-mediated heme recovery

Besides their function as hemoglobin and heme scavengers respectively, Hp and Hx are essential in the re-utilisation of heme-bound iron and represent a fundamental part of the iron-conservation mechanisms of the body (Hershko,1975; Davies,1979).

As reported above, the hemoglobin-Hp complexes are mainly taken up by macrophages through the specific receptor CD163, whereas the heme-Hx complexes enter into hepatocytes through LRP1. Once in macrophages or hepatocytes, heme is degraded by HO-1 to iron, biliverdin and CO (see next section). Iron is then stored in cells bound to ferritin or exported to the plasma and transported throughout the body. The contribution of Hp to iron recovery is further highlighted by the observation that the Hp phenotype modify iron loading in hemochromatosis both in humans and in mice (Delanghe and Langlois, 2002; Langlois et al., 2000; Tolosano et al., 2005; Van Vlierberghe et al., 2004; Van Vlierberghe et al., 2001). In addition, deletion of the Hx gene in mice results in abnormal extrahepatic iron deposits (Morello et al., 2008), thus suggesting that also in humans mutations in the Hx gene might modify iron distribution and accumulation in the body.

Other than by Hp and Hx other mechanisms have been reported to mediate hemoglobin or heme delivery to cells. Recent data suggest that in macrophages CD163 is also able to mediate the entrance of free hemoglobin through a low affinity binding. Particularly, (a)hemoglobin uptake has been observed in the absence of Hp in human macrophages and in CD163 transduced HEK293 cells but not in CD163-negative cells; (b)highly purified hemoglobin inhibits CD163 mediated uptake of labeled hemoglobin-Hp complexes or free hemoglobin, implying a common receptor binding site; (c)free hemoglobin induces transcriptional induction of HO-1, an indirect measure of hemoprotein internalization and degradation, in CD163 expressing cells in a dose dependent manner; (d)disruption of the hemoglobin interaction with Hp by chemical cross-linking of hemoglobin between its alpha chains or, alternatively, by proteolytic cleavage does not significantly affect the CD163-hemoglobin interaction.

Moreover, other than free hemoglobin, macrophages may also take up free heme, or, in other words, heme not bound to Hx. Treatment of primary macrophages or macrophage cell lines with heme resulted in the induction of HO-1 and ferritin indicating that heme enters in these cells and is degraded (Hvidberg et al., 2005; Liang et al., 2009). Moreover, Hx-deficient mice showed a prolonged HO-1 induction in Kupffer cells after acute hemolysis (Tolosano et al., 2002) and intravenous heme injection (Vinchi et al., 2008), thus suggesting that Hx limits heme delivery and thus heme-mediated HO-1 induction in these cells. Moreover, several other cell types, other than macrophages, may take up free hemoglobin and heme.

Nevertheless these alternative mechanisms do not ensure an adequate protection against oxidative damage nor an efficient iron recovery as demonstrated by the observation that, under conditions of massive hemolysis, free hemoglobin and heme accumulate in proximal tubular cells of the kidney. As mentioned in section 4.1.2,, Hp-null mice accumulated heme-derived iron in proximal tubular cells during ageing and after phenylhydrazine-induced hemolysis. This is true also for Hx-null that, after phenylhydrazine treatment show renal iron loading. Moreover, heme overloaded-Hx-null mice upregulate HO-1 and ferritins in the kidney. These data indicate that excess of free heme is recovered by the kidney, during hemolytic stress, when the buffering capacity of Hp and Hx is overwhelmed (Figure 4). (Lim et al., 1998; Tolosano et al., 1999).

In conclusion as shown in Figure 6, Hp plays a major role in mediating haemoglobin recovery in macrophages through CD163, whereas Hx promotes heme uptake by

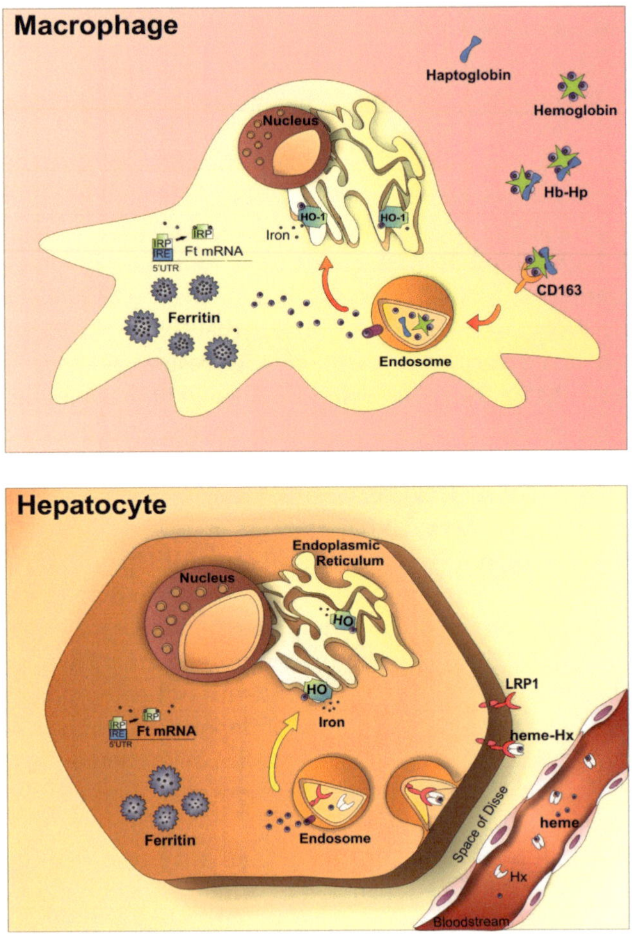

Fig. 6. Role of macrophage and hepatocyte in hemoglobin and heme recovery respectively. Macrophage takes up the hemoglobin-Hp complexes through CD163, whereas the hepatocyte recovers the heme-Hx complexes through LRP1. Once into the cell heme is degraded by HO to iron, which is bound to ferritin, CO and biliverdin (see section 4.2.2 for details). As depicted in the figure iron by itself may control the expression of ferritin (see section 4.3.2).

hepatocytes through LRP1. These mechanisms ensure an adequate protection against heme-mediated oxidative stress and mediate heme-iron reutilization. Under conditions of massive hemolysis when Hp and Hx are saturated free hemoglobin and heme may be taken up by macrophage through not well-characterized mechanisms. However, under these conditions heme pro-oxidant potential is not adequately inactivated and the vasculature and tissues are damaged.

4.2.2 Role of HO and Ferritin in heme iron recovery

Once that the hemoglobin-Hp or the heme-Hx complexes are respectively taken up by macrophages and hepatocytes, heme is released in the cytoplasm and presumably used to build new hemoproteins or catabolized by HO.

Microsomal HO is the rate-limiting enzyme in the degradation of heme and plays a key role in the protection of cells from heme-induced oxidative stress (Ferris et al., 1999). It breaks down the pro-oxidant heme into the antioxidant biliverdin, the vasodilator carbon monoxide (CO) and iron. Biliverdin is then reduced to bilirubin by the enzyme biliverdin reductase. Hitherto, three isoforms of HO have been identified: HO-1, HO-2, and HO-3.

HO-1 is highly inducible by a variety of stimuli including oxidative stress, heat shock, hypoxia, heavy metals, ischemia-reperfusion, cytokines and its substrate heme. The constitutively expressed HO-2 participates in the normal heme capturing and metabolism, while the function of HO-3 is still under investigation (Wagener et al., 2003b). HO-1 plays a crucial function in regulating heme degradation and protects against heme-mediated oxidative injury.

HO-1 can prevent the deleterious effects of free heme by several mechanisms. These include inhibiting (*a*)the release of free heme from hemoproteins, (*b*)the accumulation of free heme in cells, and/or (*c*)the pro-oxidant effects of free heme.

HO-1 can prevent heme release from hemoproteins by producing CO, a final product of heme degradation. Once bound to the heme groups of hemoproteins, CO inhibits heme-iron oxidation, thus limiting the oxidation of hemoproteins and preventing heme release. It has been recently demonstrated that by this mechanism HO-1 inhibits the accumulation of free heme in plasma following Plasmodium infection, thus preventing the onset of severe malaria in mice (Ferreira et al., 2008; Pamplona et al., 2007; Pamplona et al., 2009; Seixas et al., 2009).

Analysis of HO-1-null mice has shown that these animals accumulated, with age, hepatic and renal iron that contributed to oxidative damage, tissue injury and chronic inflammation. On the other hand, HO-1-null mice presented low serum iron concentration and developed anemia (Koizumi, 2007; Yachie et al., 1999). These data demonstrated that, although HO-1 is a stress-induced protein, it is important under basal conditions to protect liver and kidney from oxidative damage and that it is an essential regulator of iron metabolism and homeostasis.

Overexpression of HO-1 is associated to the resolution of inflammation through the generation of beneficial molecules like CO, bilirubin, and ferritin resulting from catabolism of toxic heme (Kapturczak et al., 2004; Wagener et al., 2001b). Some of the end products of heme catabolism by HO-1 might prevent the pro-oxidant effects of free heme. This is probably the case for biliverdin, which has antioxidant properties by itself but in addition can be converted by biliverdin reductase into the potent lipid-soluble antioxidant bilirubin. Owing to its lipophilic nature, free heme might act as a pro-oxidant primarily within cellular membranes. This deleterious effect may be inhibited by lipophilic bilirubin, that efficiently scavenges peroxyl radicals, thereby inhibiting lipid peroxidation and attenuating heme-induced endothelial activation. This mechanism would explain the ability of HO-1 to inhibit, via the production of bilirubin, lipid peroxidation in cells exposed to free heme and TNF. CO controls the activity of several heme proteins and causes vasodilation. It also exerts anti-inflammatory effects by inhibiting the expression of pro-inflammatory cytokines through a pathway involving the mitogen-activated protein kinases (Ndisang et al., 2002). In the last years several studies have shown the therapeutic potentialities of HO-1 and its products in counteracting the toxic effect of heme associated to pathologic conditions (Farombi and Surh, 2006; Lindenblatt et al., 2004).

Heme catabolism by HO-1 should also prevent the accumulation of free heme within cells. This cytoprotective mechanism must, however, be coupled to the induction of ferritin (Ft) expression to avoid the pro-oxidant effects of labile iron produced via heme catabolism. This notion is consistent with the observation that overexpression of Ft can mimic the cytoprotective effects of HO-1.

Ft is the major intracellular depot of non-metabolic iron and acts as a heme-detoxification system by scavenging free iron and protecting cells from its adverse effects. Ft is a multimeric protein composed of 24 subunits of two types, the heavy chain (H-Ft) and the light chain (L-Ft) and has a very high capacity for storing iron (up to 4500 mol of iron per mol of Ft). In the Ft shell, the proportion of heavy and light subunits depends on the iron status of the cell or tissue and varies among organs and species. H-Ft manifests ferroxidase activity that catalyses the oxidation of ferrous iron to ferric iron to allow intracellular iron storage in L-Ft, which acts as intracellular iron deposit (Arosio and Levi, 2002). Iron released during heme catabolism has been demonstrated to be rapidly stored in Ft (Davies et al., 1979).

Together, HO and Ft allow rapid iron shifting from heme into Ft core where iron is less available to catalyze deleterious reactions. Hence their potent antioxidant role. By increasing the expression of HO-1 and Ft, cells can survive lethal heme-induced oxidative stress (Balla et al., 2005).

Interestingly, in vivo work showed that Hx-null mice failed to up-regulate Ft in the liver after heme overload, thus demonstrating that the lack of Hx decreases the ability of the liver to recover heme-iron, under heme overload condition. Conversely, up-regulation of Ft in wild-type liver indicates a strong iron detoxifying capacity and an active iron storage and demonstrates, once again, that Hx is crucial to mediate heme delivery to hepatocytes.

4.3 Regulation of gene expression by hemoglobin-Haptoglobin and heme-Hemopexin complexes.

4.3.1 Haptoglobin mediated regulation of Ferroportin expression

Recent studies suggest an important role of Hp in modulating iron export from the duodenum. Hp-null mice showed increased iron export from the duodenum compared to wild-type mice, while iron uptake was normal (Marro et al., 2007). Iron export out of the duodenum was due to the increased expression of the iron exporter Ferroportin.

Following the injection of a low dose of hemoglobin into wild-type and Hp-null mice, a little amount of hemoglobin is delivered to the duodenum, suggesting the existence of a yet unknown mechanism for hemoglobin uptake into duodenal cells (Fagoonee et al., 2005). So, it has been proposed that hemoglobin taken up into duodenal cells could regulate Ferroportin transcription.

In vitro data on macrophages, showed that hemoglobin and heme directly activate the transcription of Ferroportin through the transcription factors Bach1 and Nrf2 (Marro et al., 2010). Thus, Hp, by controlling plasma levels of hemoglobin, participates in the regulation of ferroportin expression, thus contributing to the regulation of iron export. In the same way it is possible to speculate that Hx by controlling heme uptake by the cells may contribute to the control of ferroportin expression.

4.3.2 Hemopexin-mediated regulation of genes involved in iron recycling and cell survival

By its ability to mediate heme uptake into the liver, Hx promotes an increase in intracellular concentrations of heme, that directly affects the surface expression of transferrin receptor (TfR) and the expression level of HO-1 and ferritin. Heme has been shown to regulate the expression of several genes, including HO-1, by inhibiting the transcriptional repressor Bach1. Moreover, when intracellular heme increases, a rapid downregulation of TfR on the plasma membrane and concomitant induction of ferritin synthesis occur. It has been demonstrated that incubation of mouse Hepa cells with heme-Hx causes a rapid dose- and time-dependent decrease in the level of TfR mRNA. These regulatory effects have been observed not only in hepatic cells but also in human promyelocitic HL-60 cells (Alam and Smith, 1989), in human leukemic U937 cells and in HeLa cells (Taketani et al., 1990). Down-regulation of TfR on the plasma membrane was the result of multiple steps: a rapid redistribution of the protein between the plasma and intracellular membrane compartments and a decrease in the biosynthesis of the receptor. The latter is due to iron released from heme, that affects the stability of iron regulatory proteins (IRP), which regulate TfR mRNA stability and ferritin mRNA translation by binding to the iron responsive elements (IRE) in their 3′ and 5′ UTRs, respectively (Hentze et al., 2004). In this manner heme-derived iron enhance the expression of the iron storage protein ferritin and down-regulates the uptake of inorganic iron.

Furthermore, binding of heme–Hx to the plasma membrane Hx receptor stimulates the expression of metallothionein (MT)-1 (Alam and Smith, 1992; Ren and Smith, 1995) . Metallothioneins are cysteine-rich proteins thought to play a role in heavy metal detoxification, zinc and copper homeostasis, and cellular adaptation to stress. Upon incubation with heme-Hx, MT-1 mRNA steady state levels rapidly increase in both mouse hepatoma and human HL-60 cells. Regulation is controlled primarily at the level of MT-1 gene transcription in Hepa cells. Non protein-bound heme, although an effective inducer of HO gene transcription, was found to be a poor inducer of MT-1. This indicated that occupation of the Hx receptor itself by the heme-Hx complex is necessary for efficient accumulation of MT-1 transcripts. Activation of MT-1 gene transcription as a consequence of Hx-mediated heme transport may occur during endocytosis or via an indirect mechanism triggered by the interaction of heme-Hx with the Hx receptor on the cell surface. Recently Smith et al. demonstrated that the correct hypothesis was the first one: mainly copper, than the heme-Hx complex has been found to have an essential role in MT-1 induction (Smith et al., 2008). Copper endocytosis together with that of heme-Hx provides a mean to facilitate heme release from Hx in the maturing endosomes, by preventing the rebinding of heme to Hx. In this manner copper promotes heme export from endosomes and renders it available for HO-1 degradation. On the other hand, MT-1 induction is proposed to take place in response to a rise in cytosolic copper that directly contribute to MT-1 gene transcription. Therefore, cytosolic copper provide a link for the simultaneous regulation of HO-1 and MT-1 by heme-Hx.

5. Haptoglobin and Hemopexin function in the nervous system

Heme is an essential cofactor for many proteins involved in the normal function of neuronal tissue, such as enzymes required for neurotransmitter synthesis and myelination of axons (Connor and Menzies, 1996). On the other hand, excess of heme is usually associated to pathologic conditions as intracerebral or subarachnoid hemorrhages and ischemia reperfusion injury. In addition, some neurodegenerative disorders like Alzheimer's and Parkinson's diseases, are associated with iron accumulation in specific brain regions (Berg and Youdim, 2006; Zecca et al., 2004). As the central nervous system is separated from the body by the blood-brain barrier, it has evolved mechanisms of local heme and iron management.

5.1 Haptoglobin and Hemopexin expression in the central nervous system

Both Hp and Hx were found in the human cerebrospinal fluid and their expression increases in several pathologic conditions including Parkinson's disease, Alzheimer's disease and Guillain-Barré syndrome (Arguelles et al.; Roher et al., 2009; Yang et al., 2008).

Hp was found to be expressed in human gliobastoma cell lines, in reactive astrocytes after transient forebrain ischemia in rats and in oligodendroglia in mice (Lee et al., 2002). Hx expression was demonstrated in cortical neurons and astrocytes (Morris et al., 1993). Moreover, detection of beta-galactosidase activity on brain sections from Hx-null mice, carrying the lacZ gene into the Hx genomic locus, demonstrated that Hx was expressed primarily by ependymal cells lining the ventricular system and hippocampal neurons (Morello et al., 2008). Finally, both Hp and Hx are expressed in the neural retina (Chen et al., 1998).

5.2 Neuroprotective roles of both Haptoglobin and Hemopexin

In humans Hp haplotypes were found to be correlated with the extent of cerebral deep white matter lesions in hypertensive patients and with cerebrovascular disease, thus suggesting that the efficiency of hemoglobin scavenging may be crucial for the resolution of neuronal injury.

Moreover, by using a mouse model of intracerebral hemorrhage, Zhao and co-authors demonstrated that Hp plays an important role in defending neurons from damage induced by hemolysis (Zhao et al., 2009). *In vitro* studies demonstrated that oligodendroglia-released Hp protects neurons and oligodendrocytes against hemoglobin-mediated toxicity (Zhao et al., 2009).

A protective role against intracerebral hemorrhage has also been reported for Hx by Chen and co-authors that demonstrated increased striatal injury and behavioral deficits in Hx-null mice subjected to intracerebral hemorrhage (Chen et al.). Moreover, it has recently been reported that, in a mouse model of transient ischemia, Hx is protective as neurologic deficits and infarct volumes were significantly greater in Hx-null than in wild-type mice (Li et al., 2009). Exogenous free heme was shown to decrease cell survival in primary mouse cortical neuron cultures, whereas the heme bound to Hx was not toxic and protection was achieved through heme-Hx-mediated induction of HO-1 (Li et al., 2009).

6. Other functions

Recent works highlighted a role for Hp and Hx in the control of the immune response, mainly achieved through their ability to control inflammation. Hp modulates both innate and adaptive immune responses. Hp has been demonstrated to bind activated neutrophils, to inhibit several of their functions and to suppress secretion of TNF-α, IL-10, and IL-12p70 by macrophages upon LPS triggering (Arredouani et al., 2005; Rossbacher et al., 1999). CD11b has been identified as a macrophage receptor for Hp (El Ghmati et al., 1996). The binding of hemoglobin-Hp complex to the CD163 molecule on macrophages leads to anti-inflammatory cytokine secretion (Nielsen and Moestrup, 2009). Hp acts on Langerhans cells of the skin, preventing their differentiation and function during in vitro culture and affects proliferation and cytokine production by stimulated T cells and B cells (Huntoon et al., 2008; Xie et al., 2000). Recently, Galicia et al. demonstrated that, in a model of experimental autoimmune encephalomyelitis, Hp-null mice suffered from a more severe disease that was associated with increased expression of IL-17A, IL-6, and interferon (IFN)-γ mRNA in the CNS and with a denser cellular infiltrate in the spinal cord. During the recovery phase, a significantly higher number of myeloid DC, $CD8^+$ cells, $IL\text{-}17^+$ $CD4^+$ and $IFN\text{-}\gamma^+$ $CD4^+$ cells persisted in the CNS of Hp-null mice. Absence of Hp affected the priming and differentiation of T cells after induced encephalomyelitis (Galicia et al., 2009).

On the other hand, Hx-null mice produced significantly less autoantibodies and had less immune complex deposits than their wild-type counterpart in a model of mercury-induced autoimmunity and this response has been correlated to a blunted response of $CD4^+$ T cells from Hx-null mice to IFNγ. Some data suggested that Hx, by controlling heme-iron availability to T lymphocytes may control the expression of IFNγR at the cell membrane thus regulating IFNγ responsiveness (Fagoonee et al., 2008). However, other data demonstrated that Hx, like Hp, down-regulates LPS-induced proinflammatory cytokines from macrophages and suppresses neutrophil adhesion and phagocytosis by a mechanism unrelated to heme-binding (Liang et al., 2009). Furthermore, Spiller et al. have recently reported that Hx by inhibiting neutrophil migration leads to increased mortality in septic mice (Spiller et al., 2010).

All these results suggest that Hp and Hx play a modulatory role on the immune response likely by controlling cytokine production.

7. Conclusion

As discussed in the previous sections, Hp and Hx, by acting as plasma scavengers of hemoglobin and heme respectively, play a major role in the protection against heme-mediated oxidative stress and in preventing heme-iron loss during the acute phase response associated to massive intravascular hemolysis. In addition, they play a "local" role in the nervous system by limiting the pro-oxidant effect of heme after ischemia or intracerebral hemorrhage. Finally, they have a modulatory role in the immune system by regulating the inflammatory response.

Most of the work in the past decades has been focused on the definition of the mechanisms underlying the Hp- and Hx-mediated protection against heme toxicity. Nevertheless, recently, Schaer and co-authors investigated the potential of Hp supplementation as a strategy to counteract the intrinsic hypertensive and oxidative toxicities of free hemoglobin and demonstrated that the induction of Hp synthesis in dogs by glucocorticoid treatment prevented free hemoglobin-mediated hypertension. In a similar way, the co-infusion of exogenous Hp and hemoglobin in guinea pig prevents hemoglobin peroxidative activity and oxidative tissue damage (Boretti et al., 2009).

Thus, it is time to speculate that therapeutics that could increase Hp and/or Hx levels or act as Hp/Hx agonists might help to limit heme toxic effects in pathologic conditions associated to massive hemolysis as hemolytic anemia, sickle cell disease, ischemia-reperfusion injury.

8. Acknowledgment

We wish to thank people that in the past years worked with us and contributed to our knowledge in the field, Sharmila Fagoonee, Samuele Marro and Noemi Morello, and Fiorella Altruda for helpful discussion.

9. References

Adams, E.C., and Weiss, M.R. (1969). Calorimetric studies of the haemoglobin-haptoglobin reaction. The Biochemical journal 115, 441-447.

Ahn, H., Li, C.S., and Wang, W. (2005). Sickle cell hepatopathy: clinical presentation, treatment, and outcome in pediatric and adult patients. Pediatric blood & cancer 45, 184-190.

Alam, J., and Smith, A. (1989). Receptor-mediated transport of heme by hemopexin regulates gene expression in mammalian cells. J Biol Chem 264, 17637-17640.

Alam, J., and Smith, A. (1992). Heme-hemopexin-mediated induction of metallothionein gene expression. J Biol Chem 267, 16379-16384.

Arguelles, S., Venero, J.L., Garcia-Rodriguez, S., Tomas-Camardiel, M., Ayala, A., Cano, J., and Machado, A. Use of haptoglobin and transthyretin as potential biomarkers for the preclinical diagnosis of Parkinson's disease. Neurochem Int 57, 227-234.

Arosio, P., and Levi, S. (2002). Ferritin, iron homeostasis, and oxidative damage. Free radical biology & medicine 33, 457-463.

Arredouani, M.S., Kasran, A., Vanoirbeek, J.A., Berger, F.G., Baumann, H., and Ceuppens, J.L. (2005). Haptoglobin dampens endotoxin-induced inflammatory effects both in vitro and in vivo. Immunology 114, 263-271.

Ascenzi, P., Bocedi, A., Visca, P., Altruda, F., Tolosano, E., Beringhelli, T., and Fasano, M. (2005). Hemoglobin and heme scavenging. IUBMB life 57, 749-759.

Aydinli, M., and Bayraktar, Y. (2007). Budd-Chiari syndrome: etiology, pathogenesis and diagnosis. World J Gastroenterol 13, 2693-2696.

Balla, J., Balla, G., Jeney, V., Kakuk, G., Jacob, H.S., and Vercellotti, G.M. (2000). Ferriporphyrins and endothelium: a 2-edged sword-promotion of oxidation and induction of cytoprotectants. Blood 95, 3442-3450.

Balla, J., Vercellotti, G.M., Jeney, V., Yachie, A., Varga, Z., Eaton, J.W., and Balla, G. (2005). Heme, heme oxygenase and ferritin in vascular endothelial cell injury. Molecular nutrition & food research 49, 1030-1043.

Bayraktar, U.D., Seren, S., and Bayraktar, Y. (2007). Hepatic venous outflow obstruction: three similar syndromes. World J Gastroenterol 13, 1912-1927.

Belcher, J.D., Bryant, C.J., Nguyen, J., Bowlin, P.R., Kielbik, M.C., Bischof, J.C., Hebbel, R.P., and Vercellotti, G.M. (2003). Transgenic sickle mice have vascular inflammation. Blood 101, 3953-3959.

Berg, D., and Youdim, M.B. (2006). Role of iron in neurodegenerative disorders. Top Magn Reson Imaging 17, 5-17.

Bode, W. (1995). A helping hand for collagenases: the haemopexin-like domain. Structure 3, 527-530.

Boretti, F.S., Buehler, P.W., D'Agnillo, F., Kluge, K., Glaus, T., Butt, O.I., Jia, Y., Goede, J., Pereira, C.P., Maggiorini, M., et al. (2009). Sequestration of extracellular hemoglobin within a haptoglobin complex decreases its hypertensive and oxidative effects in dogs and guinea pigs. The Journal of clinical investigation 119, 2271-2280.

Boucher, P., Gotthardt, M., Li, W.P., Anderson, R.G., and Herz, J. (2003). LRP: role in vascular wall integrity and protection from atherosclerosis. Science (New York, NY 300, 329-332.

Chen, L., Zhang, X., Chen-Roetling, J., and Regan, R.F. Increased striatal injury and behavioral deficits after intracerebral hemorrhage in hemopexin knockout mice. J Neurosurg.

Chen, W., Lu, H., Dutt, K., Smith, A., Hunt, D.M., and Hunt, R.C. (1998). Expression of the protective proteins hemopexin and haptoglobin by cells of the neural retina. Experimental eye research 67, 83-93.

Christensen, E.I., and Birn, H. (2001). Megalin and cubilin: synergistic endocytic receptors in renal proximal tubule. Am J Physiol Renal Physiol 280, F562-573.

Connor, J.R., and Menzies, S.L. (1996). Relationship of iron to oligodendrocytes and myelination. Glia 17, 83-93.

Dampier, C., Setty, B.N., Eggleston, B., Brodecki, D., O'Neal, P., and Stuart, M. (2004). Vaso-occlusion in children with sickle cell disease: clinical characteristics and biologic correlates. J Pediatr Hematol Oncol 26, 785-790.

Davies, D.M., Smith, A., Muller-Eberhard, U., and Morgan, W.T. (1979). Hepatic subcellular metabolism of heme from heme-hemopexin: incorporation of iron into ferritin. Biochem Biophys Res Commun 91, 1504-1511.

Delanghe, J.R., and Langlois, M.R. (2002). Haptoglobin polymorphism and body iron stores. Clin Chem Lab Med 40, 212-216.

El Ghmati, S.M., Van Hoeyveld, E.M., Van Strijp, J.G., Ceuppens, J.L., and Stevens, E.A. (1996). Identification of haptoglobin as an alternative ligand for CD11b/CD18. J Immunol 156, 2542-2552.

Eskew, J.D., Vanacore, R.M., Sung, L., Morales, P.J., and Smith, A. (1999). Cellular protection mechanisms against extracellular heme. heme-hemopexin, but not free heme, activates the N-terminal c-jun kinase. J Biol Chem 274, 638-648.

Fagoonee, S., Caorsi, C., Giovarelli, M., Stoltenberg, M., Silengo, L., Altruda, F., Camussi, G., Tolosano, E., and Bussolati, B. (2008). Lack of plasma protein hemopexin dampens mercury-induced autoimmune response in mice. J Immunol 181, 1937-1947.

Fagoonee, S., Gburek, J., Hirsch, E., Marro, S., Moestrup, S.K., Laurberg, J.M., Christensen, E.I., Silengo, L., Altruda, F., and Tolosano, E. (2005). Plasma protein haptoglobin modulates renal iron loading. The American journal of pathology 166, 973-983.

Farombi, E.O., and Surh, Y.J. (2006). Heme oxygenase-1 as a potential therapeutic target for hepatoprotection. J Biochem Mol Biol 39, 479-491.

Ferreira, A., Balla, J., Jeney, V., Balla, G., and Soares, M.P. (2008). A central role for free heme in the pathogenesis of severe malaria: the missing link? J Mol Med 86, 1097-1111.

Ferris, C.D., Jaffrey, S.R., Sawa, A., Takahashi, M., Brady, S.D., Barrow, R.K., Tysoe, S.A., Wolosker, H., Baranano, D.E., Dore, S., et al. (1999). Haem oxygenase-1 prevents cell death by regulating cellular iron. Nature cell biology 1, 152-157.

Galicia, G., Maes, W., Verbinnen, B., Kasran, A., Bullens, D., Arredouani, M., and Ceuppens, J.L. (2009). Haptoglobin deficiency facilitates the development of autoimmune inflammation. Eur J Immunol 39, 3404-3412.

Gardiner, M.E., and Morgan, E.H. (1974). Transferrin and iron uptake by the liver in the rat. The Australian journal of experimental biology and medical science 52, 723-736.

Gauldie, J., Richards, C., Harnish, D., Lansdorp, P., and Baumann, H. (1987). Interferon beta 2/B-cell stimulatory factor type 2 shares identity with monocyte-derived hepatocyte-stimulating factor and regulates the major acute phase protein response in liver cells. Proceedings of the National Academy of Sciences of the United States of America 84, 7251-7255.

Gburek, J., Verroust, P.J., Willnow, T.E., Fyfe, J.C., Nowacki, W., Jacobsen, C., Moestrup, S.K., and Christensen, E.I. (2002). Megalin and cubilin are endocytic receptors involved in renal clearance of hemoglobin. J Am Soc Nephrol 13, 423-430.

Grinberg, L.N., O'Brien, P.J., and Hrkal, Z. (1999). The effects of heme-binding proteins on the peroxidative and catalatic activities of hemin. Free radical biology & medicine 27, 214-219.

Grinshtein, N., Bamm, V.V., Tsemakhovich, V.A., and Shaklai, N. (2003). Mechanism of low-density lipoprotein oxidation by hemoglobin-derived iron. Biochemistry 42, 6977-6985.

Gutteridge, J.M., and Smith, A. (1988). Antioxidant protection by haemopexin of haem-stimulated lipid peroxidation. The Biochemical journal 256, 861-865.

Hentze, M.W., Muckenthaler, M.U., and Andrews, N.C. (2004). Balancing acts; molecular control of Mammalian iron metabolism. Cell 117, 285-297.

Higa, Y., Oshiro, S., Kino, K., Tsunoo, H., and Nakajima, H. (1981). Catabolism of globin-haptoglobin in liver cells after intravenous administration of hemoglobin-haptoglobin to rats. J Biol Chem 256, 12322-12328.

Hillmen, P., Lewis, S.M., Bessler, M., Luzzatto, L., and Dacie, J.V. (1995). Natural history of paroxysmal nocturnal hemoglobinuria. The New England journal of medicine 333, 1253-1258.

Huntoon, K.M., Wang, Y., Eppolito, C.A., Barbour, K.W., Berger, F.G., Shrikant, P.A., and Baumann, H. (2008). The acute phase protein haptoglobin regulates host immunity. J Leukoc Biol 84, 170-181.

Hvidberg, V., Maniecki, M.B., Jacobsen, C., Hojrup, P., Moller, H.J., and Moestrup, S.K. (2005). Identification of the receptor scavenging hemopexin-heme complexes. Blood 106, 2572-2579.

Immenschuh, S., Song, D.X., Satoh, H., and Muller-Eberhard, U. (1995). The type II hemopexin interleukin-6 response element predominates the transcriptional regulation of the hemopexin acute phase responsiveness. Biochem Biophys Res Commun 207, 202-208.

Jeney, V., Balla, J., Yachie, A., Varga, Z., Vercellotti, G.M., Eaton, J.W., and Balla, G. (2002). Pro-oxidant and cytotoxic effects of circulating heme. Blood 100, 879-887.

Kapturczak, M.H., Wasserfall, C., Brusko, T., Campbell-Thompson, M., Ellis, T.M., Atkinson, M.A., and Agarwal, A. (2004). Heme oxygenase-1 modulates early inflammatory responses: evidence from the heme oxygenase-1-deficient mouse. The American journal of pathology 165, 1045-1053.

Kino, K., Tsunoo, H., Higa, Y., Takami, M., and Nakajima, H. (1982). Kinetic aspects of hemoglobin.haptoglobin-receptor interaction in rat liver plasma membranes, isolated liver cells, and liver cells in primary culture. J Biol Chem 257, 4828-4833.

Koizumi, S. (2007). Human heme oxygenase-1 deficiency: a lesson on serendipity in the discovery of the novel disease. Pediatr Int 49, 125-132.

Kovtunovych, G., Eckhaus, M.A., Ghosh, M.C., Ollivierre-Wilson, H., and Rouault, T.A. (2010) Dysfunction of the heme recycling system in heme oxygenase 1-deficient mice: effects on macrophage viability and tissue iron distribution. Blood 116, 6054-6062.

Kristiansen, M., Graversen, J.H., Jacobsen, C., Sonne, O., Hoffman, H.J., Law, S.K., and Moestrup, S.K. (2001). Identification of the haemoglobin scavenger receptor. Nature 409, 198-201.

Kumar, S., and Bandyopadhyay, U. (2005). Free heme toxicity and its detoxification systems in human. Toxicology letters 157, 175-188.

Kushner, I. (1982). The phenomenon of the acute phase response. Ann N Y Acad Sci 389, 39-48.

LaBadie, J.H., Chapman, K.P., and Aronson, N.N., Jr. (1975). Glycoprotein catabolism in rat liver: Lysosomal digestion of iodinated asialo-fetuin. The Biochemical journal 152, 271-279.

Langlois, M.R., Martin, M.E., Boelaert, J.R., Beaumont, C., Taes, Y.E., De Buyzere, M.L., Bernard, D.R., Neels, H.M., and Delanghe, J.R. (2000). The haptoglobin 2-2 phenotype affects serum markers of iron status in healthy males. Clin Chem 46, 1619-1625.

Law, M.L., Cai, G.Y., Hartz, J.A., Jones, C., and Kao, F.T. (1988). The hemopexin gene maps to the same location as the beta-globin gene cluster on human chromosome 11. Genomics 3, 48-52.

Lee, M.Y., Kim, S.Y., Choi, J.S., Lee, I.H., Choi, Y.S., Jin, J.Y., Park, S.J., Sung, K.W., Chun, M.H., and Kim, I.S. (2002). Upregulation of haptoglobin in reactive astrocytes after transient forebrain ischemia in rats. J Cereb Blood Flow Metab 22, 1176-1180.

Li, R.C., Saleem, S., Zhen, G., Cao, W., Zhuang, H., Lee, J., Smith, A., Altruda, F., Tolosano, E., and Dore, S. (2009). Heme-hemopexin complex attenuates neuronal cell death and stroke damage. J Cereb Blood Flow Metab 29, 953-964.

Liang, X., Lin, T., Sun, G., Beasley-Topliffe, L., Cavaillon, J.M., and Warren, H.S. (2009). Hemopexin down-regulates LPS-induced proinflammatory cytokines from macrophages. J Leukoc Biol 86, 229-235.

Lillis, A.P., Mikhailenko, I., and Strickland, D.K. (2005). Beyond endocytosis: LRP function in cell migration, proliferation and vascular permeability. J Thromb Haemost 3, 1884-1893.

Lim, S.K., Kim, H., bin Ali, A., Lim, Y.K., Wang, Y., Chong, S.M., Costantini, F., and Baumman, H. (1998). Increased susceptibility in Hp knockout mice during acute hemolysis. Blood 92, 1870-1877.

Lindenblatt, N., Bordel, R., Schareck, W., Menger, M.D., and Vollmar, B. (2004). Vascular heme oxygenase-1 induction suppresses microvascular thrombus formation in vivo. Arterioscler Thromb Vasc Biol 24, 601-606.

Marinkovic, S., and Baumann, H. (1990). Structure, hormonal regulation, and identification of the interleukin-6- and dexamethasone-responsive element of the rat haptoglobin gene. Mol Cell Biol 10, 1573-1583.

Marro, S., Barisani, D., Chiabrando, D., Fagoonee, S., Muckenthaler, M.U., Stolte, J., Meneveri, R., Haile, D., Silengo, L., Altruda, F., et al. (2007). Lack of haptoglobin affects iron transport across duodenum by modulating ferroportin expression. Gastroenterology 133, 1261-1271.

Marro, S., Chiabrando, D., Messana, E., Stolte, J., Turco, E., Tolosano, E., and Muckenthaler, M.U. (2010). Heme controls ferroportin1 (FPN1) transcription involving Bach1, Nrf2 and a MARE/ARE sequence motif at position -7007 of the FPN1 promoter. Haematologica 95, 1261-1268.

Mehta, D., and Malik, A.B. (2006). Signaling mechanisms regulating endothelial permeability. Physiological reviews 86, 279-367.

Miller, Y.I., Smith, A., Morgan, W.T., and Shaklai, N. (1996). Role of hemopexin in protection of low-density lipoprotein against hemoglobin-induced oxidation. Biochemistry 35, 13112-13117.

Morello, N., Tonoli, E., Logrand, F., Fiorito, V., Fagoonee, S., Turco, E., Silengo, L., Vercelli, A., Altruda, F., and Tolosano, E. (2008). Hemopexin affects iron distribution and ferritin expression in mouse brain. Journal of cellular and molecular medicine.

Morris, C.M., Candy, J.M., Edwardson, J.A., Bloxham, C.A., and Smith, A. (1993). Evidence for the localization of haemopexin immunoreactivity in neurones in the human brain. Neuroscience letters 149, 141-144.

Muller-Eberhard, U., Javid, J., Liem, H.H., Hanstein, A., and Hanna, M. (1968). Plasma concentrations of hemopexin, haptoglobin and heme in patients with various hemolytic diseases. Blood 32, 811-815.

Narisada, M., Kawamoto, S., Kuwamoto, K., Moriwaki, K., Nakagawa, T., Matsumoto, H., Asahi, M., Koyama, N., and Miyoshi, E. (2008). Identification of an inducible factor secreted by pancreatic cancer cell lines that stimulates the production of fucosylated haptoglobin in hepatoma cells. Biochem Biophys Res Commun 377, 792-796.

Ndisang, J.F., Zhao, W., and Wang, R. (2002). Selective regulation of blood pressure by heme oxygenase-1 in hypertension. Hypertension 40, 315-321.

Nielsen, M.J., and Moestrup, S.K. (2009). Receptor targeting of hemoglobin mediated by the haptoglobins: roles beyond heme scavenging. Blood 114, 764-771.

Nikkila, H., Gitlin, J.D., and Muller-Eberhard, U. (1991). Rat hemopexin. Molecular cloning, primary structural characterization, and analysis of gene expression. Biochemistry 30, 823-829.

Ogita, H., and Liao, J. (2004). Endothelial function and oxidative stress. Endothelium 11, 123-132.

Oliviero, S., and Cortese, R. (1989). The human haptoglobin gene promoter: interleukin-6-responsive elements interact with a DNA-binding protein induced by interleukin-6. The EMBO journal 8, 1145-1151.

Oliviero, S., Morrone, G., and Cortese, R. (1987). The human haptoglobin gene: transcriptional regulation during development and acute phase induction. The EMBO journal 6, 1905-1912.

Pamplona, A., Ferreira, A., Balla, J., Jeney, V., Balla, G., Epiphanio, S., Chora, A., Rodrigues, C.D., Gregoire, I.P., Cunha-Rodrigues, M., et al. (2007). Heme oxygenase-1 and carbon monoxide suppress the pathogenesis of experimental cerebral malaria. Nature medicine 13, 703-710.

Pamplona, A., Hanscheid, T., Epiphanio, S., Mota, M.M., and Vigario, A.M. (2009). Cerebral malaria and the hemolysis/methemoglobin/heme hypothesis: shedding new light on an old disease. Int J Biochem Cell Biol 41, 711-716.

Papanikolaou, G., and Pantopoulos, K. (2005). Iron metabolism and toxicity. Toxicol Appl Pharmacol 202, 199-211.

Poli, V., Altruda, F., and Silengo, L. (1986). Differential transcriptional pattern of the hemopexin gene. Ital J Biochem 35, 355-360.

Poli, V., Silengo, L., Altruda, F., and Cortese, R. (1989). The analysis of the human hemopexin promoter defines a new class of liver-specific genes. Nucleic Acids Res 17, 9351-9365.

Potter, D., Chroneos, Z.C., Baynes, J.W., Sinclair, P.R., Gorman, N., Liem, H.H., Muller-Eberhard, U., and Thorpe, S.R. (1993). In vivo fate of hemopexin and heme-hemopexin complexes in the rat. Archives of biochemistry and biophysics 300, 98-104.

Poznanovic, G., Vidakovic, M., Ivanovic-Matic, S., and Grujic, V. (1999). Identification of nuclear matrix and associated proteins that bind the haptoglobin gene cis-element. IUBMB life 48, 277-282.

Ren, Y., and Smith, A. (1995). Mechanism of metallothionein gene regulation by heme-hemopexin. Roles of protein kinase C, reactive oxygen species, and cis-acting elements. J Biol Chem 270, 23988-23995.

Roher, A.E., Maarouf, C.L., Sue, L.I., Hu, Y., Wilson, J., and Beach, T.G. (2009). Proteomics-derived cerebrospinal fluid markers of autopsy-confirmed Alzheimer's disease. Biomarkers 14, 493-501.

Rossbacher, J., Wagner, L., and Pasternack, M.S. (1999). Inhibitory effect of haptoglobin on granulocyte chemotaxis, phagocytosis and bactericidal activity. Scand J Immunol 50, 399-404.

Seixas, E., Gozzelino, R., Chora, A., Ferreira, A., Silva, G., Larsen, R., Rebelo, S., Penido, C., Smith, N.R., Coutinho, A., et al. (2009). Heme oxygenase-1 affords protection against noncerebral forms of severe malaria. Proceedings of the National Academy of Sciences of the United States of America 106, 15837-15842.

Senzolo, M., Germani, G., Cholongitas, E., Burra, P., and Burroughs, A.K. (2007). Veno occlusive disease: update on clinical management. World J Gastroenterol 13, 3918-3924.

Ship, N.J., Toprak, A., Lai, R.P., Tseng, E., Kluger, R., and Pang, K.S. (2005). Binding of acellular, native and cross-linked human hemoglobins to haptoglobin: enhanced distribution and clearance in the rat. Am J Physiol Gastrointest Liver Physiol 288, G1301-1309.

Smith, A., and Ledford, B.E. (1988). Expression of the haemopexin-transport system in cultured mouse hepatoma cells. Links between haemopexin and iron metabolism. The Biochemical journal 256, 941-950.

Smith, A., and Morgan, W.T. (1978). Transport of heme by hemopexin to the liver: evidence for receptor-mediated uptake. Biochem Biophys Res Commun 84, 151-157.

Smith, A., and Morgan, W.T. (1979). Haem transport to the liver by haemopexin. Receptor-mediated uptake with recycling of the protein. The Biochemical journal 182, 47-54.

Smith, A., and Morgan, W.T. (1981). Hemopexin-mediated transport of heme into isolated rat hepatocytes. J Biol Chem 256, 10902-10909.

Smith, A., and Morgan, W.T. (1984). Hemopexin-mediated heme uptake by liver. Characterization of the interaction of heme-hemopexin with isolated rabbit liver plasma membranes. J Biol Chem 259, 12049-12053.

Smith, A., Rish, K.R., Lovelace, R., Hackney, J.F., and Helston, R.M. (2008). Role for copper in the cellular and regulatory effects of heme-hemopexin. Biometals.

Spiller, F., Costa, C., Souto, F.O., Vinchi, F., Mestriner, F.L., Laure, H.J., Alves-Filho, J.C., Freitas, A., Rosa, J.C., Ferreira, S.H., et al. (2011). Inhibition of Neutrophil Migration by Hemopexin Leads to Increased Mortality Due to Sepsis in Mice. Am J Respir Crit Care Med, 183(7): 922-931.

Stocker, R., and Keaney, J.F., Jr. (2004). Role of oxidative modifications in atherosclerosis. Physiological reviews 84, 1381-1478.

Stuart, M.J., and Nagel, R.L. (2004). Sickle-cell disease. Lancet 364, 1343-1360.

Takahashi, N., Takahashi, Y., and Putnam, F.W. (1984). Structure of human hemopexin: O-glycosyl and N-glycosyl sites and unusual clustering of tryptophan residues. Proceedings of the National Academy of Sciences of the United States of America 81, 2021-2025.

Taketani, S., Kohno, H., Sawamura, T., and Tokunaga, R. (1990). Hemopexin-dependent down-regulation of expression of the human transferrin receptor. J Biol Chem 265, 13981-13985.

Tam, S.C., and Wong, J.T. (1988). Impairment of renal function by stroma-free hemoglobin in rats. The Journal of laboratory and clinical medicine 111, 189-193.

Timmins, G.S., Davies, M.J., and Muller-Eberhard, U. (1995). A study of the effects of complexation of heme by hemopexin upon its reactions with organic peroxides. Biochemical Society transactions 23, 244S.

Tolosano, E., and Altruda, F. (2002). Hemopexin: structure, function, and regulation. DNA and cell biology 21, 297-306.

Tolosano, E., Cutufia, M.A., Hirsch, E., Silengo, L., and Altruda, F. (1996). Specific expression in brain and liver driven by the hemopexin promoter in transgenic mice. Biochem Biophys Res Commun 218, 694-703.

Tolosano, E., Fagoonee, S., Garuti, C., Valli, L., Andrews, N.C., Altruda, F., and Pietrangelo, A. (2005). Haptoglobin modifies the hemochromatosis phenotype in mice. Blood 105, 3353-3355.

Tolosano, E., Fagoonee, S., Hirsch, E., Berger, F.G., Baumann, H., Silengo, L., and Altruda, F. (2002). Enhanced splenomegaly and severe liver inflammation in haptoglobin/hemopexin double-null mice after acute hemolysis. Blood 100, 4201-4208.

Tolosano, E., Fagoonee, S., Morello, N., Vinchi, F., and Fiorito, V. (2010). Heme scavenging and the other facets of hemopexin. Antioxid Redox Signal 12, 305-320.

Tolosano, E., Hirsch, E., Patrucco, E., Camaschella, C., Navone, R., Silengo, L., and Altruda, F. (1999). Defective recovery and severe renal damage after acute hemolysis in hemopexin-deficient mice. Blood 94, 3906-3914.

Tsiftsoglou, A.S., Tsamadou, A.I., and Papadopoulou, L.C. (2006). Heme as key regulator of major mammalian cellular functions: molecular, cellular, and pharmacological aspects. Pharmacol Ther 111, 327-345.

Van Vlierberghe, H., Langlois, M., and Delanghe, J. (2004). Haptoglobin polymorphisms and iron homeostasis in health and in disease. Clin Chim Acta 345, 35-42.

Van Vlierberghe, H., Langlois, M., Delanghe, J., Horsmans, Y., Michielsen, P., Henrion, J., Cartuyvels, R., Billiet, J., De Vos, M., and Leroux-Roels, G. (2001). Haptoglobin phenotype 2-2 overrepresentation in Cys282Tyr hemochromatotic patients. J Hepatol 3511, 707-711.

Vincent, S.H., Grady, R.W., Shaklai, N., Snider, J.M., and Muller-Eberhard, U. (1988). The influence of heme-binding proteins in heme-catalyzed oxidations. Archives of biochemistry and biophysics 265, 539-550.

Vinchi, F., Gastaldi, S., Silengo, L., Altruda, F., and Tolosano, E. (2008). Hemopexin prevents endothelial damage and liver congestion in a mouse model of heme overload. The American journal of pathology 173, 289-299.

Wagener, F.A., Abraham, N.G., van Kooyk, Y., de Witte, T., and Figdor, C.G. (2001a). Heme-induced cell adhesion in the pathogenesis of sickle-cell disease and inflammation. Trends in pharmacological sciences 22, 52-54.

Wagener, F.A., Eggert, A., Boerman, O.C., Oyen, W.J., Verhofstad, A., Abraham, N.G., Adema, G., van Kooyk, Y., de Witte, T., and Figdor, C.G. (2001b). Heme is a potent inducer of inflammation in mice and is counteracted by heme oxygenase. Blood 98, 1802-1811.

Wagener, F.A., van Beurden, H.E., von den Hoff, J.W., Adema, G.J., and Figdor, C.G. (2003a). The heme-heme oxygenase system: a molecular switch in wound healing. Blood 102, 521-528.

Wagener, F.A., Volk, H.D., Willis, D., Abraham, N.G., Soares, M.P., Adema, G.J., and Figdor, C.G. (2003b). Different faces of the heme-heme oxygenase system in inflammation. Pharmacological reviews 55, 551-571.

Weinstein, M.B., and Segal, H.L. (1984). Uptake of free hemoglobin by rat liver parenchymal cells. Biochem Biophys Res Commun 123, 489-496.

Xie, Y., Li, Y., Zhang, Q., Stiller, M.J., Wang, C.L., and Streilein, J.W. (2000). Haptoglobin is a natural regulator of Langerhans cell function in the skin. J Dermatol Sci 24, 25-37.

Yachie, A., Niida, Y., Wada, T., Igarashi, N., Kaneda, H., Toma, T., Ohta, K., Kasahara, Y., and Koizumi, S. (1999). Oxidative stress causes enhanced endothelial cell injury in human heme oxygenase-1 deficiency. The Journal of clinical investigation 103, 129-135.

Yang, Y.R., Liu, S.L., Qin, Z.Y., Liu, F.J., Qin, Y.J., Bai, S.M., and Chen, Z.Y. (2008). Comparative proteomics analysis of cerebrospinal fluid of patients with Guillain-Barre syndrome. Cell Mol Neurobiol 28, 737-744.

Zecca, L., Youdim, M.B., Riederer, P., Connor, J.R., and Crichton, R.R. (2004). Iron, brain ageing and neurodegenerative disorders. Nature reviews 5, 863-873.

Zhao, X., Song, S., Sun, G., Strong, R., Zhang, J., Grotta, J.C., and Aronowski, J. (2009). Neuroprotective role of haptoglobin after intracerebral hemorrhage. J Neurosci 29, 15819-15827.

13

Haptoglobin is an Exercise-Responsive Acute-Phase Protein

Cheng-Yu Chen[1,2], Wan-Ling Hsieh[3], Po-Ju Lin[3], Yung-Liang Chen[4] and Simon J. T. Mao[3]
[1]*Institute of Clinical Medicine, National Yang-Ming University, Taipei,*
[2]*Department of Medical Research and Education, National Yang-Ming University Hospital, Ilan,*
[3]*Research Institute of Biochemical Engineering, Department of Biological Science and Technology, National Chiao Tung University, Hsinchu,*
[4]*Department of Medical Laboratory Science and Biotechnology, Yuanpei University, Hsinchu, Taiwan*

1. Introduction

The nomenclature of haptoglobin (Hp) was from the character of conjugation [hapto] with hemoglobin [globin] of red blood cells. Human Hp is one of the largest proteins in the plasma originally synthesized as a single polypeptide and has been thought to be derived primarily in liver, adipose tissue, brain, lung, and kidney (Peters & Alper, 1966). Following post-translational protease cleavage of Hp, α- and β-chains are formed and then linked by disulfide bridges to generate the matured Hp form (Kurosky et al., 1980). Human Hp gene located in chromosome 16q22.1 is characterized by two common alleles *Hp 1* and *Hp 2* respectively corresponding to α1-β and α2-β chain, and resulting in three main phenotypes: Hp 1-1, 2-1 and 2-2. All the phenotypes share the same β-chain containing 245 amino-acid residues. As shown in Figure 1A, the α1-chain contains 83 amino-acid residues possessing two "free" –SH groups. The one at the –COOH-terminus always cross-linked with a β-chain to form a basic α-β unit, and the other at the NH_2-terminus linked with another $(\alpha\text{-}\beta)_1$ resulting in a Hp dimer $(\alpha1\text{-}\beta)_2$ or a Hp 1-1 molecule. In contrast, the α2-chain containing a tandem-repeat of residues 12-70 of α1 with 142 amino-acid residues is "trivalent" providing an additional free –SH (Cys-15) that is able to interact with another α-β unit. As such, α2-chains can bind to either α1-β or α2-β units to form large polymers $[(\alpha1\text{-}\beta)_2\text{-}(\alpha2\text{-}\beta)_n$ in Hp2-1 and $(\alpha2\text{-}\beta)_n$ in Hp2-2] as shown in Figure 1B (Wejman et al., 1984).

Hp is a highly conserved acute phase protein (responsive to infection and inflammation) that is present in the plasma of all mammals (Raijmakers et al., 2003, Wang et al., 2001, Yerbury et al., 2005). A recent study has found that Hp also exists in lower vertebrates, bony fish but not in frogs and chickens (Wicher & Fries, 2006). The human *Hp 2* allele has been proposed to be evolved from *Hp 1* about 2 million years ago and then gradually displaced *Hp 1* as a consequence of a non-homologous crossing-over between the structural alleles (*Hp 1*) during meiosis, which is remarkable for being the first example in partial gene duplication of human plasma proteins (Maeda, 1985, Maeda et al., 1984, McEvoy & Maeda,

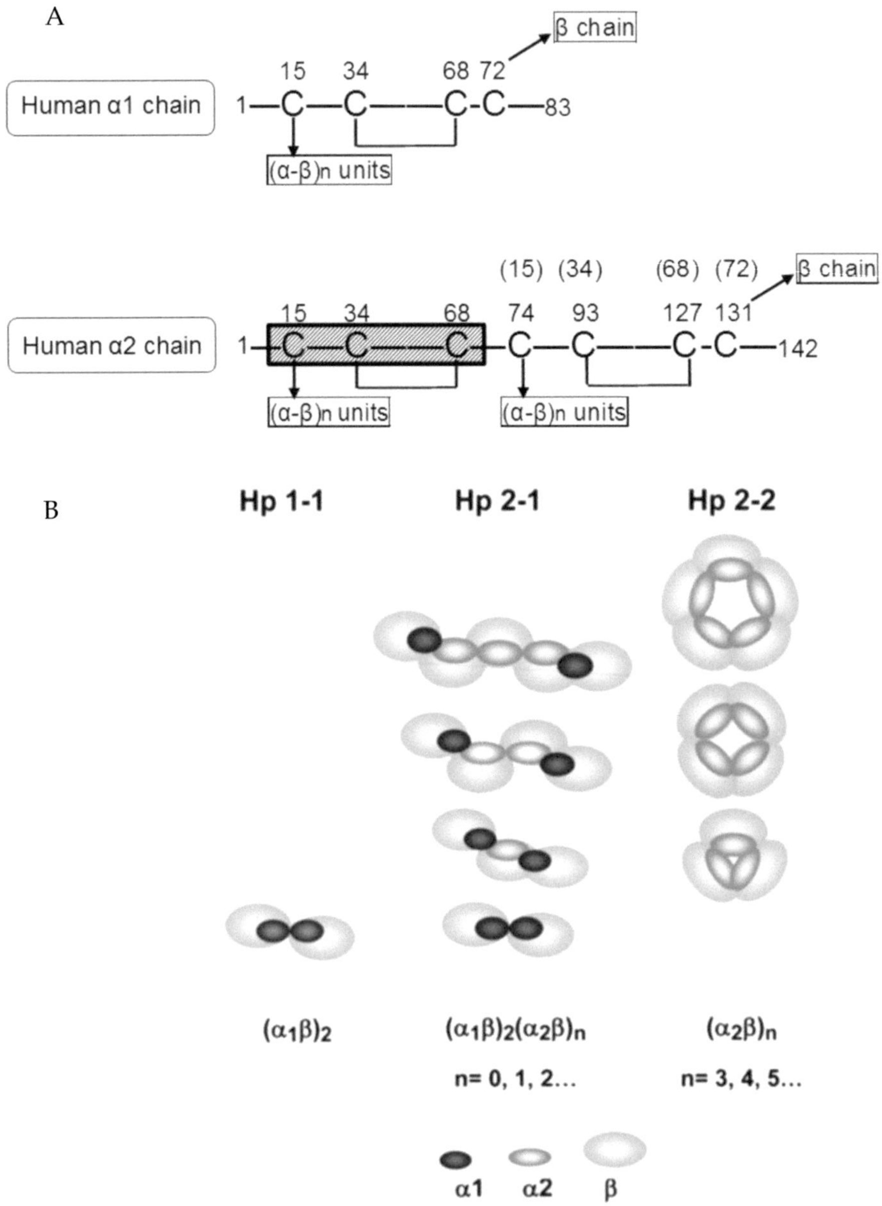

Fig. 1. A schematic model illustrating the structure of human Hp phenotypes. Panel A depicts the backbone of the amino acid sequence for α1-chain with 83 amino-acid residues and for α2-chain with 142 residues containing a 59 amino-acid tandem repeat (residues 12-70) (shown in shaded block). Panel B shows the secondary structures of Hp: Hp 1-1 represents a homodimer, the simplest combination of dimeric α1β chains $(\alpha 1\beta)_2$; Hp 2-2 is heterogeneous in size, starting with cyclic trimeric α2β chains, $(\alpha 2\beta)_3$, and other cyclic polymers; Hp 2-1 is also heterogeneous, but composed of simple homodimer $(\alpha 1\beta)_2$, a linear trimeric αβ chain, $(\alpha 1\beta)_2(\alpha 2\beta)$, and other linear polymers. All types share a common structure of the β chain.

1988). Thus, only humans possess additional Hp 2-1 and 2-2 phenotypes. However, more recently we have found that all the ruminants belong to Hp 2-2 phenotype, which was evolved during at least 20 million years (Lai et al., 2008). In general, individuals with polymeric structure of Hp 2-2 are dramatically more prevalent in certain clinical disorders, such as diabetes and inflammation-related diseases (Hochberg et al., 2002, Langlois & Delanghe, 1996, Levy et al., 2002, Miyoshi et al., 1991). Because Hp 1-1 molecule inhibits the inflammatory cascades more effectively than Hp 2-2, it is commonly assumed that patients with Hp 2-2 phenotype would expose to higher risk for poorer outcomes once suffered from diabetes and inflammation related diseases. Extrahepatic source of Hp has recently been recognized to be present in the body fluids; its regulation could be totally different from the liver -secreted Hp. For example, mononuclear cells secrete Hp when stimulated with all trans-retinoic acid (ATRA) to activate protein kinase C-δ, one of the major signal transductions (Kim et al., 2001). While tumor necrosis factor-α (TNF-α) can induce Hp release in neutrophils during the precursor stage (promyelocyte) at the condition of acute inflammation (Nakagawa-Tosa et al., 1995, Theilgaard-Monch et al., 2006).

The most-noted biological functions of Hp are to capture released hemoglobin (Hb) for accelerating the Hb degredation during an excessive hemolysis and participate in scavenging free radicals during oxidative stress (Bernard et al., 2003, Langlois & Delanghe, 1996). More recently, we have shown that Hp is an extremely potent antioxidant, which directly prevents low-density-lipoprotein (LDL) from Cu2+-induced oxidation. The potency is markedly superior to probucol, one of the most potent therapeutic antioxidants (Lai et al., 2007, Tseng et al., 2004). Transfection of Hp cDNA into Chinese hamster ovary (CHO) cells protects them against oxidative stress (Tseng et al., 2004). This finding can explain, at least in part, that the hypoxia-inducible factor-1α may enhance Hp expression (Oh et al., 2011).

Meanwhile, the concentration measurement of different Hp phenotypes is somewhat difficult hence there are limited reports showing the correlation between the Hp levels and inflammatory-related diseases in human subjects. Using an ELISA with phenotype-matched Hp standards, it becomes possible to accurately measure the Hp 1-1, 2-1, and 2-2 plasma levels and to define the response pattern to several diseases such as in patients with atherosclerosis (Cheng et al., 2007). Furthermore, the reference levels of Hp were significantly different in patients with different phenotypes. Increasing plasma Hp levels up to 2-4 times upon the inflammation or infection are considered to be a sound acute response. A human study of 10 healthy volunteers recently disclosed an elevation of Hp levels in bronchoalveolar lavage fluid (BALF) from the lung stimulated with lipopolysaccharide (LPS). We demonstrated that Hp 1 is a more dominant allele than Hp 2 based on the Hp mRNA expression (Cheng et al., 2007). Thus, subjects with Hp 1-1 and 2-1 have higher baseline levels of plasma Hp and possess stronger antioxidant activity relative to those Hp 2-2 individuals (Tseng et al., 2004).

Some conditions that commonly lead to substantial increase in plasma Hp include infection, trauma, surgery, burns, tissue infarction, various immunologically mediated inflammations, and some advanced malignant tumors. However, reports with respect to the relationship between exercise and Hp levels are rarely limited. Spitler et al. disclosed a significantly lower Hp level and a higher turnover rate of erythrocytes in subjects practicing high frequency fitness as compared to those with low frequency of practice. One reasonable explanation is that exercise induces a chronic hemolytic response (Spitler et al., 1984). It was thought that the stress due to exercise caused intra-vascular hemolysis with the consumption of Hp. This notion is consistent with reported observation that Hp was decreased after a 10-month period of repetitive treadmill program that included 11 male medium-distance runners (Wolf et al., 1987). Nevertheless, there are still controversial debates about the exercise effect on Hp expression. Hp levels remained unchanged in 12 healthy male volunteers undergoing a maximal aerobic capacity (Vo2 max) every week for 3 weeks (Cordova et al., 1992). Further, the transcriptional levels of Hp and proinflammatory cytokine genes after exercise have never been reported. We attempted to explore a possible effect of a single short-term exercise on the plasma levels of Hp in the present study.

2. Changes of human plasma Hp levels after exercise

2.1 One-time explosive running and jogging accompanied with the elevation of human plasma Hp levels

First, we conducted a preliminary study to determine whether a physical endurance jogging or an explosive run may affect the plasma Hp levels. Twelve males (phenotypes Hp 2-1 and 2-2) with age matched were recruited (Hp 1-1 were excluded in this study due to the rare population in our local area, generally < 7%) and examined by performing these exercises. Jogging was performed as a single time for 60 min, while explosive run was to race 100-m also as a single time for about 15 sec. These two types of exercise were conducted among the same individuals with a resting period of 30 days apart. To determine the time-course changes in Hp levels after one-time exercise, the fasting blood samples were collected at days 5, 10 and 25 and Hp was then measured using an appropriated ELISA (Cheng et al. , 2007).

Our preliminary data revealed that Hp is elicited in response to exercise, depending on the type of exercise. It should be noted that the basal levels of Hp were different with respect to the Hp phenotype of the subjects, i.e. low in Hp 2-2 and high in Hp 2-1 subjects similar to a previous report (Cheng et al., 2007). Both Hp 2-1 and 2-2 subjects exhibited a significant Hp elevation in plasma under an explosive exercise (100-m run). Although the overall basal levels of Hp were low in Hp 2-2 subjects, their Hp levels were increased substantially by about 20 fold after explosive running. Interestingly, 60-min jogging seems not to cause marked changes in Hp levels as compared to 100-m racing over the Hp 2-2 subjects (Figure 2). Meanwhile, these exercises did not cause overall loss of body weight or adipose tissue mass (data not shown). It is of interest to note that in general the elevation of Hp responsive to exercise is rather slow being observed after 5 days with one-shot exercise.

Recent studies indicate that acute-phase proteins changes in exercise are associated with low-grade oxidative stress (Petibois & Deleris, 2003). Since Hp is an extremely potent antioxidant (Tseng et al., 2004), we anticipated that elevated Hp expression level may potentially play a protective role reducing the oxidative stress during the exercise. The mechanism involved in such exercise-induced Hp elevation is discussed below.

2.2 High levels of plasma Hp is advantageous in patients with acute respiratory distress syndrome

Acute respiratory distress syndrome (ARDS) is a life-threatening severe inflammatory process in response to pneumocyte damages, including those mediated by free radicals. Because Hp is an anti-inflammatory and antioxidant molecule, it may be relevant in preventing against inflammation in patients with severe oxidative damage. To test whether plasma Hp levels are associated with the outcome in ARDS patients, we evaluated 88 patients with ARDS. Of remarkable interest, we have observed (unpublished data) that plasma Hp levels are greatly increased in patients affected with ARDS. Hp 2-1 patients with high Hp basal levels appear to have a much better prognosis relative to those with Hp 2-2 (Figure 3). Low Hp levels were found to be associated with multiple-organ dysfunction and independently predict 28-day mortality of those patients with ARDS. Hp 2-2 patients have unfavorable ARDS outcomes.

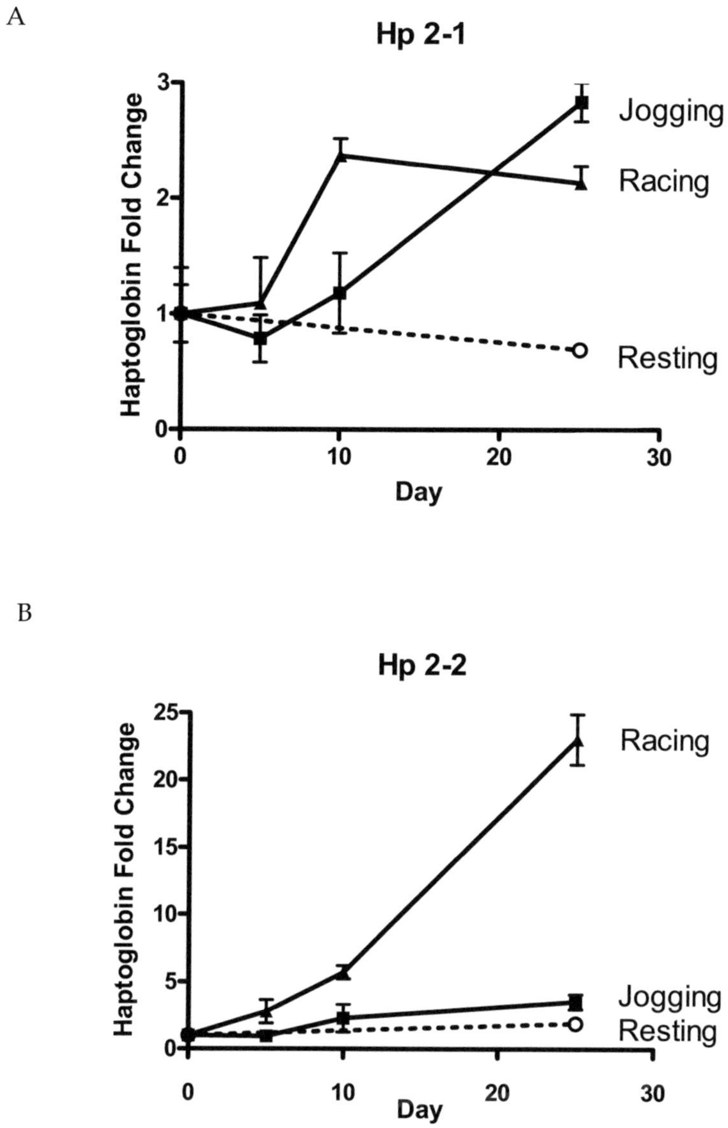

Fig. 2. Changes of plasma Hp levels in fold after one single exercise. Twelve males received a running program with endurance exercises (jogging for 60 min) with a 30-day resting period and followed by an exposing run (100-m for about 15 seconds). In 6 individuals with Hp2-1 (A), the Hp basal levels were relatively higher than those with Hp 2-2. Hp 2-1 levels increased 2.8-fold at day 25 with the mean ± SD from 1.3 ± 0.6 mg/ml for jogging ($p=0.063$). In 6 individuals with Hp 2-2 (B), the Hp basal levels were relatively low, but markedly increased by about 20-fold at day 25 from 0.09 ± 0.13 mg/ml for racing ($p<0.001$).

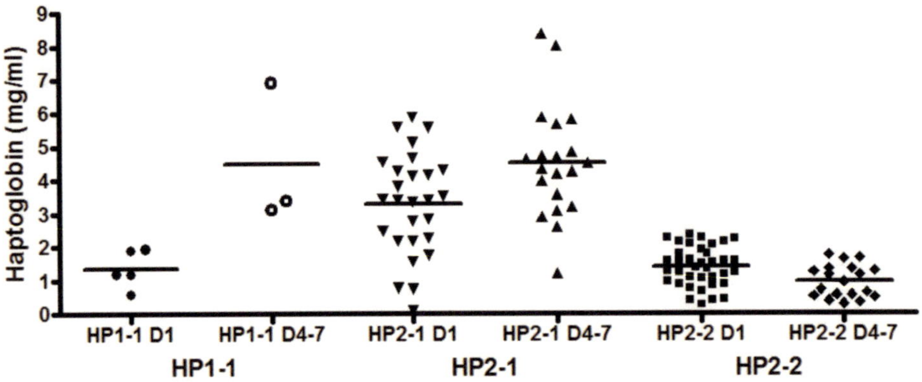

Fig. 3. Hp levels are various in septic patients with different phenotypes. Hp levels in 88 patients with sepsis-related acute respiratory distress syndrome measured on day 1 and days 4-7 are shown. Horizontal bar indicates the mean values. Patients with Hp 1-1 and 2-1 have higher Hp levels at days 4-7 relative to those with Hp 2-2 at the same period.

3. Source of elevated Hp levels in plasma and its underline mechanism involved after exercise

The rationale by which exercise induces the increase in plasma Hp is not clear. Initially, we attempted to address the source of elevated plasma Hp after exercise. By immunocytochemical staining, we show that neutrophils and monocytes in plasma, but not lymphocytes, are the two major cell types to express Hp (Figure 4). We therefore hypothesized peripheral white blood cells being responsible for the increased Hp levels at least in part.

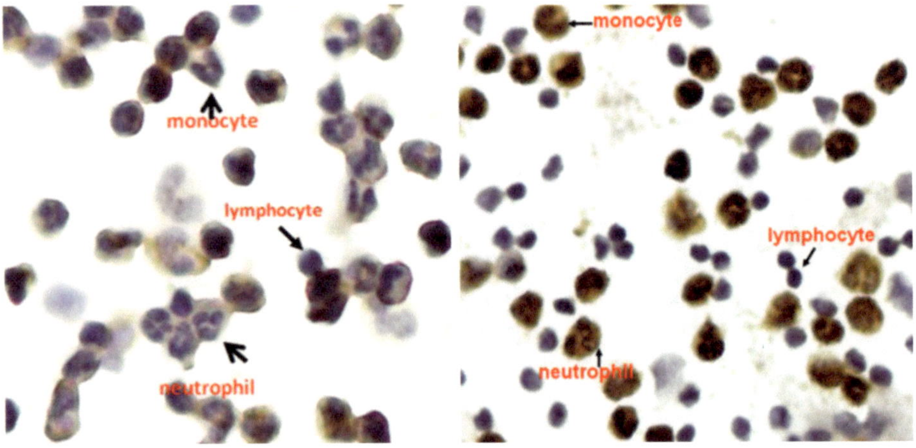

Fig. 4. Immunocytochemical analysis of Hp expression in human leukocytes. A representative staining of 3 healthy human subjects is shown. Left panel (control) displays the cells stained with hematoxylin and normal mouse serum. Right panel displays the cells stained with hematoxylin and a mouse anti-human Hp monoclonal antibody. Intracellular Hp is primarily expressed in mononuclear cells and neutrophils instead of lymphocytes.

3.1 Exercise using mice as an animal model

Since all the animal species belong to Hp 1-1 phenotype except ruminants (Lai et al., 2008), the response of Hp levels following the exercise should be more uniform in animals than that in human subjects as mentioned above. To this end, mice were chosen as an animal model to substantiate the hypothesis mentioned above. First, we tested whether exercise may raise the Hp levels in mice. They were divided as four groups (n=24 in total). The control group (n=6) received no exercise, while the rest of the tested groups (n=6 in each) received a passive exercise with mild horizontal movement at a frequency of 60 times per min for 30 min, twice a day and last for one, two, and three weeks, respectively. All the groups were kept for the same period of time (3 weeks) and simultaneously sacrificed at day 21. For examples, the one-week group started to exercise at day 14 and ended at day 21, while the 3-week group started at day 0 and ended at day 21 as shown in Table 1. The body weight of each respective group (including the control) increased progressively over 21 days, but there was no significant difference between each group during the exercise period.

Days	Exercised Group			
	Week 0	Week 1	Week 2	Week 3
0	31.4 ± 2.4	31.4 ± 0.7	33.3 ± 1.0	31.4 ± 0.8
7	34.9 ± 1.8	33.9 ± 1.4	35.8 ± 1.0	33.0 ± 0.9
14	36.8 ± 2.5	35.6 ± 1.5	37.3 ± 1.0	34.2 ± 1.2
21	37.0 ± 2.8	36.3 ± 1.1	37.8 ± 1.0	36.4 ± 1.0

Shaded area represents the time to start the exercise

Table 1. Body weight of the mice underwent passive exercise. There was no significant difference during the 3-week period when compared between the mouse groups (week 0-3) at the same day.

3.2 Elevation of plasma Hp in mice after exercise

Using the Hp-hemoglobin complex formation method (Yueh et al., 2007), we show plasma Hp levels after exercise being progressively increased over time (Figure 5). At week 3, the levels significantly went up to about 2.67 fold ($p<0.005$). The data are consistent to the denseness measurements using a Western blot analysis (data not shown). By RT-PCR analysis, the Hp mRNA levels in total white blood cells were also significantly elevated at week 3 with about 6 fold (Figure 6) ($p<0.005$). Thus, it suggests that the Hp increase in plasma is contributed from the white blood cells at least in part. Figure 6 also shows that the Hp mRNA levels in response to exercise is rather slow and consistent to that human study (Figure 2).

3.3 Changes in cytokine levels of leukocytes in mice after exercise

Since IL-6 has been reported to be a factor to stimulate the Hp biosynthesis in cultured hepatocytes, we tested whether there was a change in IL-6 of leukocytes following the exercise. Figure 7 shows that both IL-6 and IL-1β mRNA levels were increased in some extent, but not IL-10 and TNF-α, using a RT-PCR analysis. The finding postulates that there might be other factors involved in stimulating the biosynthesis of leukocyte's Hp.

A

B

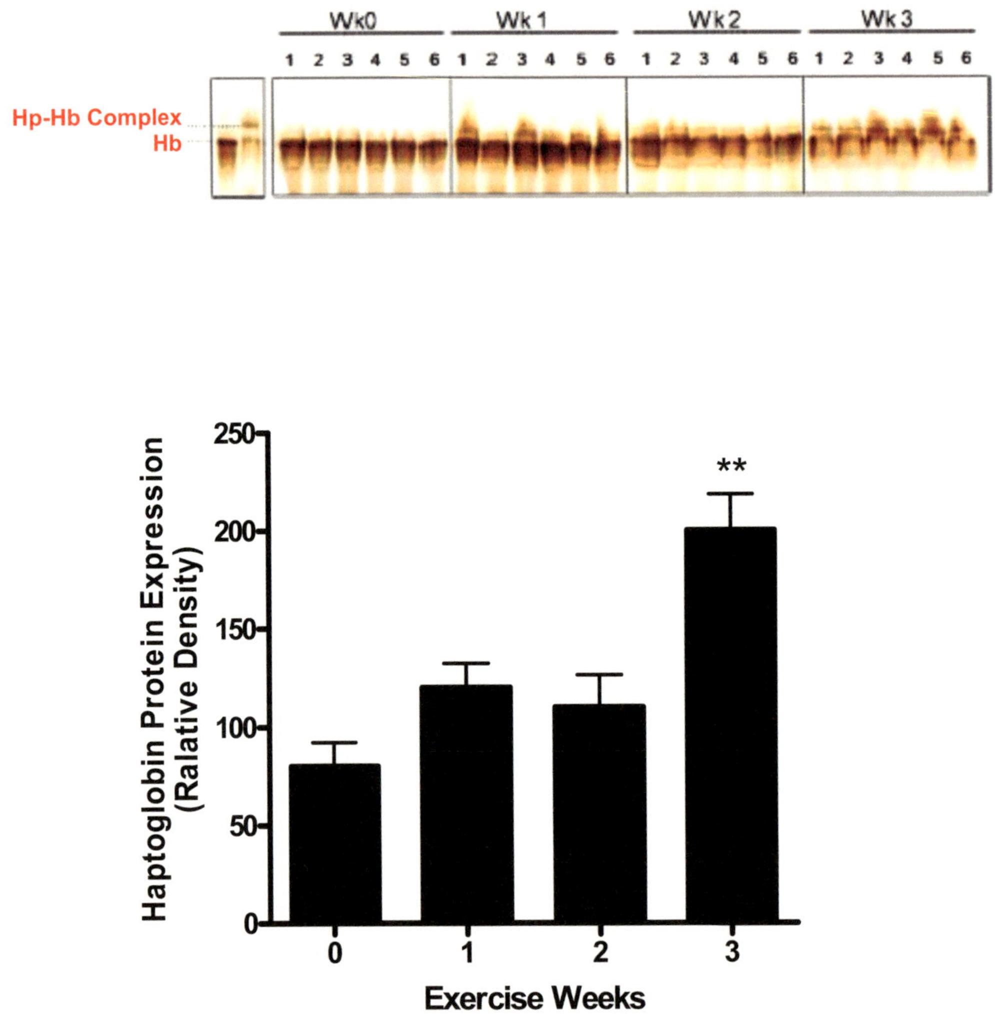

Fig. 5. Hp levels in mice with and without exercise. A: Representative native gel showing complex formation between mouse plasma Hp and added hemoglobin (Hb).
B: Chromogenity of formed Hp-Hb complex determined by a scanning densitometry.
**Hp levels in mice exercised at week 3 reveals a significant elevation relative to week 0 ($P<0.005$).

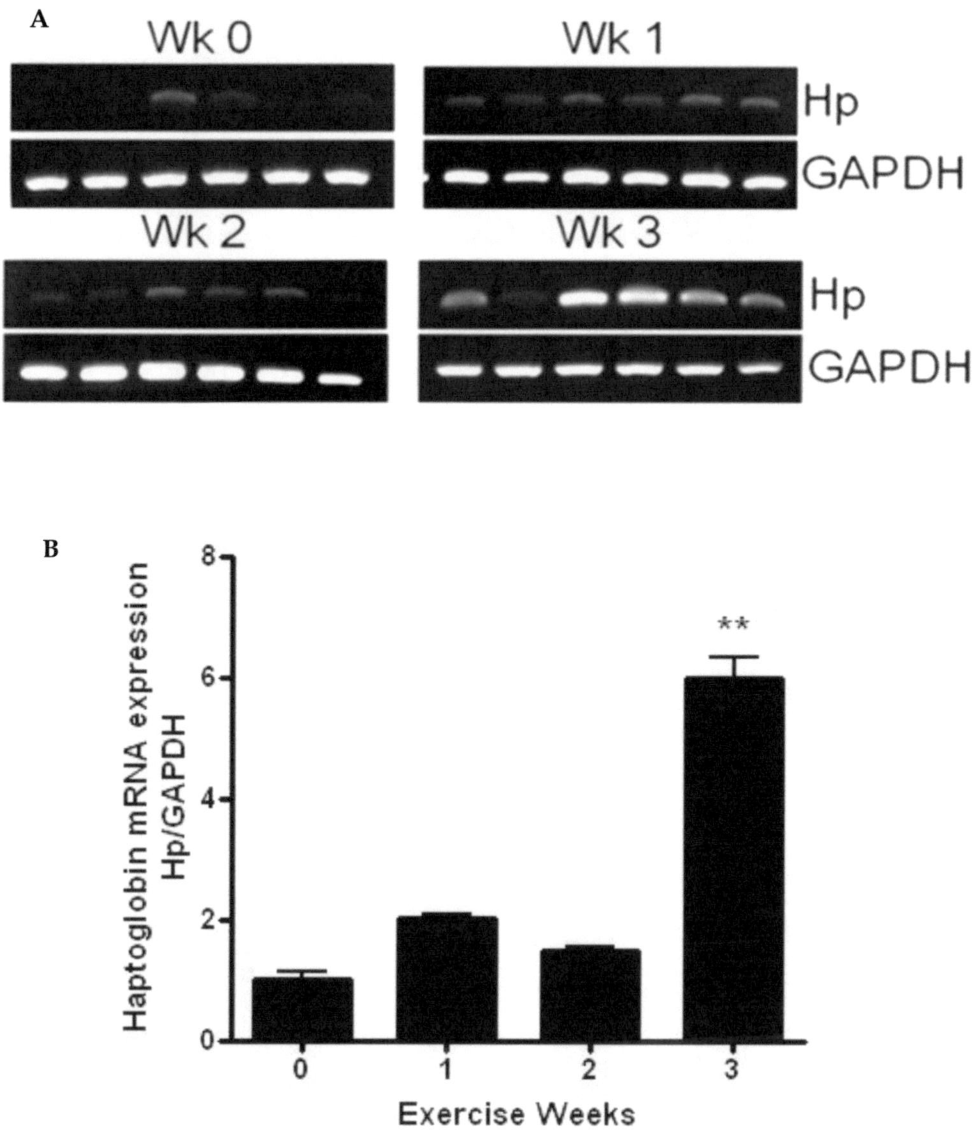

Fig. 6. Effect of exercise on Hp mRNA expression in leukocytes from different mouse groups assessed by a RT-PCR. A: Hp mRNA expression from each group (n=6). B: Mean ± SD of the density from RT-PCR results (from A) determined by a scanning densitometry. A significant increase in Hp mRNA expression levels is observed after 3 weeks of exercise ($p<0.005$). Each group was sacrificed at the same day.

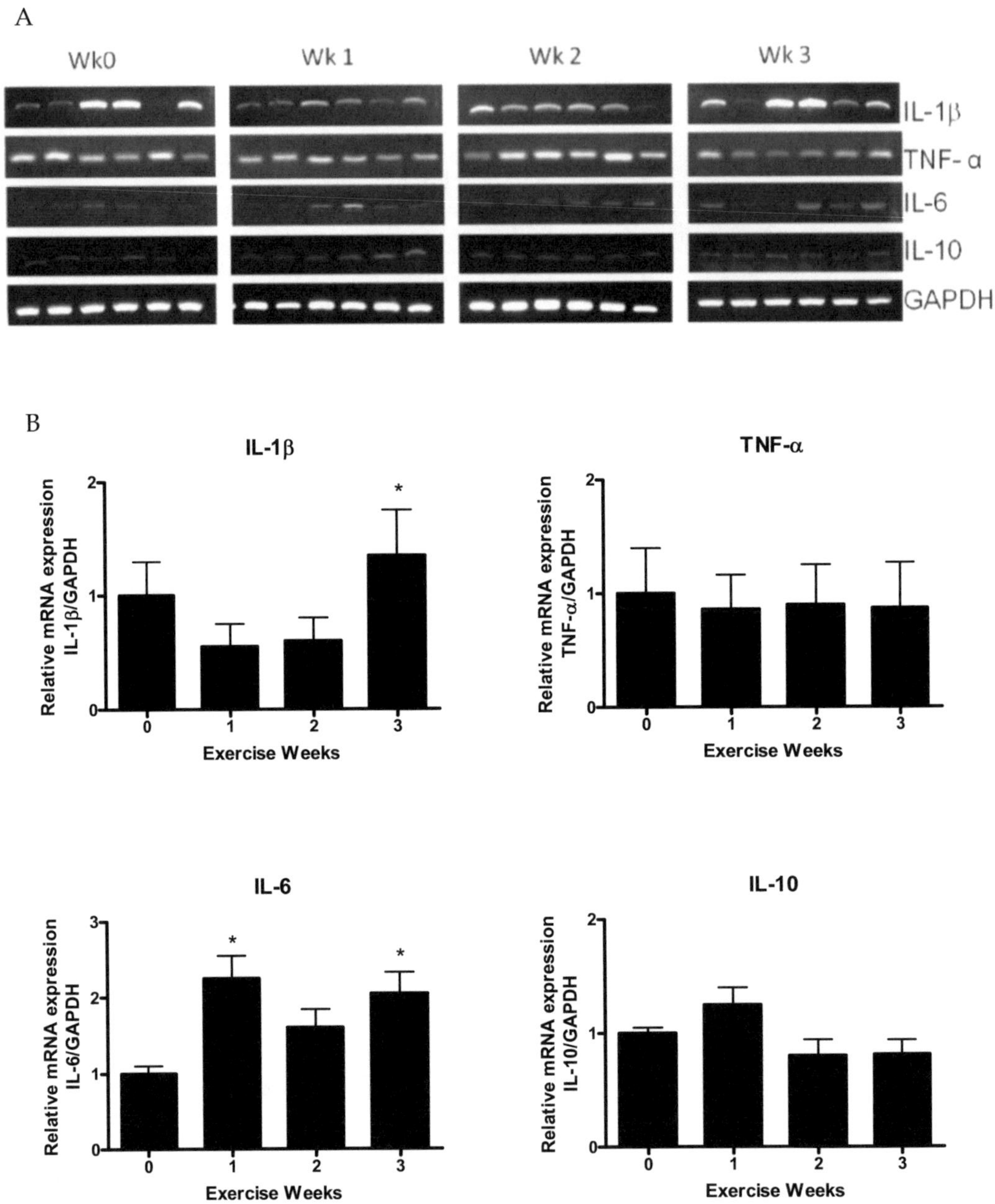

Fig. 7. Effect of exercise on mRNA expression of the cytokines, IL-1β, TNF-α, IL-6, and IL-10 in mouse leukocytes. A: mRNA levels corresponding to each cytokine after exercise (n=6 for each respective group). B: Mean ± SD of the density from RT-PCR results (from A) determined by a scanning densitometry. *$p<0.05$ as compared to week 0. Each group was sacrificed at the same day.

3.4 Hp mRNA levels of liver remaining unchanged in mice after exercise

To test whether exercise can affect the expression of hepatic Hp mRNA levels over time, we analyzed the mouse liver samples using a RT-PCR. Figure 8 shows that Hp mRNA levels were not altered during the three-week exercise suggesting that the elevated levels of plasma Hp were not derived from the livers.

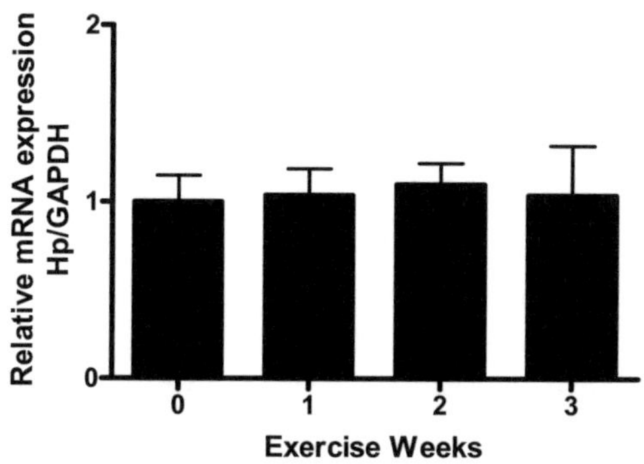

Fig. 8. Effect of exercise on mouse hepatic Hp mRNA expression over time. There are no significantly different between each group (n=6 for each respective group). $p>0.05$

3.5 Neutrophils is a major moiety responsible for the elevation of Hp in mice after exercise

Lymphocytes, neutrophils, and monocytes are taken account for the major types of white blood cells in plasma. Finally, we found only the number of plasma neutrophils being mostly increased after exercise, but not that of lymphocytes and monocytes (Figure 9). Thus,

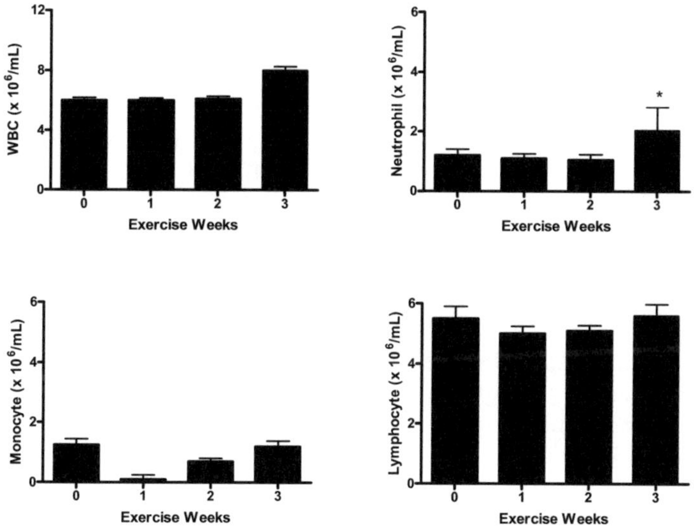

Fig. 9. Effect of exercise on the number of total leukocytes, neutrophils, monocytes, and lymphocytes in mice. Only neutrophils from the leukocytes are significantly increased as compared with the other cell types after 3-week exercise. *$p<0.05$ as compared with the week 0. Each group was sacrificed at the same day.

our results point out that the increase in neutrophils over the circulation is accompanied with the elevation of plasma Hp shown in Figures 5 and 6. Such correlation can be rationalized by the fact that exercise can induce a marked increase in blood neutrophils in human studies (Gavrieli et al., 2008, Laing et al., 2008, Weight et al., 1991). These neutrophils are then attributed for the release of Hp into the plasma shown in our study. A similar study was conducted by us in cows with mastitis, large accumulation of neutrophils in mammary glands resulted in a marked Hp increase in milk (Lai et al., 2009). We suggest that neutrophils are responsible for the elevated Hp levels in plasma following the exercise.

4. Conclusions

From the human study, we show that one short-term jogging and explosive run are able to induce the Hp plasma elevation, while the animal study revealed that a mild exercise induces marked increase in plasma Hp and neutrophil-dervied Hp mRNA or in leukocytes, but not in the hepatocytes. It is conceivable that although liver is a major organ responsible for the Hp biosynthesis, the net increase in plasma Hp, may be directly originated from the leukocytes (at least in part) following exercise. Clinically, increase in leukocytes count, particularly neutrophils, after microbial infection is very common. The present study provides evidence that a substantial elevation of Hp is associated with the neutrophil increase (mobilized from the lymphatic pool). These findings could be relevant for most inflammatory responses when neutrophils level increases in the circulation. It also suggests that Hp levels could be the marker for the neutrophil functional activity.
Given the ability of neutrophil to secret the anti-inflammatory molecule Hp into circulation, we suggest that neutrophil mobilization from the lymphatic system or bone marrow may play a role as a physiologic repair mechanism to inflammatory tissue injury. The application of mild exercise to actively elicit the plasma Hp expression in preventing infections or in reducing chronic inflammation needs further investigations.

5. Acknowledgments

This work was supported by grants of NHRI-EX94-9229SI from National Health Research Institute (SJTM), NSC 95-2313-B-009-003-MY2 (SJTM) and NSC 100-2314-B-010-001-MY2 from National Science Council (CYC), and a Translational Medicine Scholarship from Institute of Biomedical Sciences, Academia Sinica, Taiwan (CYC).

6. References

Bernard, D., Christophe, A., Delanghe, J., Langlois, M., De Buyzere, M. & Comhaire, F. (2003) The effect of supplementation with an antioxidant preparation on ldl-oxidation is determined by haptoglobin polymorphism. *Redox Rep,* Vol.8, No.1, pp. 41-46, ISSN 1351-0002

Cheng, T. M., Pan, J. P., Lai, S. T., Kao, L. P., Lin, H. H. & Mao, S. J. T. (2007) Immunochemical property of human haptoglobin phenotypes: Determination of plasma haptoglobin using type-matched standards. *Clin Biochem,* Vol.40, No.13-14, pp. 1045-1056, ISSN 0009-9120

Cordova Martinez, A. & Escanero, J. F. (1992) Iron, transferrin, and haptoglobin levels after a single bout of exercise in men. *Physiol Behav,* Vol.51, No.4, pp. 719-722, ISSN 0031-9384

Gavrieli, R., Ashlagi-Amiri, T., Eliakim, A., Nemet, D., Zigel, L., Berger-Achituv, S., Falk, B. & Wolach, B. (2008) The effect of aerobic exercise on neutrophil functions. *Med Sci Sports Exerc,* Vol.40, No.9, pp. 1623-1628, ISSN 1530-0315

Hochberg, I., Roguin, A., Nikolsky, E., Chanderashekhar, P. V., Cohen, S. & Levy, A. P. (2002) Haptoglobin phenotype and coronary artery collaterals in diabetic patients. *Atherosclerosis,* Vol.161, No.2, pp. 441-446, ISSN 0021-9150

Kim, I. S., Lee, I. H., Lee, J. H. & Lee, S. Y. (2001) Induction of haptoglobin by all-trans retinoic acid in thp-1 human monocytic cell line. *Biochem Biophys Res Commun,* Vol.284, No.3, pp. 738-742, ISSN 0006-291X

Kurosky, A., Barnett, D. R., Lee, T. H., Touchstone, B., Hay, R. E., Arnott, M. S., Bowman, B. H. & Fitch, W. M. (1980) Covalent structure of human haptoglobin: A serine protease homolog. *Proc Natl Acad Sci U S A,* Vol.77, No.6, pp. 3388-3392, ISSN 0027-8424

Lai, I. H., Tsao, J. H., Lu, Y. P., Lee, J. W., Zhao, X., Chien, F. L. & Mao, S. J. T.(2009) Neutrophils as one of the major haptoglobin sources in mastitis affected milk. *Vet Res,* Vol.40, No.3, pp. 17, ISSN 0928-4249

Lai, I. H., Lin, K. Y., Larsson, M., Yang, M. C., Shiau, C. H., Liao, M. H. & Mao, S. J. T. (2008) A unique tetrameric structure of deer plasma haptoglobin--an evolutionary advantage in the hp 2-2 phenotype with homogeneous structure. *FEBS J,* Vol.275, No.5, pp. 981-993, ISSN 1742-464X

Lai, Y. A., Lai, I. H., Tseng, C. F., Lee, J. & Mao, S. J. T. (2007) Evidence of tandem repeat and extra thiol-groups resulted in the polymeric formation of bovine haptoglobin: A unique structure of hp 2-2 phenotype. *J Biochem Mol Biol,* Vol.40, No.6, pp. 1028-1038, ISSN 1225-8687

Laing, S. J., Jackson, A. R., Walters, R., Lloyd-Jones, E., Whitham, M., Maassen, N. & Walsh, N. P. (2008) Human blood neutrophil responses to prolonged exercise with and without a thermal clamp. *J Appl Physiol,* Vol.104, No.1, pp. 20-26, ISSN 8750-7587

Langlois, M. R. & Delanghe, J. R. (1996) Biological and clinical significance of haptoglobin polymorphism in humans. *Clin Chem,* Vol.42, No.10, pp. 1589-1600, ISSN 0009-9147

Levy, A. P., Hochberg, I., Jablonski, K., Resnick, H. E., Lee, E. T., Best, L. & Howard, B. V. (2002) Haptoglobin phenotype is an independent risk factor for cardiovascular disease in individuals with diabetes: The strong heart study. *J Am Coll Cardiol,* Vol.40, No.11, pp. 1984-1990, ISSN 0735-1097

Maeda, N. (1985) Nucleotide sequence of the haptoglobin and haptoglobin-related gene pair. The haptoglobin-related gene contains a retrovirus-like element. *J Biol Chem,* Vol.260, No.11, pp. 6698-6709, ISSN 0021-9258

Maeda, N., Yang, F., Barnett, D. R., Bowman, B. H. & Smithies, O. (1984) Duplication within the haptoglobin hp2 gene. *Nature,* Vol.309, No.5964, pp. 131-135, ISSN 0028-0836

Mcevoy, S. M. & Maeda, N. (1988) Complex events in the evolution of the haptoglobin gene cluster in primates. *J Biol Chem,* Vol.263, No.30, pp. 15740-15747, ISSN 0021-9258

Miyoshi, H., Ohshiba, S., Matsumoto, A., Takada, K., Umegaki, E. & Hirata, I. (1991) Haptoglobin prevents renal dysfunction associated with intravariceal infusion of ethanolamine oleate. *Am J Gastroenterol,* Vol.86, No.11, pp. 1638-1641, ISSN 0002-9270

Nakagawa-Tosa, N., Morimatsu, M., Kawasaki, M., Nakatsuji, H., Syuto, B. & Saito, M. (1995) Stimulation of haptoglobin synthesis by interleukin-6 and tumor necrosis factor, but not by interleukin-1, in bovine primary cultured hepatocytes. *J Vet Med Sci,* Vol.57, No.2, pp. 219-223, ISSN 0916-7250

Oh, M. K., Park, H. J., Kim, N. H., Park, S. J., Park, I. Y. & Kim, I. S. (2011) Hypoxia-inducible factor-1{alpha} enhances haptoglobin gene expression by improving binding of stat3 to the promoter. *J Biol Chem,* Vol.286, No.11, pp. 8857-8865, ISSN 1083-351X

Peters, J. H. & Alper, C. A. (1966) Haptoglobin synthesis. Ii. Cellular localization studies. *J Clin Invest,* Vol.45, No.3, pp. 314-320, ISSN 0021-9738

Petibois, C. & Deleris, G. (2003) Effects of short- and long-term detraining on the metabolic response to endurance exercise. *Int J Sports Med,* Vol.24, No.5, pp. 320-325, ISSN 0172-4622

Raijmakers, M. T., Roes, E. M., Te Morsche, R. H., Steegers, E. A. & Peters, W. H. (2003) Haptoglobin and its association with the hellp syndrome. *J Med Genet,* Vol.40, No.3, pp. 214-216, ISSN 1468-6244

Spitler, D. L., Alexander, W. C., Hoffler, G. W., Doerr, D. F. & Buchanan, P. (1984) Haptoglobin and serum enzymatic response to maximal exercise in relation to physical fitness. *Med Sci Sports Exerc,* Vol.16, No.4, pp. 366-370, ISSN 0195-9131

Theilgaard-Monch, K., Jacobsen, L. C., Nielsen, M. J., Rasmussen, T., Udby, L., Gharib, M., Arkwright, P. D., Gombart, A. F., Calafat, J., Moestrup, S. K., Porse, B. T. & Borregaard, N. (2006) Haptoglobin is synthesized during granulocyte differentiation, stored in specific granules, and released by neutrophils in response to activation. *Blood,* Vol.108, No.1, pp. 353-361, ISSN 0006-4971

Tseng, C. F., Huang, H. Y., Yang, Y. T. & Mao, S. J. T. (2004) Purification of human haptoglobin 1-1, 2-1, and 2-2 using monoclonal antibody affinity chromatography. *Protein Expr Purif,* Vol.33, No.2, pp. 265-273, ISSN 1046-5928

Tseng, C. F., Lin, C. C., Huang, H. Y., Liu, H. C. & Mao, S. J. T. (2004) Antioxidant role of human haptoglobin. *Proteomics,* Vol.4, No.8, pp. 2221-2228, ISSN 1615-9853

Wang, Y., Kinzie, E., Berger, F. G., Lim, S. K. & Baumann, H. (2001) Haptoglobin, an inflammation-inducible plasma protein. *Redox Rep,* Vol.6, No.6, pp. 379-385, ISSN 1351-0002

Weight, L. M., Alexander, D. & Jacobs, P. (1991) Strenuous exercise: Analogous to the acute-phase response? *Clin Sci (Lond),* Vol.81, No.5, pp. 677-683, ISSN 0143-5221

Wejman, J. C., Hovsepian, D., Wall, J. S., Hainfeld, J. F. & Greer, J. (1984) Structure and assembly of haptoglobin polymers by electron microscopy. *J Mol Biol,* Vol.174, No.2, pp. 343-368, ISSN 0022-2836

Wicher, K. B. & Fries, E. (2006) Haptoglobin, a hemoglobin-binding plasma protein, is present in bony fish and mammals but not in frog and chicken. *Proc Natl Acad Sci U S A,* Vol.103, No.11, pp. 4168-4173, ISSN 0027-8424

Wolf, P. L., Lott, J. A., Nitti, G. J. & Bookstein, R. (1987) Changes in serum enzymes, lactate, and haptoglobin following acute physical stress in international-class athletes. *Clin Biochem,* Vol.20, No.2, pp. 73-77, ISSN 0009-9120

Yerbury, J. J., Rybchyn, M. S., Easterbrook-Smith, S. B., Henriques, C. & Wilson, M. R. (2005) The acute phase protein haptoglobin is a mammalian extracellular chaperone with an action similar to clusterin. *Biochemistry,* Vol.44, No.32, pp. 10914-10925, ISSN 0006-2960

Yueh, S. C., Lai, Y. A., Chen, W. L., Hsu, H. H. & Mao, S. J. T. (2007) An improved method for haptoglobin 1-1, 2-1, and 2-2 purification using monoclonal antibody affinity chromatography in the presence of sodium dodecyl sulfate. *J Chromatogr B Analyt Technol Biomed Life Sci,* Vol.845, No.2, pp. 210-217, ISSN 1570-0232

14

Acute Phase Proteins in Prototype Rheumatic Inflammatory Diseases

Katja Lakota[1], Mojca Frank[1], Olivio Buzan[2], Matija Tomsic[1], Blaz Rozman[1] and Snezna Sodin-Semrl[1]
[1]University Medical Centre-Ljubljana, Department of Rheumatology,
[2]Health Center Sezana, Diagnostic laboratory,
Slovenia

1. Introduction

The term "acute phase" was first coined by the group of Avery (Abernethy and Avery 1941; Macleod and Avery 1941) in reference to serum of an acutely ill patient with an infectious disease. At first, C-reactive protein (CRP) was described as one of the major components of this phase (as reviewed in Pepys and Baltz, 1983 (Pepys and Baltz 1983), however since then a more detailed description of the acute phase has emerged. Today, it is regarded to include a broad scope of processes and mechanisms comprising of neuroendocrine, hematopoietic, metabolic and hepatic changes, as well as modulations in nonprotein plasma constituents (Gabay and Kushner 1999).

The acute phase response (APR) is caused by the triggering of environmental factors, such as bacteria, viruses, injury and wound repair, autoimmunity, neoplasia in combination with stress, systemic and cellular senescence. The organism reacts to disrupted homeostasis with an influx of local cells involved in inflammation (such as polymorphonuclear leukocytes, monocytes, macrophages, lymphocytes) secreting a number of cytokines (most notably interleukins IL-1, IL-6 and tumour necrosis factor -α (TNF-α)) and chemokines (such as IL-8) into the bloodstream. This stimulates production of acute phase proteins (APPs) by the liver and their secretion into the blood circulation, all of which constitute the APR. Resolution of this response brings about, among other processes, wound healing, bacterial and viral clearance, removal of antigen-autoantibody complexes, breakdown and removal of cellular debris, and ultimately leads to the return of APPs to basal levels. APPs can be divided (based on their levels of production and detection in the circulation) into 4 groups (Table I).

1.1 Major APPs

Proteins with a > 5-fold change in their serum levels during APR are considered as major APPs (Table I). In humans the two **major** APPs are CRP and serum amyloid A (SAA), the levels of which start elevating approximately 4 hours after the initial stimulus (e.g.infection), and can reach up to 1000x greater than physiological levels following 24-72hs (Gabay and Kushner 1999). CRP is the standard inflammatory biomarker measured in humans routinely. SAA levels correlate to CRP in the majority of diseases, however, when CRP is low (even when inflammation is present) SAA can be used as an excellent alternative clinical marker (Malle and De Beer 1996). In addition to being markers of disease detection, both

CRP and SAA are also thought to actively participate in disease progression (with cytokine-like and chemoattractant properties, stimulation of matrix metalloproteinases, among other processes), and/or during the resolution phases of the APR (such as serving as opsonins). SAA is an evolutionarily conserved protein involved in innate immunity (Uhlar and Whitehead 1999). In addition to being a major APP, SAA has been reported to be a marker of rheumatoid arthritis (RA) (Cunnane, Grehan et al. 2000) and a predictive and prognostic marker of certain cardiovascular diseases and cancers (Katayama, Nakashima et al. 2005), (Morrow, Rifai et al. 2000), (Johnson, Kip et al. 2004), (Malle, Sodin-Semrl et al. 2009). SAA is used routinely in veterinary sciences (Murata, Shimada et al. 2004), and also plays a role as a major APP in mice, which enables the use of mouse models.

1.2 Moderate APPs

The concentrations of most **moderate** APPs begin elevating at 24-48 hours following the APR and peaking at 2-5-fold of their physiological levels. Following a 7-14 day period they return to physiological levels. Some examples of moderate APPs are α1-acid glycoprotein/orosomucoid, haptoglobin, fibrinogen, α1-antichymotrypsin and α1-antitrypsin. Moderate APPs could play a vital function in APR, in providing support to the major CRP and SAA, and their roles, while at the same time playing distinct roles of their own such as protease inhibition, clot formation, limiting iron loss and acting as a steroid carrier.

1.3 Minor APPs

Minor APPs, such as ceruloplasmin, complement components C3 and C4, and ferritin increase their levels approximately 0.5-1-fold in the APR (Arnett, Edworthy et al. 1988; Mackiewicz, Kushner et al. 1993). However there are exceptions. In certain diseases, such as adult Still's disease (a rare systemic inflammatory disease of unknown etiology that is characterized by spiking high-fever usually exceeding 39°C, skin rash, and arthralgia), ferritin can increase to extremely high values (Schwarz-Eywill 1992, Jandus 2010).

1.4 Negative APPs

Interestingly, some APPs termed as **negative** APPs, lower their concentrations during the acute phase in the circulation. There is a multitude of negative APPs, such as transferin, albumin, transerythrin/prealbumin, antithrombin. For example, albumin's serum levels decrease in order to stabilize oncotic pressure because of massive overproduction of the major positive APPs.

1.5 Functions of APPs

By function, APPs are involved in different processes (Table I), such as

a. host defense (major APPs CRP and SAA, minor APPs such as C3, C4)
b. wound healing role (with the major CRP and SAA having central roles and most other APPs playing multiple tasks)
c. carrier/scavenger/transportation conserving vital substances, transport of metabolites/breakdown of cell debris, limiting available nutrients for bacterial growth, metal binding, antioxidant (ceruloplasmin, haptoglobin and transferin)
d. elimination of cell debris, opsonization (most notably CRP)
e. protease inhibitors (moderate APPs such as α1-antichymotrypsin and α1-antitrypsin inhibit enzymes released from activated leukocytes and modulate cytokine activities)

f. blood clotting (such as fibrinogen and von Willebrand factor)

APPs have also been previously divided into different types based on their regulators/stimulators yielding Type I APPs, which require both IL-1 and IL-6 synergistic stimulation for maximal production of CRP, SAA and α1-acid glycoprotein, and Type II APPs, which require only IL-6 for maximal synthesis (haptoglobin, fibrinogen, and others).

1.6 Time span of APP level changes leading to disease chronicity

In the lifespan of an organism the APR occurs immediately following hits (Scheme 1). This brings about highly elevated levels of major APPs, such as CRP and SAA in the circulation. Following repair mechanisms, the resolution (which can take anywhere from 3 to 14 days) of the APR gradually returns the APPs to baseline levels. During resolution it is thought that, among other processes, clearance of cell debris, opsonization and elimination of the large quantities of major APPs take place. There are postulations about how this complicated process can take place. Certain reports have indicated that antibodies against the major APPs might be involved (Arnett, Edworthy et al. 1988; Shoenfeld, Szyper-Kravitz et al. 2007; Lakota, Thallinger et al. 2011) in binding and clearing the mass quantities of APPs. These autoantibodies might act as natural antibodies involved in homeostasis.

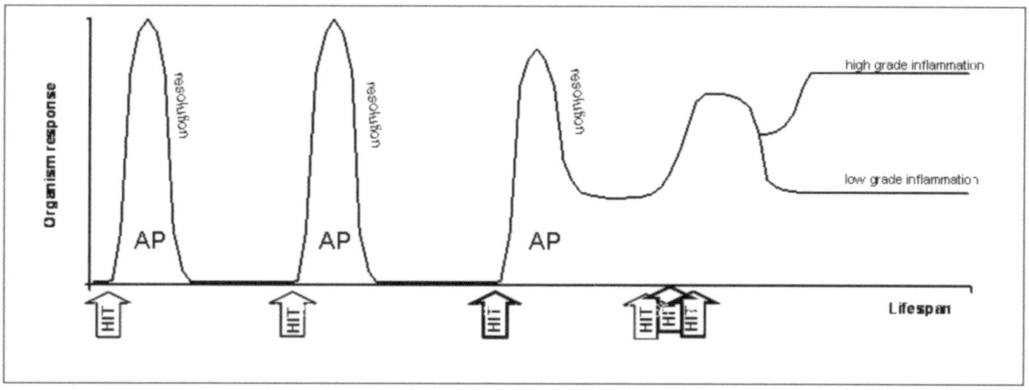

Scheme Legend: **AP**; acute phase, **HIT**; represents injuries, infections, neoplasia and/or inflammation. During the lifespan of an organism acute phases occur following hits yielding high concentrations of major APPs, influx of inflammatory cells and higher production of inflammatory cytokines and chemokines to the site all acting in defense of the organism. The process is resolved through a complex mechanism yielding physiological levels of APPs. If, however, there are too many hits, leading to an acute phase which cannot be resolved, this may lead to irreversible chronicity with high, medium or low grade inflammation.

Scheme 1. Hypothetical patient's outline of major APP level changes throughout his/her life, resolution phases and multiple hits leading to the irreversible vicious chronic inflammatory stage.

Whenever multiple hits occur simultaneously or consecutively in a short span of time or continuously throughout a longer span of time, recovery of the organism is no longer possible, nor is re-establishment of homeostasis. Throughout an organism's lifetime (with aging and general senescence prevailing), the ability of establishing an APR, as well as that of returning to homeostasis becomes weakened/diminished. In healthy individuals multiple hits could lead to a less prominent APR, and in certain proned individuals, multiple hits leading to the acute response could bring about a persistency of elevated APPs leading to chronic inflammation. In the absence of the resolution phase, a "domino effect" could occur, with APPs exerting long term degradative effects, specifically tissue and organ damage. Genetic predisposition of each individual plays a large role in determining if and when this happens. The challenge facing clinicians today is to treat patients early enough to prevent the irreversible cycle of chronicity, degradative tissue and organ damage. It is crucial to measure systemic markers in combination with monitoring local tissue and cell-specific changes "pre-chronically". Thus, longitudinal studies represent an important part for gathering data on early disease progression, however they are usually limited in time and number of patients.

1.7 Methodology description

Our report was limited to examples of rheumatic inflammatory diseases, patient population-based studies and APPs. Our initial search criteria included listing the specific "APPs" in the specific "disease" in PubMed and then narrowing the searches to patient population studies, human sera samples and protein levels (excluding genetic studies and mouse models). A division based on representative rheumatic inflammatory diseases, their disease stages, organ involvement (where applicable) and APPs (ordered by major, moderate, minor and negative APPs) has been selected in order to determine connections between them.

Table I has been constructed in order to give an overview and describe well-characterized APPs divided into groups (depending on their circulation concentrations during the acute phase) and their physiological levels during homeostasis along with potential and solely representative functions.

Only brief mention was given to the regulation of APPs, due to the complexity of different modulating molecules involved and their effects on APPs. Genetic predispositions and single nucleotide polymorphisms also largely fell outside the focus of this chapter. Understanding the mechanisms that modify APPs is an important step in developing new strategies in diagnosing and treating autoimmune diseases.

2. APPs indicating rheumatic disease pathology

The term "rheumatic diseases" comprises of a multitude (over 150) of different connective tissue diseases, syndromes, among them we have focused particularly on the most prevalent ones and characterized APPs in these diseases. Among the most noteworthy were: RA, ankylosing spondylitis (AS), systemic lupus erythematosus (SLE), primary Sjogren's syndrome (pSS) and systemic vasculitis.

2.1 Rheumatoid arthritis (RA)

RA is a chronic systemic inflammatory autoimmune disease with prevalence of 0.8% (range 0.3–2.1%) of the population worldwide leading to severe disability and premature mortality. The most notable hallmark of RA is inflammation of the synovial joints, cartilage degradation and ultimately bone resorption, resulting in joint destruction. Secondary chronic inflammatory sites are also found in vessel walls resulting in accelerated atherosclerosis. As many as 40% of RA patients may have extraarticular manifestations, such as rheumatoid nodules, vasculitis, pleuropulmonaly manifestations, pericarditis and (epi)scleritis. As a rule, these occur in patients with high titers of rheumatoid factor or antibodies against cyclic citrullinated peptides (anti-CCP) and are associated with increased mortality as compared to other RA patients or age-matched control subjects. RA is associated with an increased incidence of lymphoma, especially large B cell lymphoma, particularly in patients with persistent inflammatory disease.

The 1987 American Colleague of Rheumatology (ACR) classification criteria are useful for established RA, however are not sufficiently reliable when applied to patients with early RA (Arnett, Edworthy et al. 1988). In 2010 new RA Classification Criteria have been developed by ACR/European League Against Rheumatism Collaborative Initiative, focusing on identifying among patients newly presenting with undifferentiated inflammatory synovitis, factors that best discriminate between those who were and were not at high risk for persistent and/or erosive disease. Elevated APR defined by measuring erythrocyte sedimentation rate (ESR) and CRP levels is included in 2010 RA classification criteria as one of four scoring domains for classifying joint disease as definite RA (score ≥6/10) in patients with clinically confirmed synovitis of at least 1 joint and an absence of alternative diagnosis to explain synovitis.

2.2 Comparison of APPs in RA with healthy people and other diseases

In 66 patients with RA there was a significant elevation of CRP, ESR and von Willebrand factor above controls (Foster, Carruthers et al. 2010). SAA, apolipoprotein A, haptoglobin, ceruloplasmin were over-expressed when sera isolated from 6 RA patients and 6 healthy volunteers were screened and two-dimensional gel electrophoresis performed. ELISA confirmed that ceruloplasmin was expressed remarkably higher and the negative APP transthyretin was found to be under expressed in 32 RA patients as compared to the control group (Li, 2010). However, these differences were largely still within the normal range. Noe et al. (1995) found that 40% of 124 RA patients had an underlying iron deficiency (defined by ferritin values ≤ 60 ng/ml) (Noe, Augustin et al. 1995).

Surrall et al (1987, Clin Rheumatol) compared ceruloplasmin in RA, osteoarthritis, psoriatic arthritis and ceruloplasmin was significantly elevated in all disease groups (Surrall, Bird et al. 1987). Ceruloplasmin levels in 45 RA patients were significantly higher than in 50 osteoarthritic patients (Stojan and Hasler 1977). The same was shown in 32 RA patients as compared to 32 blood donors (Li, Zheng et al. 2010).

2.3 Comparison of different APPs in RA

A comprehensive study of 774 RA patients showed that CRP was an even better marker of disease activity than ESR (Wolfe 1997). There was good correlation also found between ESR, haptoglobin, fibrinogen, CRP, SAA and IL-6 in the serum (n=26). They found especially strong correlations between CRP and SAA and between ESR and fibrinogen (Arvidsson, Gudbjornsson et al. 1998).

2.4 APPs in RA synovial fluid

In synovial fluid levels of ferritin, CRP and SAA were higher than serum levels in RA patients and correlated to degrees of joints inflammation in RA. Ferritin levels correlated with CRP and SAA in 34 synovial fluid samples but not in serum (Kumon, Suehiro et al. 1999).

2.5 APPs during RA disease stages

Acute phase reactants were included as one of the 3 most important variables, beside tender and swollen joint counts, in defining remission of RA at initial ACR/EULAR Consensus

Conference (van Tuyl, Vlad et al. 2009) and normal CRP and ESR levels are one of the three criteria defining disease inactivity in juvenile RA.

Patients with 25 very active RA had significantly higher SAA levels in the serum than 23 patients with moderately/mildly active or inactive disease (Maury, Teppo et al. 1982). SAA has been shown to correlate better with clinical markers of RA activity (as compared to ESR and/or CRP) (Hilliquin 1995). In over 120 patients with recent onset arthritis, very high levels of SAA occurred exclusively in 64 RA patients, as compared to psoriatic arthritis, undifferentiated arthritis and other forms of arthritis (Cunnane, Grehan et al. 2000). SAA might be the optimal systemic marker to test for early rheumatoid arthritis. Our group is currently involved in testing this hypothesis. Early RA (n=79) patients also had higher levels of von Willebrand factor, soluble intercellular adhesion molecule-1 and monocyte chemotactic protein-1 as compared with controls (Sodergren, Karp et al. 2010).

Larsson et al. followed radiographic parameters in 200 patients with RA, which were correlated with laboratory parameters. CRP, α1-acid glycoprotein and haptoglobin showed a significant association with the severity and progression of radiographic parameters (Larsen 1988). Serum levels of α-1 acid glycoprotein, α-1 antichymotrypsin and antithrombin proteins in 25 RA patients were all higher at the onset of disease as compared with healthy controls. These decreased during the course of the disease and a positive correlation was shown with radiological progression (Lacki, Porawska et al. 1994). Markatseli et al. studied long-term clinical and radiological outcomes and predictive factors of radiological damage in RA at the 10-year follow up in a cohort of 144 northwestern Greek RA patients. Despite a significant clinical improvement, associated with a decrease of inflammatory markers along the timepoints, the radiologic progression of RA continued over time as defined with increased Larsen score and the number of erosive joints. Baseline radiographic damage (Larsen score and number of erosive joints), anti-CCP antibodies, and time-averaged levels of CRP constituted the main predictive factors of poor radiologic outcome in the long term (Markatseli, Voulgari et al. 2011). Lower expression of terminal sugars in synovial fibronectin was mainly associated with the early degenerative processes of RA. The higher expression levels of fibronectin terminal sugars could be associated with repair and adaptation processes. Such alterations may be applicable as a stage-specific marker for diagnosis and therapy of 58 RA patients (Przybysz, Maszczak et al. 2007).

Elevated fibrinogen levels have been observed in a number of inflammatory diseases, including RA and were shown to parallel RA disease activity assesed by DAS-28 and acute-phase markers ESR and CRP. In a study by Rooney et al. circulating fibrinogen levels were reported to be significantly higher in RA patients (n=105) compared to controls (n=62) and correlated positively and significantly with markers of inflammation (CRP, ESR, SAA, IL-6), composite and individual disease activity measures (DAS28-CRP/ESR, Simplified Disease Activity Index (SDAI) and the Clinical Disease Activity Index (CDAI)) (Rooney, Scherzer et al. 2011).

In RA patients, the value of serum α1-acid glycoprotein correlated with disease activity (Nakamura, Board et al. 1993). Both 35 men and 96 women with RA had increased α1-acid glycoprotein glycosylation (specifically fucosylation) as compared to healthy individuals in sera and synovia, which suggests a hepatic origin of synovial α1-acid glycoprotein as well (Havenaar, Dolhain et al. 1997). A weak correlation between α1-acid glycoprotein fucosylation and DAS28 was found only in 131 men (Ryden, Pahlsson et al. 2002), while Cylwik et al. reported that in 27 RA women α1-acid glycoprotein follows disease activity significantly, as do also CRP, transferrin, haptoglobin and α1-antitrypsin (Cylwik, Chrostek et al. 2010).

Serum α-1 antichymotrypsin concentrations were confirmed to be significantly elevated in 47 RA patients (Kosaka and Tazawa 1976) and reflected disease activity in 20 RA patients (Chard, Calvin et al. 1988).

Although hypocomplementemia is likely to occur in immune complex-mediated diseases such as RA, increases in C3, C4, C5a occur in active disease (Low and Moore 2005). The study that showed anti-CCP concentrations to be positively correlated to C3 levels in anti-CCP positive was performed in 123 RA patients (Xun and Zhao 2011). Complement activation was shown to be mediated via anti-CCP, as well as via CRP in RA. Elevated split products of C3, C4 were found in many associated studies in RA patients with C9 being more consistently elevated in active disease than CRP or ESR (Rumfeld, Morgan et al. 1986).

A limited retrospective study of RA patients found that serum levels of secreted phospholipase A2 activity correlated with disease activity (Pruzanski, Keystone et al. 1988). To assess the strength of this relationship the group investigated prospectively 212 patients with RA using a double blind approach. 65 patients were assessed on one occasion and 147 on multiple occasions (a mean of 2.41 visits/patient). Serum secreted phospholipase A2 activity was confirmed to correlate with disease activity in this expanded study, and secreted phospholipase A2 activity was shown to significantly correlate with the Lansbury index, active and effused joints, ESR, platelet count, and hemoglobin) (Lin, Farewell et al. 1996). Antithrombin-III levels were significantly increased in RA. Antithrombin-III depended upon disease activity and duration (from 25 to 44% patients with increased levels) (Zorina, Zorina et al. 2008).

Two other studies in 2009 measured ferritin levels and reported lower levels of serum ferritin in 61 RA patients with anti-CCP antibodies (Onder et al., 2009) or unchanged serum ferritin levels in 30 RA patients or with disease activity (Pallinti et al., 2009).

The levels of negative APPs decrease during the APR, while in disease states this can be significantly modulated. Helliwell et al. showed in 1984, that transerythrin was significantly decreased in the 54 RA patients with little relationship to disease activity as assessed clinically. RA patients with reduced transerythrin had an increased frequency of associated anthropometric and serum visceral protein abnormalities indicating nutritional impairment (Helliwell, Coombes et al. 1984).

Interestingly, increased serum levels of the negative APP leucin rich-α2-glycoprotein were identified by proteomic analysis of 326 proteins in RA patients prior to therapy. Serum leucin rich-α2-glycoprotein concentrations were significantly elevated in RA patients as compared to healthy controls and decreased after anti-tumour necrosis factor therapy. Furthermore, serum leucin rich-α2-glycoprotein concentrations correlated with disease activity in RA (Serada, Fujimoto et al. 2010).

2.6 APPs and RA vascular involvement

There was an inverse correlation reported between serum levels of SAA and reduced small artery and large artery elasticity in 52 patients (Wong, Toh et al. 2003). These correlations could be clinically important in detecting, monitoring and predicting vascular disease in RA. The hyperproduction of von Willebrand factor antigen was found to be associated with skin vasculitis symptoms in 43 RA patients (Baranov, Shilkina et al. 1993).

As shown for hs-CRP, compared to controls, fibrinogen levels remained significantly elevated even in RA patients with no joint disease activity and the degree of fibrinogen elevation was consistent with a significant contribution to cardiovascular disease risk (1.8-fold increase). This is important as fibrinogen predicts coronary heart disease independently of inflammatory markers and cardiovascular disease is now widely accepted as the leading cause of death in RA (Rooney, Scherzer et al. 2011).

A study found a higher prevalence of atherosclerosis in RA patients, with von Willebrand factor serum levels significantly elevated in 66 of these patients as compared to control patients and von Willebrand factor levels correlated with intima media thickness of the left common carotid artery in 55 of the RA patients (Daza, Aguirre et al. 2007). Several studies have reported that lipoprotein (a) also associates with early atherosclerosis in RA. Significantly higher lipoprotein (a) values were found in RA patients than in controls (n=184 patients (Yoo 2004), n=87 patients (Dursunoglu, Evrengul et al. 2005), n=122 patients (Garcia-Gomez, Nolla et al. 2009)), while one study in 69 RA patients and 491 controls did not confirm this finding (Solomon, Curhan et al. 2004). Lipoprotein (a) concentrations in active RA were higher than those in both inactive RA and controls as measured in 54 RA patients (Wang, Hu et al. 2008).

3. Spondyloarthropaties (SpA)

SpA patients are characterized by axial and peripheral arthritis, associated with enthesitis, dactylitis and extra-articular manifestations such as uveitis and skin rash (Ehrenfeld, Shoenfeld et al. 2008).

Ankylosing spondylitis (AS), a prototypic form of spondyloarthritis, is a chronic systemic inflammatory disorder affecting mainly the axial skeleton (spondylitis) and sacroiliac joints (sacroiliitis) and shows significant inherited susceptibility. Arthritis of peripheral joints, usually asymmetric, occurs in up to 30% patients and acute anterior uveitis is the most common extraarticular manifestation. In AS, the entheses are affected, with inflammation (enthesitis), bone destruction and syndesmophyte formation being principal disease mechanisms, resulting in ankylosis of spine and considerable disability. Bath Ankylosing Spondylitis Disease Activity Index (BASDAI) and Bath Ankylosing Spondylitis Functional Index (BASFI) are clinical scores used to assess disease activity. A new activity index, Ankylosing Spondylitis Disease Activity Score (ASDAS) also considers ESR and CRP as biomarkers. Novel promising candidates are emerging such as SAA, matrix metalloproteinase 3, type II collagen neoepitopes, c-propeptide of type II collagen, aggrecan 846 epitope, macrophage colony stimulating factor and IL-6, among others (Romero-Sanchez, Londono et al. 2010).

In 72 AS patients, there were two valuable surrogate markers of disease activity, namely ESR and CRP, and an established clinical activity score (BASDAI). Serum levels of SAA were correlated to CRP, ESR and BASDAI in AS patients (Lange, Boss et al. 2000). The same was later confirmed with 38 AS patients (Jung, Park et al. 2007). Elevated baseline CRP and SAA levels revealed the highest predictive value for responsiveness to anti-TNFα treatment in 155 AS patients (de Vries, van Eijk et al. 2009). Among many measured APP values only α1-antitrypsin was shown to be significantly lower in remission or partial remission group (Ozgocmen, Godekmerdan et al. 2007). SAA, apolipoprotein A-IV and its precursor, haptoglobin, ceruloplasmin and immunoglobulin superfamily 22 were all consistently over-expressed by more than 3-fold in the sera of AS patients as compared to healthy volunteers. This study used two-dimensional electrophoresis in combination with mass spectrometry to search for disease-associated proteins in the sera of 6 AS patients (Li, Zheng et al. 2010).

In 1989, a comprehensive study tested sera from 45 patients with AS for correlation of serum IgA and six APPs: CRP, α1-antitrypsin, α1-antichymotrypsin, ceruloplasmin, α1-acid glycoprotein and haptoglobin. Serum IgA significantly positively correlated with CRP, α1-antitrypsin, α1-acid glycoprotein, and haptoglobin, suggesting that gastrointestinal immunostimulation plays a role in the pathogenesis of inflammation in AS. Since microheterogenity in glycosylation was found reactivity of α1-acid glycoprotein with concavalin A was used for measuring this modification and coefficient of reactive variants versus nonreactive was calculated. In AS patients, α1-acid glycoprotein reactivity coefficient was significantly decreased as compared to healthy controls, while increasing in infection, remaining the same in SLE, and decreasing in RA (Mackiewicz, Khan et al. 1989).

Ankylosing spondylarthritis has been associated with haptoglobin 2-2 subtype (Soliev, Arifzhanov et al. 2002). In sera of AS analyzed by ESI-Q-TOF MS/MS highly expressed isoforms of haptoglobin precursor were found. Bioinformatic analysis revealed epitopes derived from haptoglobin precursor with high affinity binding to HLA-B(*)2705, a primary subtype associated with AS. These indicate that haptoglobin precursor might be involved in the pathogenesis of AS (Liu, Zhu et al. 2007).

In addition to AS, there have been reports of APP studies found in psoriatic arthritic and enteropathic SpA patients. Higher values of ceruloplasmin were demonstrated in 45 psoriatic arthritis sera as compared to 63 psoriasis sera alone or 60 healthy individuals (Oriente, Scarpa et al. 1984) with the number of synovial joints affected, significantly correlating to changes in this serum parameter.

Plasma levels of fibronectin and two spliced isoforms, Ed-A and Ed-B, in 10 patients with SpA showed an increase in plasma levels of fibronectin and Ed-B fibronectin as compared with 10 RA patients and 21 healthy volunteers, which could not be attributed solely to systemic inflammation. No significant correlation was observed in SpA patients between fibronectin level and clinical activity, ESR or CRP levels. (Claudepierre, Allanore et al. 1999).

Following colonoscopy, 38 undifferentiated SpA patients all had microscopic inflammatory lesions which were clinically silent. Direct immunofluorescence demonstrated the presence of C3, C4 and fibrinogen in 75% of the specimens examined and it was suggested that local activation of the immune system due to intestinal microbial antigens or toxins, with impaired elimination or increased exposition, may have a part in the pathogenesis of SpA (Altomonte, Zoli et al. 1994).

4. Systemic lupus erythematosus (SLE)

SLE is a prototype of a chronic systemic autoimmune disease with multiple organ involvement and the presence of antinuclear autoantibodies. SLE is characterized by a variety of clinical/laboratory abnormalities, such as fever, arthritis, rash, nephritis, neurological disease, serositis, alopecia, leucopenia and thrombocytopenia. The course of disease is characterized by exacerbations - flares interspersed with periods of relative remission but permanent complete remission is rare. Systemic symptoms, particularly fatique and myalgias/artralgias are present most of the time. Nephritis is the most serious manifestation, being along with infections the leading cause of mortality in the first decade of disease. Worsening of characteristic butterfly rash often accompanies a flare of a systemic disease. SLE is associated with an increased risk of myocardial infarction due to accelerated atherosclerosis (which probably results from chronic inflammation/ oxidative damage) but also the presence of antiphospholipid antibodies. The diagnosis of SLE is based on characteristic clinical features (≥4 out of 11 diagnostic criteria for SLE) and the presence of autoantibodies with antinuclear antibodies being diagnostically most important (positive in

>95% of patients). Anti-dsDNA and anti-Sm antibodies are specific for SLE and an increase in anti-dsDNA antibody titers may herald a flare, particularly of nephritis or vasculitis. There is a great interest toward identifying new additional markers of SLE activity or its response to therapy among them complement proteins, interferon gamma-inducible genes, soluble interleukin 2 and urinary adiponectin or monocyte chemotactic protein 1. The APR in SLE is not very pronounced or is even suppressed (Bertouch, 1983), as represented by low CRP values which have no implication in diagnostic procedure. In contrast to CRP, SAA, the second major APP, is significantly higher in SLE (n=109 patients) than in the control group (n=78 (Rho, Chung et al. 2008); n=42 (Esmat, El-Sherif et al. 2005), n=26 (Lakota, Thallinger et al. 2011)). Raised SAA concentrations may indicate disease activity, as well as lupus nephritis in SLE, but cannot be used for monitoring responses in patients on systemic corticosteroid therapy.

4.1 Possible mechanisms of low APR response

The potential nonresponsiveness of certain APPs (specifically CRP, α1-acid glycoprotein and α1-antichymotrypsin) to cytokine (IL-1, IL-10, TNF-α, IL-6) stimulation has been proposed and the results suggest a rare independence of APPs from cytokine regulation in most instances of this disease ((Gabay, Roux-Lombard et al. 1993); (Lacki, Samborski et al. 1997)). However in one report, both IL-10, as well as α1-acid glycoprotein, were found to be significantly elevated in SLE. Since IL-10 has potent immunosuppressive characteristics, it was surprising that it did not negatively correlate with APPs. Based on the obtained data, the group suggested that IL-10 may play a central role in inflammatory connective tissue diseases (Lacki, Samborski et al. 1997). Aditionaly the attempt to address the question of why CRP is not elevated overall in SLE, Liou et al. (2003) proposed that SLE has two types of monocytes responding either to lipopolysaccharides or immune complexes, while in RA monocytes respond to both stimuli (Liou 2003). Many studies were conducted in order to determine whether anti-CRP antibodies are responsible for the low CRP. They concluded that there was no correlation between anti-CRP antibodies with their CRP antigen in sera of SLE patients and this, in combination with no fluid phase inhibition, leads one to suspect an unlikely role of antibodies involved in the clearance of native antigen, with autoantibody titer following SLE activity (reviewed in (Sjowall and Wettero 2007)). With the availablility of high-sensitivity assays for CRP, its detection can become more evident in certain cases of SLE.

4.2 Comparison of APPs with healthy controls, and other diseases

Ruiz-Argüelles et al. (1991) reported that plasminogen activator inhibitor type 1 had abnormally high concentrations, with fibrinogen and plasminogen levels also significantly elevated in 18 SLE patients than in normal controls, even though both the latter were generally within normal range (Ruiz-Arguelles, Ruiz-Arguelles et al. 1991).
Significantly raised α1-acid glycoprotein levels were measured in all clinical periods in three SLE patients in 19 clinical periods. There was no association found between significantly raised α1-acid glycoprotein levels in SLE and TNF-α and IL-6, or between TNF-α, IL-6 and and levels of CRP and α1-acid glycoprotein. These data could not be explained by changes in disease course or therapy influences. It was concluded that other factors (other than TNF-α and IL-6) may play a role in the regulatory pathway of the APR in SLE (Meijer, Huysen et al. 1993).

Mannose-binding lectin, the protein responsible for activation of complement through lectin pathway levels was reported to be higher in SLE patients sera (Schafranski, Stier et al. 2004), (Scalzi, Hadi et al. 2010) on contrary low levels of mannose-binding lectin predispose patients to various infectious and inflammatory disorders and have been reported to be associated with idiopathic recurrent early and late miscarriages (Christiansen, Nielsen et al. 2009) which can also be seen in SLE.

Surrall et al (1987, Clin Rheumatol) studied ceruloplasmin in SLE and found that, contrary to RA, ceruloplasmin was not found to be significantly elevated in this disease (Surrall, Bird et al. 1987).

Alpha2-HS-glycoprotein is a negative APP and is a human homologue of the carrier protein fetuin-A. Serum α2-HS-glycoprotein concentrations in 63 SLE patients were determined, and found to be significantly lower as compared to those of 59 healthy blood donors (Kalabay, Jakab et al. 1990).

4.3 APPs during SLE disease stages

Spronk et al. (1992) studied 16 SLE cases with disease exacerbation. CRP levels were elevated in isolated cases, dependently upon higher IL-6 levels (which occured mainly in serositis) (Spronk, Limburg et al. 1995). This was confirmed in a report where CRP was recently proposed as a therapeutical agent in lupus and also, as a biomarker in order to distinguish between SLE with and without serositis (de Carvalho, Hanaoka et al. 2007).

Increased fibrinogen levels were observed in 35% of 115 SLE patients without relating to disease activity (Beyan, Beyan et al. 2007). Plasma levels of von Willebrand factor were elevated in SLE patients (n=40 (Curiel, Bhagati et al. 2008), n=36 (Mannucci, Vanoli et al. 2003)) and in these, the degree of red blood cell fragmentation correlated with lupus disease activity over time. Therefore, inflammation in SLE is likely to be associated with endothelial injury (Curiel, Bhagati et al. 2008).

Ferritin is a storage protein for iron and its serum levels were found to correlate with higher disease activity scores (with higher >10 SLE disease activity index (SLEDAI)), than in SLE patients with lower disease activity. Changes in SLEDAI scores before and after treatment positively and significantly correlated with serum ferritin levels and inversely to C3 and C4 levels (n=128 (Lim, Lee et al. 2001), n=72, (Beyan, Beyan et al. 2003), n=36 (Nishiya and Hashimoto 1997)), which have also been reported to be useful for measuring SLE activity (Spronk, Limburg et al. 1995). Hyperferritinemia was detected in 23% of 138 SLE patients (Orbach, Zandman-Goddart et al. 2007) On the other hand, there was also study reporting high increase in some cases and no increases in others in ferritin levels during flares (follow up 10 SLE patients, 4,8 years) (Hesselink, Aarden et al. 2003).

Fibronectin levels in patients with active SLE were significantly higher than in patients with non-active SLE or in normal subjects (Nishinarita, Yamamoto et al. 1990).

4.4 APPs and SLE organ involvement

Sturfelt et al. (1984) reported on 33 SLE patients who were assigned to three groups representing mild SLE, more severe or extrarenal SLE, and SLE with significant renal involvement. In patients with extrarenal disease, the inflammatory plasma protein response was often pronounced during exacerbation, as evidenced by markedly increased concentrations of CRP, α1-antichymotrypsin, α1-antitrypsin, and α1-acid glycoprotein. CRP responses were rare in patients with renal involvement, despite the increased concentrations of other acute-phase reactants in some of these patients (Sturfelt and Sjoholm 1984).

In 98 lupus nephritis pediatric patients and 30 juvenile idiopathic arthritis, urinary acute phase biomarkers were evaluated including transferrin, ceruloplasmin, α1-acid glycoprotein and albumin. All tested urinary proteins were significantly higher in active vs. inactive lupus nephritis or no lupus nephritis. Significant increases of urinary transferrin and α1-acid glycoprotein occurred as early as 3 months before the clinical diagnosis of worsening lupus nephritis, indicating that these proteins are biomarkers of lupus nephritis activity and may help anticipate the future course of lupus nephritis (Suzuki, Wiers et al. 2009).

C3, C4 levels in active SLE or renal/extrarenal involvement have been studied with contradicting results and are reviewed by Liu (Liu, Ahearn et al. 2004). Hypocomplementemia was detected in 62% SLE patients (n=597) and showed a higher prevalence of female gender, fever, nephropathy, cutaneous vasculitis, positive anti-dsDNA antibodies and cryoglobulinemia, a higher prevalence of antiphospholipid syndrome-related features such as hemolytic anemia and antiphospholipid antibodies, but not with the accumulated number of lupus flares or with the survival after a five year follow-up (Ramos-Casals, Campoamor et al. 2004). In contrast, a study of 605 SLE patients reported C3 to be increased and associated with carotid plaques (Maksimowicz-McKinnon, Magder et al. 2006).

The complex of immunoglobulin A and α1-antitrypsin was found to be elevated in a number of rheumatic diseases. In 50% of SLE and RA patients the levels of complex are increased, strikingly and especially in those with current central nervous system involvement. Their presence correlates with the progression of the disease (Lacki, Schochat et al. 1995).

Fibrinogen in 96 SLE patients median baseline levels were higher than in 39 controls, particularly in patients with thromboses and in patients with longer disease duration as compared to other patient groups. Plasma fibrinogen increases in patients with SLE throughout follow-ups regardless of disease activity, mimicking age-related increments observed in population-based studies. The rapidity of the increment may reflect the prematurity of vascular disease typical of SLE (Ames, Alves et al. 2000). Hyperfibrinogenemia was more common in patients with skin/mucosal involvements in 115 SLE patients (Beyan, Beyan et al. 2007).

Antithrombin, protein C and protein S, natural anticoagulants, weren't significantly changed in SLE patients (Tomas, Alberca et al. 1998) and are independent of a history of thrombosis, however their levels could change in patients using prednisone (Costallat, Ribeiro et al. 1998). This is confirmed with a study by Afeltra et al. (2005) which reported that antithrombin, protein C and fibrinogen were all found to be signficantly higher in 57 SLE patients, all of whom were receiving prednisone, however they did not find any correlations with thromboses (Afeltra, Vadacca et al. 2005).

Atherosclerosis is known to be accelerated in long-term well-controlled SLE. SAA was significantly increased in pre - and post-menopausal SLE patients and intima-media thickness was found to be associated with increased SAA in pre-menopausal SLE patients (Sato, Miida et al. 2007).

Osteonecrosis was significantly associated with elevated levels of plasminogen activator inhibitor type 1 activity in 26 SLE patients which causes imbalance between protein and its inhibitor (Sheikh, Retzinger et al. 1998).

5. Primary Sjogren's syndrome (pSS)

Primary Sjögren's syndrome is a chronic autoimmune disease characterized by enlargement of the major salivary glands (e.g parotid gland), xerostomia and *keratoconjunctivitis sicca.*

Salivary glands are infiltrated in more than two thirds of patients with CD4+ T cells which produce inflammatory cytokines while other exocrine glands are involved less frequently. Extraglandular (systemic) manifestations, such as arthralgias/arthritis, Raynaud's phenomenon, lymphadenopathy, lung, kidney or liver involvement and vasculitis are present in one-third of patients. Autoantibodies directed against Ro/SS-A and La/SS-B antigens, are ofently present usually at the time of diagnosis and associated with earlier disease onset, longer duration, salivary gland enlargement, more severe lymphocytic infiltration of minor salivary glands, and certain extraglandular manifestations. The high ESR and highly expressed dysprotinemia are the hallmarks of disease but without any valuable influence on disease diagnosis. Malignant lymphoma, mostly extranodal, low-grade marginal zone B cell lymphoma, is a well-known manifestation with incidence of 6%, usually presenting later in the disease. Persistent parotid gland enlargement, purpura, leukopenia, cryoglobulinemia, and low C4 complement levels suggest the development of lymphoma and are associated with increased mortality.

In the early 1980s it was pointed out that CRP is usually low in patients with pSS (Moutsopoulos, HM 1983). Recently, only modestly elevated CRP levels were found in 74 pSS patients (Pertovaara, Jylhava et al. 2009). Levels of SAA are increased in 74 patients with pSS as compared to 56 controls and immunological markers in patients with pSS are associated with variation in SAA levels. In pSS patients, SAA concentrations correlated significantly with age, leukocyte count, CRP, interleukin 6, and C4. Unlike CRP, there was a significant inverse correlation between SAA and serum IgG levels and anti-ribonucleoprotein SSA antibody titers, as well as a trend towards an inverse correlation between SAA and antinuclear antibody and rheumatoid factor titers. This implies that high SAA production could constitute a protective element in pSS with explanation that high SAA levels inhibit in particular various signs of B cell hyperreactivity, i.e., IgG and autoantibody production. SAA levels were significantly higher in pSS patients with myalgic symptoms as compared to those without, and in patients with neurological symptoms as compared to those without. However, median SAA levels did not differ significantly between patients with pSS and subjects with nonimmunologically-derived sicca symptoms. A subgroup of patients suffering from pSS displayed unexplainably low levels of complement components C3 and/or C4 which were associated with an increased risk of non-Hodgkin's lymphoma (Pertovaara, Jylhava et al. 2009).

6. Systemic vasculitis

Vasculitis is a generalized inflammation of blood vessels with numerous polymorphonuclear cells in acute lesions and lymphocytes in chronic lesions. Inflammation affects different layers of vessels and resolves usually with fibrosis and hypertrophy. Most immediate damage occurs when inflammation narrows arteries, forms clots which all cause tissue ischemia and necrosis. Systemic vasculitis spans from autoimmune diseases to nonautoimmune disorders affecting different vascular compartments by size and leading to a multitude of different subcategories some of them presented in this chapter. ESR and CRP are usually significantly elevated, however serve as nonspecific markers for systemic vasculitis.

6.1 Polymialgia rheumatica and giant-cell arteritis

Polymyalgia rheumatica and giant cell arteritis are closely associated disorders and may represent differing clinical spectrums of a single disease process. Polymyalgia rheumatica is

characterized by stiffness and pain in the proximal muscles and most commonly occurs in isolation, but may be seen in 40–50% of patients with giant cell arteritis. In polymialgia rheumatica, SAA levels were more sensitive and always elevated in determining disease activity as compared to CRP or ESR measurements which stayed at baseline levels (Hachulla, Saile et al. 1991). In addition, in polmyalgia rheumatica patients despite glucocorticoid treatment, the levels of only some APPs fell below the initial measurements at the outbreak of disease (CRP, haptoglobin, α1-acid glycoprotein, fibrinogen), while plasminogen activator inhibitor type 1 and von Willebrand factor stayed increased despite clinical remission (Uddhammar, Rantapaa-Dahlqvist et al. 1992).
Giant cell arteritis, is a systemic vasculitis, affecting medium- and large-sized arteries, most offently one or more branches of the carotid artery, particularly the temporal artery (cranial or temporal arteritis). It is characterized by fever, high ESR, anemia and headaches in a patient over 50 years with most dreaded complication being an ischemic optic neuropathy. Giant-cell arteritis frequently posses diagnostic and therapeutic challenges. Although the ESR, CRP and platelet count continue to be the primary markers, others, such as interleukin-6 and fibrinogen can provide additional information (Hall 2008). Not all patients with giant cell arteritis had increased levels of CRP, haptoglobin and fibrinogen (Gudmundsson, Nordborg et al. 1993), but CRP and fibrinogen levels fell to normal levels quickest after starting glucocorticoid treatment (67% patients in two weeks), while ESR followed later and haptoglobin being the slowest (Andersson, Malmvall et al. 1986). In contrast to CRP and ESR, which lowered after prednisolone treatment, α 1-antichymotrypsin may be useful as an indicator of underlying disease activity (Pountain, Calvin et al. 1994). A prospective clinical study on 23 patients with giant-cell arteritis concluded that SAA measurements are more sensitive than CRP in determining disease activity. The specificity of SAA was greater than ESR in the determination of inactive disease. In some cases in clinically active disease, ESR and CRP were normal, whereas SAA was always elevated, so SAA measurements in combination with clinical data and other laboratory parameters could be useful in the management of giant-cell arteritis (Hachulla, Saile et al. 1991).

6.2 Takayasu arteritis

Takayasu's arteritis is an inflammatory and stenotic arterial disease (panarteritis) involving medium- and large-sized arteries with a strong predilection for the aortic arch and its branches. It affects mainly young women with an estimated annual incidence rate of 1.2–2.6 cases per million. Plasma of acute and chronic Takayasu's arteritis and healthy people, each consisting of 20 individuals were investigated for differential expression using two-dimensional electrophoresis, mass spectrometry, and circulating levels were then determined by enzyme immunosorbent assay. Levels of SAA and C4 binding protein were significantly increased (Luo, Wu et al. 2010). In a similar study, SAA and C4 binding protein were significantly elevated in 43 active Takayasu arteritis patients as compared to nonactive patients and controls, among all other APPs measured, including CRP (Ma, Luo et al. 2010).

6.3 Kawasaki disease

Kawasaki disease, an acute, febrile, mucocutaneous lymph node syndrome, of children, can be complicated with vasculitis of the coronary arteries, resulting in coronary artery aneurysms. In Kawasaki disease, SAA is significantly elevated (Cabana, Gidding et al. 1997). There was association found between both elevated SAA and CRP and the persistence of coronary sequelae late after Kawasaki disease, associated with coronary vascular events

(Mitani, Sawada et al. 2005). Haptoglobin genotype significantly influenced the presentation of clinical signs of Kawasaki disease with haptoglobin 2-1 allele patients having delayed or incomplete presentation of clinical symptoms of 47 patients with Kawasaki disease (Lee, Hwang et al. 2000). In attempt to distinguish Kawasaki disease from other febrile illneses sera from 218 children were analyzed (among them, 64 with Kawasaki disease, and other children with diseases such as bacterial pneumonia, upper respiratory tract infection and others). Haptoglobin/apolipoprotein A-I ratio were significantly higher for the Kawasaki disease patients than the rest and with cut-off ratio of 2, with a sensitivity of 89.7% and a specificity of 85.6% for detecting Kawasaki disease (Huang, Gupta-Malhotra et al. 2010).

The proteome profiling of Kawasaki disease serum on 2D-PAGE and ELISA showed higher fibrinogen-related proteins (fibrinogen, α1-antitrypsin, clusterin, and CD5L), along with a lower level of the immunoglobulin free light chains that involve fibrin degradation in Kawasaki disease. This unique proteomic profiling with abnormal fibrinogen cascade may provide a good biomarker of Kawasaki disease and a better strategy to prevent cardiovascular complications of Kawasaki disease by correcting abnormal fibrin deposition or degradation (Yu, Kuo et al. 2009). In 36 Kawasaki disease children plasma fibrinogen levels in patients with coronary artery lesions were significantly higher than those in patients without coronary artery lesions or in the control group (Gao, Wang et al. 2010).

Predictive factors of coronary aneurysm in Kawasaki disease were reported to be multiple APPs, with special emphasis on the correlation between coronary arterial lesions and serum albumin, prealbumin, retinol-binding protein and immature neutrophils (Nakano 1987).

7. Behçet's disease

Behçet's disease, a systemic perivasculitis, is characterized by recurrent oral and genital ulcerations as well as ocular involvement (iritis, posterior uveitis, panuveitis). Differentialy expressed proteins were searched for in the serum of Behçet's disease. SAA and haptoglobin were determined to be significantly increased by MALDI-TOF/TOF MS in sera of active Behçet's disease, with haptoglobin only in active Behçet's disease and SAA in 72% of all Behçet's disease and 10% of controls (Mao, Dong et al. 2008). A more recent study found higher haptoglobin levels in patients with Behçet's as compared to healthy controls, but no differences in active/nonactive uveitis among the Behçet's disease patients (Yalcindag, Yalcindag et al. 2008). A report of 33 patients with Behçet's disease indicated that patients with active Behçet's disease had higher ESR, CRP and lipoprotein (a) levels, and lower apolipoprotein A and high density lipoprotein-C levels as compared to patients with inactive Behçet's disease and healthy controls (Musabak, Baylan et al. 2005).

Similarly, plasma lipoprotein (a) and CRP concentrations were significantly higher in the study group than in the controls. These concentrations were also higher during the active period of the disease than during the inactive phase. Lipoprotein (a) concentrations were significantly correlated with concentrations of other acute phase reactants, however there was a suggestion that plasma levels of lipoprotein (a) might be an indicator of disease activity in Behçet's disease. No difference was found between the groups with and without thrombotic complications for any of these measurements. There is no correlation between lipoprotein (a) levels and thrombotic sequela in inactive Behçet's disease (Gurbuz, Ozdemir et al. 2001).

APP groups during APR (Fold increase/decrease)	Name	Concentration in homeostasis (mg/l) unless otherwise stated	Representative Function/s
Major APP, >5-fold increase	Serum amyloid A	<10[1]	Cytokine-like, chemoattractant, induction of matrix metalloproteinases, adhesion molecules, lipid metabolism
	C-reactive protein	<5[1]	Opsonization
Moderate APP, ~2-5 fold increase	Haptoglobin	400-1800[1]	Binds hemoglobin, limits iron loss
	α1-Acid glycoprotein	400-1050[2]	Carrier of lipophilic components, steroid carrier, immunosuppressive for lymphocytes
	Mannose binding lectin	1.4 (±0.4) [3]	Pathogen recognition molecule, opsonising microorganisms, initiating the complement cascade
	α1-Antichymotrypsin	300-1600[1]	Protease inhibitor
	α1-Antitrypsin	2000-4000[2]	Protease inhibitor, induction of cell proliferation, synthesis of collagen, chemoattractant
	Fibrinogen	1000-4000[2]	Clot formation
	Secretory phospholipase A2	15.1-32.1 U/ml [4]	Increases expression of inflammatory cytokines, associates with lipoprotein
	Fibronectin	234 (±21) [5]	Binds to extracelular matrix and integrins, important in cell adhesion, migration, wound healing, forms immunecomplex with C1q, fibrin clot formation
	von Willebrand factor	107 U/dl[6]	Marker of endothelial injury/activation coagulation protein, role in collagen binding, platelet glycoprotein Ib binding, and factor VIII stabilization.
	Plasminogen activator inhibitor-1	47.1 (±4.6) ng/ml[7]	Principal inhibitor of fibrinolysis (Inhibitor of plasminogen activators and plasmin production), serine protease inhibitor
	Lipoprotein (a)	11.1-78.1 mg/dl [8]	Atherosclerogenic and thrombogenic plasma protein
Minor APP, increases ~0.5-fold	Ceruloplasmin	200-400[2]	Cu^{2+} binding, oxidation of Fe^{2+}
	Complement component 3	600-1400[2]	Opsonization (chemotaxis)
	Complement component 4	150-650[1]	Opsonization
	Ferritin	12-300 μg/l[2] higher in men	Oxdizes Fe^{2+}, stores Fe^{3+}
Negative APP, decreases	Transferrin	1,17-2,5g/l[2]	Iron binding
	Transerythrin	0,2-0,4g/l[2]	Retinol binding protein and thyroxin
	Antithrombin	0.15 g/l[9]	Inhibition of coagulation enzymes, which is potentiated by heparin

Legend: Table 1. bibliography:

[1] Mackiewicz, A. et al. (1993). Acute Phase Proteins Molecular Biology, Biochemistry, And Clinical Applications CRC PRESS, ISBN 9780849369131 United Kingdom

[2] McPherson, R. A.Pincus, M. R. (2007). Henry's Clinical Diagnosis and Management by Laboratory Methods (21), Saunders Elsevier, ISBN 978-1-4160-0287-1, PA, USA
[3] Olivier Van Till, J.W. et al. (2006). Variable Mannose-Binding Lectin Expression during Postoperative Acute-Phase Response. Surgical Infections 7(5), 443-452. doi:10.1089/sur.2006.7.443.
[4] Lima, L.M. et al. (2010). Secretory phospholipase A2 in patients with coronary artery disease. J Thromb Thrombolysis 29(3), 276-81.
[5] Nishinarita, S. et al. (1990). Increased plasma fibronectin in patients with systemic lupus erythematosus. Clin Rheumatol 9, 2, 214-219. 0770-3198 (Print)
[6] De Oliveira, C.O. et al. (2007). Plasma von Willebrand factor levels correlate with clinical outcome of severe traumatic brain injury. J Neurotrauma 24(8):1331-8.
[7] Collet, J.P. et al. (2003). Acute release of plasminogen activator inhibitor-1 in ST-segment elevation myocardial infarction predicts mortality. Circulation 108(4):391-4.
[8] Karatay, S. et al. (2010). Increased serum concentrations of homocysteine and lipoprotein (a) in familial Mediterranean fever. Ann Clin Lab Sci 40(1):10-4.
[9] Conard J. et al. (1983). Molar antithrombin concentration in normal human plasma. Haemostasis 13(6):363-8.

Table 1. Overview of selected APPs, their typical homeostatic concentrations and representative functions

Acute phase C9 was a sensitive index of disease activity; however, it failed to discriminate between the three types of recurrent oral ulcers and four types of Behçet's disease. The level of α1-acid glycoprotein and lysozyme were significantly increased predominantly in the ocular type, whereas the component of complement factor B was significantly increased especially in the neurological type of Behçet's disease. It is suggested that the changes in the concentrations of some plasma proteins may help our understanding of tissue involvement in Behçet's disease, as well as in the selection of therapeutic agents in this disease (Lehner and Adinolfi 1980). In patients with active disease, serum ferritin levels were increased and did not reflect serum iron levels, which could be especially helpful as there is no disease activity index for this disease (Odabas, Karakuzu et al. 2002), (Gonul, Gul et al. 2010). Patients with Behçet's disease had significantly lower median serum mannose-binding lectin levels compared to controls and more severe disease was more often in low mannose-binding lectin group (Inanc, Mumcu et al. 2005).

8. Conclusion and future views

Only examples of rheumatic inflammatory diseases (most of them with autoimmune background) were described and selected based on their prevalence and descriptions of APPs, which play crucial roles in enabling the protection and ultimately, the survival of the patient. There is a redundancy (known in biological systems) among APPs, with molecules having similar synthesis/production curves and providing similar functions, (such as CRP and SAA, or even more so, many moderate and minor APPs). This redundancy enables survival following infections, injuries and inflammation. However, the lack of a CRP high response found in the majority of cases of SLE and pSS implies its importance in homeostasis. SAA has not been measured as extensively as CRP in the past, however a pattern of its protein absence in the described diseases has not emerged in our study, leading to a speculation that SAA could be crucial in host protection and wound healing. Based on this, it is our recommendation that SAA be measured routinely, alongside with CRP, especially in diseases with inflammatory components, but negative or low CRP values.

In parallel, the balance/imbalance between pro- and anti-inflammatory, inhibitory and stimulatory, protective and degradative molecules, as well as antibody and antigen regulation, tilts/shifts the organism towards either a physiological, homeostatic condition or a pathological one. It seems that CRP and SAA are not only "major" (or highly abundant) in their concentrations in the APR, but also in their functions. And the moderate, minor and negative APPs play crucial supporting roles in allowing/enabling the modulation of the APR, alongside with their other roles (Arvidsson, Gudbjornsson et al. 1998).

Categorizing APPs in groups (ranging from major to minor) can be at times misleading, due to the fact that they can (in the majority of diseases) appear, for instance, as minor APP, however in rare diseases can be greatly elevated, such as ferritin in adult Still disease.

In general, earlier diagnoses require the detection of multiple markers, which can also differ based on disease staging, organ involvement or even patient development stages (ranging from neonatal, new-born, juvenile, adult and elderly). So, designing a more optimal approach/protocol for the clinician's critical decision making process is a constant requirement. More studies targeting earlier disease development with a greater number of patients are necessary, along with a more personalized view of a patient's physiology, especially to be able to compare diseased states with homeostatic ones.

In conclusion, APPs are not only disease markers, but also active players in physiology and pathology and can additionally represent one of the multiple hits that influence disease exacerbation, activity and outcome. Understanding mechanisms that modify the APR is an important step in developing new strategies for early detection, prevention and treatment of debilitating autoimmune diseases.

9. References

Abernethy, T. J. and O. T. Avery (1941). The Occurrence during Acute Infections of a Protein Not Normally Present in the Blood : I. Distribution of the Reactive Protein in Patients' Sera and the Effect of Calcium on the Flocculation Reaction with C Polysaccharide of Pneumococcus. *J Exp Med* 73(2): pp. 173-182, ISSN: 0022-1007

Afeltra, A., M. Vadacca, et al. (2005). Thrombosis in systemic lupus erythematosus: congenital and acquired risk factors. *Arthritis Rheum* 53(3): pp. 452-459, ISSN: 0004-3591

Altomonte, L., A. Zoli, et al. (1994). Clinically silent inflammatory gut lesions in undifferentiated spondyloarthropathies. *Clin Rheumatol* 13(4): pp. 565-570, ISSN: 0770-3198

Ames, P. R., J. Alves, et al. (2000). Fibrinogen in systemic lupus erythematosus: more than an acute phase reactant? *J Rheumatol* 27(5): pp. 1190-1195, ISSN: 0315-162X

Andersson, R., B. E. Malmvall, et al. (1986). Acute phase reactants in the initial phase of giant cell arteritis. *Acta Med Scand* 220(4): pp. 365-367, ISSN: 0001-6101

Arnett, F. C., S. M. Edworthy, et al. (1988). The American Rheumatism Association 1987 revised criteria for the classification of rheumatoid arthritis. *Arthritis Rheum* 31(3): pp. 315-324, ISSN: 0004-3591

Arvidsson, N. G., B. Gudbjornsson, et al. (1998). Concordant message of different inflammatory markers in patients with rheumatoid arthritis. *Ups J Med Sci* 103(1): pp. 35-42, ISSN: 0300-9734

Baranov, A. A., N. P. Shilkina, et al. (1993). [The von Willebrand factor antigen in systemic vasculitis]. *Ter Arkh* 65(5): pp. 15-19, ISS: 0040-3660

Bertouch, J. V., P. J. Roberts-Thompson, et al. (1983). C-reactive protein and serological indices of disease activity in systemic lupus erythematosus. Ann Rheum Dis 42(6): pp. 655-658, ISS: 0003-4967

Beyan, E., C. Beyan, et al. (2003). The relationship between serum ferritin levels and disease activity in systemic lupus erythematosus. *Scand J Rheumatol* 32(4): pp. 225-228, ISSN: 0300-9742

Beyan, E., C. Beyan, et al. (2007). Hematological presentation in systemic lupus erythematosus and its relationship with disease activity. *Hematology* 12(3): pp. 257-261, ISSN: 1607-8454

Cabana, V. G., S. S. Gidding, et al. (1997). Serum amyloid A and high density lipoprotein participate in the acute phase response of Kawasaki disease. *Pediatr Res* 42(5): pp. 651-655, ISSN: 0031-3998

Chard, M. D., J. Calvin, et al. (1988). Serum alpha 1 antichymotrypsin concentration as a marker of disease activity in rheumatoid arthritis. *Ann Rheum Dis* 47(8): pp. 665-671, ISSN: 0003-4967

Christiansen, O. B., H. S. Nielsen, et al. (2009). Mannose-binding lectin-2 genotypes and recurrent late pregnancy losses. *Hum Reprod* 24(2): pp. 291-299, ISSN: 1460-2350

Claudepierre, P., Y. Allanore, et al. (1999). Increased Ed-B fibronectin plasma levels in spondyloarthropathies: comparison with rheumatoid arthritis patients and a healthy population. *Rheumatology (Oxford)* 38(11): pp. 1099-1103, ISSN: 1462-0324

Costallat, L. T., C. C. Ribeiro, et al. (1998). Antithrombin, protein S and protein C and antiphospholipid antibodies in systemic lupus erythematosus. *Sangre (Barc)* 43(5): pp. 345-348, ISSN: 0036-4355

Cunnane, G., S. Grehan, et al. (2000). Serum amyloid A in the assessment of early inflammatory arthritis. *J Rheumatol* 27(1): pp. 58-63, ISSN: 0315-162X

Curiel, R. V., R. Bhagati, et al. (2008). Von Willebrand factor, red cell fragmentation, and disease activity in systemic lupus erythematosus. *HSS J* 4(2): pp. 170-174, ISSN: 1556-3316

Cylwik, B., L. Chrostek, et al. (2010). Relationship between serum acute-phase proteins and high disease activity in patients with rheumatoid arthritis. *Adv Med Sci* 55(1): pp. 80-85, ISSN: 1898-4002

Daza, L., M. Aguirre, et al. (2007). Common carotid intima-media thickness and von Willebrand factor serum levels in rheumatoid arthritis female patients without cardiovascular risk factors. *Clin Rheumatol* 26(4): pp. 533-537, ISSN: 0770-3198

de Carvalho, J. F., B. Hanaoka, et al. (2007). C-Reactive protein and its implications in systemic lupus erythematosus. *Acta Reumatol Port* 32(4): pp. 317-322, ISSN: 0303-464X

de Vries, M. K., I. C. van Eijk, et al. (2009). Erythrocyte sedimentation rate, C-reactive protein level, and serum amyloid a protein for patient selection and monitoring of anti-tumor necrosis factor treatment in ankylosing spondylitis. *Arthritis Rheum* 61(11): pp. 1484-1490, ISSN: 0004-3591

Dursunoglu, D., H. Evrengul, et al. (2005). Lp(a) lipoprotein and lipids in patients with rheumatoid arthritis: serum levels and relationship to inflammation. *Rheumatol Int* 25(4): pp. 241-245, ISSN: 0172-8172

Ehrenfeld M. (2008). Spondyloarthropathies, In: Diagnostic Criteria in Autoimmune Diseases, Y. Shoenfeld (eds.), pp. (195-200), Humana Press, ISBN: 978-1-60327-285-8, Totowa, NJ

Esmat, S. M., H. E. El-Sherif, et al. (2005). Serum amyloid a protein level, and its significance in systemic lupus erythematosus patients. *Egyptian Dermatology Online Journal* 1(2): pp. 11, ISSN: 1687-3831.

Foster, W., D. Carruthers, et al. (2010). Inflammatory cytokines, endothelial markers and adhesion molecules in rheumatoid arthritis: effect of intensive anti-inflammatory treatment. *J Thromb Thrombolysis* 29(4): pp. 437-442, ISSN: 1573-742X

Gabay, C. and I. Kushner (1999). Acute-phase proteins and other systemic responses to inflammation. *N Engl J Med* 340(6): pp. 448-454, ISSN: 0028-4793

Gabay, C., P. Roux-Lombard, et al. (1993). Absence of correlation between interleukin 6 and C-reactive protein blood levels in systemic lupus erythematosus compared with rheumatoid arthritis. *J Rheumatol* 20(5): pp. 815-821, ISSN: 0315-162X

Gao, J., H. Y. Wang, et al. (2010). [Relationship between fibrinogen Bss-148C/T polymorphism and coronary artery lesions in children with Kawasaki disease]. *Zhongguo Dang Dai Er Ke Za Zhi* 12(7): pp. 518-520, ISSN: 1008-8830

Garcia-Gomez, C., J. M. Nolla, et al. (2009). Conventional lipid profile and lipoprotein(a) concentrations in treated patients with rheumatoid arthritis. *J Rheumatol* 36(7): pp. 1365-1370, ISSN: 0315-162X

Gonul, M., U. Gul, et al. (2010). Serum iron and ferritin levels in Behcet's disease. *Indian J Dermatol Venereol Leprol* 76(1): pp. 85, ISSN: 0973-3922

Gudmundsson, M., E. Nordborg, et al. (1993). Plasma viscosity in giant cell arteritis as a predictor of disease activity. *Ann Rheum Dis* 52(2): pp. 104-109, ISSN: 0003-4967

Gurbuz, O., Y. Ozdemir, et al. (2001). Lipoprotein (a) in Behcet's disease as an indicator of disease activity and in thrombotic complications. *Eur J Ophthalmol* 11(1): pp. 62-65, ISSN: 1120-6721

Hachulla, E., R. Saile, et al. (1991). Serum amyloid A concentrations in giant-cell arteritis and polymyalgia rheumatica: a useful test in the management of the disease. *Clin Exp Rheumatol* 9(2): pp. 157-163, ISSN: 0392-856X

Hall, J. K. (2008). Giant-cell arteritis. *Curr Opin Ophthalmol* 19(6): pp. 454-460, ISSN: 1531-7021

Havenaar, E. C., R. J. Dolhain, et al. (1997). Do synovial fluid acute phase proteins from patients with rheumatoid arthritis originate from serum? *Glycoconj J* 14(4): pp. 457-465, ISSN: 0282-0080

Helliwell, M., E. J. Coombes, et al. (1984). Thyroxine-binding prealbumin--an index of disease activity or nutritional status in rheumatoid arthritis? *Br J Rheumatol* 23(3): pp. 190-194, ISSN: 0263-7103

Hesselink, D. A., L. A. Aarden, et al. (2003). Profiles of the acute-phase reactants C-reactive protein and ferritin related to the disease course of patients with systemic lupus erythematosus. *Scand J Rheumatol* 32(3): pp. 151-155, ISSN: 0300-9742

Hilliquin, P. (1995). Biological markers in inflammatory rheumatic diseases. *Cell Mol Biol (Noisy-le-grand)* 41(8): pp. 993-1006, ISSN: 0145-5680

Huang, M. Y., M. Gupta-Malhotra, et al. (2010). Acute-phase reactants and a supplemental diagnostic aid for Kawasaki disease. *Pediatr Cardiol* 31(8): pp. 1209-1213, ISSN: 1432-1971

Inanc, N., G. Mumcu, et al. (2005). Serum mannose-binding lectin levels are decreased in behcet's disease and associated with disease severity. *J Rheumatol* 32(2): pp. 287-291, ISSN: 0315-162X

Jandus P., w. Wang, et al. (2010), High Serum Ferritin in Adult-Onset Still's Disease Int. J. Clinical Medicine, (1), pp. 81-83, Available from URL (http://www.SciRP.org/journal/ijcm)

Johnson, B. D., K. E. Kip, et al. (2004). Serum amyloid A as a predictor of coronary artery disease and cardiovascular outcome in women: the National Heart, Lung, and Blood Institute-Sponsored Women's Ischemia Syndrome Evaluation (WISE). *Circulation* 109(6): pp. 726-732, ISSN: 1524-4539

Jung, S. Y., M. C. Park, et al. (2007). Serum amyloid a as a useful indicator of disease activity in patients with ankylosing spondylitis. *Yonsei Med J* 48(2): pp. 218-224, ISSN: 0513-5796

Kalabay, L., L. Jakab, et al. (1990). Correlations between serum alpha 2-HS-glycoprotein concentration and conventional laboratory parameters in systemic lupus erythematosus. *Acta Med Hung* 47(1-2): pp. 53-64, ISSN: 0236-5286

Katayama, T., H. Nakashima, et al. (2005). Prognostic value of serum amyloid A protein in patients with acute myocardial infarction. *Circ J* 69(10): pp. 1186-1191, ISSN: 1346-9843

Kosaka, S. and M. Tazawa (1976). Alpha1-antichymotrypsin in rheumatoid arthritis. *Tohoku J Exp Med* 119(4): pp. 369-375, ISSN: 0040-8727

Kumon, Y., T. Suehiro, et al. (1999). Ferritin correlates with C-reactive protein and acute phase serum amyloid A in synovial fluid, but not in serum. *Amyloid* 6(2): pp. 130-135, ISSN: 1350-6129

Lacki, J. K., W. Porawska, et al. (1994). Acute-phase response in early refractory rheumatoid arthritis: long-term follow-up study. *J Investig Allergol Clin Immunol* 4(4): pp. 168-171, ISSN: 1018-9068

Lacki, J. K., W. Samborski, et al. (1997). Interleukin-10 and interleukin-6 in lupus erythematosus and rheumatoid arthritis, correlations with acute phase proteins. *Clin Rheumatol* 16(3): pp. 275-278, ISSN: 0770-3198

Lacki, J. K., T. Schochat, et al. (1995). IgA-alpha-1-antitrypsin complex in systemic lupus erythematosus: preliminary report. *Lupus* 4(3): pp. 221-224, ISSN: 0961-2033

Lakota, K., G. G. Thallinger, et al. (2011). Could antibodies against serum amyloid A function as physiological regulators in humans? *Autoimmunity* 44(2): pp. 149-158, ISSN: 1607-842X

Lange, U., B. Boss, et al. (2000). Serum amyloid A--an indicator of inflammation in ankylosing spondylitis. *Rheumatol Int* 19(4): pp. 119-122, ISSN: 0172-8172

Larsen, A. (1988). The relation of radiographic changes to serum acute-phase proteins and rheumatoid factor in 200 patients with rheumatoid arthritis. *Scand J Rheumatol* 17(2): pp. 123-129, ISSN: 0300-9742

Lee, W. C., K. P. Hwang, et al. (2000). Late diagnosis of Kawasaki disease is associated with haptoglobin phenotype. *Eur J Clin Invest* 30(5): pp. 379-382, ISSN: 0014-2972

Lehner, T. and M. Adinolfi (1980). Acute phase proteins, C9, factor B, and lysozyme in recurrent oral ulceration and Behcet's syndrome. *J Clin Pathol* 33(3): pp. 269-275, ISSN: 0021-9746

Li, T. W., B. R. Zheng, et al. (2010). Screening disease-associated proteins from sera of patients with rheumatoid arthritis: a comparative proteomic study. *Chin Med J (Engl)* 123(5): pp. 537-543, ISSN: 0366-6999

Lim, M. K., C. K. Lee, et al. (2001). Serum ferritin as a serologic marker of activity in systemic lupus erythematosus. *Rheumatol Int* 20(3): pp. 89-93, ISSN: 0172-8172

Lin, M. K., V. Farewell, et al. (1996). Secretory phospholipase A2 as an index of disease activity in rheumatoid arthritis. Prospective double blind study of 212 patients. *J Rheumatol* 23(7): pp. 1162-1166, ISSN: 0315-162X

Liou, L. B. (2003). Different monocyte reaction patterns in newly diagnosed, untreated rheumatoid arthritis and lupus patients probably confer disparate C-reactive protein levels. *Clin Exp Rheumatol* 21(4): pp. 437-444, ISSN: 0392-856X

Liu, C. C., J. M. Ahearn, et al. (2004). Complement as a source of biomarkers in systemic lupus erythematosus: past, present, and future. *Curr Rheumatol Rep* 6(2): pp. 85-88, ISSN: 1523-3774

Liu, J., P. Zhu, et al. (2007). Identification of disease-associated proteins by proteomic approach in ankylosing spondylitis. *Biochem Biophys Res Commun* 357(2): pp. 531-536, ISSN: 0006-291X

Low, J. M. and T. L. Moore (2005). A role for the complement system in rheumatoid arthritis. *Curr Pharm Des* 11(5): pp. 655-670, ISSN: 1381-6128

Luo, X. Y., Q. H. Wu, et al. (2010). [Preliminary study on differential expression of plasma proteins of patients with Takayasu's arteritis in different stage]. *Zhonghua Yi Xue Za Zhi* 90(3): pp. 157-160, ISSN: 0376-2491

Ma, J., X. Luo, et al. (2010). Circulation levels of acute phase proteins in patients with Takayasu arteritis. *J Vasc Surg* 51(3): pp. 700-706, ISSN: 1097-6809

Mackiewicz, A., M. A. Khan, et al. (1989). Serum IgA, acute phase proteins, and glycosylation of alpha 1-acid glycoprotein in ankylosing spondylitis. *Ann Rheum Dis* 48(2): pp. 99-103, ISSN: 0003-4967

Mackiewicz, A., I. Kushner, et al. (1993). *Acute Phase Proteins Molecular Biology, Biochemistry, And Clinical Applications* CRC PRESS, ISBN 9780849369131 United Kingdom

Macleod, C. M. and O. T. Avery (1941). The Occurrence during Acute Infections of a Protein Not Normally Present in the Blood : Iii. Immunological Properties of the C-Reactive Protein and Its Differentiation from Normal Blood Proteins. *J Exp Med* 73(2): pp. 191-200, ISSN: 0022-1007

Maksimowicz-McKinnon, K., L. S. Magder, et al. (2006). Predictors of carotid atherosclerosis in systemic lupus erythematosus. *J Rheumatol* 33(12): pp. 2458-2463, ISSN: 0315-162X

Malle, E. and F. C. De Beer (1996). Human serum amyloid A (SAA) protein: a prominent acute-phase reactant for clinical practice. *Eur J Clin Invest* 26(6): pp. 427-435, ISSN: 0014-2972

Malle, E., S. Sodin-Semrl, et al. (2009). Serum amyloid A: an acute-phase protein involved in tumour pathogenesis. *Cell Mol Life Sci* 66(1): pp. 9-26, ISSN: 1420-9071

Mannucci, P. M., M. Vanoli, et al. (2003). Von Willebrand factor cleaving protease (ADAMTS-13) in 123 patients with connective tISSNue diseases (systemic lupus erythematosus and systemic sclerosis). *Haematologica* 88(8): pp. 914-918, ISSN: 1592-8721

Mao, L., H. Dong, et al. (2008). MALDI-TOF/TOF-MS reveals elevated serum haptoglobin and amyloid A in Behcet's disease. *J Proteome Res* 7(10): pp. 4500-4507, ISSN: 1535-3893

Markatseli, T. E., P. V. Voulgari, et al. (2011). Prognostic Factors of Radiological Damage in Rheumatoid Arthritis: A 10-year Retrospective Study. *J Rheumatol* 38(1): pp. 44-52, ISSN: 0315-162X

Maury, C. P., A. M. Teppo, et al. (1982). Relationship between urinary sialylated saccharides, serum amyloid A protein, and C-reactive protein in rheumatoid arthritis and systemic lupus erythematosus. *Ann Rheum Dis* 41(3): pp. 268-271, ISSN: 0003-4967

Meijer, C., V. Huysen, et al. (1993). Profiles of cytokines (TNF alpha and IL-6) and acute phase proteins (CRP and alpha 1AG) related to the disease course in patients with systemic lupus erythematosus. *Lupus* 2(6): pp. 359-365, ISSN: 0961-2033

Mitani, Y., H. Sawada, et al. (2005). Elevated levels of high-sensitivity C-reactive protein and serum amyloid-A late after Kawasaki disease: association between inflammation and late coronary sequelae in Kawasaki disease. *Circulation* 111(1): pp. 38-43, ISSN: 1524-4539

Morrow, D. A., N. Rifai, et al. (2000). Serum amyloid A predicts early mortality in acute coronary syndromes: A TIMI 11A substudy. *J Am Coll Cardiol* 35(2): pp. 358-362, ISSN: 0735-1097

Murata, H., N. Shimada, et al. (2004). Current research on acute phase proteins in veterinary diagnosis: an overview. *Vet J* 168(1): pp. 28-40, ISSN: 1090-0233

Musabak, U., O. Baylan, et al. (2005). Lipid profile and anticardiolipin antibodies in Behcet's disease. *Arch Med Res* 36(4): pp. 387-392, ISSN: 0188-4409

Nakamura, T., P. G. Board, et al. (1993). Alpha 1-acid glycoprotein expression in human leukocytes: possible correlation between alpha 1-acid glycoprotein and inflammatory cytokines in rheumatoid arthritis. *Inflammation* 17(1): pp. 33-45, ISSN: 0360-3997

Nakano, M. (1987). Predictive factors of coronary aneurysm in Kawasaki disease--correlation between coronary arterial lesions and serum albumin, cholinesterase activity, prealbumin, retinol-binding protein and immature neutrophils. *Prog Clin Biol Res* 250: pp. 535-537, ISSN: 0361-7742

Nishinarita, S., M. Yamamoto, et al. (1990). Increased plasma fibronectin in patients with systemic lupus erythematosus. *Clin Rheumatol* 9(2): pp. 214-219, ISSN: 0770-3198

Nishiya, K. and K. Hashimoto (1997). Elevation of serum ferritin levels as a marker for active systemic lupus erythematosus. *Clin Exp Rheumatol* 15(1): pp. 39-44, ISSN: 0392-856X

Noe, G., J. Augustin, et al. (1995). Serum erythropoietin and transferrin receptor levels in patients with rheumatoid arthritis. *Clin Exp Rheumatol* 13(4): pp. 445-451, ISSN: 0392-856X

Odabas, A. R., A. Karakuzu, et al. (2002). Increased serum ferritin levels in active Behcet's disease. *Int J Clin Pract* 56(4): pp. 310-311, ISSN: 1368-5031

Onder, B., A. Kurtaran, et al. (2009). Association of anti-CCP positivity with serum ferritin and DAS-28. *Rheumatol Int*, ISSN: 1437-160X

Orbach, H., G. Zandman-Goddard, et al. (2007). Novel biomarkers in autoimmune diseases: prolactin, ferritin, vitamin D, and TPA levels in autoimmune diseases. *Ann N Y Acad Sci* 1109: pp. 385-400, ISSN: 0077-8923

Oriente, P., R. Scarpa, et al. (1984). Supportive laboratory findings in psoriatic arthritis. *Clin Rheumatol* 3(2): pp. 189-193, ISSN: 0770-3198

Ozgocmen, S., A. Godekmerdan, et al. (2007). Acute-phase response, clinical measures and disease activity in ankylosing spondylitis. *Joint Bone Spine* 74(3): pp. 249-253, ISS: 1778-7254

Pallinti, V., N. Ganesan, et al. (2009). Serum biochemical markers in rheumatoid arthritis. *Indian J Biochem Biophys* 46(4): pp. 342-344, ISS: 0301-1208

Pepys, M. B. and M. L. Baltz (1983). Acute phase proteins with special reference to C-reactive protein and related proteins (pentaxins) and serum amyloid A protein. *Adv Immunol* 34: pp. 141-212, ISS: 0065-2776

Pertovaara, M., J. Jylhava, et al. (2009). Serum amyloid A and C-reactive protein concentrations are differently associated with markers of autoimmunity in patients with primary Sjogren's syndrome. *J Rheumatol* 36(11): pp. 2487-2490, ISSN: 0315-162X

Pountain, G. D., J. Calvin, et al. (1994). Alpha 1-antichymotrypsin, C-reactive protein and erythrocyte sedimentation rate in polymyalgia rheumatica and giant cell arteritis. *Br J Rheumatol* 33(6): pp. 550-554, ISSN: 0263-7103

Pruzanski, W., E. C. Keystone, et al. (1988). Serum phospholipase A2 correlates with disease activity in rheumatoid arthritis. *J Rheumatol* 15(9): pp. 1351-1355, ISSN: 0315-162X

Przybysz, M., D. Maszczak, et al. (2007). Relative sialylation and fucosylation of synovial and plasma fibronectins in relation to the progression and activity of rheumatoid arthritis. *Glycoconj J* 24(9): pp. 543-550, ISSN: 0282-0080

Ramos-Casals, M., M. T. Campoamor, et al. (2004). Hypocomplementemia in systemic lupus erythematosus and primary antiphospholipid syndrome: prevalence and clinical significance in 667 patients. *Lupus* 13(10): pp. 777-783, ISSN: 0961-2033

Rho, Y. H., C. P. Chung, et al. (2008). Novel cardiovascular risk factors in premature coronary atherosclerosis associated with systemic lupus erythematosus. *J Rheumatol* 35(9): pp. 1789-1794, ISSN: 0315-162X

Romero-Sanchez, C., J. Londono, et al. (2010). [Biomarkers for spondyloarthropathies. State of the art]. *Rev Med Chil* 138(9): pp. 1179-1185, ISSN: 0034-9887

Rooney, T., R. Scherzer, et al. (2011). Levels of plasma fibrinogen are elevated in well-controlled rheumatoid arthritis. *Rheumatology (Oxford)*, ISSN: 1462-0332

Ruiz-Arguelles, G. J., A. Ruiz-Arguelles, et al. (1991). Disturbances in the tISSNue plasminogen activator/plasminogen activator inhibitor (TPA/PAI) system in systemic lupus erythematosus. *Am J Hematol* 37(1): pp. 9-13, ISSN: 0361-8609

Rumfeld, W. R., B. P. Morgan, et al. (1986). The ninth complement component in rheumatoid arthritis, Behcet's disease and other rheumatic diseases. *Br J Rheumatol* 25(3): pp. 266-270, ISSN: 0263-7103

Ryden, I., P. Pahlsson, et al. (2002). Fucosylation of alpha1-acid glycoprotein (orosomucoid) compared with traditional biochemical markers of inflammation in recent onset rheumatoid arthritis. *Clin Chim Acta* 317(1-2): pp. 221-229, ISSN: 0009-8981

Sato, H., T. Miida, et al. (2007). Atherosclerosis is accelerated in patients with long-term well-controlled systemic lupus erythematosus (SLE). *Clin Chim Acta* 385(1-2): pp. 35-42, ISSN: 0009-8981

Scalzi, V., H. A. Hadi, et al. (2010). Anti-endothelial cell antibodies in rheumatic heart disease. *Clin Exp Immunol* 161(3): pp. 570-575, ISSN: 1365-2249

Schafranski, M. D., A. Stier, et al. (2004). Significantly increased levels of mannose-binding lectin (MBL) in rheumatic heart disease: a beneficial role for MBL deficiency. *Clin Exp Immunol* 138(3): pp. 521-525, ISSN: 0009-9104

Schwarz-Eywill, M., B. Heilig, et al. (1992). Evaluation of serum ferritin as a marker for adult Still's disease activity. Ann Rheum Dis 51(5): pp. 683-685, ISS: 0003-4967

Serada, S., M. Fujimoto, et al. (2010). iTRAQ-based proteomic identification of leucine-rich alpha-2 glycoprotein as a novel inflammatory biomarker in autoimmune diseases. *Ann Rheum Dis* 69(4): pp. 770-774, ISSN: 1468-2060

Sheikh, J. S., G. S. Retzinger, et al. (1998). Association of osteonecrosis in systemic lupus erythematosus with abnormalities of fibrinolysis. *Lupus* 7(1): pp. 42-48, ISSN: 0961-2033

Shoenfeld, Y., M. Szyper-Kravitz, et al. (2007). Autoantibodies against protective molecules--C1q, C-reactive protein, serum amyloid P, mannose-binding lectin, and apolipoprotein A1: prevalence in systemic lupus erythematosus. *Ann N Y Acad Sci* 1108: pp. 227-239, ISSN: 0077-8923

Sjowall, C. and J. Wettero (2007). Pathogenic implications for autoantibodies against C-reactive protein and other acute phase proteins. *Clin Chim Acta* 378(1-2): pp. 13-23, ISSN: 0009-8981

Sodergren, A., K. Karp, et al. (2010). Atherosclerosis in early rheumatoid arthritis: very early endothelial activation and rapid progression of intima media thickness. *Arthritis Res Ther* 12(4): pp. R158, ISSN: 1478-6362

Soliev, T. S., K. R. Arifzhanov, et al. (2002). [Haptoglobin phenotype in patients with spondyloarthritis and healthy individuals]. *Klin Lab Diagn*(4): pp. 41-42, ISSN: 0869-2084

Solomon, D. H., G. C. Curhan, et al. (2004). Cardiovascular risk factors in women with and without rheumatoid arthritis. *Arthritis Rheum* 50(11): pp. 3444-3449, ISSN: 0004-3591

Spronk, P. E., P. C. Limburg, et al. (1995). Serological markers of disease activity in systemic lupus erythematosus. *Lupus* 4(2): pp. 86-94, ISSN: 0961-2033

Stojan, B. and F. Hasler (1977). [Immunological findings in serum and synovial fluid in patients with rheumatoid arthritis (author's transl)]. *Wien Klin Wochenschr* 89(21): pp. 713-716, ISSN: 0043-5325

Sturfelt, G. and A. G. Sjoholm (1984). Complement components, complement activation, and acute phase response in systemic lupus erythematosus. *Int Arch Allergy Appl Immunol* 75(1): pp. 75-83, ISSN: 0020-5915

Surrall, K. E., H. A. Bird, et al. (1987). Caeruloplasmin, prealbumin and alpha 2-macroglobulin as potential indices of disease activity in different arthritides. *Clin Rheumatol* 6(1): pp. 64-69, ISSN: 0770-3198

Suzuki, M., K. Wiers, et al. (2009). Initial validation of a novel protein biomarker panel for active pediatric lupus nephritis. *Pediatr Res* 65(5): pp. 530-536, ISSN: 1530-0447

Tomas, J. F., I. Alberca, et al. (1998). Natural anticoagulant proteins and antiphospholipid antibodies in systemic lupus erythematosus. *J Rheumatol* 25(1): pp. 57-62, ISSN: 0315-162X

Uddhammar, A., S. Rantapaa-Dahlqvist, et al. (1992). Plasminogen activator inhibitor and von Willebrand factor in polymyalgia rheumatica. *Clin Rheumatol* 11(2): pp. 211-215, ISSN: 0770-3198

Uhlar, C. M. and A. S. Whitehead (1999). Serum amyloid A, the major vertebrate acute-phase reactant. *Eur J Biochem* 265(2): pp. 501-523, ISSN: 0014-2956

van Tuyl, L. H., S. C. Vlad, et al. (2009). Defining remISSNion in rheumatoid arthritis: results of an initial American College of Rheumatology/European League Against Rheumatism consensus conference. *Arthritis Rheum* 61(5): pp. 704-710, ISSN: 0004-3591

Wang, J., B. Hu, et al. (2008). Native, oxidized lipoprotein(a) and lipoprotein(a) immune complex in patients with active and inactive rheumatoid arthritis: plasma concentrations and relationship to inflammation. *Clin Chim Acta* 390(1-2): pp. 67-71, ISSN: 0009-8981

Wolfe, F. (1997). Comparative usefulness of C-reactive protein and erythrocyte sedimentation rate in patients with rheumatoid arthritis. *J Rheumatol* 24(8): pp. 1477-1485, ISSN: 0315-162X

Wong, M., L. Toh, et al. (2003). Reduced arterial elasticity in rheumatoid arthritis and the relationship to vascular disease risk factors and inflammation. *Arthritis Rheum* 48(1): pp. 81-89, ISSN: 0004-3591

Xun, C. and Y. Zhao (2011). Comparison of serological markers between ACPA(+) and ACPA (-) of RA patients. *Rheumatol Int*, ISSN: 1437-160X

Yalcindag, F. N., A. Yalcindag, et al. (2008). Serum haptoglobin levels in ocular Behcet disease and acute phase proteins in the course of Behcet disease. *Eur J Ophthalmol* 18(5): pp. 787-791, ISSN: 1120-6721

Yoo, W. H. (2004). Dyslipoproteinemia in patients with active rheumatoid arthritis: effects of disease activity, sex, and menopausal status on lipid profiles. *J Rheumatol* 31(9): pp. 1746-1753, ISSN: 0315-162X

Yu, H. R., H. C. Kuo, et al. (2009). A unique plasma proteomic profiling with imbalanced fibrinogen cascade in patients with Kawasaki disease. *Pediatr Allergy Immunol* 20(7): pp. 699-707, ISSN: 1399-3038

Zorina, V. N., R. M. Zorina, et al. (2008). [Some proteins of acute phase of inflammation in differential diagnostics of rheumatoid arthritis]. *Klin Med (Mosk)* 86(6): pp. 58-61, ISSN: 0023-2149

15

Role of Fetuin-A in Injury and Infection

Haichao Wang, Wei Li, Shu Zhu, Ping Wang and Andrew E. Sama
Departments of Emergency Medicine and Surgery, North Shore University Hospital,
Hofstra North Shore – LIJ School of Medicine at the Hofstra University
Laboratories of Emergency Medicine and Surgical Research,
The Feinstein Institute for Medical Research, NY
USA

1. Introduction

Injury and infection, seemingly unrelated conditions, converge on a common process - inflammation, which is mediated partly by innate immune cells including macrophages and monocytes. These innate immune cells are equipped with pattern recognition receptors (such as TLR2, TLR4, and TLR9) (Brightbill *et al.* 1999; Poltorak *et al.* 1998; Hemmi *et al.* 2000), and can recognize both damage- and pathogen-associated molecular patterns (DAMPs, such as HMGB1; and PAMPs, such as endotoxin) (Andersson *et al.* 2000; Chen *et al.* 2009;Krieg 2002;Wang *et al.* 1999;Ivanov *et al.* 2007). In response to various PAMPs or DAMPs, innate immune cells release proinflammatory cytokines (such as TNF, IL-1, IFN-γ or HMGB1) to mount inflammatory responses. If dysregulated, an uncontrolled inflammation may adversely lead to detrimental consequences. To orchestrate the inflammatory response to infection and injury, the liver strategically re-prioritizes the synthesis and systemic release of a group of proteins collectively termed "acute phase proteins" (APPs). For instance, fetuin-A, also called the alpha-2-HS-glycoprotein for the human homologue (Christie *et al.* 1987), has been implicated as an anti-inflammatory protein during injury or infections. In this book chapter, we summarize emerging evidence to support fetuin-A as an acute phase protein capable of attenuating injury- or infection-elicited inflammatory responses.

2. Fetuin-A as a negative or positive APP

Fetuin-A was first isolated by Pederson more than sixty years ago as a major plasma protein in the fetus (Pedersen 1944). During fetal development, it is expressed in most organs including the liver, kidney, gastrointestinal tract, skin and brain (Terkelsen *et al.* 1998; Kitchener *et al.* 1997; Dziegielewska *et al.* 2000; Kitchener *et al.* 1999). In adults however, fetuin-A is produced primarily by the liver, and its synthesis is divergently regulated during injury or infection, classifying it as a negative or positive APP.

2.1 Regulators of hepatic Fetuin-A expression

Although fetuin-A is constitutively expressed in hepatocytes, its expression is negatively regulated by several proinflammatory cytokines. For instance, the fetuin-A expression levels in human HepG2 hepatoma cells were reduced by proinflammatory cytokines such as TNF, IL-1, IL-6, and IFN-γ (Daveau *et al.* 1988;Li *et al.* 2011a). IFN-γ, at concentrations as low as 10-50 ng/ml, reduced fetuin-A expression levels by as much as 50-70% (Li *et al.* 2011a). In contrast, HMGB1 (1 μg/ml), a late proinflammatory mediator of lethal systemic inflammation (Wang *et al.* 1999; Yang *et al.* 2004; Wang *et al.* 2008), elevated fetuin-A expression levels by 2-3 folds in HepG2 cells, suggesting that different cytokines divergently regulate hepatic fetuin-A expression.

2.2 Elevation of Fetuin-A Levels during ischemia

In patients with cerebral ischemic injury (stroke), plasma fetuin-A levels were paradoxically elevated (Weikert *et al.* 2008;Tuttolomondo *et al.* 2010). The elevation of circulating fetuin-A levels correlated with an increase not only in LDL-cholesterol levels (Tuttolomondo *et al.* 2010) but also in risk of cardiovascular disorders (Weikert *et al.* 2008). Similarly, serum fetuin-A levels were increased up to 10-fold in cattle following traumatic injury (Dziegielewska *et al.* 1992), suggesting fetuin-A as a positive APP during ischemic or traumatic injury. Notably, HMGB1 can be passively leaked from injured cells (Peltz *et al.* 2009), and functions as an early mediator of traumatic or ischemic injury (Zhu *et al.* 2010; Wu *et al.* 2007; Liu *et al.* 2007b; Tsung *et al.* 2005; Tsung *et al.* 2007; Watanabe *et al.* 2005). It is thus plausible that HMGB1 participates in the up-regulation of hepatic fetuin-A expression during injury.

In an animal model of focal cerebral ischemia (i.e., permanent middle cerebral artery occlusion, MCAo), fetuin-A levels in the ischemic brain tissue were also elevated in a time-dependent manner, starting between 2-6 h, peaking around 24-48 h, and returning towards base-line at 72 h post MCAo (Wang *et al.* 2010). This time-dependent increase in cerebral fetuin-A levels parallels with the transient elevation of the blood-brain barrier (BBB) permeability (Belayev *et al.* 1996), suggesting that circulating fetuin-A can gain entry across the BBB into the ischemic brain tissue. This possibility was supported by the observation that peripherally (intravenously) administered FITC-labeled fetuin-A was found in the ischemic brain region at 24 h after MCAo (Wang *et al.* 2010).

2.3 Reduction of circulating Fetuin-A levels during infection

In animal models of endotoxemia and sepsis (induced by cecal ligation and puncture, CLP), circulating fetuin-A levels were decreased in a time-dependent fashion, starting between 2-6 h, reaching a nadir (with maximal reduction by 50-60%) around 24-48 h. Afterwards, fetuin-A levels started to increase, returning towards basal levels approximately 72 h post endotoxemia or sepsis, supporting fetuin-A as a negative APP in animal models of lethal endotoxemia and sepsis (Li *et al.* 2011a). Interestingly, disruption of expression of early proinflammatory cytokines (such as IFN-γ) impaired bacterial endotoxin-mediated down-regulation of fetuin-A expression (Li *et al.* 2011a). It thus appears that early proinflammatory cytokines (such as TNF and IFN-γ) function as negative regulators to reduce circulating fetuin-A levels during an early stage of endotoxemia or sepsis; whereas late-acting proinflammatory mediators (e.g., HMGB1) stimulate fetuin-A expression to restore its circulating levels at a late stage.

In patients with other inflammatory diseases such as pancreatitis (Kusnierz-Cabala *et al.* 2010), chronic kidney diseases (Metry *et al.* 2008), and rheumatoid arthritis (Sato *et al.* 2007), serum fetuin A levels were also decreased by 20-30%. In these patients, circulating fetuin-A levels were not only inversely correlated with levels of inflammatory cytokines (such as IL-6) (Kusnierz-Cabala *et al.* 2010), but also associated with increased mortality rates (Metry *et al.* 2008). Collectively, these observations classify fetuin-A as a negative APP during infection or other inflammatory illness.

3. Biological functions of Fetuin-A

Despite its abundance, the functions of fetuin-A remain poorly understood. A wide range of biological functions have been proposed for fetuin-A based on its structural similarities to other proteins or physical interactions with biogenic molecules.

3.1 Inhibitor of insulin or TGF-β Signalling

Fetuin-A shares sequence similarity to type II TGF-β receptors (Demetriou *et al.* 1996) and insulin receptor tyrosine kinases (Mathews *et al.* 1997;Haasemann *et al.* 1991), and has thus been proposed as an inhibitor of the TGF-β or insulin signaling pathways. After binding to to TGF-β1, fetuin-A prevents TGF-β1 from binding to its receptors, thereby antagonizing TGF-β1-mediated antiproliferative effects (Demetriou *et al.* 1996). Similarly, fetuin-A can also bind to the insulin receptor, and consequently inactivate (rather than activate, as in the case for insulin) the receptor tyrosine kinase (Goustin & Abou-Samra 2010). This may partly explain why higher fetuin-A levels were associated with insulin resistance in some patients with type 2 diabetes (Ix *et al.* 2008).

3.2 Inhibition of pathological calcification

As a glycoprotein, fetuin-A carries two N-linked and three O-linked oligosaccharide chains that terminate with sialic acid residues, and can bind cationic Ca^{2+} ions. Accordingly, fetuin-A has been proposed as an endogenous inhibitor of pathological mineralization or calcification in soft tissues (Jahnen-Dechent *et al.* 2001;Schinke *et al.* 1996;Szweras *et al.* 2002;Schafer *et al.* 2003;Ketteler *et al.* 2003). Specifically, fetuin-A forms protein-mineral colloids with calcium and phosphate (Heiss *et al.* 2003;Wu *et al.* 2009), thereby preventing uncontrolled mineralization that may otherwise occur under pathological conditions (Rochette *et al.* 2009).

3.3 Inhibition of inflammation

While investigating the mechanism underlying a cationic molecule spermine-mediated anti-inflammatory actions, we serendipitously discovered that macrophages lost their responsiveness to spermine when cultured under low serum conditions (Wang *et al.* 1997). That is, despite the addition of cytokine-suppressing concentrations of spermine, the bacterial lipopolysaccharide (LPS)-induced production of TNF by these serum-starved macrophages was uninhibited. Subsequently, we discovered that these serum-starved macrophages became deprived of fetuin-A that was required for spermine to inhibit TNF production (Wang *et al.* 1997). The involvement of fetuin-A in spermine-mediated immunosuppression was confirmed by adding highly purified fetuin-A or fetuin-specific antibodies, which respectively restored or impaired spermine-mediated TNF inhibition (Wang *et al.* 1997).

It is plausible that fetuin-A functions as an opsonin for cationic spermine, and its availability to immune cells may be critical in regulating the innate immune response (Wang & Tracey 1999). Indeed, levels of fetuin-A in macrophage cultures could be altered by LPS stimulation or fetuin-A supplementation (**Figure 1A**). Intriguingly, the exogenously administered fetuin-A was predominantly localized in cytoplasmic punctate structures (**Figure 1B**), which co-localized with vesicles containing an autophagy marker (LC3) - possibly autophagosomes or amphisomes - in LPS-stimulated macrophages.

When given at higher concentrations (e.g., 3.5 mg/ml), crude fetuin-A (> 98%, Sigma-Aldrich) abrogated endotoxin-induced release of IL-1 and nitric oxide (Dziegielewska *et al.* 1998). Upon purification by gel filtration and ion-exchange chromatography, the highly purified intact fetuin-A could effectively inhibit IFN-γ- or LPS-induced release of HMGB1 (Li *et al.* 2011a), a newly identified late mediator of lethal endotoxemia and sepsis (Wang *et al.* 2008;Wang *et al.* 2009). However, even at the concentrations (e.g., 100 μg/ml) that abrogated LPS-induced HMGB1 release, fetuin-A only partly inhibited LPS-induced TNF secretion, suggesting fetuin-A as an effective inhibitor of HMGB1 release.

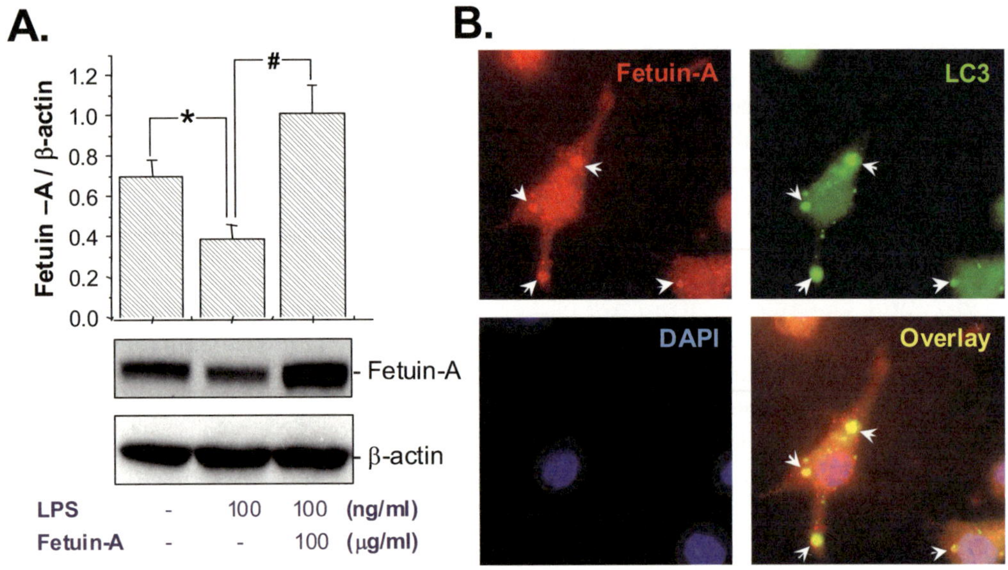

Fig. 1. **Exogenous fetuin-A was internalized into cytoplasmic vesicles in macrophage cultures**. A). Supplementation of exogenous fetuin-A prevented endotoxin-induced fetuin-A depletion. Murine macrophage-like RAW 264.7 cells were stimulated with LPS (100 ng/ml) in the absence or presence of fetuin-A (100 μg/ml) for 2 h, and cellular fetuin-A levels were determined by Western blotting. The relative fetuin-A levels, as a ratio to β-actin, were expressed as the mean ± SD of three independent experiments. *, $p < 0.05$ versus control ("+LPS"); #, $p < 0.01$ vs control ("+LPS"). B) Exogenous fetuin-A was internalized into LC3-containing cytoplasmic vesicles. GFP-LC3-transfected RAW 264.7 cells were stimulated with LPS (200 ng/ml) in the presence of fetuin-A (100 μg/ml) overnight, and immunostained with fetuin-A-specific antibodies.

4. Therapeutic potential of Fetuin-A in infection or injury

4.1 Carrageenan-induced paw edema

In an animal model of carrageenan-induced inflammation, intraperitoneal administration of fetuin-A (5 to 500 mg/kg) dose-dependently attenuated the development of paw edema (Ombrellino *et al.* 2001). The sialic acid moieties of fetuin-A might be required for its anti-inflammatory activities. When these sialic acid residues were removed by neuraminidase, the resultant asialofetuin-A failed to potentiate the anti-inflammatory activities of spermine (Wang *et al.* 1997) and failed to attenuate carrageenan-induced TNF production *in vivo*

(Ombrellino *et al.* 2001). In contrast, administration of anti-fetuin-A neutralizing antibodies in combination with carrageenan led to significantly increased paw edema, indicating that fetuin-A plays an important role in counter-regulating inflammatory responses.

4.2 Cerebral ischemic injury

Cerebral ischemia is frequently caused by an obstruction of a cerebral artery. Despite advances in acute and prophylactic therapies, stroke represents the leading cause of long-term disability (500,000-700,000 cases per year), and the third most common cause of death (with a mortality rate of 20-25%) in the United States.

4.2.1 Pathogenesis of cerebral ischemic injury

Cerebral ischemic injury consists of two stages: primary tissue damage in the ischemic core and secondary tissue injury in the surrounding penumbra. The primary injury in the ischemic core is primarily mediated by tissue ion (Ca^{2+} and Na^{+}) overload (Taylor & Meldrum 1995) and excitotoxicity (Lee *et al.* 1999); whereas the secondary injury in the surrounding penumbra is partly mediated by proinflammatory cytokines (**Figure 2**, Feuerstein *et al.* 1998).

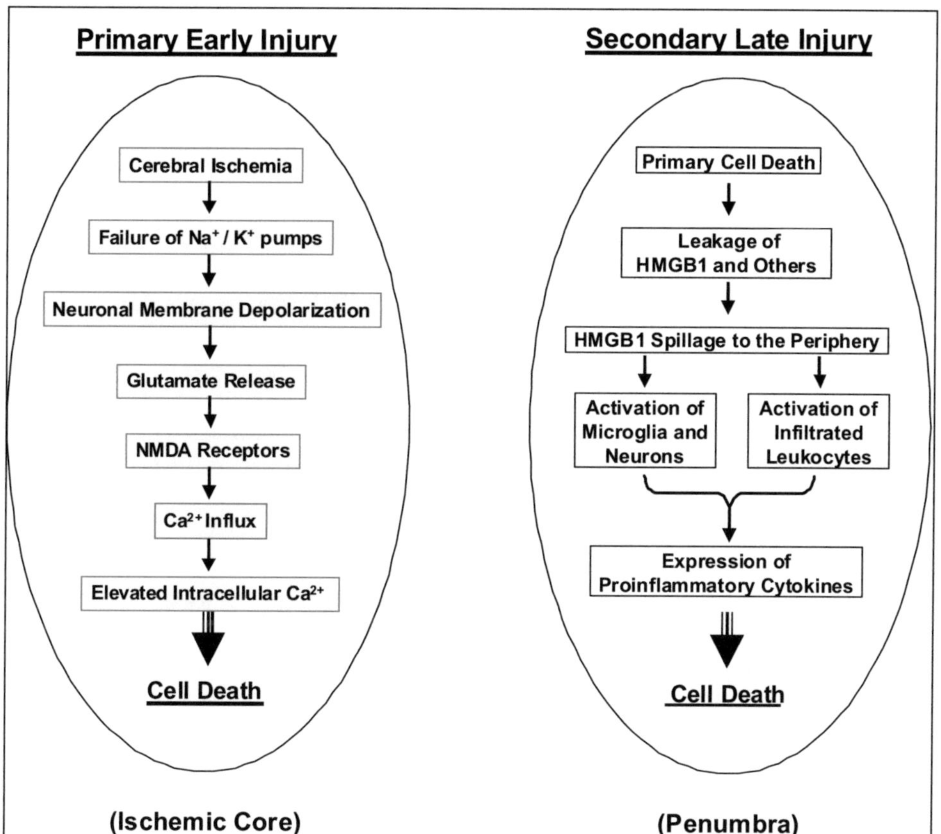

Fig. 2. **Cascade of events leading to primary injury in the ischemic core and secondary injury in the surrounding penumbra.**

4.2.1.1 Primary early injury in the core

Within seconds to minutes after cerebral ischemia, decreased ATP production leads to failure of the Na^+/K^+-ATPase pump, disruption of membrane potentials, influx of sodium and calcium, and subsequent release of excitatory amino acids (such as glutamate, **Figure 2**). Engagement of glutamate with the ionotropic N-methyl-D-aspartate receptor (NMDA) leads to Ca^{2+} influx and activation of damaging proteases (e.g., phospholipase A_2, nitric oxide synthase, endonucleases, and calpain) that compromise the functional and structural integrity of neuronal cells within 20-60 minutes (**Figure 2**). Early-stage therapeutics that block ion (Na^+ and Ca^{2+}) channels (Taylor & Meldrum 1995) and glutamate receptors (Meldrum 1990) fail in clinical trials, partly because of the impracticalities of administering such drugs at a time when those mechanisms are already activated. These failures have prompted the search for downstream targets that also mediate ischemic injury.

4.2.1.2 Secondary late injury in the penumbral zone

Outside of the ischemic core where cells are destined to die lies a penumbral zone where brain cell death continues slowly for hours and even days after the onset of ischemia (**Figure 2**). This progressive expansion of cell death in the penumbra (i.e., secondary injury) is mediated by ischemia-elicited inflammatory responses. Within a few hours, microglia and neurons become activated to produce TNF and other cytokines (Kato *et al.* 1996;Botchkina *et al.* 1997). Subsequently, polymorphonuclear cells infiltrate into the ischemic brain tissue within 12-48 hours (Akopov *et al.* 1996), followed by an influx of monocytes and macrophages over a period of one to several days. Together, these centrally- and peripherally-derived cells orchestrate a potentially injurious inflammatory response by overproducing various proinflammatory cytokines (**Figure 2**).
Many pro-inflammatory cytokines (e.g., TNF and IL-1) contribute to cerebral ischemic injury (Buttini *et al.* 1996;Zaremba & Losy 2001), because inhibition of their production (Meistrell *et al.* 1997;Bertorelli *et al.* 1998) or activity (Barone *et al.* 1997;Yang *et al.* 1999) confers protective effects. In addition, an ubiquitous nuclear protein, HMGB1, can be passively released from the ischemic core, and spilled into the surrounding periphery (Qiu *et al.* 2008). In the penumbra, it amplifies a potentially injurious inflammatory response by inducing various cytokines, chemokines, tissue factor and adhesion molecules (Andersson *et al.* 2000;Lv *et al.* 2009;Fiuza *et al.* 2003;Treutiger *et al.* 2003) (**Figure 2**). Indeed, HMGB1-specific neutralizing antibodies and antagonists (e.g., the A box) have been proven protective (Liu *et al.* 2007a;Muhammad *et al.* 2008), supporting a pathogenic role for HMGB1 in ischemic injury.

4.2.2 Divergent roles of spermine in cerebral ischemic injury

Another abundant molecule, spermine, can also be passively released by injured cells (Paschen 1992). At higher (millimolar) concentrations, spermine could be neuroprotective by binding and blocking the NMDA receptor (Araneda *et al.* 1999;Ferchmin *et al.* 2000). In addition, it counter-regulates expression of inflammatory cytokines (Zhang *et al.* 2000;Zhang *et al.* 1997;Zhang *et al.* 1999;Zhu *et al.* 2009) and scavenges free radicals (Ha *et al.* 1998;Adibhatla *et al.* 2002). However, spermine can be enzymatically converted by polyamine oxidases into cytotoxic metabolites (e.g., 3-aminopropanal) (Ivanova *et al.* 1998), which readily spreads and mediates direct cytotoxicities (Ivanova *et al.* 1998). At low (micromolar) concentrations, spermine activates the NMDA receptor (Zubrow *et al.* 2000;Ferchmin *et al.* 2000;Williams 1997), thereby augmenting glutamate-mediated neurotoxicity by overactivating Ca^{2+} fluxes and disturbances of the calcium homeostasis.

During cerebral ischemia, brain spermine levels are decreased (Paschen *et al.* 1992), owing largely to an accompanying increase in the enzymatic activity of brain polyamine oxidase (Ivanova *et al.* 1998). The loss of spermine consequently tilts the balance towards neurotoxicity through activating the NMDA receptor, and increasing susceptibility to oxidative stress as well as excessive inflammatory response.

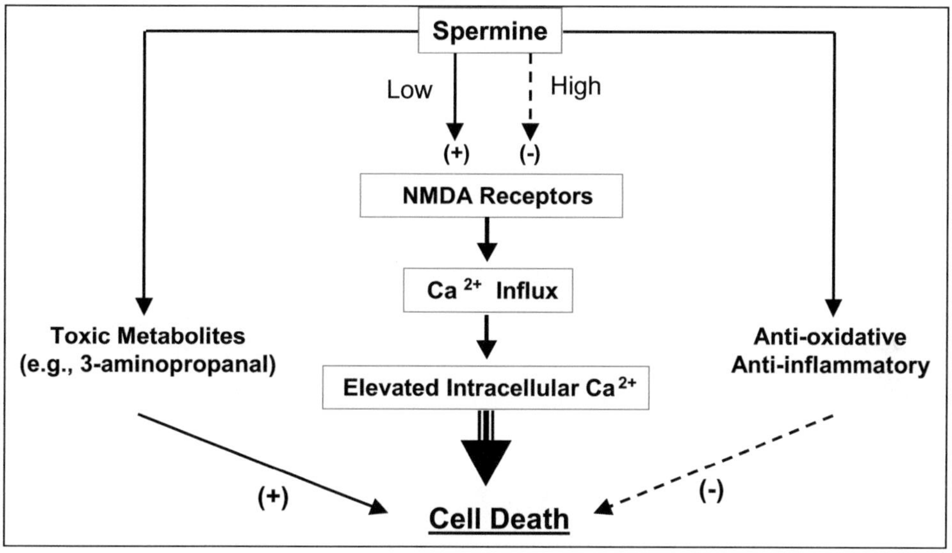

Fig. 3. **Divergent roles of spermine in cerebral ischemic injury.**

4.2.3 Peripheral administration of fetuin-A reduced cerebral ischemic injury

As mentioned earlier, when given peripherally, exogenous fetuin-A gains entry across the BBB into the ischemic brain tissue (**Figure 4**). The time-course of fetuin-A extravasation in the ischemic brain tissue parallels with the time-dependent alteration of the BBB permeability (Belayev *et al.* 1996), which was transiently elevated (5 -25 h post MCAo) followed by a return towards baseline at 72 h post MCAo (Belayev *et al.* 1996). It is possible that the temporal breakdown of the BBB is required for circulating fetuin-A to transiently gain entry into the brain. Consistently, peripheral administration of fetuin-A (50 mg/kg) promoted a dose-dependent protection against cerebral ischemic injury during an early stage of cerebral ischemia (i.e., 24 h post MCAo) (Wang *et al.* 2010). However, the fetuin-A-mediated protection was not long-lasting, and gradually diminished at a later stage (e.g., 7 days post MCAo). It is possible that the restore of BBB function at a late stage (3 days after MCAo) limits subsequent fetuin-A extravasation, thereby diminishing fetuin-A-mediated long-lasting protective effects.

Given the aforementioned pathogenic roles of Ca^{2+} and spermine in cerebral ischemia (in **section 4.2.1 and 4.2.2**), as well as the capacity of fetuin-A in binding Ca^{2+} and spermine (in **secton 3.2 and 3.3**) (Suzuki *et al.* 1994;Wang *et al.* 1997), it is plausible that fetuin-A confers protection by caging these toxic cationic molecules (Lee *et al.* 1999;Ivanova *et al.* 1998), thereby depriving them from damaging enzymes (such as Ca^{2+} -dependent proteases and polyamine oxidase). Furthermore, the fetuin-A-mediated protection is associated with a reduction of ischemia-elicited HMGB1 leakage from the ischemic core, and an inhibition of expression of proinflammatory cytokines (e.g., TNF) in the penumbra (Wang *et al.* 2010) (**Figure 4**), suggesting that fetuin-A confers protection partly by attenuating early inflammatory responses.

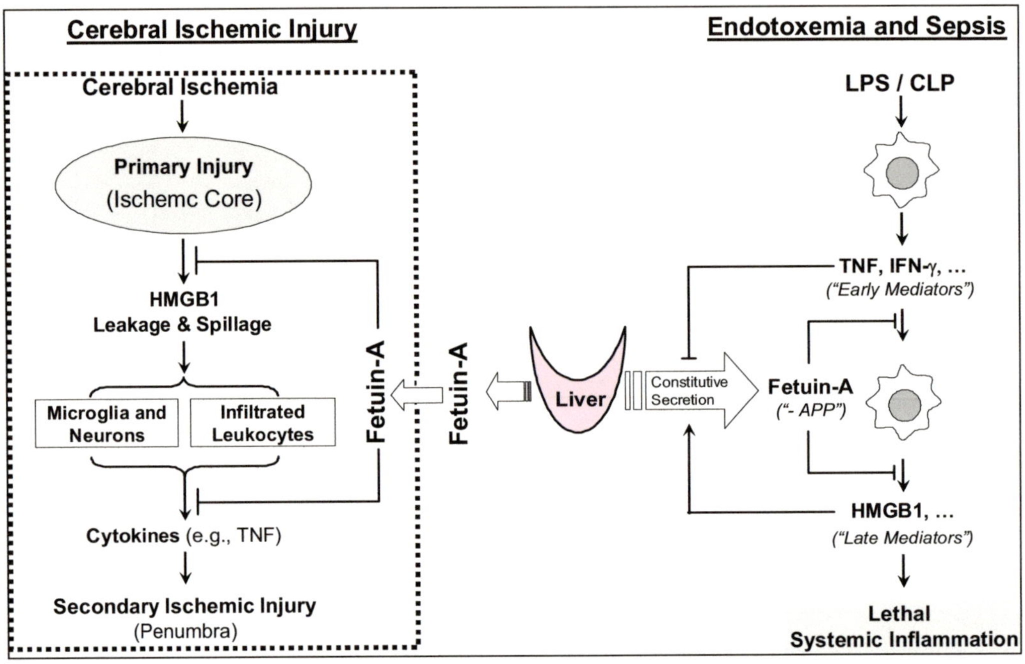

Fig. 4. **Protective roles of fetuin-A in cerebral ischemic injury and sepsis.**

4.3 Experimental sepsis

Sepsis is the most common cause of death in intensive care units, claiming approximately 225,000 victims annually in the U.S. alone. The high mortality of sepsis is in part mediated by bacterial endotoxin , which activates macrophages and monocytes to sequentially release early (e.g., TNF and IL-1) (Dinarello 1996) and late (e.g., HMGB1) proinflammatory cytokines.

4.3.1 Pathogenesis of sepsis

The pathogenesis of sepsis is partly attributable to dysregulated systemic inflammatory responses that are initiated by early proinflammatory cytokines and sustained by late-acting proinflammatory mediators. For instance, excessive accumulation of early proinflammatory cytokines, including TNF (Tracey *et al.* 1987), interleukin (IL)-1 (Dinarello & Thompson 1991), interferon (IFN)-γ (Heinzel 1990), individually or in combination, contribute to the pathogenesis of lethal systemic inflammation. Because these early cytokines are difficult to target in clinical settings, we searched for other late proinflammatory mediators that may offer a wider therapeutic window.

As aforementioned, HMGB1 is released from activated innate immune cells in response to microbial products (such as endotoxin or CpG-DNA) (Wang *et al.* 1999;Ivanov *et al.* 2007), or host cytokines (e.g., TNF or IFN-γ) (Wang *et al.* 1999;Rendon-Mitchell *et al.* 2003), and functions as a late mediator of endotoxemia and sepsis (Wang *et al.* 1999;Yang *et al.* 2004;Wang *et al.* 2008;Wang *et al.* 2009). In murine models of endotoxemia and sepsis, HMGB1 is first detectable in the circulation eight hours after the onset of diseases, subsequently increasing to plateau levels from 16 to 32 hours (Wang *et al.* 1999;Yang *et al.* 2004) (**Figure 4**). This late appearance of circulating HMGB1 parallels with the onset of animal lethality from endotoxemia or sepsis, and distinguishes itself from TNF and other early proinflammatory cytokines (Wang *et al.* 2001). Therefore, agents capable of selectively attenuating systemic HMGB1 accumulation at a late stage may hold potential in the treatment of lethal sepsis.

4.3.2 Dual roles of spermine in experimental sepsis

In light of the anti-inflammatory activities of spermine *in vitro* (Zhang *et al.* 1997;Zhu *et al.* 2009), we evaluated the effects of spermine on animal survival in animal models of sepsis. Intraperitoneal administration of spermine (1.0 -10 mg/kg, twice daily, for three days) did not protect mice against lethal endotoxemia, but confers a dose-dependent protection against lethal sepsis. This protection was associated with a significant attenuation of systemic accumulation of HMGB1 and other cytokines (e.g., IL-6, KC, MCP-1, MIP-2, TIMP-1, sTNFRI and sTNFRII) (Zhu *et al.* 2009). At a higher dose (100 mg/kg), however, spermine decreased animal survival rate from 58% to 38% at 48 h post CLP, and further decreasing it to 0% at 72 h post CLP. It is possible that spermine is enzymatically converted by polyamine oxidases into cytotoxic metabolites (e.g., 3-aminopropanal), thereby exerting these potentially toxic effects when given at higher doses.

4.3.3 Protective role of Fetuin-A in sepsis

To understand the role of fetuin-A in systemic inflammatory diseases, we determined the influence of fetuin-A disruption on endotoxemic and septic lethality. Although fetuin-A-deficient C57BL/6J mice were not more susceptible to cerebral ischemic insult than sex- and body-matched (male, 27-29 g) wild-type C57BL/6J mice (Wang *et al.* 2010), they were more susceptible to lethal endotoxemic or septic insult (Li *et al.* 2011a). It suggests that endogenous fetuin-A occupies an integral role in host defense against lethal systemic inflammation.

The protective role of fetuin-A was further supported by the observations that supplementation with exogenous fetuin-A (20-100 mg/kg) provided a dose-dependent protection against lethal endotoxemia (Li *et al.* 2011a). In an animal model of sepsis, delayed administration of fetuin-A (20 - 100 mg/kg), beginning 24 h *after* the onset of sepsis and followed by an additional dose at 48 h post CLP, dose-dependently and significantly increased long-term animal survival rates from 45% to 90% (Li *et al.* 2011a).

4.3.4 Protective mechanisms

Supplementation of fetuin-A was associated with significant reduction of circulating HMGB1 levels, suggesting that fetuin-A confers protection by inhibiting late-acting proinflammatory mediators (Li *et al.* 2011a). The mechanisms underlying fetuin-A-mediated suppression of HMGB1 release may be complex. At the concentrations (100 μg/ml) that fetuin-A attenuated LPS-induced HMGB1 release in macrophage cultures, fetuin-A stimulated autophagy and impaired LPS-induced elevation of cytoplasmic and nuclear HMGB1 levels (Li et al. 2011a). It is presently unknown whether fetuin-A reduces

cytoplasmic HMGB1 levels by stimulating its degradation in an autophagy-dependent fashion, as what has been shown for other HMGB1 inhibitors such as EGCG, the major catechin of Green tea (*Camellia sinensis*) (Li *et al.* 2011b).
Accumulating evidence has suggested the possibility that fetuin-A functions as a negative regulator of HMGB1 release during lethal systemic inflammation (**Figure 4**). First, the time-dependent decrease of circulating fetuin-A levels was accompanied by parallel but opposite changes - a time-dependent increase - of circulating HMGB1 levels in animal models of endotoxemia (Wang *et al.* 1999) or sepsis (Yang *et al.* 2004). Second, disruption of fetuin-A expression led to elevation of serum HMGB1 levels in endotoxemia and sepsis *(Li et al. 2011a)*. Lastly, supplementation of fetuin-A resulted in significant reduction of circulating HMGB1 levels during endotoxemia and sepsis *(Li et al. 2011a)*.
Nevertheless, the current study can not exclude other alternative mechanisms by which fetuin-A confers these protective effects. For instance, fetuin-A may be capable of binding bacteria (Chmiela *et al.* 1997;Dubreuil *et al.* 2002), thereby affecting macrophage-mediated pathogen elimination. Furthermore, fetuin-A may facilitate macrophages-mediated ingestion and elimination of apoptotic neutrophils (Lord 2003;Jersmann *et al.* 2003), thereby preventing secondary necrosis and passive leakage of injurious molecules (e.g., proteases, reactive oxygen species, and HMGB1) (Bell *et al.* 2006).

5. Conclusions

A liver-derived acute phase protein, fetuin-A, appears to be distinctly regulated by different proinflammatory mediators. A previously under-appreciated protective role for fetuin-A in injury and infection has been suggested by recent studies. Fetuin-A is capable of crossing the blood-brain barrier, inhibiting early inflammatory response in animal models of cerebral ischemia, thereby conferring a short-term neuroprotection against ischemic injury. Disruption of fetuin-A expression renders mice significantly more susceptible to lethal endotoxemia or sepsis; whereas repetitive administration of fetuin-A confers a dose-dependent and long-lasting protection in animal models of lethal endotoxemia and sepsis. Thus, fetuin-A occupies protective roles against injury- or infection-elicited inflammation.

6. Acknowledgment

We thank Arvin Jundoria for critical reading of the manuscript. Work in the author's laboratory was supported by the National Institute of General Medical Sciences (R01GM063075 and R01GM070817 to HW) and the National Center of Complementary & Alternative Medicine (R01AT05076 to HW).

7. References

Adibhatla R.M., Hatcher J.F., Sailor K. & Dempsey R.J. (2002) Polyamines and central nervous system injury: spermine and spermidine decrease following transient focal cerebral ischemia in spontaneously hypertensive rats. *Brain Res* 938, 81-86

Akopov S.E., Simonian N.A. & Grigorian G.S. (1996) Dynamics of polymorphonuclear leukocyte accumulation in acute cerebral infarction and their correlation with brain tissue damage. *Stroke* 27, 1739-1743

Andersson U., Wang H., Palmblad K., Aveberger A.C., Bloom O., Erlandsson-Harris H., Janson A., Kokkola R., Zhang M., Yang H. & Tracey K.J. (2000) High Mobility Group 1 Protein (HMG-1) Stimulates Proinflammatory Cytokine Synthesis in Human Monocytes. *J Exp Med* 192, 565-570

Araneda R.C., Lan J.Y., Zheng X., Zukin R.S. & Bennett M.V. (1999) Spermine and arcaine block and permeate N-methyl-D-aspartate receptor channels. *Biophys.J* 76, 2899-2911

Barone F.C., Arvin B., White R.F., Miller A., Webb C.L., Willette R.N., Lysko P.G. & Feuerstein G.Z. (1997) Tumor necrosis factor-alpha. A mediator of focal ischemic brain injury. *Stroke* 28, 1233-1244

Belayev L., Busto R., Zhao W. & Ginsberg M.D. (1996) Quantitative evaluation of blood-brain barrier permeability following middle cerebral artery occlusion in rats. *Brain Res.* 739, 88-96

Bell C.W., Jiang W., Reich C.F. & Pisetsky D.S. (2006) The Extracellular Release of HMGB1 during Apoptotic Cell Death. *Am J Physiol Cell Physiol* 291(6), C1318-1325

Bertorelli R., Adami M., Di Santo E. & Ghezzi P. (1998) MK 801 and dexamethasone reduce both tumor necrosis factor levels and infarct volume after focal cerebral ischemia in the rat brain. *Neurosci Lett* 246, 41-44

Botchkina G.I., Meistrell M.E., Botchkina I.L. & Tracey K.J. (1997) Expression of TNF and TNF receptors (p55 and p75) in the rat brain after focal cerebral ischemia. *Mol Med* 3, 765-781

Brightbill H.D., Libraty D.H., Krutzik S.R., Yang R.B., Belisle J.T., Bleharski J.R., Maitland M., Norgard M.V., Plevy S.E., Smale S.T., Brennan P.J., Bloom B.R., Godowski P.J. & Modlin R.L. (1999) Host defense mechanisms triggered by microbial lipoproteins through toll-like receptors. *Science* 285, 732-736

Buttini M., Appel K., Sauter A., Gebicke-Haerter P.J. & Boddeke H.W. (1996) Expression of tumor necrosis factor alpha after focal cerebral ischaemia in the rat. *Neuroscience* 71, 1-16

Chmiela M., Czkwianianc E., Wadstrom T. & Rudnicka W. (1997) Role of Helicobacter pylori surface structures in bacterial interaction with macrophages. *Gut* 40, 20-24

Christie D.L., Dziegielewska K.M., Hill R.M. & Saunders N.R. (1987) Fetuin: the bovine homologue of human alpha 2HS glycoprotein. *FEBS Lett* 214, 45-49

Daveau M., Christian D., Julen N., Hiron M., Arnaud P. & Lebreton J.P. (1988) The synthesis of human alpha-2-HS glycoprotein is down-regulated by cytokines in hepatoma HepG2 cells. *FEBS Lett* 241, 191-194

Demetriou M., Binkert C., Sukhu B., Tenenbaum H.C. & Dennis J.W. (1996) Fetuin/alpha2-HS glycoprotein is a transforming growth factor-beta type II receptor mimic and cytokine antagonist. *J Biol Chem* 271, 12755-12761

Dinarello C.A. (1996) Biologic basis for interleukin-1 in disease. *Blood* 87, 2095-2147

Dinarello C.A. & Thompson R.C. (1991) Blocking IL-1: interleukin 1 receptor antagonist in vivo and in vitro. *Immunol Today* 12, 404-410

Dubreuil J.D., Giudice G.D. & Rappuoli R. (2002) Helicobacter pylori interactions with host serum and extracellular matrix proteins: potential role in the infectious process. *Microbiol Mol Biol Rev* 66, 617-29, table

Dziegielewska K.M. & Andersen N.A. (1998) The fetal glycoprotein, fetuin, counteracts ill-effects of the bacterial endotoxin, lipopolysaccharide, in pregnancy. *Biol Neonate.* 74, 372-375

Dziegielewska K.M., Andersen N.A. & Saunders N.R. (1998) Modification of macrophage response to lipopolysaccharide by fetuin. *Immunol Lett* 60, 31-35

Dziegielewska K.M., Brown W.M., Gould C.C., Matthews N., Sedgwick J.E. & Saunders N.R. (1992) Fetuin: an acute phase protein in cattle. *J Comp Physiol [B]* 162, 168-171

Dziegielewska K.M., Daikuhara Y., Ohnishi T., Waite M.P., Ek J., Habgood M.D., Lane M.A., Potter A. & Saunders N.R. (2000) Fetuin in the developing neocortex of the rat: distribution and origin. *J Comp Neurol* 423, 373-388

Ferchmin P.A., Perez D. & Biello M. (2000) Spermine is neuroprotective against anoxia and N-methyl-D-aspartate in hippocampal slices. *Brain Res* 859, 273-279

Feuerstein G.Z., Wang X. & Barone F.C. (1998) The role of cytokines in the neuropathology of stroke and neurotrauma. *Neuroimmunomodulation* 5, 143-159

Fiuza C., Bustin M., Talwar S., Tropea M., Gerstenberger E., Shelhamer J.H. & Suffredini A.F. (2003) Inflammation-promoting activity of HMGB1 on human microvascular endothelial cells. *Blood* 101, 2652-2660

Goustin A.S. & Abou-Samra A.B. (2010) The "thrifty" gene encoding Ahsg/Fetuin-A meets the insulin receptor: Insights into the mechanism of insulin resistance. *Cell Signal*

Ha H.C., Sirisoma N.S., Kuppusamy P., Zweier J.L., Woster P.M. & Casero R.A., Jr. (1998) The natural polyamine spermine functions directly as a free radical scavenger. *Proc Natl Acad Sci U S A* 95, 11140-11145

Haasemann M., Nawratil P. & Muller-Esterl W. (1991) Rat tyrosine kinase inhibitor shows sequence similarity to human alpha 2-HS glycoprotein and bovine fetuin. *Biochem J* 274, 899-902

Heinzel F.P. (1990) The role of IFN-gamma in the pathology of experimental endotoxemia. *J Immunol* 145, 2920-2924

Heiss A., DuChesne A., Denecke B., Grotzinger J., Yamamoto K., Renne T. & Jahnen-Dechent W. (2003) Structural basis of calcification inhibition by alpha 2-HS glycoprotein/fetuin-A. Formation of colloidal calciprotein particles. *J Biol Chem* 278, 13333-13341

Hemmi H., Takeuchi O., Kawai T., Kaisho T., Sato S., Sanjo H., Matsumoto M., Hoshino K., Wagner H., Takeda K. & Akira S. (2000) A Toll-like receptor recognizes bacterial DNA. *Nature* 408, 740-745

Ivanov S., Dragoi A.M., Wang X., Dallacosta C., Louten J., Musco G., Sitia G., Yap G.S., Wan Y., Biron C.A., Bianchi M.E., Wang H. & Chu W.M. (2007) A novel role for HMGB1 in TLR9-mediated inflammatory responses to CpG-DNA. *Blood.* 110, 1970-1981

Ivanova S., Botchkina G.I., Al-Abed Y., Meistrell M., Batliwalla F., Dubinsky J.M., Iadecola C., Wang H., Gregersen P.K., Eaton J.W. & Tracey K.J. (1998) Cerebral ischemia enhances polyamine oxidation: identification of enzymatically formed 3-aminopropanal as an endogenous mediator of neuronal and glial cell death. *J Exp Med* 188, 327-340

Ix J.H., Wassel C.L., Kanaya A.M., Vittinghoff E., Johnson K.C., Koster A., Cauley J.A., Harris T.B., Cummings S.R. & Shlipak M.G. (2008) Fetuin-A and incident diabetes mellitus in older persons. *JAMA* 300, 182-188

Jahnen-Dechent W., Schafer C., Heiss A. & Grotzinger J. (2001) Systemic inhibition of spontaneous calcification by the serum protein alpha 2-HS glycoprotein/fetuin. *Z Kardiol* 90 Suppl 3, 47-56

Jersmann H.P., Dransfield I. & Hart S.P. (2003) Fetuin/alpha2-HS glycoprotein enhances phagocytosis of apoptotic cells and macropinocytosis by human macrophages. *Clin Sci (Lond)* 105, 273-278

Kato H., Kogure K., Liu X.H., Araki T. & Itoyama Y. (1996) Progressive expression of immunomolecules on activated microglia and invading leukocytes following focal cerebral ischemia in the rat. *Brain Res.* 734, 203-212

Ketteler M., Bongartz P., Westenfeld R., Wildberger J.E., Mahnken A.H., Bohm R., Metzger T., Wanner C., Jahnen-Dechent W. & Floege J. (2003) Association of low fetuin-A (AHSG) concentrations in serum with cardiovascular mortality in patients on dialysis: a cross-sectional study. *Lancet* 361, 827-833

Kitchener P.D., Dziegielewska K.M., Hutton E.J., Hinrichsen C.F. & Saunders N.R. (1999) Fetuin in neurons of the retina and cerebellum during fetal and postnatal development of the rat. *Int J Dev Neurosci* 17, 21-30

Kitchener P.D., Dziegielewska K.M., Knott G.W., Miller J.M., Nawratil P., Potter A.E. & Saunders N.R. (1997) Fetuin expression in the dorsal root ganglia and trigeminal ganglia of perinatal rats. *Int J Dev Neurosci* 15, 717-727

Krieg A.M. (2002) CpG motifs in bacterial DNA and their immune effects. *Annu Rev Immunol* 20, 709-760

Kusnierz-Cabala B., Gurda-Duda A., Panek J., Fedak D., Dumnicka P., Solnica B. & Kulig J. (2010) Serum fetuin A concentrations in patients with acute pancreatitis. *Clin Lab* 56, 191-195

Lee J.M., Zipfel G.J. & Choi D.W. (1999) The changing landscape of ischaemic brain injury mechanisms. *Nature* 399 Supplement, A7-A14

Li W., Zhu S., Li J., Huang Y., Zhou R., Fan X., Yang H., Gong X., Eissa N.T., Jahnen-Dechent W., Wang P., Tracey K.J., Sama A.E. & Wang H. (2011a) A hepatic protein, fetuin-A, occupies a protective role in lethal systemic inflammation. *PLoS ONE* 6(2), e16945

Li, W., Zhu S., Li J., Assa A., Xu J., Fan S., Eissa N.T., Tracey K.T., Sama A.E., & Wang H. (2011b). EGCG induces autophagy and reduced cytoplasmic HMGB1 levels in endotoxin-stimulated macrophages. *Biochem Pharmacol* 81(9), 1152-1163.

Liu K., Mori S., Takahashi H.K., Tomono Y., Wake H., Kanke T., Sato Y., Hiraga N., Adachi N., Yoshino T. & Nishibori M. (2007a) Anti-high mobility group box 1 monoclonal antibody ameliorates brain infarction induced by transient ischemia in rats. *FASEB J* 21, 3904-3916

Liu K., Mori S., Takahashi H.K., Tomono Y., Wake H., Kanke T., Sato Y., Hiraga N., Adachi N., Yoshino T. & Nishibori M. (2007b) Anti-high mobility group box 1 monoclonal antibody ameliorates brain infarction induced by transient ischemia in rats. *FASEB J* 21, 3904-3916

Lord J.M. (2003) A physiological role for alpha2-HS glycoprotein: stimulation of macrophage uptake of apoptotic cells. *Clin Sci (Lond)* 105, 267-268

Lv B., Wang H., Tang Y., Fan Z., Xiao X. & Chen F. (2009) High-mobility group box 1 protein induces tissue factor expression in vascular endothelial cells via activation of NF-kappaB and Egr-1. *Thromb Haemost* 102, 352-359

Mathews S.T., Srinivas P.R., Leon M.A. & Grunberger G. (1997) Bovine fetuin is an inhibitor of insulin receptor tyrosine kinase. *Life Sci* 61, 1583-1592

Meistrell M.E., Botchkina G.I., Wang H., Di Santo E., Cockroft K.M., Bloom O., Vishnubhakat J.M., Ghezzi P. & Tracey K.J. (1997) Tumor necrosis factor is a brain damaging cytokine in cerebral ischemia. *Shock* 8, 341-348

Meldrum B. (1990) Protection against ischaemic neuronal damage by drugs acting on excitatory neurotransmission. *Cerebrovasc Brain Metab Rev* 2, 27-57

Metry G., Stenvinkel P., Qureshi A.R., Carrero J.J., Yilmaz M.I., Barany P., Snaedal S., Heimburger O., Lindholm B. & Suliman M.E. (2008) Low serum fetuin-A concentration predicts poor outcome only in the presence of inflammation in prevalent haemodialysis patients. *Eur J Clin Invest* 38, 804-811

Muhammad S., Barakat W., Stoyanov S., Murikinati S., Yang H., Tracey K.J., Bendszus M., Rossetti G., Nawroth P.P., Bierhaus A. & Schwaninger M. (2008) The HMGB1 receptor RAGE mediates ischemic brain damage. *J Neurosci* 28, 12023-12031

Ombrellino M., Wang H., Yang H., Zhang M., Vishnubhakat J., Frazier A., Scher L.A., Friedman S.G. & Tracey K.J. (2001) Fetuin, a negative acute phase protein, attenuates TNF synthesis and the innate inflammatory response to carrageenan. *Shock* 15, 181-185

Paschen W. (1992) Polyamine metabolism in reversible cerebral ischemia. *Cerebrovasc Brain Metab Rev* 4, 59-88

Paschen W., Csiba L., Rohn G. & Bereczki D. (1991) Polyamine metabolism in transient focal ischemia of rat brain. *Brain Res* 566, 354-357

Paschen W., Widmann R. & Weber C. (1992) Changes in regional polyamine profiles in rat brains after transient cerebral ischemia (single versus repetitive ischemia): evidence for release of polyamines from injured neurons. *Neurosci Lett* 135, 121-124

Pedersen KO. (1944) Fetuin, a new globulin isolated from serum. *Nature* 154, 575-576

Peltz E.D., Moore E.E., Eckels P.C., Damle S.S., Tsuruta Y., Johnson J.L., Sauaia A., Silliman C.C., Banerjee A. & Abraham E. (2009) HMGB1 is markedly elevated within 6 hours of mechanical trauma in humans. *Shock* 32, 17-22

Poltorak A., He X., Smirnova I., Liu M.Y., Huffel C.V., Du X., Birdwell D., Alejos E., Silva M., Galanos C., Freudenberg M., Ricciardi-Castagnoli P., Layton B. & Beutler B. (1998) Defective LPS signaling in C3H/HeJ and C57BL/10ScCr mice: mutations in Tlr4 gene. *Science* 282, 2085-2088

Qin S., Wang H., Yuan R., Li H., Ochani M., Ochani K., Rosas-Ballina M., Czura C.J., Huston J.M., Miller E., Lin X., Sherry B., Kumar A., Larosa G., Newman W., Tracey K.J. & Yang H. (2006) Role of HMGB1 in apoptosis-mediated sepsis lethality. *J Exp Med* 203, 1637-1642

Qiu J., Nishimura M., Wang Y., Sims J.R., Qiu S., Savitz S.I., Salomone S. & Moskowitz M.A. (2008) Early release of HMGB-1 from neurons after the onset of brain ischemia. *J Cereb Blood Flow Metab* 28, 927-938

Rendon-Mitchell B., Ochani M., Li J., Han J., Wang H., Yang H., Susarla S., Czura C., Mitchell R.A., Chen G., Sama A.E., Tracey K.J. & Wang H. (2003) IFN-gamma Induces High Mobility Group Box 1 Protein Release Partly Through a TNF-Dependent Mechanism. *J Immunol* 170, 3890-3897

Rochette C.N., Rosenfeldt S., Heiss A., Narayanan T., Ballauff M. & Jahnen-Dechent W. (2009) A shielding topology stabilizes the early stage protein-mineral complexes of fetuin-A and calcium phosphate: a time-resolved small-angle X-ray study. *Chembiochem* 10, 735-740

Sato H., Kazama J.J., Wada Y., Kuroda T., Narita I., Gejyo F., Gao P. & Yamashita H. (2007) Decreased levels of circulating alpha2-Heremans-Schmid glycoprotein/Fetuin-A (AHSG) in patients with rheumatoid arthritis. *Intern Med* 46, 1685-1691

Schafer C., Heiss A., Schwarz A., Westenfeld R., Ketteler M., Floege J., Muller-Esterl W., Schinke T. & Jahnen-Dechent W. (2003) The serum protein alpha 2-Heremans-Schmid glycoprotein/fetuin-A is a systemically acting inhibitor of ectopic calcification. *J Clin Invest* 112, 357-366

Schinke T., Amendt C., Trindl A., Poschke O., Muller-Esterl W. & Jahnen-Dechent W. (1996) The serum protein alpha2-HS glycoprotein/fetuin inhibits apatite formation in vitro and in mineralizing calvaria cells. A possible role in mineralization and calcium homeostasis. *J Biol Chem* 271, 20789-20796

Suzuki M., Shimokawa H., Takagi Y. & Sasaki S. (1994) Calcium-binding properties of fetuin in fetal bovine serum. *J Exp Zoology* 270, 501-507

Szweras M., Liu D., Partridge E.A., Pawling J., Sukhu B., Clokie C., Jahnen-Dechent W., Tenenbaum H.C., Swallow C.J., Grynpas M.D. & Dennis J.W. (2002) alpha 2-HS glycoprotein/fetuin, a transforming growth factor-beta/bone morphogenetic protein antagonist, regulates postnatal bone growth and remodeling. *J Biol Chem* 277, 19991-19997

Taylor C.P. & Meldrum B.S. (1995) Na+ channels as targets for neuroprotective drugs. *Trends Pharmacol Sci* 16, 309-316

Terkelsen O.B., Jahnen-Dechent W., Nielsen H., Moos T., Fink E., Nawratil P., Muller-Esterl W. & Mollgard K. (1998) Rat fetuin: distribution of protein and mRNA in embryonic and neonatal rat tissues. *Anat Ebryol (Berl)* 197, 125-133

Tracey K.J., Fong Y., Hesse D.G., Manogue K.R., Lee A.T., Kuo G.C., Lowry S.F. & Cerami A. (1987) Anti-cachectin/TNF monoclonal antibodies prevent septic shock during lethal bacteraemia. *Nature* 330, 662-664

Treutiger C.J., Mullins G.E., Johansson A.S., Rouhiainen A., Rauvala H.M., Erlandsson-Harris H., Andersson U., Yang H., Tracey K.J., Andersson J. & Palmblad J.E. (2003) High mobility group 1 B-box mediates activation of human endothelium. *J Intern Med* 254, 375-385

Tsung A., Klune J.R., Zhang X., Jeyabalan G., Cao Z., Peng X., Stolz D.B., Geller D.A., Rosengart M.R. & Billiar T.R. (2007) HMGB1 release induced by liver ischemia involves Toll-like receptor 4 dependent reactive oxygen species production and calcium-mediated signaling. *J Exp Med* 204, 2913-2923

Tsung A., Sahai R., Tanaka H., Nakao A., Fink M.P., Lotze M.T., Yang H., Li J., Tracey K.J., Geller D.A. & Billiar T.R. (2005) The nuclear factor HMGB1 mediates hepatic injury after murine liver ischemia-reperfusion. *J Exp Med* 201, 1135-1143

Tuttolomondo A., Di Raimondo D., Di Sciacca R., Casuccio A., Bivona G., Bellia C., Barreca L., Serio A., D'Aguanno G., Ciaccio M., Licata G. & Pinto A. (2010) Fetuin-A and CD40 L plasma levels in acute ischemic stroke: differences in relation to TOAST subtype and correlation with clinical and laboratory variables. *Atherosclerosis.* 208, 290-296

Wang H., Bloom O., Zhang M., Vishnubhakat J.M., Ombrellino M., Che J., Frazier A., Yang H., Ivanova S., Borovikova L., Manogue K.R., Faist E., Abraham E., Andersson J., Andersson U., Molina P.E., Abumrad N.N., Sama A. & Tracey K.J. (1999) HMG-1 as a late mediator of endotoxin lethality in mice. *Science* 285, 248-251

Wang H., Li W., Zhu S., Li J., D'Amore J., Ward M.F., Yang H., Wu R., Jahnen-Dechent W., Tracey K.J., Wang P. & Sama A.E. (2010) Peripheral administration of fetuin-A attenuates early cerebral ischemic injury in rats. J Cereb Blood Flow Metab 30, 493-504

Wang H., Liao H., Ochani M., Justiniani M., Lin X., Yang L., Al Abed Y., Wang H., Metz C., Miller E.J., Tracey K.J. & Ulloa L. (2004) Cholinergic agonists inhibit HMGB1 release and improve survival in experimental sepsis. *Nat Med* 10, 1216-1221

Wang H. & Tracey K.J. (1999) Fetuin opsonizes macrophage-deactivating cations. In: *Update in Intensive Care and Emergency Medicine: Immune Response in the Critically Ill* (eds Marshall J.C. & Cohen J.), pp. 155-163. SpringerVerlag Press.

Wang H., Ward M.F. & Sama A.E. (2009) Novel HMGB1-inhibiting therapeutic agents for experimental sepsis. *Shock.* 32, 348-357

Wang H., Yang H., Czura C.J., Sama A.E. & Tracey K.J. (2001) HMGB1 as a Late Mediator of Lethal Systemic Inflammation. *Am J Respir Crit Care Med* 164, 1768-1773

Wang H., Zhang M., Soda K., Sama A. & Tracey K.J. (1997) Fetuin protects the fetus from TNF [letter]. *Lancet* 350, 861-862

Wang H., Zhu S., Zhou R., Li W. & Sama A.E. (2008) Therapeutic potential of HMGB1-targeting agents in sepsis. *Expert Rev Mol Med* 10:e32.

Watanabe T., Kubota S., Nagaya M., Ozaki S., Nagafuchi H., Akashi K., Taira Y., Tsukikawa S., Oowada S. & Nakano S. (2005) The role of HMGB-1 on the development of necrosis during hepatic ischemia and hepatic ischemia/reperfusion injury in mice. *J Surg Res* 124, 59-66

Weikert C., Stefan N., Schulze M.B., Pischon T., Berger K., Joost H.G., Haring H.U., Boeing H. & Fritsche A. (2008) Plasma fetuin-a levels and the risk of myocardial infarction and ischemic stroke. *Circulation* 118, 2555-2562

Williams K. (1997) Modulation and block of ion channels: a new biology of polyamines. *Cell Signal* 9, 1-13

Wu C.Y., Martel J., Young D. & Young J.D. (2009) Fetuin-A/albumin-mineral complexes resembling serum calcium granules and putative nanobacteria: demonstration of a dual inhibition-seeding concept. *PLoS.One.* 4, e8058

Wu H., Chen G., Wyburn K.R., Yin J., Bertolino P., Eris J.M., Alexander S.I., Sharland A.F. & Chadban S.J. (2007) TLR4 activation mediates kidney ischemia/reperfusion injury. *J.Clin.Invest* 117, 2847-2859

Yang G.Y., Gong C., Qin Z., Liu X.H. & Lorris B.A. (1999) Tumor necrosis factor alpha expression produces increased blood-brain barrier permeability following temporary focal cerebral ischemia in mice. *Brain Res Mol Brain Res* 69, 135-143

Yang H., Ochani M., Li J., Qiang X., Tanovic M., Harris H.E., Susarla S.M., Ulloa L., Wang H., DiRaimo R., Czura C.J., Wang H., Roth J., Warren H.S., Fink M.P., Fenton M.J., Andersson U. & Tracey K.J. (2004) Reversing established sepsis with antagonists of endogenous high-mobility group box 1. *Proc Natl Acad Sci U S A* 101, 296-301

Zaremba J. & Losy J. (2001) Early TNF-alpha levels correlate with ischaemic stroke severity. *Acta Neurol Scand* 104(5), 288-295

Zhang M., Borovikova L.V., Wang H., Metz C. & Tracey K.J. (1999) Spermine inhibition of monocyte activation and inflammation. *Mol Med* 5, 595-605

Zhang M., Caragine T., Wang H., Cohen P.S., Botchkina G., Soda K., Bianchi M., Ulrich P., Cerami A., Sherry B. & Tracey K.J. (1997) Spermine inhibits proinflammatory cytokine synthesis in human mononuclear cells: a counterregulatory mechanism that restrains the immune response. *J Exp Med* 185, 1759-1768

Zhang M., Wang H. & Tracey K.J. (2000) Regulation of macrophage activation and inflammation by spermine: a new chapter in an old story. *Crit Care Med* 28, N60-N66

Zhu S., Ashok M., Li J., Li W., Yang H., Wang P., Tracey K.J., Sama A.E. & Wang H. (2009a) Spermine protects mice against lethal sepsis partly by attenuating surrogate inflammatory markers. *Mol Med* 15, 275-282

Zhu S., Li W., Ward M.F., Sama A.E. & Wang H. (2010) High mobility group box 1 protein as a potential drug target for infection- and injury-elicited inflammation. *Inflamm.Allergy Drug Targets.* 9, 60-72

Zubrow A.B., Numagami Y., Fritz K.I., Mishra O.P. & Delivoria-Papadopoulos M. (2000) Spermine dependent activation of the N-methyl-D-aspartate receptor and the effect of nitric oxide synthase inhibition during hypoxia in the cerebral cortex of newborn piglets. *Brain Res* 854, 11-18

16

Neutrophil Gelatinase Associated Lipocalin: Structure, Function and Role in Human Pathogenesis

Subhankar Chakraborty[1], Sukhwinder Kaur[1], Zhimin Tong[2], Surinder K. Batra[1] and Sushovan Guha[2]
[1]*University of Nebraska Medical Center, Omaha, NE*
[2]*The University of Texas MD Anderson Cancer Center, Houston, Texas*
USA

1. Introduction

Glycoproteins have a unique position in the pathogenesis of human diseases. Most of the commonly employed protein biomarkers are glycoproteins. Examples include CA19-9 (carbohydrate antigen 19-9) to follow-up patients with pancreatic cancer, CEA (carcinoembryonic antigen) for multiple solid tumors and CA125 (carbohydrate antigen 125) used in the diagnosis, follow-up and therapy of patients with ovarian cancer. Most of these glycoproteins are large molecules. However, there is a family of smaller, secreted glycoproteins (called lipocalins) that are important in the maintenance of health and in combating diseases effectively. A prototype of this family is a small, secreted glycoprotein called Neutrophil gelatinase associated lipocalin or NGAL. In recent years, NGAL has emerged as a novel biomarker in several benign and malignant diseases. Further, studies in cultured cells and in murine models have revealed a pivotal role for this molecule in several physiological processes and pathological conditions. In this Chapter, we review the biology of lipocalins, focusing specifically on NGAL and its role in human health and disease.

2. The lipocalin family

Lipocalins are a family of small (160-180 amino acids long) secreted proteins that mediate (among other functions) a common functional role- i.e., transportation of small hydrophobic ligands. Most protein families are classified on the basis of similarity in amino acid sequences, domain architecture and three-dimensional protein structure. The lipocalins however are a unique exception in that the percentage of sequence identity among different members of the lipocalin family is sometimes even lower than the minimum (20%) identity required to call it a reliable alignment (Flower *et al.*, 2000; Flower, 1996; Flower, 1995; Flower, 1994). Despite this lack of a sequence similarity, the lipocalins share three short stretches of amino acid sequences (or motifs) that are part of the structural conservation among different lipocalin sequences. These motifs, which are aptly termed as "structurally conserved regions or SCRs" are used to classify this large family into two main sub-families-the "kernel" and the "outlier" lipocalins (**Table 1**). The kernel lipocalins contain all three motifs while the outlier lipocalins contain only one or two of these (but not all three) SCRs.

Abbreviation	Protein name
Kernel Lipocalins	
Alpha 1M	Alpha 1-microglobulin
ApoD	Apolipoprotein D
A2U	α2micro-Globulin
BBP	Bilin binding protein
Blg	β1-Lactoglobulin
C8γ	C8γ
CPP	Choroid plexus protein
CRABP2	Cellular Retinoic acid binding protein
ACC	α-Crustacyanin
MUP	Major Urinary Protein
NGAL	Neutrophil gelatinase associated Lipocalin
PGDS	Prostaglandin D synthase
PP14	Pregnancy protein 14
PURP	Purpurin
	Lazarillo
Outlier Lipocalins	
AAAG	Alpha 1-Acid glycoprotein
	Aphrodisin
OBP	Odorant binding protein
	Probasin
VEGP	von Ebner's-gland protein

Table 1. List of known Kernel and Outlier Lipocalin proteins

The secondary and tertiary structure of the lipocalin family members is very similar and is characterized by the presence of a "lipocalin fold"- a symmetrical structure comprised almost entirely of β-pleated sheets closed at the two ends by two α helices (**Figure 1)**. There are eight antiparallel β sheets linked to each other by seven short loops. The N-terminal region of the protein forms the ligand binding cavity which is closed by a conserved 3_{10} helix. The cup-shaped cavity of the lipocalins enclosed within the β-pleated sheets is well adapted for binding to a wide array of hydrophobic ligands- for instance, while retinol binding protein (RBP) binds primarily to its endogenous ligand retinol, it can also bind to several other hydrophobic ligands including β-ionone, β-carotene, cholesterol, terpenoids and long chain esters of retinol and retinoic acid.

Many lipocalins have also been shown to bind to specific receptors including RBP, alpha1-microglobulin, major urinary protein (MUP) and Odorant-binding protein (OBP). A third property of lipocalins is their tendency to form complexes with soluble macromolecules. Some of the well-known protein-protein complexes involving the lipocalin family members include the complex of RBP with transthyretin, NGAL with human neutrophil gelatinase, C8γ with C8α as part of the membrane attack complex (MAC) and α1-microglobulin (A1M) with immunoglobulin A (IgA). These associations may either serve to transport proteins

(RBP), stabilize the interactor (NGAL), protect normal cells from damage (C8γ) or alter the biological activity of the interacting protein (A1M).

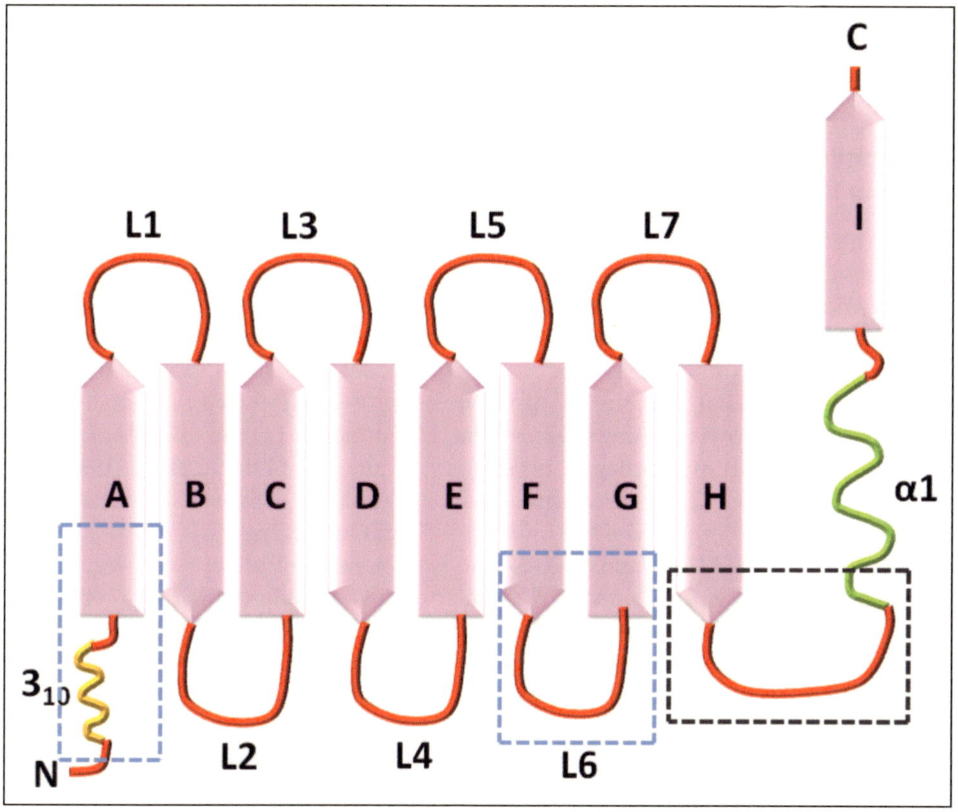

Fig. 1. Schematic representation of the lipocalin fold. The characteristic feature of lipocalins is the "lipocalin fold" which comprises of an N-terminal 3-10 helix followed by eight beta sheets (A-I) arranged in an antiparallel orientation. The eighth beta sheet is connected to an alpha helix (denoted as α1), which is in turn connected to a C-terminal beta sheet. The beta sheets are connected by loops (L1-L7). Loops L1,L3,L5 and L7 form the open end of the molecule (i.e. the opening to the ligand binding site of NGAL). The portion of the lipocalin fold that are structurally conserved between different lipocalins is indicated by the blue boxed regions while the region that shows significant conservation in amino acid sequence is indicated by the black boxed region.

Functionally, the lipocalins are generally well known as transport proteins that exist in the extracellular space. The prototypical lipocalin involved in transport of cargo in the body is RBP which binds to and transports retinol (Vitamin A) from the liver to various organs. Binding to RBP not only protects retinol from being excreted by the kidneys but also from being oxidized within the body. Further, it also permits the transport of a relatively insoluble retinol in the form of a soluble complex to the tissues to mediate its effects. Other functions attributed to lipocalins including regulation of cell ageing, survival and differentiation (probasin and purpurin), modulation of immune response (NGAL, AGP, PP14 and AIM), prostaglandin synthesis (glutathione-independent PGD2 synthase), coloration (insecticyanin, BBP and crusticyanin), smell (OBP), taste (VEGP) and as sex hormones or pheromones (MUP and Aphrodisin) (Flower *et al.*, 2000; Flower, 1996; Flower, 1995; Flower, 1994). We will examine the role of a member of the lipocalin family (NGAL) that has been extensively studied particularly as a potential marker for diagnosis and prognosis in several human diseases. We will investigate its biology, functions and clinical applications both in benign and malignant diseases.

3. Neutrophil gelatinase associated lipocalin (NGAL)-genomic organization and protein structure

Neutrophil gelatinase associated lipocalin (NGAL) also known as migration stimulating factor inhibitor (MSFI), human neutrophil lipocalin (HNL), alpha-1 microglobulin related protein, siderocalin or uterocalin is a 198 amino acid glycoprotein encoded by a gene located on the chromosome locus 3p11. It was first isolated from mouse kidney cells infected with a simian virus (SV-40) (Hraba-Renevey *et al.*, 1989). Triebel and colleagues identified a novel association between NGAL and the gelatinolytic enzyme MMP-9 (matrix metalloproteinase 9 or gelatinase B) known to degrade several components of the basement membrane including type I gelatin and collagen types I, IV, V and XI (Triebel *et al.*, 1992). Human NGAL protein (or LCN2) is represented in upper case, while the murine and rat homologues are usually represented in lower case (Ngal or Lcn2).

Structurally, human NGAL contains a 20-amino acid signal peptide at the N-terminal end of the protein followed by the "lipocalin" domain. This domain which is responsible for binding of lipocalins to their ligands, is structurally comprised of an eight stranded β barrel with its loops running in an antiparallel direction. A comparison of the amino acid sequence between NGAL homologues in different species reveals that human NGAL is highly similar to the homologue present in chimpanzees (98% identity) but shows much less identity to the mouse and rat homologues (62% and 63% identity respectively). Despite the limited identity of their amino acid sequences, the mouse and human homologue are remarkably similar in their domain architecture (**Figure 2**) and three-dimensional structure. This feature, i.e. marked structural identity in the absence of significant sequence identity is a common feature of the lipocalin-family of proteins and underlies the conserved function of the lipocalin domain. Studies carried out on mouse Ngal (also called mLcn2) have revealed that it can bind hydrophobic ligands like retinol, cholesterol oleate and oleic acid (Chu *et al.*, 1998). NMR (nuclear magnetic resonance) studies have revealed that the NGAL molecule contains eight antiparallel β strands that form a barrel shaped structure (Coles *et al.*, 1999). Three β bulges present in this barrel (one formed by the 1st and two by the 6th β strand) have been suggested to contribute to the ligand binding site of NGAL. Hydrophobic residues (Tryptophan, Valine and Phenylalanine) present at the base of this barrel-like structure have been shown to be involved in direct binding to the ligand. A patch of positively charged amino acid residues (Lysine and Arginine) present near the mouth of the barrel and projecting into the open end of the molecule has also been suggested to be also important in binding to ligands. Further, a negatively charged "pit" present at the base of the barrel formed by the amino acids Aspartate and Glutamate and a nearby unpaired Cysteine residue have been suggested to be crucial for binding of NGAL to the gelatinase MMP-9. Based on whether NGAL is free or bound to a ligand, it is termed as "apo" or "holo" NGAL respectively. The conformational change between these two forms of the protein is affected by a conformation change occurring at the open end of the NGAL protein.

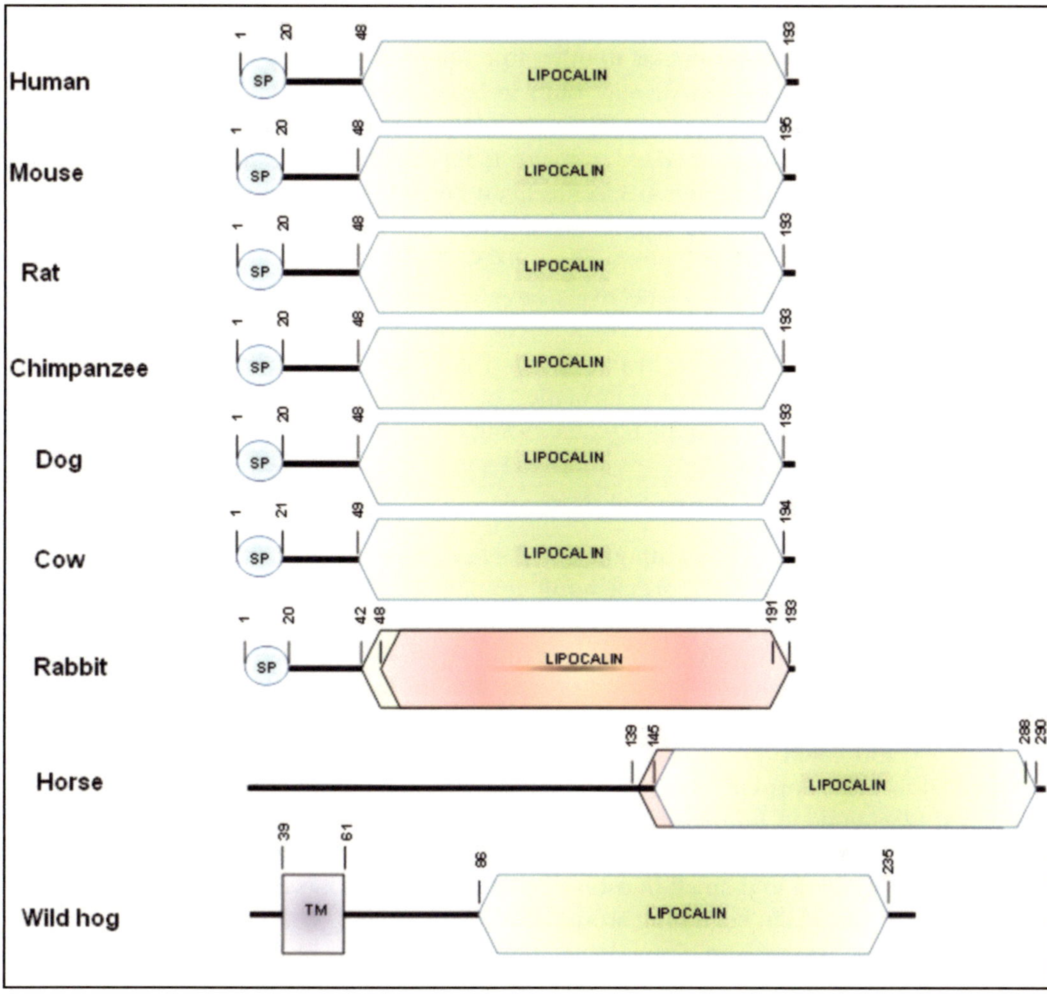

Fig. 2. Domain architecture of human NGAL and its homologues. Human NGAL and its homologues are characterized by a high degree of similarity in their domain architecture. All NGAL homologues (with the exception of the horse and wild hog) contain an N-terminal signal peptide which is cleaved prior to secretion of the protein. This is followed by the lipocalin domain (IPR000566 Lipocln_cytosolic_FA-bd) which makes up most of the length of the protein. This domain which has the consensus sequence [DENG] - {A} - [DENQGSTARK] - x(0,2) - [DENQARK] - [LIVFY] - {CP} - G - {C} - W - [FYWLRH] - {D} - [LIVMTA] is characteristic of proteins belonging to the lipocalin family. Structurally, the lipocalin domain is an eight stranded antiparallel beta barrel enclosing a ligand binding site which can bind to small hydrophobic molecules (e.g. steroids, retinoids, bilins and lipids). The rabbit and horse NGAL proteins also contain a second domain called the "lipocalin-2" domain (Accession number: IPR013208 Lipocalin_2). This domain is present in a small number of proteins (calycin, apolipoprotein D and Lipocalin 2) and is believed to be involved in the transport of hydrophobic ligands (Source: http://www.ebi.ac.uk/interpro/).

Recent data on the ligand binding pocket of NGAL has revealed that it is significantly larger and more polar than a similar pocket in other lipocalin proteins (Goetz *et al.*, 2000). This has led to the speculation that NGAL may bind to large, macromolecular and relatively less hydrophobic ligands including mammalian proteins. However, the identity of one or more of these mammalian ligands for NGAL remains to be elucidated. However, NGAL has been shown to bind to bacterial proteins. Specifically, it binds to iron-chelating proteins released by both gram negative bacteria (i.e. enterobacteria) and mycobacteria (e.g. *Mycobacterium tuberculosis*) (Nairz *et al.*, 2009; Holmes *et al.*, 2005). These proteins, termed as enterochelin and carboxymycobactin (CMB) respectively have been shown to bind to the ligand binding cavity of NGAL. The latter (i.e. CMBs) however, forms a better fit into the ligand binding pocket of NGAL. This has been in part attributed to the larger number of hydrophobic residues in CMBs which permits the formation of a larger number of hydrogen bonds and Van Der Walls interactions with the ligand binding cavity of NGAL.

3. Expression of NGAL in normal tissues

Although first discovered as a component of the late granules of neutrophils, NGAL is also strongly expressed in several normal adult human tissues including the non-neoplastic breast ducts, kidney, liver, lungs, trachea, small intestine, bone marrow, thymus, prostate, adipose tissue and macrophages. A weak to no expression of NGAL is observed in the normal pancreas, endometrial glands, and the thymus and peripheral blood leucocytes. NGAL is however completely absent from the normal brain, heart, skeletal muscle, spleen, testes, ovary and colon (Le, V *et al.*, 1997; Seth *et al.*, 2002; Moreno-Navarrete *et al.*, 2010; Cowland *et al.*, 2003; Furutani *et al.*, 1998; Cowland and Borregaard, 1997).

Limited studies done in human fetal tissues reveal that NGAL is expressed in trophoblast cells of the placenta, cartilage forming cells (chondrocytes) and in the epithelial cells present in the developing lung and small intestine. NGAL expression has also been reported in the epidermis of the fetal skin beginning around the 20th week of gestation. With increasing age of the fetus, the expression spreads to the lower layers of the skin and becomes progressively concentrated around the hair follicles (Mallbris *et al.*, 2002).

4. Altered expression of NGAL in benign and malignant diseases

4.1 Inflammatory diseases

The expression of NGAL is altered in several benign disease conditions including inflammatory and metabolic disorders. Inflammatory conditions associated with an increase in NGAL expression include pancreatitis, meningitis, myocarditis, psoriasis and periodontitis.

Acute pancreatitis (AP) is a reversible, acute inflammation of the pancreas that affects nearly 210,000 patients every year in the United States alone (Banks and Freeman, 2006). While nearly 85% of these patients have a mild form of the illness (termed as mild acute pancreatitis or MAP) and make an uneventful recovery, about 15%-20% of them develop features of severe acute pancreatitis (SAP) (Carroll *et al.*, 2007). SAP is associated with significant morbidity and mortality primarily owing to multi-organ failure (MOF, usually in the first week following onset of disease) and infected pancreatic necrosis (2 weeks or later after onset of disease). We have reported that compared to healthy individuals and those with MAP, plasma NGAL levels are significantly elevated (nearly 15-fold) within 48 hours (of onset of symptoms) in patients with SAP (Chakraborty *et al.*, 2010). The NGAL levels showed a tendency to decline when measured in blood samples collected at later time points (i.e. 72 hrs, 96 hrs and 120 hrs). To get a better idea of the time course of the rise in NGAL levels in the blood, we induced either mild or severe acute pancreatitis in mice and followed the change in plasma Ngal levels over time. We found that Ngal levels in mice rose early (within 6 hours following induction of AP) and remained elevated in those with SAP while trending down to levels in control mice (no pancreatitis) and in those with MAP.

Meningitis, particularly that caused by gram negative bacteria can cause a systemic inflammatory response syndrome (SIRS) associated with sepsis and significant mortality. A key mediator of this inflammatory response is lipopolysaccharide (LPS), a structural biomolecule present in the outer wall of gram negative bacteria. LPS is a potent stimulator of the immune response and a central player in septic shock in patients with gram negative bacterial infections. Ngal mRNA levels were found to be significantly induced in the choroid plexus (a structure in the ventricles of the brain that produces cerebrospinal fluid) within 12 hours following intraperitoneal injection of LPS while the levels of circulating Ngal (in the cerebrospinal fluid) was strongly induced within 6 hours after injection of LPS (Marques *et al.*, 2008).

A significant increase in the level of circulating Ngal was also noted in rats induced to develop features of autoimmune myocarditis by injection of purified porcine myosin (Ding *et al.*, 2010). However, compared to the acute inflammations described earlier, the elevation in Ngal in the rats was significantly delayed, being first evident 9 days following immunization with the foreign protein. A significant increase in NGAL mRNA levels has also been reported in the heart tissues from patients with myocarditis (Ding *et al.*, 2010).

Psoriasis, a chronic inflammatory disease of the skin is characterized by the formation of plaques covered by variable amount of scales. NGAL mRNA levels were shown to be significantly upregulated (nearly 10-fold) in the psoriatic lesions (Nomura *et al.*, 2003; Mallbris *et al.*, 2002). Further, NGAL levels were also upregulated in lesions that like psoriasis, exhibited a dysregulation in the process of keratinocyte differentiation (termed as parakeratosis). These diseases include pityriasis rubra pilaris, porokeratosis and chronic (not acute) eczema. Significantly, NGAL expression (from the affected areas of skin) disappeared once the psoriatic lesions had healed with treatment, suggesting that NGAL may play a role in the pathogenesis of diseases with dysregulated epidermal differentiation.

NGAL levels were significantly elevated in gum (i.e. alveolar mucosa) tissue from patients affected with localized juvenile periodontitis (LJP), a chronic inflammatory disease of the gums affecting young adults and associated with severe destruction of both soft tissues and bone (Van Dyke *et al.*, 1985). In addition to bacterial infections, NGAL, particularly circulating levels are significantly altered in certain viral infections. For instance, circulating NGAL levels were significantly lower in patients infected with the human immune deficiency virus (HIV) who had not received any therapy (i.e. treatment naïve) compared to non-HIV controls. Significantly, treatment of these patients with the highly active anti-retroviral therapy (HAART) was associated with a progressive increase in circulating NGAL levels (Landro *et al.*, 2008). In vitro studies using neutrophils isolated from the three groups of patient revealed that in healthy and HAART-treated HIV positive patients, the neutrophils released NGAL normally into the culture medium. However, in untreated HIV positive patients, this process was defective suggesting that the release of NGAL from neutrophils is inhibited by HIV infection and can be restored following therapy. What proteins of the virus mediate this inhibition, and if there is a prognostic significance of the restoration of NGAL levels following HAART therapy remain unanswered questions.

4.2 Metabolic diseases

Metabolic diseases associated with a dysregulation in NGAL expression include obesity, pre-eclampsia and kidney disease.

Obesity, defined as a body mass index (BMI) of $\geq 30 kg/m^2$ is now recognized to be associated with low grade chronic inflammation and insulin resistance (Pi-Sunyer, 2002). Studies have shown that NGAL levels are significantly elevated in the adipose tissues of both overweight mice and obese human subjects (Wang *et al.*, 2007). Studies in healthy human subjects have revealed that insulin can significantly increase the level of circulating NGAL in the blood (Tan *et al.*, 2009). Similar results have emerged from studies in pregnant women with gestational diabetes who had significantly higher levels of circulating NGAL than those without this complication of pregnancy (D'Anna *et al.*, 2009a).

Another pregnancy associated complication associated with a rise in circulating NGAL levels is pre-eclampsia. This condition, characterized by the development of hypertension in or after the 20th week of pregnancy is associated with significant maternal and fetal complications. The elevated levels of NGAL in pre-eclampsia were positively correlated with both systolic and diastolic blood pressure and presence of proteinuria but showed a significant negative correlation with maternal age, pre-pregnancy BMI and weight (D'Anna *et al.*, 2008; D'Anna *et al.*, 2009b). Other conditions where NGAL levels are significantly elevated include atherosclerosis (Anwaar *et al.*, 1998; Elneihoum *et al.*, 1997; te Boekhorst *et al.*, 2011) and hepatitis (Bu *et al.*, 2006). Both hyperlipidemia and chronic alcohol ingestion are associated with significant metabolic perturbations and the aforementioned correlative studies suggest that NGAL has a role to play in the pathogenesis of these diseases. With the development of animal models to study the function of NGAL (discussed later), it is expected that the mechanisms by which NGAL modulates metabolic pathways in health and disease will become better delineated in the near future.

The kidney is essential for our survival as it performs the crucial function of maintaining the fluid and mineral balance in our body. This in turn maintains the osmolarity of inter and intracellular fluids crucial for cellular metabolism. Both acute and chronic damage to the kidneys causes metabolic perturbations associated with a significant increase in the expression of NGAL.

Chronic kidney disease (CKD) is a disease characterized by a progressive decline in renal function and associated with significant morbidity. Studies in a mouse model that mimics the pathophysiology of CKD in humans revealed that NGAL is the most highly upregulated gene in the kidneys of mice with severe CKD (Viau *et al.*, 2010). It appears that the damaged kidneys synthesize a significantly higher amount of NGAL than usual, particularly in the proximal convoluted tubules (PCT) and the ascending limb of the loop of Henle. NGAL being a secreted protein is then released into the ultrafiltrate and subsequently excreted in urine. The level of Ngal expression in the diseased kidneys correlated positively with the severity of renal lesions (in mice) suggesting that Ngal may promote renal damage in CKD (Viau *et al.*, 2010). A similar observation was also noted in an animal model of autosomal polycystic kidney disease (ADPKD), another cause of CKD in humans (Lau *et al.*, 2000).

NGAL levels are elevated in acute kidney injury (AKI) resulting from a wide variety of insults to the kidney ranging from ischemia to toxins. This rise occurs early and depends on both the cause and the extent of renal damage. For instance, following ischemic injury, NGAL levels in the kidney tissue rises by nearly 10-fold within only 3 hours (Mishra *et al.*, 2003). Further, the rise appears to be sustained, being evident for several days following the initial insult. This pattern, an early rise and persistence, makes NGAL a highly sensitive marker of early AKI. Like in CKD, the kidney is the major source of NGAL release in AKI. However, other sources of NGAL that have been suggested include organs that synthesize and release mediators of an acute inflammatory response (e.g. the liver) and immune cells that contain NGAL in their granules (neutrophils and macrophages) (Hvidberg *et al.*, 2005).

4.3 Malignant diseases

The expression of NGAL is significantly increased in several solid and hematological tumors and been shown to correlate with both tumor characteristics and disease outcome. Solid tumors that express high levels of NGAL arise in a variety of organs including the digestive (e.g. esophagus, stomach, liver, bile ducts and pancreas), respiratory (lungs), endocrine (thyroid gland and ovaries), reproductive (breast and endometrium) organs and even in the skin.

Pancreatic cancer (PC) is the most lethal of all malignant solid tumors in humans (Chakraborty *et al.*, 2011). Several groups including ours have now shown that while NGAL is either completely absent or weakly expressed in the normal pancreatic ducts, a strong expression of NGAL is seen in the malignant cells (Moniaux *et al.*, 2008; Furutani *et al.*, 1998; Tong *et al.*, 2008; Tong *et al.*, 2011). We also observed that the expression of NGAL first appears in pre-malignant lesions (termed as Pancreatic intraepithelial neoplasia or PanINs), with a progressive increase from low to high grade dysplasia. In invasive pancreatic cancer, NGAL expression was significantly higher in well-differentiated PC while poorly differentiated cancer cells showed no expression of the protein (Moniaux *et al.*, 2008). Functional studies to investigate the role of NGAL in PC (discussed later) suggest that it plays a role in the progression of this deadly malignancy. Further, quantitative measurement of NGAL levels in plasma revealed that there was a significant increase in the levels of NGAL in the plasma compared to healthy individuals. These results suggest that NGAL might be potentially useful as a novel biomarker for the diagnosis of PC. Similar to PC, NGAL was weakly expressed by the normal liver cells but strongly expressed in hepatocellular carcinoma (Lee *et al.*, 2011). In gastric cancer however, NGAL expression remains controversial with two groups reporting opposing results- one reporting overexpression and the other a significant downregulation of NGAL in pre-malignant and malignant gastric tissues (Alpizar *et al.*, 2009; Wang *et al.*, 2010).

Ngal, the mouse homologue of human NGAL was strongly upregulated in mice that overexpress Insulin like growth factor (IGF-2), a major growth promoting hormone that acts during *in utero* development. These mice developed lung tumors spontaneously which showed a significant upregulation of Ngal mRNA.

Among the endocrine tumors, papillary, follicular and anaplastic thyroid cancers all express NGAL (Iannetti *et al.*, 2008). Notably, the expression of NGAL increases with the loss of tumor differentiation. While NGAL is not detected in the normal ovarian follicles and weakly expressed in benign ovarian tumors, a strong expression of NGAL is noted in borderline and grade 1 (well differentiated) malignant ovarian tumors (Lim *et al.*, 2007). Interestingly, its expression decreased in grade 2 (moderately differentiated) and 3 (poorly differentiated) ovarian cancer (Cho and Kim, 2009).

Of the malignancies arising from reproductive organs, ductal carcinoma of the breast and endometrial cancer express high levels of NGAL (Miyamoto *et al.*, 2011; Bauer *et al.*, 2008).

NGAL appears to promote the progression of breast cancer, being higher in actively proliferating cells, in lymph node metastasis and cells positive for the human epidermal growth factor receptor-2 (HER-2/ErbB2). Studies in cell lines suggest that NGAL expression in breast cancer may be regulated by HER-2 (Stoesz and Gould, 1995). In fact, another name for the Ngal protein in rats is Neu-related lipocalin (Neu being the other name for HER-2).

Microarray analysis using microdissected normal and malignant endometrial glands revealed that NGAL was strongly upregulated in the malignant endometrial glands . Immunohistochemical analysis of formalin fixed and paraffin embedded tissues also revealed that while the normal endometrium showed a weak expression of NGAL, a strong expression was noted in the areas of endometrial carcinoma (Miyamoto *et al.*, 2011).

NGAL is also secreted by the malignant cells in hematological malignancies. Studies done on the murine homolog of NGAL (24p3/Ngal) suggest that in leukemias, particularly those where the cells expresses BCR-ABL, *24p3/Ngal* is strongly expressed by the malignant cells (Devireddy *et al.*, 2005; Arlinghaus and Leng, 2008). BCR-ABL is a fusion protein that is found in association with certain leukemias, chiefly chronic myelogenous leukemia (CML) and to a lesser extent in acute lymphoblastic leukemia (ALL) and rarely in acute myelogenous leukemia (AML). This fusion results from a reciprocal translocation event occurring between the long arms of chromosomes 9 and 22. The resultant protein encodes for a protein kinase, specifically a tyrosine kinase that is constitutively active (i.e. does not require any external activation signal). As shown in **Figure 3**, normal hematopoietic cells (but not the BCR-ABL positive leukemia cells) in mice express the receptor for Ngal (called NgalR or 24p3R). The leukemia cells release large quantities of 24p3/Ngal into the bloodstream which acts via its receptor to induce cell death in the normal hematopoietic cells. Since the leukemic cells do not express the receptor, they remain unaffected. This

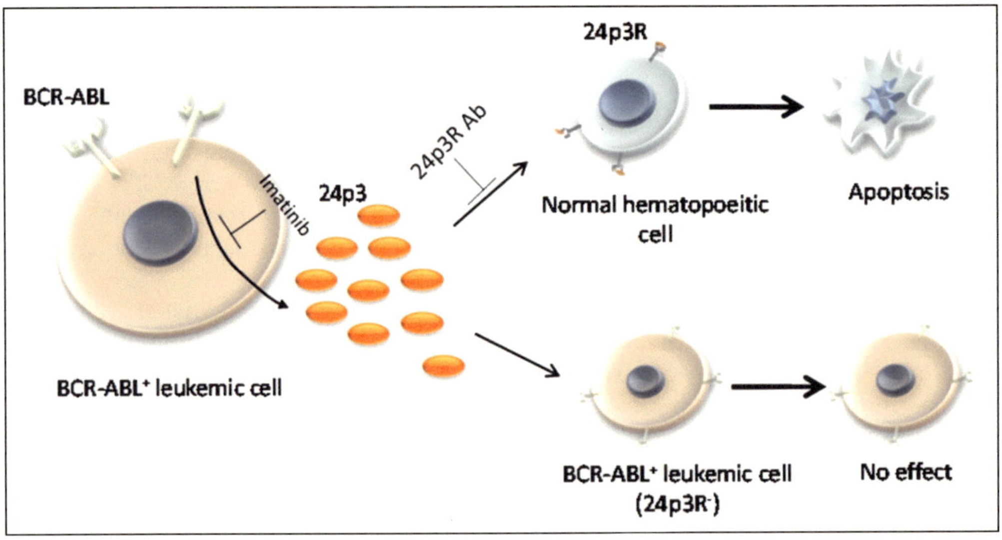

Fig. 3. Role of NGAL in hematopoietic malignancies: 24p3, the mouse homologue of human NGAL is secreted from BCR-ABL expressing mouse leukemic blast cells, a process that can be blocked using Imatinib, a specific inhibitor of the BCR-ABL tyrosine kinase activity. The 24p3 in the conditioned medium induces apoptosis in normal hematopoietic cells (express the 24p3 receptor or 24p3R) but not in the BCR-ABL+ leukemic cells that are devoid of 24p3R.

mechanism has been suggested to be responsible for the spread of leukemia cells through the healthy bone marrow (Hu *et al.*, 2009; Leng *et al.*, 2008; Lin *et al.*, 2005). Further, studies in mice also suggest that while 24p3/Ngal is required for the establishment of BCR-ABL$^+$ leukemia cells in the spleen and bone marrow, it is the *BCR-ABL* but not *Ngal* was the gene ultimately driving the progression of the disease. Studies in CML patients have confirmed the findings in mice. Both NGAL mRNA and plasma levels are significantly elevated in patients with CML (Leng *et al.*, 2008; Villalva *et al.*, 2008). Further, patients who responded to treatment with Imatinib (a specific inhibitor of BCR-ABL tyrosine kinase) showed a significant decrease in NGAL mRNA (but not in plasma NGAL levels). (Owen *et al.*, 2008)

5. Functions of NGAL

An important function of NGAL under physiological conditions is to act as bacteriostatic agent, thus protecting the body against both gram negative bacteria and mycobacterial infection. It mediates this function by binding with strong affinity to bacterial iron binding proteins called siderophores. Iron, particularly ferrous form is required by bacteria for their growth. However, the extremely low levels of free iron in the body make it an essential nutrient required by bacterial cells. To circumvent this requirement for iron, bacteria have evolved a mechanism involving the expression of proteins (termed siderophores) that bind to free iron (present in the intestinal fluid and inside macrophages) particularly in its ferric form. NGAL has a strong affinity to bind to siderophores, both when free and when laden with iron. Upon binding to these proteins, the NGAL siderophore complex is taken up by cells expressing the cognate receptor for NGAL and thus these iron laden proteins are sequestered away. In this way, by depriving bacteria of an essential nutrient, NGAL inhibits their proliferation (Nairz *et al.*, 2009; Holmes *et al.*, 2005).

The recent discovery that catechols, a family of plant derived metabolites present in our diet, can bind NGAL has opened new possibilities for the functional role of human NGAL in health and disease. Interestingly, while catechols itself bound weakly to NGAL, their binding was significantly enhanced in the presence of iron, specifically ferric iron. More detailed studies have revealed that three catechol molecules form a complex (a triscatecholate complex) with iron acting as a stabilizing agent through formation of pi interactions and electrostatic interactions with the catechol molecules. This ferric-triscatecholate complex then binds to the ligand binding cavity (calyx) of NGAL. In mice, it has been observed that this complex of Ngal and iron-catechol is filtered through the kidneys before being re-absorbed in the proximal convoluted tubules through specific Ngal receptors (Bao *et al.*, 2010; Backhed *et al.*, 2005). However, the function of these complexes alone and in combination with Ngal still remains to be elucidated.

Other functions attributed to Ngal include acting as a chemoattractant for neutrophils and as an inhibitor of cellular oxidative stress. The former function is based on observations that mice in which the Ngal gene is knocked out show a significant decrease in the number of neutrophils infiltrating transplanted heart tissue (compared to wild type mice with both copies of the gene intact). This suggests that neutrophils, the primary effectors of acute inflammatory response in the body, require NGAL to home in to the target organs (in this case the transplanted heart). The latter role is suggested from observations made in both Chinese hamster ovary (CHO) and human embryonic kidney (HEK) cells that an aberrant expression of 24p3/Ngal leads to a significant upregulation in the expression of the antioxidant enzymes superoxide dismutase (SOD) and heme oxygenase (HO) (Bahmani *et al.*, 2010; Roudkenar *et al.*, 2007; Roudkenar *et al.*, 2008c; Roudkenar *et al.*, 2008a; Roudkenar *et al.*, 2008b).

NGAL also appears to play a role in wound healing. In a study of patients with chronic venous ulcers (CVUs), an analysis of the exudate from the wounds of those with either healing (H) or non-healing (NH) CVUs revealed that the former (H-CVU) group had a significant decline the level of exudate-NGAL levels compared to the latter (NH-CVU) group of patients (Pukstad *et al.*, 2010).

NGAL also appears to modulate proliferation and synthesis of cartilage by murine chondrocytes and promotes proliferation of renal tubular epithelial cells (Owen *et al.*, 2008). Apart from healthy cells, NGAL also modulates proliferation and survival of certain types of malignant cells (thyroid cancer and hepatocellular carcinoma). In the former type of cancer cells, NGAL appears to promote proliferation and survival, while it had the opposite effect in hepatocellular carcinoma cells (Iannetti *et al.*, 2008; Lee et al., 2011). In other types of cancer cells (e.g. pancreatic, breast and colon cancer) however, NGAL does not seem to have any effect on proliferation. Instead, it significantly inhibits the ability of these cancer cells to invade and metastasize (Tong *et al.*, 2008; Lee *et al.*, 2006). Two possible mechanisms have been suggested to explain this anti-invasive effect of NGAL. One mechanism involves inhibition of the non-receptor tyrosine kinase FAK (focal adhesion kinase). FAK interacts with Src (another non-receptor tyrosine kinase) and provides a scaffold for activation of the Ras-MAPK (Mitogen activated protein kinase pathway), a key mediator of metastasis in cancer cells. NGAL, by inhibiting FAK would in turn inhibit the Ras-MAPK pathway and thus block both invasion and metastasis of cancer cells. A second mechanism, based on studies by our group, suggests that E-cadherin when ectopically expressed can increase expression of NGAL (Tong *et al.*, 2011). E-cadherin is a calcium dependent cell adhesion molecule that is expressed in and promotes epithelial cells to adhere to one another (thus preventing metastasis). Further, studies by us in human pancreatic cancer cells also suggest that NGAL inhibits angiogenesis (formation of blood vessels) (Tong *et al.*, 2008). A clue to the underlying mechanism comes from observations that conditioned media from pancreatic cells in which endogenous NGAL had been silenced (using short hairpin RNAs) significantly decrease formation of capillary like structures by human vascular endothelial (HUVEC) cells *in vitro*. This is associated with a significant decrease in the release of vascular endothelial growth factor (VEGF), a key promoter of angiogenesis from the NGAL silenced cells.

Knockout of both copies of the murine Ngal homologue (i.e. Ngal$^{-/-}$ mice) did not result in any phenotypic abnormalities in the knockout mice compared to their wild type littermates. However, the Ngal knockout mice were significantly more sensitive to infection with gram negative bacteria, exhibiting a nearly 1000-fold greater bacteremia (upon infection with *Escherichia coli*, a gram negative enteric pathogen) compared to their wild type littermates. Further investigation revealed that there was no difference in the absolute number of different leukocyte subpopulations between the wild type (Ngal$^{+/+}$) and knockout mice (Ngal$^{-/-}$) (Flo *et al.*, 2004). As discussed earlier, Ngal is crucial to prevent growth of bacteria, particularly within the macrophages and also for homing of neutrophils to sites of acute inflammation (including bacterial infection). Both these mechanisms would be severely affected in the *Ngal* knockout mice, thus contributing to the enhanced bacteremia and resulting mortality. These observations suggest that lack of Ngal produces a qualitative rather than a quantitative defect in the immune system that in turn leads to an increased susceptibility to gram negative sepsis.

6. Regulation of NGAL expression

Given the observation that NGAL is differentially expressed in a wide array of benign and malignant diseases, it is extremely important to investigate the mechanisms that regulate its expression. Most studies have focused on the regulation of transcription of its mRNA. Several cytokines, hormones, vitamins, minerals, synthetic drugs and growth factors have been shown to influence the expression of NGAL (**Table 2**). Each of these probably acts in a context dependent manner to influence the expression of this glycoprotein.

NF-κB , a transcription factor and regulator of several key pathways in the cell has emerged as a front runner in the regulation of NGAL gene expression. The NF-κB family comprises five transcription factors (p50, p52, p65 (or RelA) and c-Rel and RelB). These proteins are related to one another by the presence of the Rel homology domain (RHD), present in the N-terminal region of each member of this family. The C-terminal region contains either a transcription activation domain (TAD, in case of RelA, c-Rel and RelB) or a transcription repression domain (TRD in case of p50 and p52). These proteins form homo or heterodimers with each other through the RHD domain and then bind to short (9-10 bases long) sequence in the promoter or enhancer regions of target genes (termed as kB response elements). RelA, c-Rel and RelB activate gene expression (owing to presence of the TAD) while p50 and p52 inhibit gene expression (through the TRD) unless they associate with another member that has a TAD in its C-terminus. NGAL too has κB elements in its promoter region and has been shown to be positively regulated by agents that induce NF-κB (like insulin, IL-1β and TLRs). Another pathway that has been shown to promote NGAL expression is the JNK (c-jun N-terminal kinase) MAPK pathway. Cytokines like IL-1 and IL-17 can both activate the JNK pathway. A cross talk between the JNK and NF-κB has been suggested to act together to upregulate NGAL expression (Florin *et al.*, 2004; Yang *et al.*, 2008; Park *et al.*, 2005). Dexamethasone, a synthetic corticosteroid induces NGAL mRNA expression acting through the glucocorticoid receptor (GRs) and glucocorticoid response elements (GREs) present in the promoter region of NGAL (Garay-Rojas *et al.*, 1996).

The epidermal growth factor receptor (EGFR) when activated initiates signaling events that promote cell proliferation, survival and enhance migration and invasiveness of a variety of cancer cells. We have reported that EGF treatment decreases the expression of NGAL mRNA. This was associated with a significant downregulation of the epithelial marker E-cadherin. Mechanistically, EGF mediated downregulation of NGAL expression occurs by inhibition of the NF-κB pathway (Tong *et al.*, 2011). However, the role of EGF in regulating NGAL appears to be dependent on the cell type. For instance, treatment of mouse renal tubular epithelial cells with EGF led to a significant upregulation of *Ngal* expression. The mechanism of upregulation of *Ngal* by EGF (in mice renal cells) appears not to be through the NF-κB pathway but rather through stabilization of the transcription factor HIF-1α (hypoxia inducible factor-1 α).

Epigenetic mechanisms have been shown to be central to the process of *de novo* induction or repression of genes. Treatment of endometrial cancer cells that express a low level of NGAL with a demethylating agent 5-aza cytidine led to a significant upregulation of NGAL mRNA. However, the same agent had no effect on cells that had a high basal level of NGAL (Miyamoto *et al.*, 2011). This suggests that methylation may be a mechanism to differentially turn on or off the expression of NGAL in disease states including cancer.

Factors	Comments	Effect on NGAL expression
Cytokines		
GM-CSF	Granulocyte Monocyte colony stimulating factor	↑
IL-1α	Interleukin 1 alpha	↑
IL-1β	Interleukin 1 beta	↑
IL-6	Interleukin 6	↔
IL-17	Interleukin 17	↑
IL-22	Interleukin 22	↑
TGF-α	Transforming growth factor alpha	↑
TNF-α	Tumor necrosis factor alpha	↔/↓ [a]
bFGF	Basic fibroblast growth factor	↔
Growth factors		
IGF-1	Insulin like growth factor-1	↑
EGF	Epidermal growth factor	↓/↑ [a]
Synthetic drugs		↑
Dexamethasone	Synthetic corticosteroid	↑
Deferoxamine	Iron-chelator	↑
Diethylstilbestrol	Synthetic nonsteroidal estrogen	↑
5-aza cytidine	Demethylating agent	↑
Hormones		
Insulin		↑
Estrogen		↓/↑ [a]
Progesterone		↔
Bacterial components		
LPS	Lipopolysaccharide (TLR-4 ligand)	↑
Lipotechoic acid	Gram +ve bacterial cell wall component	↑
Peptidoglycan	Gram +ve bacterial cell wall component	↑
Others		
HIV-tat	HIV virus tat protein	↑
Pam3CSK4	TLR-1/2 ligand	↑
Flagellin	TLR-5 ligand	↑
pIC	Polyinosinic polycytidylic acid (TLR-3 ligand)	↑
CpG	Unmethylated CpG oligonucleotides (TLR-9 ligand)	↑
Calcium	Promotes cell differentiation	↑

Footnote 1 ↑ Indicates upregulation, ↓ indicates downregulation and ↔ indicates no effect on NGAL expression. [a] The same factor can have opposite effects on NGAL expression in a context dependent manner. HIV (Human Immune deficiency virus), TLR (Toll like receptor).

Table 2. Summary of factors regulating NGAL expression

These reports taken together suggest that multiple stimuli, acting through a relatively small number of pathways regulate the expression of NGAL. However, many of these studies have been done *in vitro* and need to be examined *in vivo* particularly using knockout mouse models. Nonetheless, they shed important light on the complex regulation of this protein and will be important in future attempts to modulate its expression for therapeutic purposes.

7. Role of NGAL as a diagnostic and prognostic marker

The differential expression of NGAL in disease states has been utilized as a rationale to investigate the potential of NGAL as a biomarker in the diagnosis of these diseases. Among benign diseases, acute kidney injury (AKI) represents the disease where this secreted protein has been most extensively studied for its diagnostic performance. In one study, urine NGAL levels rose significantly within as early as 6 hours following elective cardiac surgery in patients admitted to the intensive care units (ICU) who met the criteria for AKI, suggesting that it is an early marker of renal injury (Koyner *et al.*, 2010). Further, corrected urine NGAL levels (corrected for serum creatinine) when measured at the time of the patient's arrival to the ICU was a good predictor of severe AKI post-cardiac surgery (Area under the curve or AUC being 0.88, 95% CI: 0.73-0.99). Another study found that among post-cardiac surgery patients, plasma NGAL levels rose upto 24 hours prior to patients meeting the current clinical criteria for AKI (i.e. the RIFLE or Risk, Injury, Failure, Loss and End stage renal disease criteria) (Cruz *et al.*, 2010). Further, plasma NGAL was a good predictor of the need for renal replacement therapy (RRT) during the stay of the patients in the ICU (AUC 0.82, 95% CI 0.70-0.95). NGAL is also an early predictor of DGD (delayed graft dysfunction), a type of renal dysfunction in kidney transplant recipients that often develops within a week after transplant and is often severe enough to require dialysis (Korbely *et al.*, 2011; Shapiro *et al.*, 2010).

Pre-renal azotemia refers to reversible renal injury which is completely reversible within 24-72 hours if the cause is removed. Distinguishing pre-renal azotemia from AKI is one of the major challenges for nephrologists and critical care physicians today. A comparison of urine NGAL levels between patients with pre-renal azotemia and AKI revealed that urine NGAL levels were significantly higher in patients with AKI (mean±SEM level being 416+387 µg/g of creatinine) compared to those with pre-renal azotemia (mean±SEM being 30+92 µg/g creatinine) (Nickolas *et al.*, 2008). The results were validated in another independent cohort of 107 patients, 32 of whom had pre-renal azotemia (Singer *et al.*, 2011).

Diagnosis of AKI in children presents a special challenge. Owing to the incomplete development of their nephrons, they have higher baseline levels of creatinine than adults. Hence, serum creatinine may not be an appropriate marker to detect AKI in these patients. A comparison of NGAL and creatinine in pediatric patients (both neonates and older patients) revealed that urine NGAL levels were elevated within 2 hours following cardiopulmonary bypass (CPB) surgery and remained elevated for even upto 48 hours. Significantly, urine NGAL >185 ng/ml or a plasma NGAL >95 ng/ml was 100% sensitive (88% for plasma) and 93% specific (both urine and plasma) in identifying AKI in neonatal patients. The corresponding cut-off for older children was >45ng/ml (urine) or >48ng/ml (plasma). The corresponding sensitivity and specificity were 85% (90% for plasma) and 86% (88% for plasma) respectively (Krawczeski *et al.*, 2011).

Elevation in NGAL, particularly in combination with an elevation in the levels of IL-1 receptor and protein C was the best predictor of the risk of developing severe sepsis among a panel of nine potential markers in a cohort of 506 patients admitted with systemic inflammatory response syndrome (SIRS) (AUC 0.75, 95% CI 0.72-0.78 vs. those who did not develop severe sepsis). This panel of three markers was also fairly accurate in predicting both septic shock (AUC 0.77) and death (AUC 0.79) within 24 hours of hospital admission in critically ill patients (Endre *et al.*, 2011).

In addition to its role as a diagnostic marker, NGAL has also emerged as an important prognostic indicator in several diseases. Studies in obese type-2 diabetics revealed that serum NGAL levels were negatively correlated with the levels of total cholesterol, an important determinant of coronary artery disease (CAD). Further, the level of serum NGAL was an independent predictor of insulin resistance and hyperglycemia in these patients. In patients with acute decompensated heart failure (ADHF), serum NGAL levels (at admission) were significantly higher in those patients who had worsening of renal function (WRF) compared to those whose renal function was intact. At a cut-off of ≥140 ng/ml, serum NGAL was 86% sensitive and 54% specific in predicting the development of WRF in these patients (Chertow *et al.*, 1998).

NGAL has been widely investigated as a prognostic indicator in AKI from various causes. In patients undergoing cardiovascular surgery, AKI is always a potential complication predominantly due to ischemia during the procedure. Urine NGAL levels have been shown to be fairly accurate (AUC 0.59-0.65) in early identification (within 3 hours) of AKI following CPB surgery (Shapiro *et al.*, 2009). We have demonstrated that an elevated plasma NGAL level among patients with SAP is associated with a significantly poor outcome (i.e. increased risk of death). This effect appears to be specific to SAP as no such correlation was observed in MAP patients. Further, in a small study, NGAL appeared to perform equal or better than other established clinical prognostic indicators in SAP (i.e. serum creatinine, Ranson's score and the APACHE-II score) (Chakraborty *et al.*, 2010).

As techniques continue to evolve, it is expected that assays for NGAL will become increasingly sensitive. One study comparing ELISA (enzyme linked immunosorbent assay) with RIA (radioimmunoassay) found that the latter was between 5-10 fold more sensitive than ELISA in detecting a rise in NGAL among patients undergoing cardiac surgery, with the sensitivity being the highest in the first 2 hours (Aghel *et al.*, 2010).

NGAL has also emerged as a potential biomarker in several epithelial malignancies. In gastric cancer patients, serum NGAL could distinguish patients with cancer from non-cancer patients with an AUC of 0.93 (Wang et al., 2010). NGAL was better than either CA19-9 or CEA (carcinoembryonic antigen) in identifying early gastric cancer (i.e. Stage 1 and 2) patients suggesting that it could be a potential biomarker for early stage gastric cancer. NGAL was also fairly accurate in discriminating between benign and malignant biliary obstruction (AUC 0.76 with a sensitivity and specificity of 96% and 56%) (Klapper *et al.*, 2008). In ovarian cancer however, NGAL was 72% sensitive but only 50% specific in distinguishing ovarian cancer from non-cancer patients. In comparison, CA125 was 80% sensitive and 79% specific in distinguishing between the two groups (Argani *et al.*, 2001).

NGAL also appears to correlate with prognosis of cancer patients. For instance, patients whose tumors expressed NGAL had a significantly shorter survival (both disease specific and disease free) compared to those with NGAL non-expressing tumors (12.2 years in NGAL expressing vs. 17.1 years in NGAL non-expressing tumors). Multivariate analysis revealed that NGAL was an independent predictor of disease free survival (hazard ratio 1.85). In gastric cancer too, patients whose tumors expressed NGAL had a significantly shorter survival compared to tumors whose tumors did not express any NGAL (35.6 .months vs. 54.4 months respectively) (Alpizar *et al.*, 2009).

8. Conclusions

The preceding discussion suggests that NGAL, despite its low molecular weight is an important protein particularly from the standpoint of protecting against bacterial infections. Further, it appears that NGAL has other novel functions in disease states, particularly in epithelial malignancies where it can modulate cell proliferation, cell death, invasion and metastasis of cancer cells. In other diseases, particularly in renal injury, the role of NGAL remains to be elucidated.

NGAL expression appears to be regulated by a variety of stimuli through mainly the NF-κB pathway although epigenetic modifications may be important, particularly in initiating its *de novo* expression during diseases like cancer. NGAL has also emerged as a biomarker with immense clinical potential, both in benign and malignant diseases. Further, while limited studies exist, it also appears to be capable of predicting the outcome of patients with multiple diseases.

All these features make NGAL an important diagnostic target. An interesting observation is that the Ngal knockout mice do not exhibit any obvious defects. However, they are extremely sensitive to infection by gram negative bacteria. These results clearly suggest that NGAL may be an important protective agent in gram negative bacterial infections. Further studies using these mice will be crucial to delineate its role in determining sensitivity to other inflammatory and malignant diseases. Taken together, NGAL has emerged as a clinically important member of the lipocalin family and holds immense potential for diagnostic and therapeutic applications in the future.

9. Acknowledgements

Surinder K Batra, Subhankar Chakraborty and Sukhwinder Kaur are supported in part by grants from the US Department of Defense (BC074631, BC083295 and PC074289) and the NIH (RO1 CA78590, UO1 CA111294, RO1 CA131944, RO1 CA133774, RO1 CA 138791 and P50 CA127297). Sushovan Guha is supported by grants from MDACC McNair Foundation Scholar Award and the Cyrus Scholar Award. The authors have no other relevant affiliations or financial involvement with any organization or entity with a financial interest in or financial conflict with the subject matter or materials discussed in the manuscript apart from those disclosed. No writing assistance was utilized in the production of this manuscript.

10. References

Aghel A, Shrestha K, Mullens W, Borowski A, Tang WH (2010) Serum neutrophil gelatinase-associated lipocalin (NGAL) in predicting worsening renal function in acute decompensated heart failure. *J Card Fail* 16, 49-54

Alpizar YA, Ramirez BS, Fernandez DR, Capote AR, Hidalgo GG, Rodriguez RP, Molina LE (2009) HER1-ECD vaccination dispenses with emulsification to elicit HER1-specific anti-proliferative effects. *Hum Vaccin* 5, 158-165

Anwaar I, Gottsater A, Hedblad B, Palmqvist B, Mattiasson I, Lindgarde F (1998) Endothelial derived vasoactive factors and leukocyte derived inflammatory mediators in subjects with asymptomatic atherosclerosis. *Angiology* 49, 957-966

Argani P, Rosty C, Reiter RE, Wilentz RE, Murugesan SR, Leach SD, Ryu B, Skinner HG, Goggins M, Jaffee EM, Yeo CJ, Cameron JL, Kern SE, Hruban RH (2001) Discovery of new markers of cancer through serial analysis of gene expression: prostate stem cell antigen is overexpressed in pancreatic adenocarcinoma. *Cancer Res* 61, 4320-4324

Arlinghaus R, Leng X (2008) Requirement of lipocalin 2 for chronic myeloid leukemia. *Leuk Lymphoma* 49, 600-603

Backhed F, Ley RE, Sonnenburg JL, Peterson DA, Gordon JI (2005) Host-bacterial mutualism in the human intestine. *Science* 307, 1915-1920

Bahmani P, Halabian R, Rouhbakhsh M, Roushandeh AM, Masroori N, Ebrahimi M, Samadikuchaksaraei A, Shokrgozar MA, Roudkenar MH (2010) Neutrophil gelatinase-associated lipocalin induces the expression of heme oxygenase-1 and superoxide dismutase 1, 2. *Cell Stress Chaperones* 15, 395-403

Banks PA, Freeman ML (2006) Practice guidelines in acute pancreatitis. *Am J Gastroenterol* 101, 2379-2400

Bao G, Clifton M, Hoette TM, Mori K, Deng SX, Qiu A, Viltard M, Williams D, Paragas N, Leete T, Kulkarni R, Li X, Lee B, Kalandadze A, Ratner AJ, Pizarro JC, Schmidt-Ott KM, Landry DW, Raymond KN, Strong RK, Barasch J (2010) Iron traffics in circulation bound to a siderocalin (Ngal)-catechol complex. *Nat Chem Biol* 6, 602-609

Bauer M, Eickhoff JC, Gould MN, Mundhenke C, Maass N, Friedl A (2008) Neutrophil gelatinase-associated lipocalin (NGAL) is a predictor of poor prognosis in human primary breast cancer. *Breast Cancer Res Treat* 108, 389-397

Bu DX, Hemdahl AL, Gabrielsen A, Fuxe J, Zhu C, Eriksson P, Yan ZQ (2006) Induction of neutrophil gelatinase-associated lipocalin in vascular injury via activation of nuclear factor-kappaB. *Am J Pathol* 169, 2245-2253

Carroll JK, Herrick B, Gipson T, Lee SP (2007) Acute pancreatitis: diagnosis, prognosis, and treatment. *Am Fam Physician* 75, 1513-1520

Chakraborty S, Baine MJ, Sasson AR, Batra SK (2011) Current status of molecular markers for early detection of sporadic pancreatic cancer. *Biochim Biophys Acta* 1815, 44-64

Chakraborty S, Kaur S, Muddana V, Sharma N, Wittel UA, Papachristou GI, Whitcomb D, Brand RE, Batra SK (2010b) Elevated serum neutrophil gelatinase-associated lipocalin is an early predictor of severity and outcome in acute pancreatitis. *Am J Gastroenterol* 105, 2050-2059

Chertow GM, Levy EM, Hammermeister KE, Grover F, Daley J (1998) Independent association between acute renal failure and mortality following cardiac surgery. *Am J Med* 104, 343-348

Cho H, Kim JH (2009) Lipocalin2 expressions correlate significantly with tumor differentiation in epithelial ovarian cancer. *J Histochem Cytochem* 57, 513-521

Chu ST, Lin HJ, Huang HL, Chen YH (1998) The hydrophobic pocket of 24p3 protein from mouse uterine luminal fluid: fatty acid and retinol binding activity and predicted structural similarity to lipocalins. *J Pept Res* 52, 390-397

Coles M, Diercks T, Muehlenweg B, Bartsch S, Zolzer V, Tschesche H, Kessler H (1999) The solution structure and dynamics of human neutrophil gelatinase-associated lipocalin. *J Mol Biol* 289, 139-157

Cowland JB, Borregaard N (1997) Molecular characterization and pattern of tissue expression of the gene for neutrophil gelatinase-associated lipocalin from humans. *Genomics* 45, 17-23

Cowland JB, Sorensen OE, Sehested M, Borregaard N (2003) Neutrophil gelatinase-associated lipocalin is up-regulated in human epithelial cells by IL-1 beta, but not by TNF-alpha. *J Immunol* 171, 6630-6639

Cruz DN, de CM, Garzotto F, Perazella MA, Lentini P, Corradi V, Piccinni P, Ronco C (2010) Plasma neutrophil gelatinase-associated lipocalin is an early biomarker for acute kidney injury in an adult ICU population. *Intensive Care Med* 36, 444-451

D'Anna R, Baviera G, Corrado F, Giordano D, Recupero S, Di BA (2009a) First trimester serum neutrophil gelatinase-associated lipocalin in gestational diabetes. *Diabet Med* 26, 1293-1295

D'Anna R, Baviera G, Giordano D, Russo S, Dugo N, Santamaria A, Corrado F (2009b) First trimester serum PAPP-A and NGAL in the prediction of late-onset pre-eclampsia. *Prenat Diagn* 29, 1066-1068

D'Anna R, Baviera G, Giordano D, Todarello G, Corrado F, Buemi M (2008) Second trimester neutrophil gelatinase-associated lipocalin as a potential prediagnostic marker of preeclampsia. *Acta Obstet Gynecol Scand* 87, 1370-1373

Devireddy LR, Gazin C, Zhu X, Green MR (2005) A cell-surface receptor for lipocalin 24p3 selectively mediates apoptosis and iron uptake. *Cell* 123, 1293-1305

Ding L, Hanawa H, Ota Y, Hasegawa G, Hao K, Asami F, Watanabe R, Yoshida T, Toba K, Yoshida K, Ogura M, Kodama M, Aizawa Y (2010) Lipocalin-2/neutrophil gelatinase-B associated lipocalin is strongly induced in hearts of rats with autoimmune myocarditis and in human myocarditis. *Circ J* 74, 523-530

Elneihoum AM, Falke P, Hedblad B, Lindgarde F, Ohlsson K (1997) Leukocyte activation in atherosclerosis: correlation with risk factors. *Atherosclerosis* 131, 79-84

Endre ZH, Pickering JW, Walker RJ, Devarajan P, Edelstein CL, Bonventre JV, Frampton CM, Bennett MR, Ma Q, Sabbisetti VS, Vaidya VS, Walcher AM, Shaw GM, Henderson SJ, Nejat M, Schollum JB, George PM (2011) Improved performance of urinary biomarkers of acute kidney injury in the critically ill by stratification for injury duration and baseline renal function. *Kidney Int, in press*

Flo TH, Smith KD, Sato S, Rodriguez DJ, Holmes MA, Strong RK, Akira S, Aderem A (2004) Lipocalin 2 mediates an innate immune response to bacterial infection by sequestrating iron. *Nature* 432, 917-921

Florin L, Hummerich L, Dittrich BT, Kokocinski F, Wrobel G, Gack S, Schorpp-Kistner M, Werner S, Hahn M, Lichter P, Szabowski A, Angel P (2004) Identification of novel AP-1 target genes in fibroblasts regulated during cutaneous wound healing. *Oncogene* 23, 7005-7017

Flower DR (1994) The lipocalin protein family: a role in cell regulation. *FEBS Lett* 354, 7-11

Flower DR (1995) Multiple molecular recognition properties of the lipocalin protein family. *J Mol Recognit* 8, 185-195

Flower DR (1996) The lipocalin protein family: structure and function. *Biochem J* 318 (Pt 1), 1-14

Flower DR, North AC, Sansom CE (2000) The lipocalin protein family: structural and sequence overview. *Biochim Biophys Acta* 1482, 9-24

Furutani M, Arii S, Mizumoto M, Kato M, Imamura M (1998) Identification of a neutrophil gelatinase-associated lipocalin mRNA in human pancreatic cancers using a modified signal sequence trap method. *Cancer Lett* 122, 209-214

Garay-Rojas E, Harper M, Hraba-Renevey S, Kress M (1996) An apparent autocrine mechanism amplifies the dexamethasone- and retinoic acid-induced expression of mouse lipocalin-encoding gene 24p3. *Gene* 170, 173-180

Goetz DH, Willie ST, Armen RS, Bratt T, Borregaard N, Strong RK (2000) Ligand preference inferred from the structure of neutrophil gelatinase associated lipocalin. *Biochemistry* 39, 1935-1941

Holmes MA, Paulsene W, Jide X, Ratledge C, Strong RK (2005) Siderocalin (Lcn 2) also binds carboxymycobactins, potentially defending against mycobacterial infections through iron sequestration. *Structure* 13, 29-41

Hraba-Renevey S, Turler H, Kress M, Salomon C, Weil R (1989) SV40-induced expression of mouse gene 24p3 involves a post-transcriptional mechanism. *Oncogene* 4, 601-608

Hu L, Hittelman W, Lu T, Ji P, Arlinghaus R, Shmulevich I, Hamilton SR, Zhang W (2009) NGAL decreases E-cadherin-mediated cell-cell adhesion and increases cell motility and invasion through Rac1 in colon carcinoma cells. *Lab Invest* 89, 531-548

Hvidberg V, Jacobsen C, Strong RK, Cowland JB, Moestrup SK, Borregaard N (2005) The endocytic receptor megalin binds the iron transporting neutrophil-gelatinase-associated lipocalin with high affinity and mediates its cellular uptake. *FEBS Lett* 579, 773-777

Iannetti A, Pacifico F, Acquaviva R, Lavorgna A, Crescenzi E, Vascotto C, Tell G, Salzano AM, Scaloni A, Vuttariello E, Chiappetta G, Formisano S, Leonardi A (2008) The neutrophil gelatinase-associated lipocalin (NGAL), a NF-kappaB-regulated gene, is a survival factor for thyroid neoplastic cells. *Proc Natl Acad Sci U S A* 105, 14058-14063

Klapper JA, Downey SG, Smith FO, Yang JC, Hughes MS, Kammula US, Sherry RM, Royal RE, Steinberg SM, Rosenberg S (2008) High-dose interleukin-2 for the treatment of metastatic renal cell carcinoma : a retrospective analysis of response and survival in patients treated in the surgery branch at the National Cancer Institute between 1986 and 2006. *Cancer* 113, 293-301

Korbely R, Wilflingseder J, Perco P, Kainz A, Langer RM, Mayer B, Oberbauer R (2011) Molecular biomarker candidates of acute kidney injury in zero-hour renal transplant needle biopsies. *Transpl Int* 24, 143-149

Koyner JL, Vaidya VS, Bennett MR, Ma Q, Worcester E, Akhter SA, Raman J, Jeevanandam V, O'Connor MF, Devarajan P, Bonventre JV, Murray PT (2010) Urinary biomarkers in the clinical prognosis and early detection of acute kidney injury. *Clin J Am Soc Nephrol* 5, 2154-2165

Krawczeski CD, Woo JG, Wang Y, Bennett MR, Ma Q, Devarajan P (2011) Neutrophil Gelatinase-Associated Lipocalin Concentrations Predict Development of Acute Kidney Injury in Neonates and Children after Cardiopulmonary Bypass. *J Pediatr*,

Landro L, Damas JK, Flo TH, Heggelund L, Ueland T, Tjonnfjord GE, Espevik T, Aukrust P, Froland SS (2008) Decreased serum lipocalin-2 levels in human immunodeficiency virus-infected patients: increase during highly active anti-retroviral therapy. *Clin Exp Immunol* 152, 57-63

Lau WK, Blute ML, Weaver AL, Torres VE, Zincke H (2000) Matched comparison of radical nephrectomy vs nephron-sparing surgery in patients with unilateral renal cell carcinoma and a normal contralateral kidney. *Mayo Clin Proc* 75, 1236-1242

Le C, V, Calafat J, Borregaard N (1997) Sorting of the specific granule protein, NGAL, during granulocytic maturation of HL-60 cells. *Blood* 89, 2113-2121

Lee EK, Kim HJ, Lee KJ, Lee HJ, Lee JS, Kim DG, Hong SW, Yoon Y, Kim JS (2011) Inhibition of the proliferation and invasion of hepatocellular carcinoma cells by lipocalin 2 through blockade of JNK and PI3K/Akt signaling. *Int J Oncol* 38, 325-333

Lee HJ, Lee EK, Lee KJ, Hong SW, Yoon Y, Kim JS (2006) Ectopic expression of neutrophil gelatinase-associated lipocalin suppresses the invasion and liver metastasis of colon cancer cells. *Int J Cancer* 118, 2490-2497

Leng X, Lin H, Ding T, Wang Y, Wu Y, Klumpp S, Sun T, Zhou Y, Monaco P, Belmont J, Aderem A, Akira S, Strong R, Arlinghaus R (2008) Lipocalin 2 is required for BCR-ABL-induced tumorigenesis. *Oncogene* 27, 6110-6119

Lim R, Ahmed N, Borregaard N, Riley C, Wafai R, Thompson EW, Quinn MA, Rice GE (2007) Neutrophil gelatinase-associated lipocalin (NGAL) an early-screening biomarker for ovarian cancer: NGAL is associated with epidermal growth factor-induced epithelio-mesenchymal transition. *Int J Cancer* 120, 2426-2434

Lin H, Monaco G, Sun T, Ling X, Stephens C, Xie S, Belmont J, Arlinghaus R (2005) Bcr-Abl-mediated suppression of normal hematopoiesis in leukemia. *Oncogene* 24, 3246-3256

Mallbris L, O'Brien KP, Hulthen A, Sandstedt B, Cowland JB, Borregaard N, Stahle-Backdahl M (2002) Neutrophil gelatinase-associated lipocalin is a marker for dysregulated keratinocyte differentiation in human skin. *Exp Dermatol* 11, 584-591

Marques F, Rodrigues AJ, Sousa JC, Coppola G, Geschwind DH, Sousa N, Correia-Neves M, Palha JA (2008) Lipocalin 2 is a choroid plexus acute-phase protein. *J Cereb Blood Flow Metab* 28, 450-455

Mishra J, Ma Q, Prada A, Mitsnefes M, Zahedi K, Yang J, Barasch J, Devarajan P (2003) Identification of neutrophil gelatinase-associated lipocalin as a novel early urinary biomarker for ischemic renal injury. *J Am Soc Nephrol* 14, 2534-2543

Miyamoto T, Kashima H, Suzuki A, Kikuchi N, Konishi I, Seki N, Shiozawa T (2011) Laser-captured microdissection-microarray analysis of the genes involved in endometrial carcinogenesis: stepwise up-regulation of lipocalin2 expression in normal and neoplastic endometria and its functional relevance. *Hum Pathol, in press*

Moniaux N, Chakraborty S, Yalniz M, Gonzalez J, Shostrom VK, Standop J, Lele SM, Ouellette M, Pour PM, Sasson AR, Brand RE, Hollingsworth MA, Jain M, Batra SK (2008) Early diagnosis of pancreatic cancer: neutrophil gelatinase-associated lipocalin as a marker of pancreatic intraepithelial neoplasia. *Br J Cancer* 98, 1540-1547

Moreno-Navarrete JM, Manco M, Ibanez J, Garcia-Fuentes E, Ortega F, Gorostiaga E, Vendrell J, Izquierdo M, Martinez C, Nolfe G, Ricart W, Mingrone G, Tinahones F, Fernandez-Real JM (2010) Metabolic endotoxemia and saturated fat contribute to circulating NGAL concentrations in subjects with insulin resistance. *Int J Obes (Lond)* 34, 240-249

Nairz M, Theurl I, Schroll A, Theurl M, Fritsche G, Lindner E, Seifert M, Crouch ML, Hantke K, Akira S, Fang FC, Weiss G (2009) Absence of functional Hfe protects mice from invasive Salmonella enterica serovar Typhimurium infection via induction of lipocalin-2. *Blood* 114, 3642-3651

Nickolas TL, O'Rourke MJ, Yang J, Sise ME, Canetta PA, Barasch N, Buchen C, Khan F, Mori K, Giglio J, Devarajan P, Barasch J (2008) Sensitivity and specificity of a single emergency department measurement of urinary neutrophil gelatinase-associated lipocalin for diagnosing acute kidney injury. *Ann Intern Med* 148, 810-819

Nomura I, Gao B, Boguniewicz M, Darst MA, Travers JB, Leung DY (2003) Distinct patterns of gene expression in the skin lesions of atopic dermatitis and psoriasis: a gene microarray analysis. *J Allergy Clin Immunol* 112, 1195-1202

Owen HC, Roberts SJ, Ahmed SF, Farquharson C (2008) Dexamethasone-induced expression of the glucocorticoid response gene lipocalin 2 in chondrocytes. *Am J Physiol Endocrinol Metab* 294, E1023-E1034

Park H, Li Z, Yang XO, Chang SH, Nurieva R, Wang YH, Wang Y, Hood L, Zhu Z, Tian Q, Dong C (2005) A distinct lineage of CD4 T cells regulates tissue inflammation by producing interleukin 17. *Nat Immunol* 6, 1133-1141

Pi-Sunyer FX (2002) The obesity epidemic: pathophysiology and consequences of obesity. *Obes Res* 10 Suppl 2, 97S-104S

Pukstad BS, Ryan L, Flo TH, Stenvik J, Moseley R, Harding K, Thomas DW, Espevik T (2010) Non-healing is associated with persistent stimulation of the innate immune response in chronic venous leg ulcers. *J Dermatol Sci* 59, 115-122

Roudkenar MH, Halabian R, Ghasemipour Z, Roushandeh AM, Rouhbakhsh M, Nekogoftar M, Kuwahara Y, Fukumoto M, Shokrgozar MA (2008a) Neutrophil gelatinase-associated lipocalin acts as a protective factor against H(2)O(2) toxicity. *Arch Med Res* 39, 560-566

Roudkenar MH, Halabian R, Ghasemipour Z, Roushandeh AM, Rouhbakhsh M, Nekogoftar M, Kuwahara Y, Fukumoto M, Shokrgozar MA (2008b) Neutrophil gelatinase-associated lipocalin acts as a protective factor against H(2)O(2) toxicity. *Arch Med Res* 39, 560-566

Roudkenar MH, Halabian R, Oodi A, Roushandeh AM, Yaghmai P, Najar MR, Amirizadeh N, Shokrgozar MA (2008c) Upregulation of neutrophil gelatinase-associated lipocalin, NGAL/Lcn2, in beta-thalassemia patients. *Arch Med Res* 39, 402-407

Roudkenar MH, Kuwahara Y, Baba T, Roushandeh AM, Ebishima S, Abe S, Ohkubo Y, Fukumoto M (2007) Oxidative stress induced lipocalin 2 gene expression: addressing its expression under the harmful conditions. *J Radiat Res (Tokyo)* 48, 39-44

Seth P, Porter D, Lahti-Domenici J, Geng Y, Richardson A, Polyak K (2002) Cellular and molecular targets of estrogen in normal human breast tissue. *Cancer Res* 62, 4540-4544

Shapiro NI, Trzeciak S, Hollander JE, Birkhahn R, Otero R, Osborn TM, Moretti E, Nguyen HB, Gunnerson K, Milzman D, Gaieski DF, Goyal M, Cairns CB, Kupfer K, Lee SW, Rivers EP (2010) The diagnostic accuracy of plasma neutrophil gelatinase-associated lipocalin in the prediction of acute kidney injury in emergency department patients with suspected sepsis. *Ann Emerg Med* 56, 52-59

Shapiro NI, Trzeciak S, Hollander JE, Birkhahn R, Otero R, Osborn TM, Moretti E, Nguyen HB, Gunnerson KJ, Milzman D, Gaieski DF, Goyal M, Cairns CB, Ngo L, Rivers EP (2009) A prospective, multicenter derivation of a biomarker panel to assess risk of organ dysfunction, shock, and death in emergency department patients with suspected sepsis. *Crit Care Med* 37, 96-104

Singer E, Elger A, Elitok S, Kettritz R, Nickolas TL, Barasch J, Luft FC, Schmidt-Ott KM (2011) Urinary neutrophil gelatinase-associated lipocalin distinguishes pre-renal from intrinsic renal failure and predicts outcomes. *Kidney Int*,

Stoesz SP, Gould MN (1995) Overexpression of neu-related lipocalin (NRL) in neu-initiated but not ras or chemically initiated rat mammary carcinomas. *Oncogene* 11, 2233-2241

Tan BK, Adya R, Shan X, Syed F, Lewandowski KC, O'Hare JP, Randeva HS (2009) Ex vivo and in vivo regulation of lipocalin-2, a novel adipokine, by insulin. *Diabetes Care* 32, 129-131

te Boekhorst BC, Bovens SM, Hellings WE, van der Kraak PH, van de Kolk KW, Vink A, Moll FL, van Oosterhout MF, de Vries JP, Doevendans PA, Goumans MJ, de Kleijn DP, van Echteld CJ, Pasterkamp G, Sluijter JP (2011) Molecular MRI of murine atherosclerotic plaque targeting NGAL: a protein associated with unstable human plaque characteristics. *Cardiovasc Res* 89, 680-688

Tong Z, Chakraborty S, Sung B, Koolwal P, Kaur S, Aggarwal BB, Mani SA, Bresalier RS, Batra SK, Guha S (2011) Epidermal growth factor down-regulates the expression of neutrophil gelatinase-associated lipocalin (NGAL) through E-cadherin in pancreatic cancer cells. *Cancer*, 117, 2408-2418

Tong Z, Kunnumakkara AB, Wang H, Matsuo Y, Diagaradjane P, Harikumar KB, Ramachandran V, Sung B, Chakraborty A, Bresalier RS, Logsdon C, Aggarwal BB, Krishnan S, Guha S (2008) Neutrophil gelatinase-associated lipocalin: a novel suppressor of invasion and angiogenesis in pancreatic cancer. *Cancer Res* 68, 6100-6108

Triebel S, Blaser J, Reinke H, Tschesche H (1992) A 25 kDa alpha 2-microglobulin-related protein is a component of the 125 kDa form of human gelatinase. *FEBS Lett* 314, 386-388

Van Dyke TE, Schweinebraten M, Cianciola LJ, Offenbacher S, Genco RJ (1985) Neutrophil chemotaxis in families with localized juvenile periodontitis. *J Periodontal Res* 20, 503-514

Viau A, El KK, Laouari D, Burtin M, Nguyen C, Mori K, Pillebout E, Berger T, Mak TW, Knebelmann B, Friedlander G, Barasch J, Terzi F (2010) Lipocalin 2 is essential for chronic kidney disease progression in mice and humans. *J Clin Invest* 120, 4065-4076

Villalva C, Sorel N, Bonnet ML, Guilhot J, Mayeur-Rousse C, Guilhot F, Chomel JC, Turhan AG (2008) Neutrophil gelatinase-associated lipocalin expression in chronic myeloid leukemia. *Leuk Lymphoma* 49, 984-988

Wang HJ, He XJ, Ma YY, Jiang XT, Xia YJ, Ye ZY, Zhao ZS, Tao HQ (2010) Expressions of neutrophil gelatinase-associated lipocalin in gastric cancer: a potential biomarker for prognosis and an ancillary diagnostic test. *Anat Rec (Hoboken)* 293, 1855-1863

Wang Y, Lam KS, Kraegen EW, Sweeney G, Zhang J, Tso AW, Chow WS, Wat NM, Xu JY, Hoo RL, Xu A (2007) Lipocalin-2 is an inflammatory marker closely associated with obesity, insulin resistance, and hyperglycemia in humans. *Clin Chem* 53, 34-41

Yang XO, Chang SH, Park H, Nurieva R, Shah B, Acero L, Wang YH, Schluns KS, Broaddus RR, Zhu Z, Dong C (2008) Regulation of inflammatory responses by IL-17F. *J Exp Med* 205, 1063-1075